FACIAL CLEFTS
AND
CRANIOSYNOSTOSIS

Principles and Management

FACIAL CLEFTS AND CRANIOSYNOSTOSIS
Principles and Management

Timothy A. Turvey, D.D.S.
Professor and Chairman
Department of Oral and Maxillofacial Surgery
University of North Carolina School of Dentistry
Chapel Hill, North Carolina

Katherine W. L. Vig, B.D.S., M.S., F.D.S., D.Orth.R.C.S.
Professor and Chairman
Department of Orthodontics
The Ohio State University College of Dentistry
Columbus, Ohio

Raymond J. Fonseca, D.M.D.
Dean
University of Pennsylvania School of Dental Medicine
Philadelphia, Pennsylvania

With illustrations by
WILLIAM M. WINN

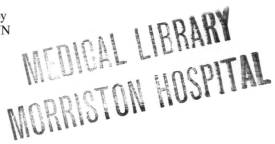

W.B. SAUNDERS COMPANY
A Division of Harcourt Brace & Company
Philadelphia   London   Toronto   Montreal   Sydney   Tokyo

W.B. SAUNDERS COMPANY
A Division of Harcourt Brace & Company

The Curtis Center
Independence Square West
Philadelphia, Pennsylvania 19106

Library of Congress Cataloging-in-Publication Data

Facial clefts and craniosynostosis: principles and management/[edited by] Timothy A.
Turvey, Katherine W. L. Vig, Raymond J. Fonseca.
   p.   cm.
Includes bibliographical references and index.
ISBN 0–7216–3783–3
1. Craniosynostoses.   2. Cleft palate.   3. Cleft lip.   4. Face—Abnormalities.   I. Turvey, Timothy
A.   II. Vig, Katherine W. L.   III. Fonseca, Raymond J.   IV. Title.
RJ482.C73T87   1996   617.5′ 2043—dc20
DNLM/DLC   95-7122

FACIAL CLEFTS AND CRANIOSYNOSTOSIS: ISBN 0–7216–3783–3
Principles and Management

Printed in the United States of America.

Last digit is the print number: 9   8   7   6   5   4   3   2   1

This book is dedicated to the authors' spouses,
Martha, Peter, and Marilyn,
and to their children,
Samantha, Amanda, Blake, and MacKenzie;
Caroline and Amanda;
and Tiffany and Gabriel.

Contributors

Frank E. Åbyholm, M.D., D.D.S.
  Professor and Head of Department of Plastic Surgery, University of Oslo;
  Rikshospitalet, National Hospital, Oslo, Norway
  Primary Closure of Cleft Lip and Palate

Alexia A. Antczak-Bouckoms, D.M.D., Sc.D., M.P.H.
  Assistant Professor of Medicine, Division of Clinical Care Research, Tufts
  University School of Medicine, Boston, Massachusetts
  A Methodologic Approach to Outcome Assessment

Michael R. Arcuri, D.D.S., M.S.
  Assistant Professor, Departments of Hospital Dentistry and Otolaryngology,
  University of Iowa Hospitals and Clinics, Iowa City, Iowa
  Prosthodontic Management

Arthur S. Aylsworth, M.D.
  Professor of Pediatrics and Director, Genetic Counseling Program, University of
  North Carolina School of Medicine, Chapel Hill, North Carolina
  Genetic Considerations in Craniofacial Birth Defects

Mary Breen, M.S., R.N.
  Craniofacial Clinical Nurse Specialist, Children's Medical Center of Dallas, Dallas,
  Texas
  Nursing Considerations for Children with Craniofacial Anomalies

Hillary L. Broder, Ph.D., M.Ed.
  Associate Professor, Division of Behavioral Sciences, Department of General and
  Hospital Dentistry, University of Medicine and Dentistry, New Jersey School of
  Dentistry, Newark, New Jersey; Consultant, Montefiore Medical Center, Center for
  Craniofacial Disorders, Bronx, New York
  *Psychosocial Considerations in Habilitation of Patients with Facial Deformity: A
  Developmental Perspective*

Vincent N. Carrasco, M.D.
  Assistant Professor of Surgery and Chief of Section of Otology, Neurotology, and
  Skull Base Surgery, University of North Carolina, Chapel Hill, North Carolina
  Management of Middle Ear Disease and Malformations

M. Michael Cohen, Jr., D.M.D., M.S.D., Ph.D., F.C.C.M.G.
  Professor of Oral and Maxillofacial Pathology, Pediatrics, Community Health and
  Epidemiology, Health Services Administration, Sociology and Social Anthropology,
  Dalhousie University; and Staff, IWK Children's Hospital and Atlantic Research
  Centre for Medical Genetics and Mental Retardation, Halifax, Nova Scotia, Canada
  Syndrome Delineation and Growth in Orofacial Clefting and Craniosynostosis

David A. Cottrell, D.M.D.
  Assistant Professor and Director of Resident Research, Department of Oral and
  Maxillofacial Surgery, Boston University School of Graduate Dentistry; Assistant
  Visiting Professor, Boston University Medical Center, Boston, Massachusetts
  End-Stage Reconstruction in the Complex Cleft Lip/Palate Patient

Ginny Curtin, M.S., R.N.C., P.N.P.
Clinical Nurse Specialist, Craniofacial Center, Children's Hospital Oakland, Oakland, California
Nursing Considerations for Children with Craniofacial Anomalies

Rodger M. Dalston, Ph.D.
Amon G. Carter Jr. Professor of Communication, University of Texas at Austin College of Communication, Austin, Texas
Speech and Hearing Considerations in Facial Clefting and Craniosynostosis

Jefferson U. Davis, D.D.S., M.D.
Former Assistant Professor, Department of Surgery, Division of Plastic Surgery, and Craniofacial Consultant, University of North Carolina, and Craniofacial Center, University of North Carolina School of Medicine, Chapel Hill, North Carolina; Attending Plastic Surgeon, Phoebe Putney Memorial Hospital, Palmyra Medical Center, Albany, Georgia
Principles and Management of the Soft Tissues in Facial Clefts

Susan E. Downey, M.D.
Assistant Professor of Plastic Surgery, University of Southern California School of Medicine, Los Angeles; Attending Surgeon, Children's Hospital Los Angeles, USC University Hospital, Kenneth Norris, Jr. Cancer Hospital, and Doheny Eye Hospital, Los Angeles, California
Surgical Management of Velopharyngeal Insufficiency: Pharyngeal Flap and Sphincter Pharyngoplasty

Amelia F. Drake, M.D., F.A.C.S.
Associate Professor, Otolaryngology/Head and Neck Surgery and Department of Pediatrics, University of North Carolina School of Medicine; Attending Physician, University of North Carolina Hospitals, Chapel Hill, North Carolina
Airway Management

James Henry Peter Ellis, M.A., Ph.D.
Senior Lecturer, University of the Western Cape, Department of Sociology, Bellville, South Africa
Comprehensive Team Management

Bruce N. Epker, D.D.S., M.S.D., Ph.D.
Staff, Department of Maxillofacial Surgery and Center for Correction of Facial Deformities, John Peter Smith Hospital, Forth Worth, Texas
Diagnosis of and Treatment Planning for Facial Asymmetries

Raymond J. Fonseca, D.M.D.
Dean, University of Pennsylvania School of Dental Medicine, Philadelphia, Pennsylvania
Orthodontic and Surgical Considerations in Bone Grafting in the Cleft Maxilla and Palate; Midface Advancement and Contouring in the Presence of Cleft Lip and Palate

Klaus W. Grätz, M.D., D.D.S.
Senior Staff Member, Department of Maxillofacial Surgery, University of Zurich Medical School, Zurich, Switzerland
Surgical Treatment of Hypertelorism

Steven K. Gudeman, M.D.
Professor and Chief of Neurosurgery, University of North Carolina at Chapel Hill School of Medicine; Chief of Neurosurgery, University of North Carolina Hospitals, Chapel Hill, North Carolina
Nonsyndromic Craniosynostosis

William Hoffman, M.D.
Associate Professor, Department of Surgery, Division of Plastic and Reconstructive Surgery, University of California at San Francisco School of Medicine, San Francisco, California
Comprehensive Surgical and Orthodontic Management of Hemifacial Microsomia

Leonard B. Kaban, D.M.D., M.D.
Walter C. Guralnick Professor and Chair, Department of Oral and Maxillofacial Surgery, Harvard School of Dental Medicine; Professor and Chair, Department of Oral and Maxillofacial Surgery, Massachusetts General Hospital, Boston, Massachusetts
Comprehensive Surgical and Orthodontic Management of Hemifacial Microsomia

Sven Kreiborg, D.D.S., Ph.D., D.Odont.
Professor, School of Dentistry, Faculty of Health Sciences, University of Copenhagen, Copenhagen, Denmark
Syndrome Delineation and Growth in Orofacial Clefting and Craniosynostosis

William E. LaVelle, D.D.S., M.S.
Professor, Department of Otolaryngology, University of Iowa Hospitals and Clinics, Iowa City, Iowa
Prosthodontic Management

H. Wolfgang Losken, M.B.Ch.B., F.C.S.(S.A.), F.R.C.S.Ed.
Associate Professor, University of Pittsburgh School of Medicine; Chief of Plastic Surgery, Children's Hospital Pittsburgh, Pittsburgh, Pennsylvania
Distraction Osteogenesis: Indications, Clinical Application, and Preliminary Case Reports

Marilyn T. Miller, M.S., M.D.
Professor of Ophthalmology and Director, Pediatric Ophthalmology and Adult Strabismus, University of Illinois at Chicago and Department of Ophthalmology, Eye and Ear Infirmary, Chicago, Illinois
Ophthalmologic Considerations in Craniosynostosis, Hypertelorism, and Facial Clefts

Fernando Molina, M.D.
Professor of Plastic Surgery, Medical School, Universidad Nacional, Autonoma de Mexico; Assisting Plastic Surgeon, Hospital General ''Dr. Manuel Gea Gonzales,'' Mexico City, Mexico
Distraction Osteogenesis: Indications, Clinical Application, and Preliminary Case Reports

Jeffrey C. Posnick, D.M.D., M.D.
Associate Professor of Plastic Surgery, Pediatrics and Otolaryngology–Head and Neck Surgery, Georgetown University School of Medicine; Chief, Craniomaxillofacial Surgery, Department of Surgery, and Director, Georgetown Craniofacial Center, Georgetown University Medical Center, Washington, DC
Craniofacial Synostosis Syndromes: A Staged Reconstructive Approach

Christopher T. Roberts, M.Sc.
Lecturer in Biostatistics, University Dental Hospital of Manchester, Manchester, England
Evaluating Treatment Alternatives: Measurement and Design

Per Rygh, D.D.S., D.Odont.
Professor and Chairman, Department of Orthopedics and Facial Orthopedics, Dental Faculty, University of Bergen, Bergen, Norway
Early Considerations in the Orthodontic Management of Skeletodental Discrepancies

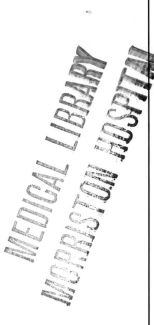

Herman F. Sailer, M.D., D.D.S.
Professor and Chairman, Department of Craniomaxillofacial Surgery, University of Zurich Medical School, Zurich, Switzerland
Surgical Treatment of Hypertelorism

Stephen A. Schendel, M.D., D.D.S., F.A.C.S.
Professor and Chairman, Department of Functional Restoration, and Chief, Division of Plastic Surgery, Stanford University School of Medicine; Director, Craniofacial Anomalies Center, Head, Division of Plastic Surgery, Lucile Salter Packard Children's Hospital at Stanford, Stanford, California
Facial Clefting Disorders and Craniofacial Synostoses: Skeletal Considerations

Gunvor Semb, D.D.S., Ph.D.
Head of Dental Unit, Department of Plastic Surgery, National Center of Logopedics; Rikshospitalet, National Hospital of Norway, Oslo, Norway
Facial Growth in Orofacial Clefting Disorders; Evaluating Treatment Alternatives: Measurement and Design

William C. Shaw, B.D.S., F.D.S., D.Orth., D.D.O., M.Sc.D., Ph.D.
Professor of Orthodontics and Dentofacial Development and Dean, Turner Dental School, The University of Manchester; Head of Orthodontic Unit, University Dental Hospital of Manchester, Manchester, England
Facial Growth in Orofacial Clefting Disorders; Surgical Management of Velopharyngeal Insufficiency: Pharyngeal Flap and Sphincter Pharyngoplasty; Evaluating Treatment Alternatives: Measurement and Design

James D. Sidman, M.D.
Clinical Professor, Department of Otolaryngology, University of Minnesota Hospitals and Clinics; Assistant Chief of Surgery and Chief Elect of Surgery, Children's Medical Center, Minneapolis, Minnesota
Airway Management

Gerald M. Sloan, M.D.
Professor of Plastic Surgery and Pediatrics, University of North Carolina School of Medicine, and Professor of Dentistry, University of North Carolina School of Dentistry; Attending Surgeon, The University of North Carolina Hospitals, Chapel Hill, North Carolina
Surgical Management of Velopharyngeal Insufficiency: Pharyngeal Flap and Sphincter Pharyngoplasty

John Paul Stella, D.D.S.
Clinical Professor of Surgery, Southwestern Medical School, Dallas; Chairman, Department of Oral and Maxillofacial Surgery, John Peter Smith Hospital, Fort Worth; Staff, Parkland Hospital, Dallas. Texas
Diagnosis of and Treatment Planning for Facial Asymmetries

Ronald P. Strauss, D.M.D., Ph.D.
Professor, Department of Dental Ecology, and Professor, Department of Social Medicine, University of North Carolina School of Dentistry; Dental Director, University of North Carolina Craniofacial Center, Chapel Hill, North Carolina
Comprehensive Team Management

Kathleen K. Sulik, Ph.D.
Professor of Cell Biology and Anatomy, University of North Carolina School of Medicine, Chapel Hill, North Carolina
Craniofacial Development

Clark O. Taylor, M.D., D.D.S.
Director, Institute of Facial Surgery, Bismarck, North Dakota; Assistant Clinical Professor of Surgery, University of Nebraska Medical Center, Omaha, Nebraska; Assistant Clinical Professor of Surgery, Oral and Maxillofacial Surgery, University of Texas Southwest Medical Center, Dallas, Texas; Parkland Hospital, Dallas, Texas; Director, Resident Training in Oral and Maxillofacial Surgery, University of North Dakota School of Medicine, Bismarck, North Dakota
Rhinoplasty for the Cleft Nasal Deformity

Paul Tessier, M.D.
Former Chief, Department of Plastic Surgery, Fôch Hospital, Paris, France
Facial Clefting Disorders and Craniofacial Synostoses: Skeletal Considerations; Management of Mandibulofacial Dysostosis

Rolf S. Tindlund, D.D.S.
Associate Professor and Director, Bergen Cleft Palate–Craniofacial Team, Department of Orthodontics and Facial Orthopedics, Dental Faculty, University of Bergen, Bergen, Norway
Early Considerations in the Orthodontic Management of Skeletodental Discrepancies

J.-F. Tulasne, M.D., D.D.S.
Private Practice, Paris, France
Facial Clefting Disorders and Craniofacial Synostoses: Skeletal Considerations; Management of Mandibulofacial Dysostosis

J. F. Camilla Tulloch, B.D.S., F.D.S., D.Orth.R.C.S.
Associate Professor, Department of Orthodontics, School of Dentistry, University of North Carolina, Chapel Hill, North Carolina
A Methodologic Approach to Outcome Assessment

Timothy A. Turvey, D.D.S.
Professor and Chairman, Department of Oral and Maxillofacial Surgery, University of North Carolina School of Dentistry; Chief of Oral and Maxillofacial Surgery, University of North Carolina Hospitals, Chapel Hill, North Carolina
Orthodontic and Surgical Considerations in Bone Grafting in the Cleft Maxilla and Palate; Midface Advancement and Contouring in the Presence of Cleft Lip and Palate; Nonsyndromic Craniosynostosis

Carol Ursich, R.N., B.S.N.
Nurse Specialist, Cleft/Craniofacial Team, Children's Hospital of Orange County, Orange, California
Nursing Considerations for Children with Craniofacial Anomalies

Karin Vargervik, D.D.S.
Professor, Growth and Development, and Adjunct Professor, Surgery, School of Dentistry/School of Medicine, University of California, San Francisco, California
Comprehensive Surgical and Orthodontic Management of Hemifacial Microsomia

Katherine W. L. Vig, B.D.S., M.S., F.D.S., D.Orth.R.C.S.
Professor and Chairman, Department of Orthodontics, The Ohio State University College of Dentistry, Columbus, Ohio
Orthodontic and Surgical Considerations in Bone Grafting in the Cleft Maxilla and Palate; Midface Advancement and Contouring in the Presence of Cleft Lip and Palate; Distraction Osteogenesis: Indications, Clinical Application, and Preliminary Case Reports

Donald W. Warren, D.D.S., M.S., Ph.D., D.Odont.(h.c.)
Kenan Professor and Director, University of North Carolina Craniofacial Center and Research Professor of Otolaryngology, School of Medicine, University of North Carolina School of Dentistry; Attending, Dental Service, University of North Carolina Hospitals, Chapel Hill, North Carolina
Speech and Hearing Considerations in Facial Clefting and Craniosynostosis

Larry M. Wolford, D.D.S.
Clinical Professor, Department of Oral and Maxillofacial Surgery, Baylor College of
Dentistry; Private Practice, Baylor University Medical Center, Dallas, Texas
End-Stage Reconstruction in the Complex Cleft Lip/Palate Patient

Foreword

Facial Clefts and Craniosynostosis: Principles and Management was conceived by the authors before 1985. The three of us crossed academic and career pathways on several occasions and share a common interest in craniofacial anomalies. We often commented on the lack of a single resource that provided an overview of the subject. The seeds of this book were sown in 1991, when we met in Philadelphia and outlined what we believed to be a useful compendium of topics. Because of the developmental, genetic, and therapeutic complexity of craniofacial anomalies, we realized that a definitive treatise would not be attainable. With the advances in craniofacial biology on the cellular, molecular, and developmental levels and in the development of new surgical procedures and techniques, knowledge of the topics discussed in this book continues to evolve rapidly. Many important topics about facial clefts and craniosynostosis are discussed in detail. Some topics, such as the fibroblast growth factor receptor genes and their association with some forms of craniofacial dysostosis, are so new that details are just now emerging and therefore are not included in depth. Other topics, such as the latest imaging techniques, are mentioned but not discussed in detail. Our primary goal of providing an overview of facial clefts and craniosynostosis has resulted in the production of *Facial Clefts and Craniosynostosis: Principles and Management*.

The American Cleft Palate–Craniofacial Association is a multidisciplinary organization that grew out of the American Cleft Palate Association after it was recognized that affected individuals with craniofacial anomalies are best treated when multiple health care disciplines participate in team care. Recognition that no single individual is completely capable of identifying and categorizing the dysmorphology, determining the pathogenesis and the genetic pathways, caring for the emotional and physical needs of the patient and family, and so forth supports the need for an interdisciplinary approach to craniofacial anomalies. The three of us have been associated with the team concept for our entire careers, and we understood from the outset the need to identify a cadre of experts to contribute their knowledge, time, and efforts to the text. The fruits of this undertaking have come from eight countries and have involved 48 contributors from a variety of health care disciplines: dentistry, developmental and cellular biology, dysmorphology and pathology, genetics and metabolism, medical illustration, neurosurgery, nursing, ophthalmology, oral and maxillofacial surgery, otolaryngology, plastic surgery, psychology, social work, and speech pathology.

The text is divided into four sections: Causes and Consequences, Diagnosis and Treatment Planning, Surgical Management, and Outcome Assessment. We find it refreshing that this book is constructed with different writing styles and opinions that are consistent with the eclectic nature of a text directed toward multiple health care disciplines. We were able to accomplish this because the contributors are experienced writers and authorities in their respective disciplines. The text is enhanced and clarified by detailed illustrations that are used liberally throughout the book.

The first section covers topics that include craniofacial development accompanied by detailed illustrations demonstrating key changes occurring at precise stages in development. Facial dysmorphology and syndrome delineation, genetic counseling, the impact of facial clefts and craniosynostosis on facial growth, and the importance of recognizing the associated skeletal abnormalities occurring with craniofacial malformations are other topics covered in this section.

The second section represents contributions dedicated to problems specific to patients with facial clefts and craniosynostosis. It includes the importance of team management, psychological findings and the need for counseling, nursing and social considerations, airway problems, ear disease, ophthalmologic abnormalities and considerations, speech problems, orthodontic considerations, prosthetic problems, and analysis and treatment planning considerations for the asymmetric face.

The third section contains chapters on contemporary surgical and orthodontic management of specific problems associated with facial clefting and craniosynostosis condition, including craniofacial dysostosis. Each of these chapters is illustrated in detail with current surgical techniques, and a variety of cases are presented and discussed.

The topics of the final section of the book are outcome assessment and a methodologic approach to delivering evidence-based care. In light of the current direction of health care, we thought it appropriate to conclude the book with these chapters.

This text is intended to provide health care participants with an overview of facial clefts and craniosynostosis. It is specifically targeted toward residents in surgical disciplines and toward orthodontists, speech pathologists, dentists, psychologists, nurses, social workers, and novices and experts interested in the subject of craniofacial anomalies.

Timothy A. Turvey
Katherine W. L. Vig
Raymond J. Fonseca

Acknowledgments

We wish to pay special tribute to those who have significantly
influenced our careers:

Dr. Robert V. Walker
Mr. Norman Lester Rowe
Dr. Paul Tessier

and to the numerous others who inspired our professional development,
including teachers, mentors, residents, and students.

Contents

I | Causes and Consequences

1 | Craniofacial Development

Kathleen K. Sulik

NORMAL CRANIOFACIAL DEVELOPMENT

Introduction

An understanding of the normal developmental events that shape the craniofacial region is implicit to beginning to comprehend those changes that result in malformations affecting this area. Data acquired as a result of the application of new research techniques in experimental animals provide an ever-expanding base of information to add to our traditional understanding of craniofacial morphogenesis. Research advances include, for example, new methods of labeling cells for lineage analyses and identification of migratory pathways; identification of genes involved in patterning; and identification of significant growth factors, extracellular matrix components, and other agents that help to orchestrate the complex changes involved in mammalian craniofacial embryogenesis. Although mammalian species are receiving increasingly more research attention, much of our information regarding developmental events has been derived from studies of other classes of vertebrates. In many cases, extrapolation from one class or species to another is appropriate, but in some cases, it leads to misconceptions. Herein, emphasis is placed, wherever possible, on results of studies utilizing mammalian species. Descriptive and illustrative material from human embryos is presented to the extent that is possible, and the majority of the remainder is derived from studies of the mouse. Scanning electron micrographs have been liberally used because their three dimension–like quality is very well suited for illustrating the morphology of embryos. The reader is encouraged to rely heavily on these illustrations and their accompanying legends for an understanding of the concepts presented herein.

Gastrulation and Neurulation

This account of craniofacial embryogenesis begins at the time in gestation when the embryo has implanted in the uterine wall and is beginning the process of gastrulation (during the third week post-fertilization in the human). At this stage of development, the embryo is establishing its definitive germ layers. The bilayered disc of cells that comprises the 2-week-old human conceptus (Fig. 1–1a) is remodeled into a trilaminar configuration as a portion of the ''upper'' or epiblast layer (that layer in contact with the amniotic cavity) of cells migrates (gastrulates) through the area of the caudal midline known as the primitive streak (Figs. 1–1b and 1–2a,b). This establishes the mesoderm and results in replacement of the original ''lower'' layer or hypoblast (that layer in contact with the yolk sac cavity) with the definitive embryonic endoderm. With the establishment of three cell (germ) layers, the term ''ectoderm'' replaces ''epiblast'' in reference to the uppermost cell layer. Gastrulation proceeds in a cranial-to-caudal sequence, with this process continuing through the fourth week of human gestation. Unlike elsewhere in the embryo, in the midsagittal region, extending forward from the cranialmost aspect of the primitive streak, only two cell layers are present. The cells subjacent to the median ectoderm constitute the prechordal (prochordal) plate and the notochordal plate (Fig. 1–2c,d). The cells that make up the notochordal plate are of mesodermal origin, but they constitute a layer of cells that is continuous laterally with the endoderm. Later, this mesodermal population separates from the endoderm, forming the notochord.[1] The anterior rim of the prechordal plate indicates the region where the primitive oral cavity, the stomodeum, will form. The prechordal plate is initially located caudal to the cardiogenic (heart-forming) region. However,

3

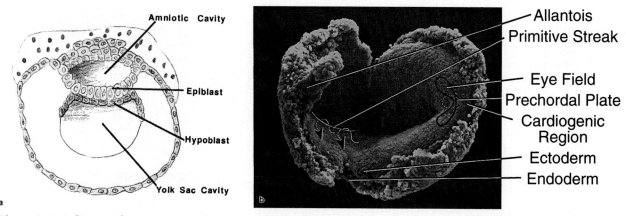

Figure 1-1. A diagram of a cross-section of a human embryo at the beginning of the third week post-fertilization illustrates that the cells are arranged as a bilayered disc. *a,* During the third week after fertilization in the human, gastrulation begins, as cells from the epiblast migrate through the primitive streak *(arrows). b,* It is significant to note the position of the prechordal plate and the eye fields at this stage of development.

relative differences in growth rate result in a ventrocaudal displacement of the cardiogenic region, carrying it below the stomodeum (Figs. 1–1 to 1–3).

Simultaneous with the gastrulation process, the ectoderm differentiates into neural and surface ectoderm with thickening of the neural ectodermal cells (i.e., these cells acquire a tall columnar form), and with thinning of the surface ectodermal cells to a squamous or cuboidal configuration. The neural ectoderm comprises the neural plate (see Figs. 1–2 and 1–3). Cells at the lateral rim of the anterior neural plate will later form the olfactory and otic placodes, the thickened ectoderm that will line the forming nasal cavities and inner ears, respectively, while cells at the anterior midline of this

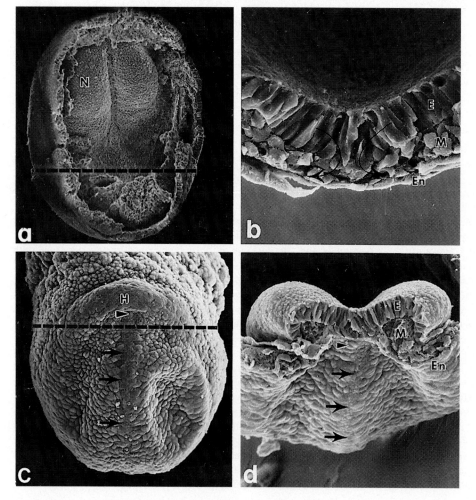

Figure 1-2. Scanning electron micrographs of gastrulation stage mouse embryos. The dorsal view *(a)* illustrates the developing neural plate (N). A cut through the caudal end of the embryo *(b)* at the position of the dotted line reveals the morphology of the primitive streak as the cells of the epiblast (E) migrate through the primitive streak to form the mesoderm (M) and endoderm (En) *(arrows).* The ventral view of the embryo *(c)* illustrates the position of the cardiogenic area (H) anterior to the prechordal plate *(arrowhead).* A cut through the anterior end of the embryo *(d)* as indicated by the dotted line reveals the morphology. It is evident that a bilayer of cells occupies the midline *(arrows).* The ectoderm (E) is columnar, the mesoderm (M) forms a relatively loose mesenchyme, and the endoderm (En) is a squamous layer. (Modified from Seibert JR, Cohen MM Jr, Sulik KK, et al: Holoprosencephaly: An Overview and Atlas of Cases. New York: Wiley-Liss, 1990.)

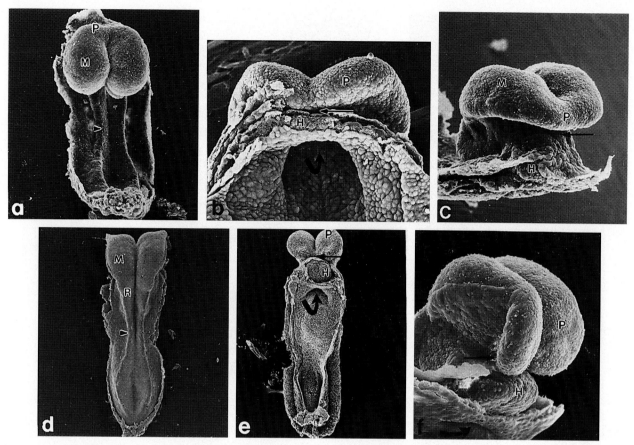

Figure 1–3. Scanning electron micrographs of neurulating mouse embryos. Three distinct regions of the developing brain—the prosencephalon (P, forebrain), mesencephalon (M, midbrain), and rhombencephalon (R, hindbrain)—become evident at a time corresponding to the fourth week after fertilization in the human. Dorsal views *(a* and *d)* illustrate the developing brain and spinal cord. The neural folds *(arrowheads)* have not yet begun to fuse. Ventral views *(b* and *e)* illustrate the relationships of the prosencephalon (P), stomodeum *(straight arrow),* heart (H), and foregut *(curved arrow).* The prosencephalon enlarges at a more rapid rate than the other regions of the brain (compare *c* and *f*). (From Seibert JR, Cohen MM Jr, Sulik KK, et al: Holoprosencephaly: An Overview and Atlas of Cases. New York: Wiley-Liss, 1990.)

rim will contribute to the anterior pituitary.[3] In addition, the presumptive optic neuroectoderm is located in the central aspect of the developing anterior neural plate at this stage (see Fig. 1–1). Changes in the shape of the neural plate, as it develops into the regions that are distinguishable as the future prosencephalon (forebrain), mesencephalon (midbrain), and rhombencephalon (hindbrain), and as it folds to form the neural tube (Figs. 1–3 and 1–4), are dependent upon differential rates of mitosis, normal cellular degeneration (physiologic cell death), and cytoskeletal and extracellular matrix components.

At these early developmental stages, the mesodermal cell population that is located just lateral to the midline (paraxial mesoderm) in the developing cranial region becomes segmented (see Fig. 1–4). These segmental units are termed somitomeres, which are analogous to the somites at more caudal levels.[4] Seven somitomeres form in a cranial-to-caudal sequence in the region of the brain rostral to the developing inner ear. The seventh somitomere is adjacent to the first of four occipital somites. Each segment is associated with a specific portion of the cranial neural plate. The sclerotomal components of the cranial somitomeres and the occipital somites form portions of the skull; the occipital somites fuse to form the basioccipital bone, whereas the basi-postsphenoid is somitomere-derived.[5] The somitomeric and somitic mesoderm also gives rise to the myoblasts of all of the voluntary muscles of the head.[6]

Cephalic neural tube closure occurs during the fourth week of human gestation, being completed by the time that approximately 20 somite pairs are present. Closure progresses both cranially and caudally, with the site of initial neural fold fusion at the level of the fourth to fifth somite (i.e., at the level of the junction of the occipital and

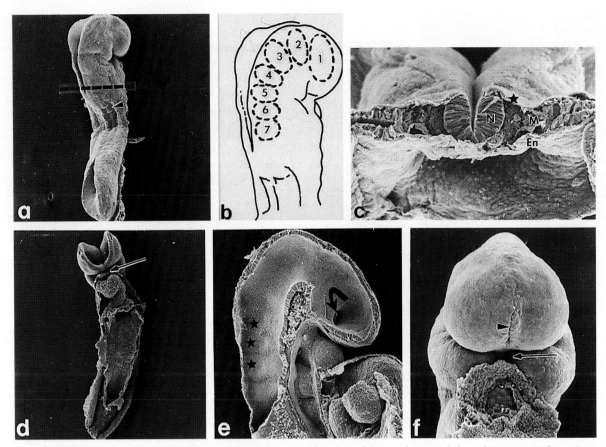

Figure 1–4. Relationships between the developing brain (neural ectoderm), surface ectoderm, and the subjacent mesoderm. In *a,* note that the neural tube has begun to close; the dashed line above the somite *(arrowhead)* is representative of the level of the cut for *c,* which shows the surface ectoderm *(star),* neural ectoderm (N), mesoderm (M), and endoderm (En). Although segmentation of the cranial paraxial mesoderm is no longer evident at the stage illustrated in *a* and *d,* the positions of the former somitomeres in relation to the brain are indicated in *b,* which is a line drawing of the cranial region in *a.* The somitomeres presage the development of morphologically distinct neuromeres *(stars),* as are evident in the rhombencephalon and illustrated in *e* in an embryo that has been cut midsagittally *(curved arrow* represents the optic stalk). *d* and *f* show the stomodeum *(straight arrow),* and *f* shows the anterior neuropore *(arrowhead).* (Modified from Seibert JR, Cohen MM Jr, Sulik KK, et al: Holoprosencephaly: An Overview and Atlas of Cases. New York: Wiley-Liss, 1990.)

cervical regions). Subdivisions of the developing brain termed neuromeres are evident before the time of complete cephalic neural tube closure (see Fig. 1–4). The neuromeres form in register with the underlying segmentation pattern that is present at earlier stages in the paraxial mesoderm. The forebrain has only one neuromere; two neuromeres are present in the midbrain; and the hindbrain is initially composed of four neuromeres that undergo further subdivision. Differentiation of the neuromeres into specific components of the brain is regulated by families of genes that are receiving a great deal of attention by developmental biologists. Among these are homeobox *(Hox)* and paired box *(Pax)* genes.[7] The protein products of these genes are sequentially expressed, with anterior boundaries of expression often coinciding with the boundaries of specific neuromeres (Fig. 1–5). Agents that control the expression of these genes have been identified and include retinoic acid, a naturally occurring "morphogen" that has its own family of nuclear receptors and cellular binding proteins. Identification of mutations in these genes is expanding our understanding of the basis for a variety of malformations. For example, type 1 Waardenburg syndrome, in which the characteristic facial features are dystopia canthorum, congenital hearing loss, and pigmentary disorders of the eye, skin, and hair, results from mutation of a paired box gene.[9] It has long been speculated that abnormality of a particular cell population, neural crest cells, accounts for the Waardenburg phenotype. Indeed, in mice that have a mutation in the homologous paired box gene *(Pax 3)* that is abnormal in patients with Waardenburg syndrome, the development of neural crest cell populations is aberrant.[10]

Cranial neural crest cell development is illustrated in Figure 1–6. As the neural folds elevate, but before their fusion at pre-otic levels in the mammal, these cells, which are located at the junction between the surface ectoderm and neural plate on each side, begin to leave the ectodermal layer, becoming mesenchymal (i.e., forming loose connective tissue). In the mouse, for the most part, the neural crest cells leave the neural folds in a cranial-to-caudal sequence, an exception being the slightly later emigration of the forebrain versus midbrain-associated crest cells. The cells from the various levels of the neural folds populate specific regions (although there may be some overlap), with those from the prosencephalon and upper mesencephalic levels populating the region of the frontonasal prominence; and those from the lower mesencephalic and upper rhombencephalic regions populating the presumptive maxillary and mandibular regions, and so on (see Fig. 1–6f).[11–15] The majority of the newly formed ectomesenchyme at cranial levels, unlike that in the trunk, is located immediately subjacent to the surface ectoderm (see Fig. 1–6c,e). In the trunk, most of the neural crest cells migrate more deeply, through the cranial half of each somite. At least some of the "displacement" of cranial neural crest cells in the mammal is the result not of active migration, but of "deposition" (i.e., as the neural folds elevate, the crest cells are left behind at their original level).[12, 16]

The neural crest cells derived from all levels of the neural folds play a significant role throughout the body as they differentiate into pigment cells, nerve cells (both sensory and motor), and glial cells; in the craniofacial region, they are of particular importance.[17–19] Unlike the trunk, where skeletal and connective tissues are mesodermally-derived, in the head, much of the skeletal and connective tissue is neural crest–derived. All of the skeletal and connective tissue components of the face (with the exception of the enamel of the teeth), including dentin, cartilage, bone, and the connective tissue surrounding blood vessels, glands, and muscle, and the dermis, smooth muscle, and adipose tissue of the skin, are neural crest–derived. In addition, the meninges, the corneal endothelium and stroma, and most of the sclera and the ciliary muscles of the eye are of neural crest origin. Using avian species, cell labeling experiments have illustrated that neural crest cells also form the entire skull rostral to the sella turcica.[5] In addition, caudal to this boundary, the parietal bone and part of the otic region of the skull is derived from neural crest, whereas the remainder of the skull is derived from mesoderm. The junction between the basi-presphenoid and basi-postsphenoid (i.e., the cranialmost level reached by the notochord) divides the ventrome-

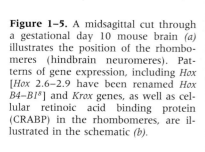

Figure 1–5. A midsagittal cut through a gestational day 10 mouse brain (a) illustrates the position of the rhombomeres (hindbrain neuromeres). Patterns of gene expression, including Hox [Hox 2.6–2.9 have been renamed Hox B4–B1[8]] and Krox genes, as well as cellular retinoic acid binding protein (CRABP) in the rhombomeres, are illustrated in the schematic (b).

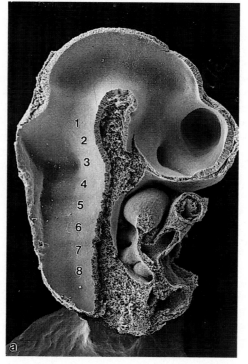

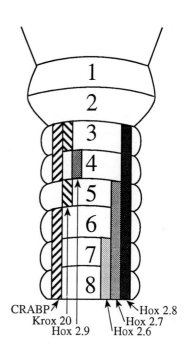

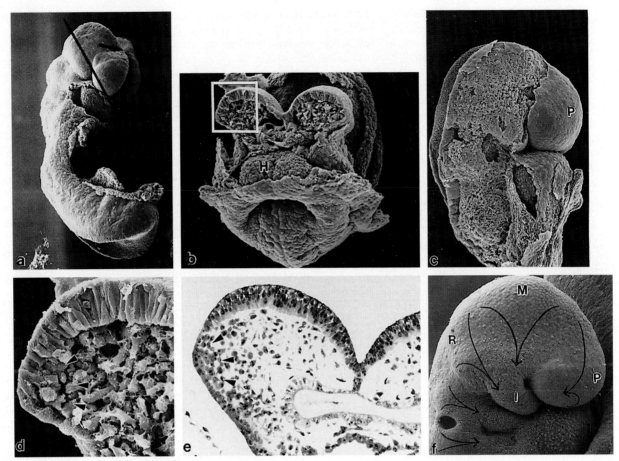

Figure 1–6. Emigration of the neural crest cells cranial to the otocyst, as opposed to that in the trunk, begins before neural tube closure in mammals. A cut made at the level of the midbrain *(a)* shows neural crest cells *(arrowheads* in *d* and *e)* leaving the open neural tube (N). The area in the box *(b)* is shown at a higher magnification in *d*. Removal of the surface ectoderm in the cranial region before neural tube closure reveals the subjacent neural crest cell population *(c);* the prosencephalic region (P) is also shown. The *arrows* in *f* indicate the general relationships between the brain level of origin and the destination of neural crest populations: the first visceral arch (I), the mesencephalic region (M), the rhombencephalic region (R), and the prosencephalic region (frontonasal prominence) (P).

dial skull in terms of its crest versus mesodermal origin; the sella turcica, therefore, is of mesodermal origin caudally and neural crest origin rostrally.

As previously noted, some of the cranial neural crest cells give rise to sensory neurons. In the head, sensory neurons are also derived from placodes (a term referring to thick surface ectoderm)—the olfactory, otic, trigeminal, and epibranchial placodes. The positions of these placodes are illustrated in Figure 1–7. The olfactory (nasal) placodes, which form on the frontonasal prominence, contribute not only the olfactory neurons, but also luteinizing hormone–releasing hormone (LHRH) cells that, during embryogenesis, migrate from the olfactory placodes to the brain.[20] The LHRH cells are later required for sexual maturation. The otic placodes, which pinch off the surface ectoderm to form vesicles on each side of the hindbrain, later differentiate into the membranous labyrinth of the inner ear. The sensory neurons of the eighth cranial nerve are derived from the otic epithelium. The trigeminal and epibranchial placodes contribute sensory neurons to cranial nerves V, VII, IX, and X (see Fig. 1–7).

Development of the Face and Visceral Arches

At the time of anterior neuropore closure, the tissue surrounding the developing forebrain, the frontonasal prominence, has a smooth, rounded external contour (see Fig. 1–4*f*). The position of the olfactory placodes is evident upon surface examination a short time later (Fig. 1–8). These two areas of thick ectoderm located on the frontolateral aspects of the frontonasal prominence are apparent as nasal pits,

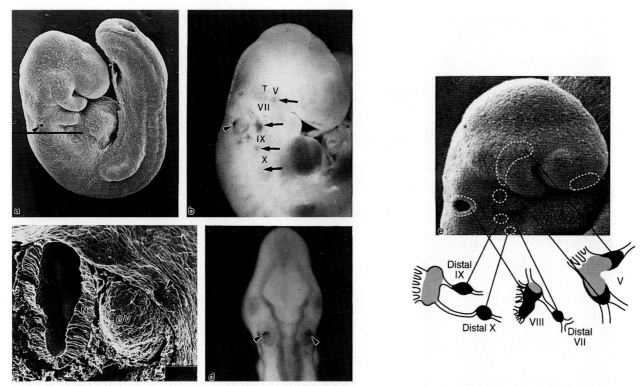

Figure 1–7. Thick surface ectoderm in the craniofacial region (placodes; circled areas in *e*) contributes sensory neurons for cranial nerves I, V, VII, VIII, IX, and X. The otic placode *(arrowhead),* which has invaginated to form a vesicle (OV) and subsequently forms the inner ear, is located lateral to the hindbrain (*a* to *e*). *c* illustrates a specimen cut at the level of the line in *a*. The positions of the trigeminal (T) and epibranchial placodes are illustrated through the use of a vital dye on the embryo in *b* and in the micrograph in *e*.

surrounded by tissue elevations termed the nasal prominences (processes). A reciprocal relationship exists between the nasal placodes and the olfactory fields of the forebrain (i.e., they are mutually dependent for normal growth and development).[21]

As their name implies, the nasal prominences develop into the nose (see Fig. 1–8). The lower portions of the medial nasal prominences also contribute to the upper lip, and form the portion of the alveolar ridge that contains the upper four incisors as well as the associated part of the hard palate that is termed the primary palate. On each side of the developing face, union of the medial nasal prominence with the lateral nasal prominence and the maxillary prominence of the first visceral arch is required for normal formation of the upper lip.

The visceral (pharyngeal, branchial) arches form in a cranial-to-caudal sequence on the ventrolateral aspect of the developing face and neck (Fig. 1–9). These bars of tissue (containing cells of both mesodermal and neural crest origin) are delineated from one another externally by grooves, and internally by pouches. The visceral arches initially serve as conduits for blood vessels, the aortic arch arteries. Four arches are visible on the external surface of the embryo. The fifth arch is rudimentary and the last, or sixth arch, is not apparent externally. Each of the arches is associated with specific cranial nerves and has specific muscular and skeletal derivatives (Table 1–1). The muscular components are mesodermally derived, whereas the connective tissue components are derived from neural crest cells.

Scanning electron microscopic views of embryos that have been cut through the first and second visceral arches in the coronal plane reveal the relationship between the visceral arches, pouches, and grooves (see Fig. 1–9). In addition, the breakdown of the buccopharyngeal membrane (tissue that is believed to be analogous to the anterior-most aspect of the prechordal plate), which results in continuity between the primitive oral cavity (stomodeum) and the pharynx, can be observed. The epithelium on the stomodeal side of this membrane is ectodermally derived, whereas that on the pharyngeal side is endodermal. The definitive position of this ectodermal-endodermal boundary is just in front of the palatine tonsils. Because the tongue is derived from the first

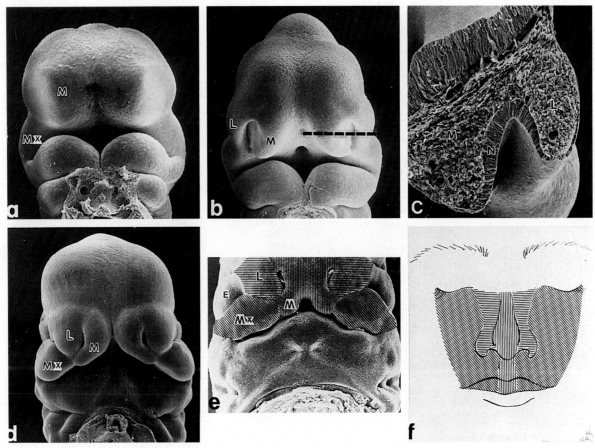

Figure 1–8. Development of the portion of the face above the oral cavity centers on formation and fusion of the medial (M) and lateral (L) nasal and maxillary (Mx) prominences (*a* to *d*). A cut through the nasal pit at the level indicated by the dotted line *(b)* illustrates the thickness of the nasal or olfactory placode (N) in relation to the surface ectoderm *(c)*. Contributions of the facial prominences to the adult face are shown in *e* and *f*. The specimen in *e* is a human embryo; the other specimens illustrated in this figure are mouse embryos. E, eyes. (From Seibert JR, Cohen MM Jr, Sulik KK, et al: Holoprosencephaly: An Overview and Atlas of Cases. New York: Wiley-Liss, 1980.)

Table 1–1. THE VISCERAL ARCHES AND POUCHES

Arch	Nerve	Muscles	Skeleton and Ligaments
1. Mandibular	V. Trigeminal	Muscles of mastication, mylohyoid, anterior belly of digastric, tensor veli palatini, tensor tympani	Meckle's cartilage, sphenomandibular ligament, malleus, incus
2. Hyoid	VII. Facial	Muscles of facial expression, posterior belly of digastric, stylohyoid, stapedius	Styloid process, stapes, stylohyoid ligament, lesser horn and upper portion of the body of the hyoid bone
3.	IX. Glossopharyngeal	Stylopharyngeus	Greater horn and lower portion of the body of the hyoid bone
4–6.	X. Vagus	Levator veli palatini, laryngeal, pharyngeal constrictors	Laryngeal cartilages

Pouch	Derivatives
First	Eustachian tube
Second	Palatine tonsils
Third	Thymus gland and inferior parathyroid glands
Fourth	Superior parathyroid glands
Fifth	Ultimobranchial bodies

four arches, its surface is covered by epithelium of ectodermal origin (the first arch component or anterior two thirds of the tongue), as well as of endodermal origin. The endoderm that lines the second to fifth visceral pouches contributes glandular elements including the tonsils, the thymus, and the parathyroid glands (see Table 1–1). The thyroid gland, however, is a midline derivative, originating from the epithelium at the junction of the first and second arch.

The first visceral arch is evident in embryos having 15 somite pairs. This arch initially appears as a single prominence of tissue (see Fig. 1–9). By the time the embryo has 30 somites, two distinct areas—the maxillary and mandibular

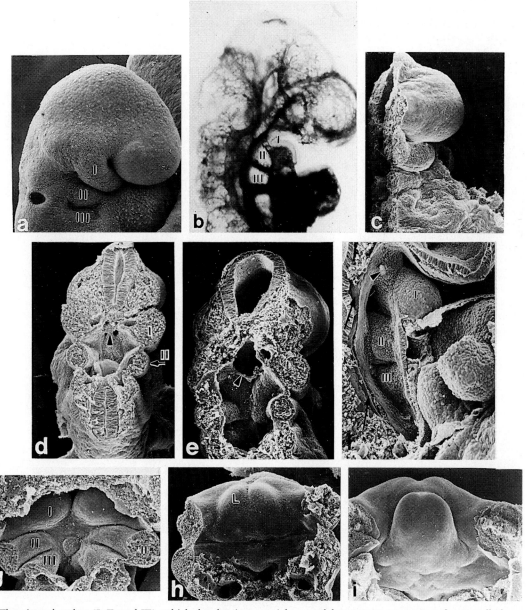

Figure 1–9. The visceral arches (I, II, and III), which develop in a cranial-to-caudal sequence, are separated externally by grooves and internally by pouches, as illustrated in *a* and *c* to *f*. They provide conduits for blood vessels, as illustrated in the India ink–perfused specimen in *b*. Frontal (*c* and *d* are the same embryo, and *e* is a slightly older specimen) as well as a midsagittal cut (*f*) through embryos at this time allow visualization of the breakdown of the buccopharyngeal membrane *(arrowheads)*, which allows continuity between the stomodeum and pharynx (*d* to *f*). In addition, the mesenchymal cores of the arches and the position of the pouches can be seen. Note the position of the notochord (*arrows* in *f*), which extends only as far forward as the remnant of the buccopharyngeal membrane. The tongue develops from the ventral aspect of the visceral arches; the first arch contributes the lateral lingual swellings (L; the anterior two thirds of the tongue), and the second to fourth arches contribute to the posterior third (*g* to *i*). (Modified from Seibert JR, Cohen MM Jr, Sulik KK, et al: Holoprosencephaly: An Overview and Atlas of Cases. New York: Wiley-Liss, 1990.)

prominences—are apparent (Fig. 1–10). These are generally (although, perhaps, inappropriately, relative to the maxillary prominences) both considered part of the first arch. Neural crest cells derived from mesencephalic and upper rhombencephalic levels initially form most, if not all, of the mesenchyme of the maxillary prominences. The mesenchymal population of the mandibular prominences initially consists of mesodermal cells. Neural crest cells from the level of the lower mesencephalon and upper rhombencephalon join the mesodermal cells to populate these prominences. The lower jaw and a large portion of the tongue are major derivatives of the mandibular prominences. The maxillary prominences contribute the majority of the tissue of the upper jaw. As previously noted, they unite with the medial nasal prominences in the course of normal development of the upper lip. The maxillary prominences also form the majority of the hard palate, the portion termed the secondary palate. The secondary palatal shelves initially grow down on each side of the tongue. Before their union in the midline, and before their union with the primary palate and the nasal septum, which occurs early in the ninth week in the human, they come to lie above the tongue (see Fig. 1–10).

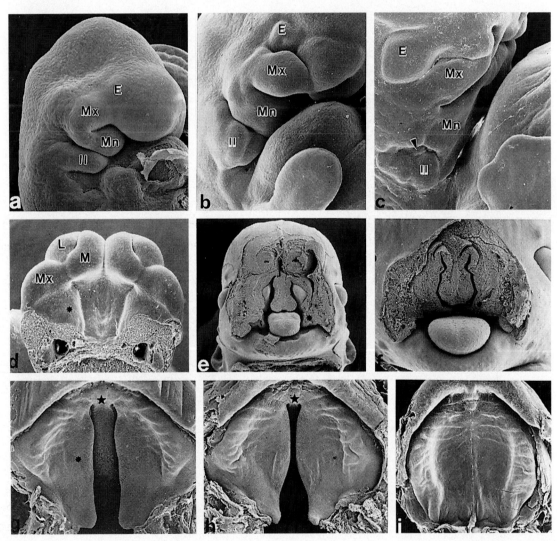

Figure 1–10. Development of the lateral surface of the head proceeds with the external ear forming from the first and second visceral arches (*a* to *c*; *arrowhead* in *c* points to the external auditory meatus, which is surrounded by the auricular hillocks). The first arch region is composed of both maxillary and mandibular prominences. A cut through the corners of the mouth (*d*) or frontally, through the nose (*e* and *f*), allows visualization of the developing palate. The primary palate (*star* in *g* and *h*) is composed of tissue from the medial nasal prominences (M), whereas the secondary palate (*asterisk* in *d* to *g*) is of maxillary prominence (Mx) origin. The secondary palatal shelves reorient to become positioned above the tongue, allowing fusion in the midline (*e* to *i*). Specimens in *c* and *g* to *i* are human and are courtesy of Dr. L. Russell. E, eye; Mn, mandibular prominence; II, second visceral arch. (Modified from Seibert JR, Cohen MM Jr, Sulik KK, et al: Holoprosencephaly: An Overview and Atlas of Cases. New York: Wiley-Liss, 1990.)

Tissues from both the first (mandibular) and second (hyoid) arches contribute to the external ears, with three auricular hillocks (on each side) forming from each (see Fig. 1–10a,b,c). The bones of the middle ear also originate from tissues of these two visceral arches, with the majority of the malleus and incus developing from Meckle's cartilage (the first arch cartilage) and the majority of the stapes from Reichert's cartilage (the second arch cartilage). The middle ear cavity is lined by the epithelium of the first pouch (the pouch between the first and second arches).

Ocular Development

The ectoderm that is destined to form the neural and pigmented retina, as well as a significant portion of the iris and ciliary body of the eye, originates, at presomite stages, in the central aspect of the anterior neural plate. In embryos having six to nine somite pairs, the optic neural ectoderm is apparent as two depressions (evaginations) termed optic sulci, each of which is centrally placed in the developing prosencephalic hemispheres (Fig. 1–11). As the anterior neural folds close, the optic evaginations, now termed optic vesicles (connected to the forebrain by the optic stalks), closely approximate the surface ectoderm. The surface ectoderm in the region of this approximation is induced to become columnar, forming the lens placode. Invagination of the optic vesicles to form the bilayered (neural and pigmented) optic cup is accompanied by invagination of the lens placode to form the lens vesicle. After separation of the lens vesicle from the surface ectoderm, the cornea develops. Although the ectoderm forms the epithelium of this structure, all of the subjacent layers of the cornea are derived from cells of neural crest origin. Neural crest–derived cells also enter the vitreous space, surrounding the vascular endothelia, which are of mesodermal origin. In addition, neural crest cells form the musculature of the ciliary apparatus, whereas

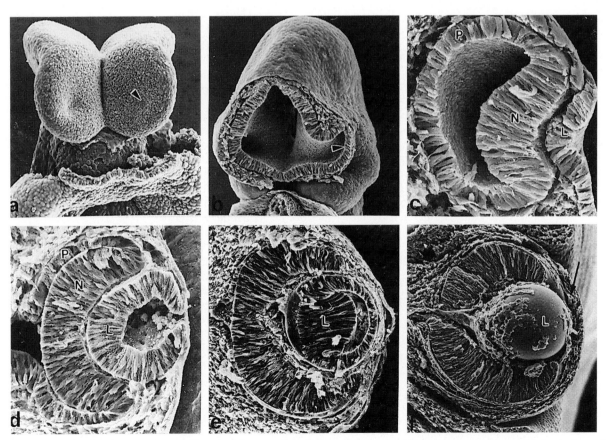

Figure 1–11. Ocular development is well-illustrated by scanning electron microscopy. This includes evagination of the optic vesicle from the prosencephalon (*arrowheads* in *a* and *b*), development and invagination of the lens (L) placode that is concurrent with optic cup formation (*c* to *f*), and formation of the cornea (*arrow* in *f*). *c* and *d* also show the neural retina (N) and the pigmented retina (P). (From Seibert JR, Cohen MM Jr, Sulik KK, et al: Holoprosencephaly: An Overview and Atlas of Cases. New York: Wiley-Liss, 1990.)

the muscles of the iris are derived directly from the neural ectoderm at the margin of the optic cup.

ABNORMAL CRANIOFACIAL DEVELOPMENT

Introduction

Teratogenic and genetic insults to the process of embryogenesis usually result in inadequate cell numbers or cellular products and/or abnormal interactions between cells or between cells and their extracellular matrix. For a malformation to occur, all tissues of the embryo would not be expected to be uniformly affected, because the result would probably be a growth-retarded but structurally normal individual. Thus a basis for the induction of malformations is the presence of selectively vulnerable cell populations. Speculation relative to selective sensitivity to teratogenic insult has focused on proliferative activity (i.e., tissues with high proliferative activity are more likely to be affected than those that proliferate slowly). However, it is apparent that others factors, such as state of cellular differentiation, production of specific gene products, the presence of specific cellular receptors, differential drug distribution, or other cellular or regional characteristics, can impart selective vulnerability.

The types of malformations that can be caused by genetic factors and environmental agents are dependent upon the developmental stage of the embryo at the time of insult. The term *critical period* is used to designate stages of vulnerability of specific organ systems to the induction of malformations. For the most part, the critical periods for most major malformations occur during the process of embryogenesis (i.e., before the ninth week postfertilization). However, because closure of the secondary palate occurs early in the fetal period, and cleft palate could result from insult just before the time of closure, a critical period for the secondary palate provides an exception. For some malformations, such as lateral (as opposed to median) cleft of the lip, as well as clefts of the secondary palate, there is more than one critical period. This is because a number of events in embryogenesis can be perturbed to result in what appears to be a common end point. Frequently, it is assumed that clefting usually results directly from failure of fusion (i.e., an abnormality in the fusion process itself) and, therefore, the critical period is at the time of fusion. Although this can be the case, other events occurring well before the normal fusion process that can, for example, lead to size deficiencies in the tissues and subsequent clefting are of major importance.

For an understanding of the typical placement and pattern of a variety of craniofacial clefts, familiarity with the contours of the developing face of the embryo is essential. Examination of human 5- and 6-week embryos reveals that the standardly described facial prominences (e.g., lateral nasal, maxillary, mandibular) are composed of smaller units that probably represent specific growth centers (Fig. 1–12). The boundaries between these regions appear to represent many of the facial clefting sites. Figure 1–12 illustrates the potential sites of clefting between apparent growth centers in the faces of human embryos and relates these sites to the craniofacial clefting classification scheme developed by Tessier.[22]

Experimental models for a number of craniofacial malformations have provided significant insight into critical periods for the induction of malformations as well as for their pathogenic basis. To provide examples of this, descriptions of models for a variety of craniofacial malformations follow. These include those that primarily affect the facial midline, including malformations associated with holoprosencephaly and anencephaly as well as some forms of frontonasal dysplasia; malformations that resemble some forms of hemifacial microsomia (oculo-auriculovertebral syndrome) and mandibulofacial dysostosis; typical clefts of the lip and palate; and abnormality of the cranial base involving abnormal union of the basioccipital and sphenoid bones.

Abnormalities Primarily Affecting the Craniofacial Midline

It is clear from studies of rodents exposed acutely to short-acting teratogens, as well as studies of genetically based models, that malformations involving the facial midline, including those associated with holoprosencephaly (those with premaxillary deficien-

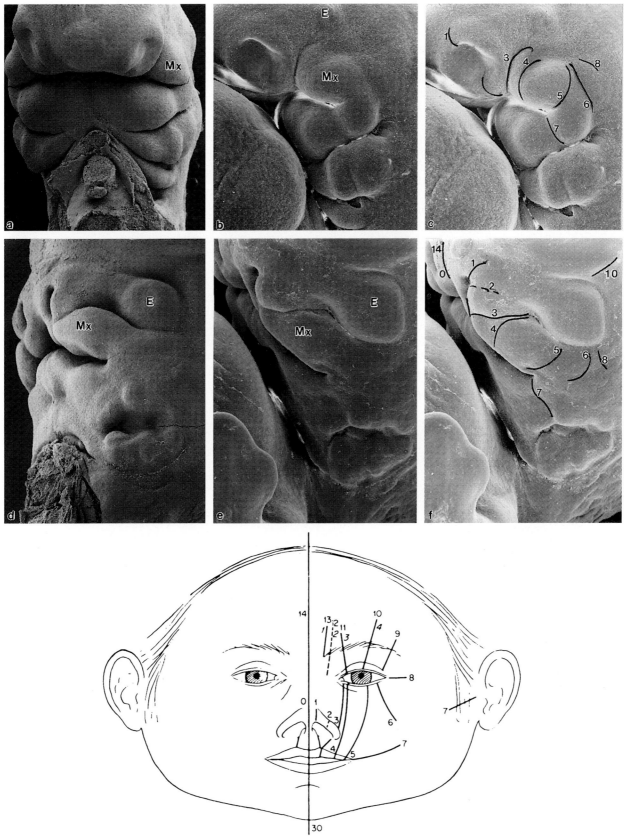

Figure 1–12. The contours notable in human embryos at 5 (*a* to *c*) and 6 (*d* to *f*) weeks of gestation can be correlated with the placement of facial clefts. Frontolateral (*a* and *d*), unlabeled lateral (*b* and *e*), and lateral views (*c* and *f*) with numbered potential clefting sites are shown. *b, d,* and *e* also show the eye *(E),* and *a, b, d,* and *e* show the maxillary prominence (Mx). (Line drawing from Tessier P [ed]: Symposium on Plastic Surgery in the Orbital Region, pp. 189–198. St. Louis: CV Mosby, 1976.)

cies), as well as some forms of frontonasal dysplasia (median facial clefts), can originate from an insult that occurs as early as the third week of human gestation. These malformations usually involve both the brain and the face. The fact that the facial malformations in the holoprosencephalies are a result of a concurrent insult to the brain and developing face has been long recognized. DeMyer and coworkers,[23] although aware of exceptions, concluded that in many cases the face, in those with midline abnormalities, predicts or reflects the coexisting brain malformations.

In mice, acute maternal treatment with ethanol administered when the embryos are in the early stages of gastrulation (gestational day 7) to early neurulation stages (gestational day 8) (approximately comparable with human days 15 to 21 of gestation), results in malformations consistent with some of those that constitute the holoprosencephaly spectrum, anterior neural tube defects including anencephaly (exencephaly), and/or facial clefting.[24-27] Sequential analysis of affected embryos following gestational day 8 ethanol exposure has illustrated a significant amount of teratogen-induced cell death within 12 hours of maternal treatment in the neural plate, particularly at its rim, followed in many specimens by diminished size of the prosencephalon and frontonasal prominence with abnormally close proximity of the olfactory placodes of the two sides (Fig. 1–13). In some specimens, the effect is notably asymmetric. Excessive cell death at the rim of the neural folds at these early stages involves the cranial premigratory neural crest cells. Reductions in this cell population are expected to play a causative role in the subsequently observed failure of neural tube closure (Fig. 1–13e,f; Fig. 1–14g,h) as well as in reduction of the size of the facial prominences. It is clear that even though the facial prominences involved in forming the nose and upper lip have not formed at the time of insult, unilateral as well as bilateral clefts of the lip can be induced (see Fig. 1–14b). In addition, a spectrum of median plane abnormalities, including median clefts through apparently normally proportioned upper lip and nasal

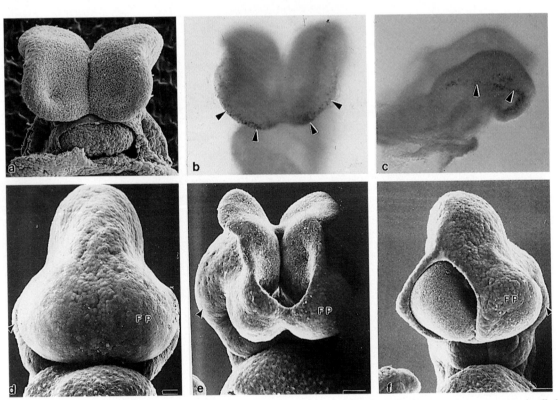

Figure 1–13. Exposure of gestational day 8 mouse embryos to large doses of ethanol results in excessive amounts of cell death 12 hours after treatment in the neural crest cells at the margin of the neural folds. This is illustrated by staining with a vital dye, Nile blue sulphate; dark stippling is indicative of dead or dying cells or cellular debris (*arrowheads* in *b* and *c*). Comparison of control (*d*) and ethanol-exposed (*e* and *f*) embryos approximately 24 hours after maternal drug administration reveals marked deficiency in the developing forebrain and frontonasal prominence (FP) in the latter two. *a* is a normal embryo that is at the same developmental stage as the treated embryo in *b*. (Modified from Kotch LE, Sulik KK: Experimental fetal alcohol syndrome: Proposed pathogenic basis for a variety of associated facial and brain anomalies. Am J Med Genet 1992; 44:168–176.)

tissues (see Fig. 1–14*e,f*) or very small and narrow nasal structures accompanied by a cleft involving only the midline of the upper lip (see Fig. 1–14*c,d*), can be induced at this treatment time. Regarding the median clefts that extend through the nose, it appears that they are related to delayed and tenuous closure of the anterior neuropore with subsequent formation of frontonasal encephalocele (see the discussion later of genetically induced frontonasal dysplasia).

After the earlier ethanol exposure time (gestational day 7), extensive studies have been conducted to examine the sequential changes that lead to varying degrees of holoprosencephaly with the associated ocular and facial malformations.[24–26,28] It is clear that narrowing of the forebrain occurs primarily at the expense of the midline. The abnormal olfactory placode positioning that results is illustrated in Figure 1–15. The location of the placodes greatly affects the development of the medial nasal prominences (MNPs), the lower aspect of the MNPs being more severely affected than the upper aspect. In severely affected individuals, the placodes may be so closely set that they converge. Minor degrees of convergence involve only the inferior-medial portion of the placodes, with elimination of the lower portion of the MNPs and subsequent loss of their philtral (intermaxillary) derivative (Fig. 1–15*b,e*). The upper lip, lacking the MNP-derived component, then consists of maxillary prominence–derived tissue and therefore appears abnormally long (from the nose to the mouth) and smooth. In these cases, the tip of the nose, which is derived from the upper portion of the MNPs, is expected to be small, but present. However, in more severely affected individuals, convergent formation of the placodes results in subsequent development in which a single nostril is surrounded by tissue from the lateral nasal prominences of each side, with little or no MNP-derived tissue being present and with subsequent expression as a cebocephalic phenotype (Fig. 1–15*a,d*). Less frequently in this animal model, complete premaxillary agenesis with median cleft lip occurs. Although not formally recognized as part of the holoprosencephaly spectrum, animal studies have illustrated that the characteristic craniofacial phenotype of the fetal alcohol syndrome

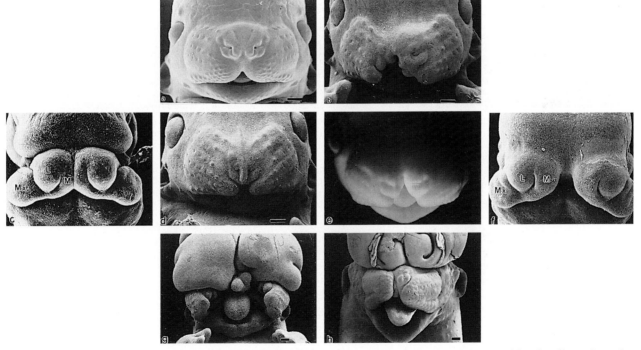

Figure 1–14. Gestational day 14 (*a, b, d, e, g,* and *h*) and day 11 (*c* and *f*) mouse embryos show a variety of facial malformations after acute maternal ethanol exposure on gestational day 8. The defects include unilateral cleft lip *(b)*; too close positioning of the medial nasal prominences (M) and nasal placodes *(c)*, resulting in a small nose *(d)*; too wide positioning of the medial nasal prominences *(f)*, resulting in a median cleft *(e)*; open neural tube with median facial cleft *(g)*; and open neural tube with a single nostril, probably resulting from the effect as illustrated in Figure 1–13*f (h)*. The specimen in *(a)* is normal. (Modified from Kotch LE, Sulik KK: Experimental fetal alcohol syndrome: Proposed pathogenic basis for a variety of associated facial and brain anomalies. Am J Med Genet 1992; 44:168–176.)

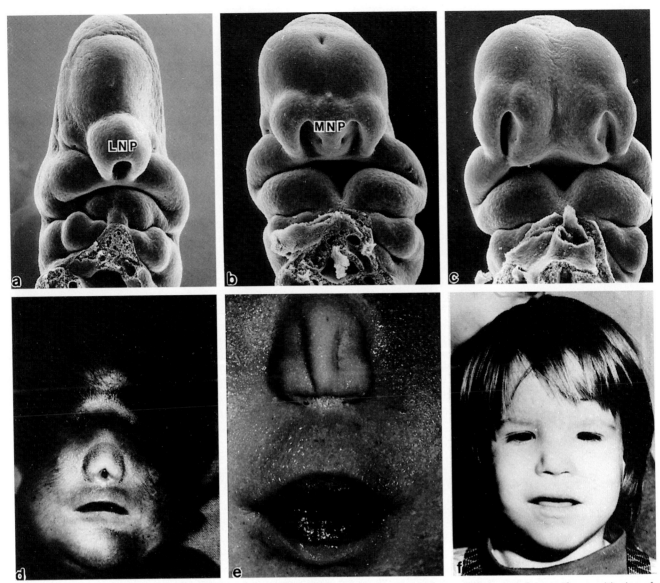

Figure 1–15. After gestational day 7 ethanol exposure, the midline of the developing face and brain is deficient. Close positioning of the nasal placodes results in abnormal development of the medial nasal prominences (MNPs) in ethanol-exposed embryos (*a* to *c*). The severity of effect varies; the nasal placodes may be so closely approximated as to become convergent (*a*). Convergence occurs first at the lower pole of the placodes, resulting in lack of development of the lower portions of the medial nasal prominences and formation of a single median structure that represents the upper portions of two medial nasal prominences (*b*). Variable degrees of severity of effect in ethanol-exposed mouse fetuses are manifested in phenotypes comparable with those in humans with cebocephaly (*d*), premaxillary agenesis (*e*), and fetal alcohol syndrome (*f*). (Modified from Sulik KK, Johnston MC: Embryonic origin of holoprosencephaly: Interrelationship of the developing brain and face. Scan Electron Microsc 1982; Part 1: 309–322.)

(FAS) could result from this same sequence of changes, with the FAS phenotype lying at the mild end of the holoprosencephaly spectrum (Fig. 1–15*c,f*).

Because the eyes originate as extensions of the forebrain, malformations involving ocular structures are expected to accompany those of the face and brain that are induced at these early developmental stages. Position (hypertelorism, hypotelorism, and synophthalmia) and structural abnormalities including anophthalmia, microphthalmia, iridial colobomata, and anterior chamber cleavage anomalies are, in fact, very common in experimental animals exposed at gastrulation and neurulation stages to ethanol[28] as well as other drugs, including retinoic acid[29] and Ochratoxin A.[30] The latter teratogen, a mycotoxin, has a much longer half-life than ethanol and, after single exposures, continues to kill selected cell populations in the embryos for several days. As a result of exposure initiated on gestational day 8, the entire frontonasal region of mouse embryos is notably diminished, with resulting holoprosencephaly (Fig. 1–16*a,b*). The eyes are less severely diminished than the forebrain and associated

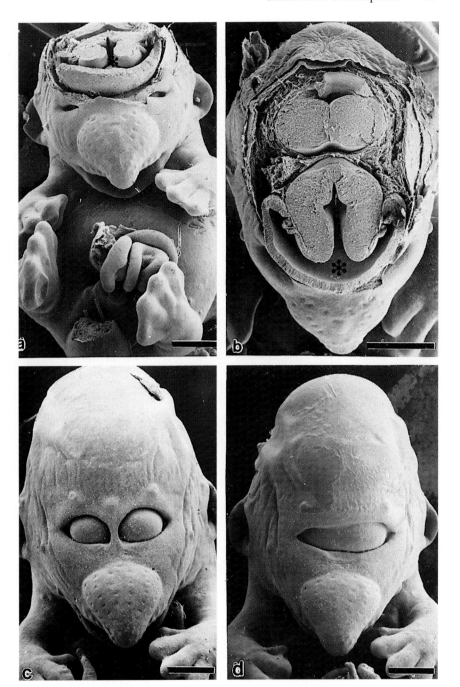

Figure 1–16. Teratogenic insult initiated in mice on gestational day 8 results in holoprosencephaly (i.e., a single cerebral vesicle; *asterisks* in *a* and *b*) and abnormal ocular positioning, including hypotelorism *(c)* and synophthalmia *(d)*. (From Wei X, Sulik KK: Pathogenesis of craniofacial and body wall malformations induced by Ochratoxin A in mice. Am J Med Genet 1993; 47:862–871.)

nasal structures, and as a result of the selective loss of the intervening tissues, they are synophthalmic (i.e., approximated in the midline) (Fig. 1–16*d*) or hypoteloric (Fig. 1–16*c*).

Abnormalities of the facial midline that fall within the spectrum of frontonasal dysplasia may be causally linked to abnormal closure of the anterior neuropore (delayed or tenuous closure), abnormal distension of the developing brain, and/or diminished mesenchymal cell populations within the frontonasal prominence. In an animal model of frontonasal dysplasia that was created as a result of a transgenetically induced mutation,[31] it was observed that the upper medial poles of the olfactory placodes do not separate from the rim of the neural plate and the upper portion of the MNPs are deficient or absent (Fig. 1–17).[32] In addition, closure of the anterior neuropore is delayed and frontonasal encephaloceles occur. This model appears to be consistent with those cases of frontonasal dysplasia that, in addition to midline defects, have clefts between the medial and lateral nasal prominence derivatives. Teratogenic exposure of mouse embryos to methotrexate close to the time of anterior neuropore

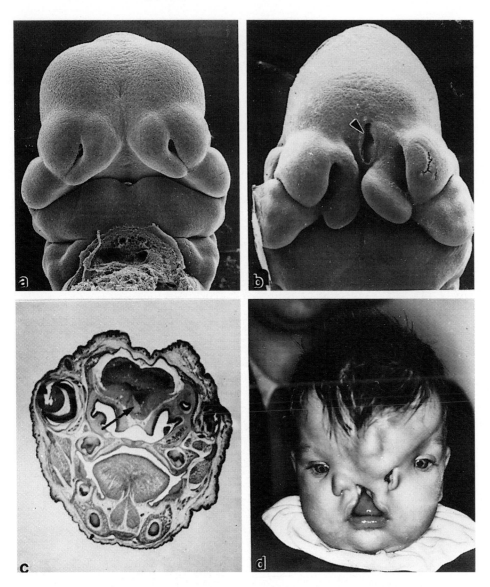

Figure 1–17. Features of frontonasal dysplasia are present in a transgenically produced mouse mutant, as illustrated in *b* and *c*. Note abnormal persistence of the anterior neuropore *(arrowhead)* and marked deficiency in the upper portions of the medial nasal prominences in the affected specimen *(b)* in comparison with a control *(a)*. Frontonasal encephalocele *(arrow in c)* follows the abnormal anterior neuropore closure. The phenotype shown in *b* is believed to correspond to that which would result in the type of facial malformation shown in *d*. (*b,c* courtesy of Dr. J. Thayer.)

closure also yields phenotypes consistent with those of frontonasal dysplasia.[33] Within a few hours of drug exposure, embryos exhibit excessive fluid accumulation that results in distension of the neural tube and formation of blisters in the frontonasal region (Fig. 1–18). Similar blister formation has been noted in a mouse mutant (6Gso) that has an unbalanced karyotype involving partial duplication of chromosome 15 and partial deletion of chromosome 19 and that presents with frontonasal dysplasia.[34]

Abnormalities Primarily Affecting the First and Second Visceral Arches

Insight from animal models into the pathogenesis associated with abnormalities resembling some forms of hemifacial microsomia (oculo-auriculovertebral syndrome) or mandibulofacial dysostosis (Treacher Collins syndrome) has been gained from a number of studies in which retinoids (vitamin A and related compounds) have been utilized. Teratogenic doses of retinoic acid administered to mice on gestational day 8 (at the early stages of neurulation; i.e., as neural crest cells first begin to leave the cranial neural folds) yield craniofacial malformations that are strikingly similar to those in children with retinoic acid embryopathy (Fig. 1–19). Abnormalities that are most notable in the second visceral arch appear to result from neural crest cell deficiencies.[35] Subsequent external ear abnormalities can be very severe, although

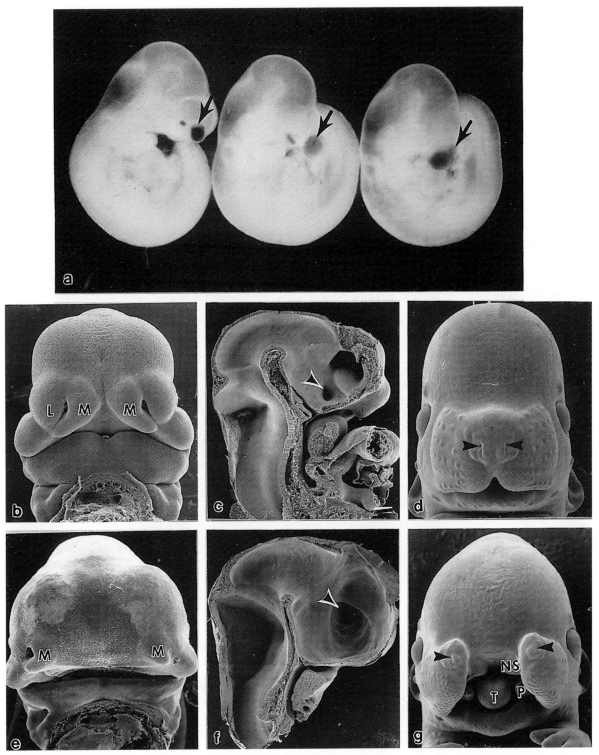

Figure 1–18. Teratogenic doses of methotrexate administered to mice on gestational day 9 (close to the normal time of anterior neuropore closure) result in abnormal fluid accumulation and distension of the brain (compare *c* and *f*) as well as vascular blebs in the frontonasal prominence (*arrows* in *a*). The resulting phenotype is illustrated in affected embryos in *e* to *g* in comparison with normal embryos in *b* to *d*. *Abbreviations:* M, medial nasal prominence; L, lateral nasal prominence; NS, nasal septum; T, tongue; P, palate. (Modified from Darab D, Sciote J, Minkoff R, et al: Pathogenesis of medial facial clefts in mice treated with methotrexate. Teratology 1987; 36:76–86.)

degrees of effect vary from individual to individual as well as on the two sides of an individual. Although this may serve as a model for some cases of hemifacial microsomia, concurrent effects on the developing brain, especially involving the cerebellum, are commonly noted, and are not a feature of most hemifacial microsomias. As

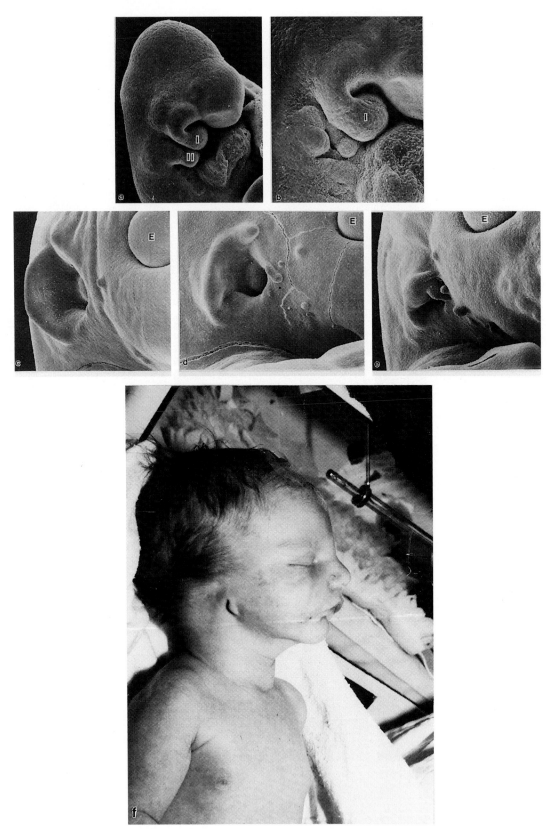

Figure 1–19. Retinoic acid exposure at early stages of development (gestational day 8 in mice; early in the fourth week after fertilization in humans) results in deficiencies that are most notable in the second arch (compare the normal specimen in part *a* with the affected specimen in *b*). Varying degrees of effect are reflected in subsequent external ear malformations (*d* and *e*; *c* is a normal specimen), which are typical in children with retinoic acid embryopathy *(f)*. (Modified from Webster WS, Johnston MC, Lammer EJ, et al: Isotretinoin embryopathy and the cranial neural crest: An in vivo and vitro study. J Craniofac Genet Dev Biol 1986; 6:211–222.)

suggested by Poswillo,[36] some forms of hemifacial microsomia may be related to vascular hemorrhage, with a limited regional effect that does not include involvement of the brain, eye, or vertebrae.

Administration of retinoids 1 day later in the mouse (gestational day 9; i.e., after neural crest cell emigration from the cranial neural folds is complete) also results in abnormalities of the external ear, although they are usually less severe than those following the earlier treatment time. Remarkable features of affected specimens include phenotypic resemblance to mandibulofacial dysostosis (Fig. 1–20). Within 12 hours of the gestational day 9 drug exposure, affected specimens have excessive amounts of cell death in the region of the epibranchial placodes. The resulting deficiency in the dorsal aspect of the maxillary prominence appears to account for subsequent abnormalities of the zygoma and the posterior part of the secondary palate.[37,38]

The adverse effects of teratogens on neural crest and epibranchial placodal cells on

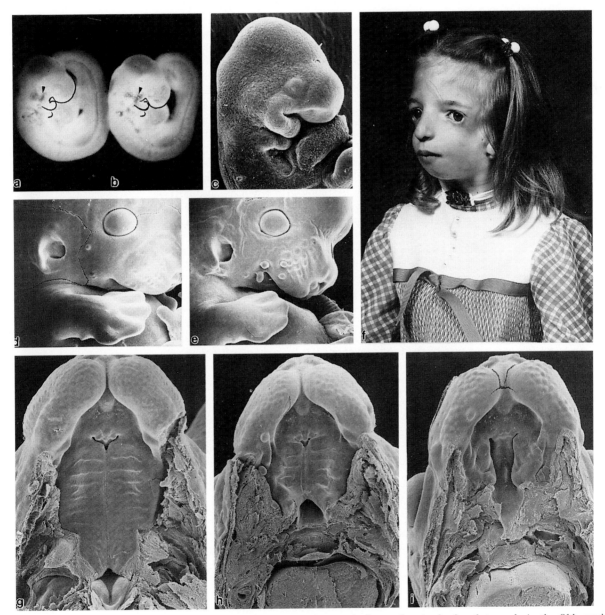

Figure 1–20. Retinoic acid administration on gestational day 9 in mice (equivalent to late in the fourth to early in the fifth week in the human) yields a phenotype similar to mandibulofacial dysostosis *(f)*. The major effects is on cells at the dorsal aspect of the first arch (those in the region of the trigeminal placode, to which arrowheads point). Abnormalities induced in the mouse model include size reduction in the region of the zygoma and mandibular ramus. In addition, the secondary palate may be reduced posteriorly *(h)* in comparison with normal *(g)* or, in severe cases, may be cleft *(i)*. *a* and *d* are also normal.

gestational days 8 to 9 in the mouse (comparable with the fourth week of human gestation) also appear to account for features that are part of the DiGeorge sequence, the CHARGE association (coloboma, heart defects, choanal atresia, retardation, genitourinary anomalies, ear anomalies), and Shprintzen syndrome.[38–40] Although a genetic basis has been established for many of the human cases, experimental teratology has illustrated the cell populations and the timing during which these cells must be adversely affected by the abnormal genome.

Cleft Lip and Palate

It has previously been pointed out that clefts of the lip occurring at the site of normal union of the medial nasal prominences with the lateral nasal and maxillary prominences (lateral or typical cleft lip) can be induced at early neurulation stages and result from excessive cell death in premigratory neural crest cell populations. However, individuals in whom cleft lip is teratogenically induced at this early developmental stage may also be expected to have notable brain abnormalities. Because this is not the case in most humans with cleft lip, it is expected that most clefts of the lip result from insult closer to the time of normal lip closure, which occurs in the sixth week of human gestation. Cleft lip has been induced in experimental animals with a variety of teratogens, including phenytoin and maternal hypoxia.[41,42] The latter induces cleft lip in animal models by diminishing the size of the nasal prominences and by killing cells in the olfactory placodes. A critical period for hypoxia-induced cleft lip in mice corresponds to the fifth week of human gestation.

In individuals with cleft lip and palate, it is generally accepted that cleft lip is the primary abnormality. The accompanying cleft palate is assumed to be caused by excessive facial width that, in turn, results from failure of the lip to close.

A great deal of the experimental work that has been conducted with regard to cleft palate has focused on the corticosteroids as inducing agents.[43,44] Secondary palate closure is normally completed by the 15th day of gestation in the mouse, and most of the teratogenesis studies have involved drug exposure just a few days before this time. Complete or incomplete isolated clefting of the secondary palate can also result from drug treatment much earlier, with deficient maxillary prominence size induced on gestational day 8 or 9 accounting for the inability of the palatal shelves to meet in the midline (Fig. 1–20c,i). It is of interest that retinoid treatment of mouse embryos on gestational day 8½ diminishes the size of the first visceral arch derivatives with accompanying microglossia and cleft palate in which the palatal shelves have very reduced size.[45] This appears to be a model for the Pierre Robin anomalad. As previously noted, retinoic acid, when administered on gestational day 9 in mice, has its major affect on the most posterior aspect of the palatal shelves, with subsequent clefting of just the posterior part of the palate or formation of a short soft palate (Fig. 1–20h).[38]

Cranial Base Abnormalities

The majority of research efforts and speculation regarding premature fusion of the craniofacial sutures involves fetal and postnatal development. For example, intrauterine constraint during fetal periods has been demonstrated as a cause of craniosynostosis in experimental animals.[46] Very few studies have been done regarding the embryogenesis associated with premature cranial suture fusion or failure of the sutures to form. The latter condition (abnormal proximity of ossification centers without formation of a proper suture) has been shown to result from insult during the embryonic period and perhaps should not be considered true craniosynostosis.

It is expected that establishment of the normal position of sutures in the craniofacies is dependent upon patterns that are set up by gene families including the Hox genes. In fact, transgenic mice with ectopic expression of the Hox 1.1 gene exhibit abnormal development of the cervical vertebral column and the cranial base.[47] Alteration of the normal patterns that result, for example, in failure of the suture formation between the occipital and sphenoid bones has also been achieved after exposures of early (gestational day 8–8.5) mouse embryos to retinoids (Fig. 1–21).[48,49] This suggests a modifying effect of retinoic acid on the patterning genes or, perhaps, a more generalized toxic effect on the cells that are involved in establishing the cranial base pattern.

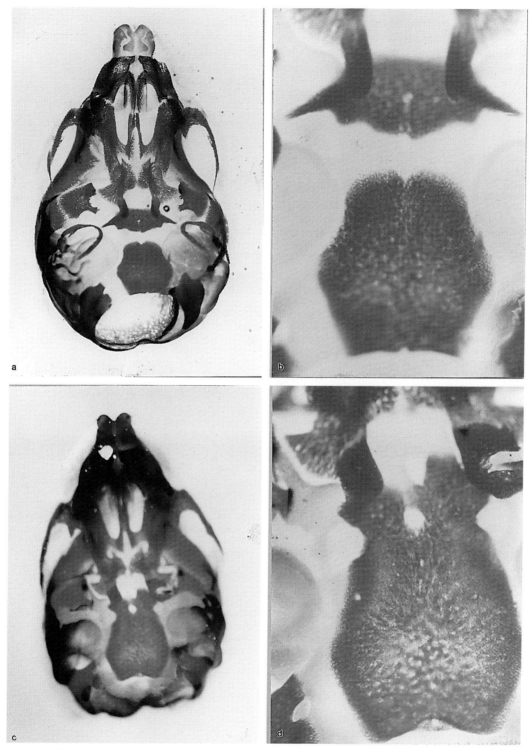

Figure 1–21. Cleared skeletal preparations illustrate the cranial base in normal (*a* and *b*) and retinoic-treated (*c* and *d*) near-term mouse fetuses. In the latter, the sphenoid and basioccipital bones are united. (Courtesy of Alles AJ, Wu TF-T, Alysworth AS, et al: Etretinate-induced abnormalities of the cranial base. Teratology 1992; 45:485.)

CONCLUSIONS

Our understanding of the pathogenesis and mechanisms of abnormal development that underly the genesis of craniofacial abnormalities is growing. This is partly the result of the development of suitable animal models for human malformations and the use of modern research methods to analyze them, coupled with our increasing base of

knowledge of normal embryology and cell biology. For the comprehensive understanding that is needed to best serve patients with craniofacial malformations, the
knowledge that can be acquired from experimental analyses of animal models must be
combined with that gained from clinical experience.

References

1. Jurand A: Some aspects of the development of the notochord in mouse embryos. J Embryol Exp Morphol 1974; 32:1–33.
2. Siebert JR, Cohen MM Jr, Sulik KK, et al: Holoprosencephaly: An Overview and Atlas of Cases. New York: Wiley-Liss, 1990.
3. Couly GF, Le Douarin NM: Mapping of the early neural primordium in quail-chick chimeras. II. The prosencephalic neural plate and the neural folds: Implications for the genesis of cephalic human congenital abnormalities. Devel Biol 1987; 120:198–214.
4. Meier S, Tam PPL: Metameric pattern development in the embryonic axis of the mouse. I. Differentiation of the cranial segments. Differentiation 1982; 21:95–108.
5. Couly GF, Coltey PM, Le Douarin NM: The triple origin of skull in higher vertebrates: A study in quail-chick chimeras. Development 1993; 117:409–429.
6. Noden DM: Vertebrate craniofacial development: The relation between ontogenetic process and morphological outcome. Brain Behav Evol 1991; 38:190–225.
7. Kessel M, Gruss P: Murine developmental control genes. Science 1990; 249:374–379.
8. Scott MP: Vertebrate homeobox gene nomenclature. Cell 1992; 71:551–553.
9. Tassabehji M, Read AP, Newton VE, et al: Waardenburg's syndrome patients have mutations in the human homologue of the Pax-3 paired box gene. Nature 1992; 355(6361):635–636.
10. Epstein DJ, Vekemans M, Gros P: Splotch (Sp^{2H}), a mutation affecting development of the mouse neural tube, shows a deletion within the paired homeodomain of Pax-3. Cell 1991; 67:767–774.
11. Nichols DH: Neural crest formation in the head of the mouse as observed using a new histological technique. J Embryol Exp Morphol 1981; 64:105–120.
12. Nichols DH: Formation and distribution of neural crest mesenchyme to the first pharyngeal arch region of the mouse embryo. Am J Anat 1986; 176:221–231.
13. Tan SS, Morriss-Kay G: The development and distribution of cranial neural crest in the rat embryo. Cell Tissue Res 1985; 240:403–416.
14. Tan SS, Morris-Kay G: Analysis of cranial neural crest cell migration and early fates in postimplantation rat chimeras. J Embryol Exp Morphol 1986; 98:21–58.
15. Serbedzija GN, Bronner-Fraser M, Fraser SE: Vital dye analysis of cranial neural crest migration in the mouse embryo. Development 1992; 116:297–307.
16. Vermeij-Keers C, Poelmann RE: The neural crest: A study on cell degeneration and improbability of cell migration in mouse embryos. Neth J Zool 1980; 30:74–81.
17. Johnston MC: A radioautographic study of the migration and fate of cranial neural crest cells in the chick embryo. Anat Rec 1966; 156:143–156.
18. Le Douarin NM: The Neural Crest. Cambridge: Cambridge University Press, 1982.
19. Noden DM: Interactions and fates of avian craniofacial mesenchyme. Development 1988; 103[Suppl]: 121–140.
20. Schwanzel-Fukuda M, Pfaff DW: Origin of luteinizing hormone releasing hormone neurons. Nature 1989; 338:161–164.
21. Bossy J: Development of olfactory and related structures in staged human embryos. Anat Embryol 1980; 161:225–226.
22. Tessier P: Anatomical classification of facial, craniofacial, and laterofacial clefts. In Tessier P (ed): Symposium on Plastic Surgery in the Orbital Region, pp 189–198. St. Louis: CV Mosby, 1976.
23. DeMyer W: Median facial malformations and their implications for brain malformations. Birth Defects 1975; 11:155–181.
24. Sulik KK, Johnston MC: Embryonic origin of holoprosencephaly: Interrelationship of the developing brain and face. Scan Electron Microsc 1982; Part 1:309–322.
25. Sulik KK, Johnston MC: Sequence of developmental alterations following acute ethanol exposure in mice: Craniofacial features of the fetal alcohol syndrome. Am J Anat 1983; 166:257–269.
26. Sulik KK, Lauder JM, Dehart DB: Brain malformations in prenatal mice following acute maternal ethanol administration. Int J Devel Neurol 1984; 2:203–214.
27. Kotch LE, Sulik KK: Experimental fetal alcohol syndrome: Proposed pathogenic basis for a variety of associated facial and brain anomalies. Am J Med Genet 1992; 44:168–176.
28. Cook CS, Nowotny AZ, Sulik KK: Fetal alcohol syndrome: Eye malformations in a mouse model. Arch Ophthalmol 1987; 105:1576–1581.
29. Sulik KK, Dehart DB, Rogers JM, et al: Teratogenicity of low doses of all-trans retinoic acid. Teratology 1993; 47:383.
30. Wei X, Sulik KK: Pathogenesis of craniofacial and body wall malformations induced by Ochratoxin A in mice. Am J Med Genet 1993; 47:862–871.
31. McNeish JD, Thayer JM, Walling K, et al: Phenotypic characterization of the transgenic mouse insertional mutation, Legless. J Exper Zool 1990; 253:151–162.
32. Thayer JM, Merker HJ, McNeish JD, et al: Pathogenesis involved in craniofacial and limb malformations in a transgenic mouse line. Teratology 1988; 37:498.
33. Darab D, Sciote J, Minkoff R, et al: Pathogenesis of medial facial clefts in mice treated with methotrexate. Teratology 1987; 36:76–86.
34. Thayer JM, Generoso WM, Cacherio NLA, et al: Pathogenesis of frontonasal dysplasia in a duplication deficiency mouse mutant. Teratology 1989; 39:486.

35. Webster WS, Johnston MC, Lammer EJ, et al: Isotretinoin embryopathy and the cranial neural crest: An in vivo and vitro study. J Craniofac Genet Dev Biol 1986; 6:211–222.
36. Poswillo D: The pathogenesis of the first and second branchial arch syndrome. Oral Surg 1973; 35:302–329.
37. Sulik KK, Johnston MC, Smiley SJ, et al: Mandibulofacial dysostosis (Treacher Collins syndrome): A new proposal for its pathogenesis. Am J Med Genet 1987; 27:359–372.
38. Sulik KK, Smiley SJ, Turvey TA, et al: Pathogenesis of cleft palate in Treacher Collins, Nager, and Miller syndromes. Cleft Palate J 1989; 26:209–216.
39. Sulik KK, Johnston MC, Daft PA, et al: Fetal alcohol syndrome and DiGeorge anomaly: Critical ethanol exposure periods for craniofacial malformations as illustrated in an animal model. Am J Med Genet 1986; [Suppl 2]:97–112.
40. Kuratani SC, Bockman DE: Inhibition of epibranchial placode-derived ganglia in the developing rat by bisdiamine. Anat Rec 1992; 233:617–624.
41. Sulik KK, Johnston MC, Ambrose LJH, et al: Phenytoin (Dilantin)-induced cleft lip and palate in A/J mice: A scanning and transmission electron microscopic study. Anat Rec 1979; 195:243–256.
42. Bronsky PT, Johnston MC, Sulik KK: Morphogenesis of hypoxia-induced cleft lip in CL/Fr mice. J Craniofac Genet Dev Biol 1986; [Suppl 2]:113–128.
43. Greene RM, Kochhar DM: Some aspects of corticosteroid-induced cleft palate: A review. Teratology 1975; 11:47–56.
44. Pratt RM, Salomon D: Biochemical basis for the teratogenic effects of glucocorticoids. In Jachau M (ed): Chemical Teratogenesis, pp 171–193. Amsterdam: Elsevier/North Holland, 1981.
45. Speight HS, Smiley SJ, Johnston MC, et al: Development of microglossia induced in mice with 13-cis retinoic acid. J Dent Res 1987; 66:240.
46. Koskinen-Moffett L: In vivo experimental model for prenatal craniosynostosis. J Dent Res [Special Issue] 1986; 65:980.
47. Kessel M, Balling R, Gruss P: Variations of cervical vertebrae after expression of a Hox-1.1 transgene in mice. Cell 1990; 61(2):301–308.
48. Kessel M: Respecification of vertebral identities by retinoic acid. Development 1992; 115:487–501.
49. Alles AJ, Wu TF-T, Alysworth AS, et al: Etretinate-induced abnormalities of the cranial base. Teratology 1992; 45:485.

Facial Growth in Orofacial Clefting Disorders | 2

Gunvor Semb and William C. Shaw

There is no question that the face of an individual with a repaired orofacial cleft differs from those of unaffected individuals. The differences typically go beyond the scarred lip and residual nasal deformity and reflect a distinctive aberrant pattern of facial growth.

FACIAL GROWTH IN THE NONCLEFT POPULATION

Three important mechanisms are involved in changing the size and shape of the craniofacial bones: (1) conversion of cartilage, (2) sutural growth, and (3) remodeling. By the end of the first year of life, only three sites of *cartilage replacement* that are significant in skull growth remain: the spheno-occipital synchondrosis, the nasal septum, and the secondary growth cartilage at the head of the mandibular condyle. *Sutural growth* occurs across the circummaxillary suture system, which lies on an inclined plane, so that maxillary translation in a downward and forward direction is permitted (Fig. 2–1). In the final stage, the process of *subperiosteal surface deposition and internal resorption* makes an important contribution to the outward shape of the face and its cavities and recesses, especially the marked differential growth for the deepening and widening of the face.[44]

Theories that changes in facial shape are driven by skeletal and especially septal cartilage growth[160] have given way to the functional matrix theory[112] (i.e., that the mechanisms of cartilage replacement, sutural growth, and remodeling are merely responsive to functional demands that are somehow conveyed by the soft tissues and capsular linings).[113, 114, 133] Enlargement of the temporal and frontal lobes of the growing cerebrum (Fig. 2–2) is perhaps the most plausible candidate as the prime mover in forward translation of the nasomaxillary complex.[44]

For all the books and chapters that have been written on facial growth, remarkably little is known about its controlling mechanisms. It is evident that the general shape of the individual bone of the normal facial skeleton is genetically predetermined. Even in vitro excised bony blastemata grown in culture assume the general shape of the appropriate normal bone. In everyday life, we observe family resemblance in facial form and can suppose that among the genetic information that parents impart to their children, some is capable of ensuring the replication of skeletal, dental, and neuromuscular features. Monozygotic twins look alike. Eskimos and Lapps live in the same environment, eat the same sort of food, and have essentially similar functional demands on their craniofacial structures; however, Eskimos have heavy skulls and facial bones with prominent muscle markings, whereas Lapps have light, delicate skulls and facial bones.

Nonetheless, the facial skeleton provides structural support for the critical functions of air movement and food indigestion necessary to sustain life. Although the precise mechanism remains obscure, evidence is increasing that adaptations in craniofacial orientation and shape are stimulated by functional demands. Some possible causal links have emerged from studies of nasal obstruction.[102, 129, 134, 139] It can be postulated that airway insufficiency leads to a backward tilt of the head, lowering of the mandible and tongue, and different stresses on the lower jaw from the platysma and suprahyoid musculature (Fig. 2–3). This apparently leads in some degree to a permanent increase in lower face height, altered mandible shape, a decrease in facial depth, upright

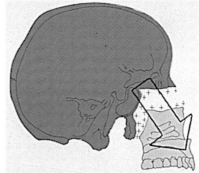

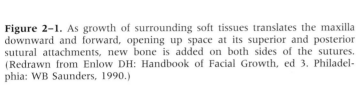

Figure 2–1. As growth of surrounding soft tissues translates the maxilla downward and forward, opening up space at its superior and posterior sutural attachments, new bone is added on both sides of the sutures. (Redrawn from Enlow DH: Handbook of Facial Growth, ed 3. Philadelphia: WB Saunders, 1990.)

incisors, and a narrow deep palate.[185,191] So far, these studies demonstrate only minor average skeletal changes in relation to nasal obstruction, but future research may discern other forms of functional adaptation.

Both jaws consist of a *basal part* that is thought to be more dependent on genetic control, and *different processes* that are dependent on their size and shape by muscle function (such as the gonial region) or that are dependent on the presence of teeth (such as the dentoalveolar processes).

Considerable doubt remains whether it is possible to induce actual change in size and shape of the basal parts of the maxilla and mandible, but a redirection and acceleration of growth that would otherwise take place at a later stage may be achieved by orthopedic forces.[133] There is general agreement that the maxilla is more easily influenced in its growth than the mandible.[87,153,198]

The dentoalveolar processes are highly influenced by external forces (e.g., pressure from the surrounding soft tissue) or orthopedic and orthodontic forces. The teeth are guided in their eruption by the tongue, lip, and cheek muscles, and they show a great ability to adapt and compensate for minor maxillomandibular discrepancies to establish an acceptable occlusion.

FACIAL GROWTH ASSOCIATED WITH REPAIRED CLEFTS

Figures 2–4 to 2–6 illustrate the principal differences in facial form for individuals with repaired clefts.[32] Numerous descriptive studies of facial form have been reported; a few of them are longitudinal.

Many reports reveal that craniofacial linear measurements in all cleft types including those of unoperated patients are smaller than in the noncleft population.[29,32,156,174] This is often explained by the smaller stature and head size and retarded skeletal maturity found in patients with cleft lip-palate (CLP).[32,40,88,156] The pubertal growth spurt occurs on average 6 months later in boys with CLP, but growth continues longer, especially in the mandible.[88,156] At any age, smaller facial dimensions can be expected in subjects with clefting. It is suggested that the reason for this is largely early feeding problems and recurrent infections of the upper airways combined with the surgical procedures.

Clefts of the Lip and the Alveolus

In patients with clefts of the lip and alveolus only (CLA), facial growth is reported to be within the normal variation for most angular variables including the maxilla and the cranial base.[32,56,62,155,156]

One consistent finding is the increased interocular width in patients with clefts of the lip and alveolus,[32,34,56,74,83,117] but there is some disagreement whether this is concurrent with increased maxillary width,[120] decreased maxillary width,[32] or the same width as the noncleft population.[56]

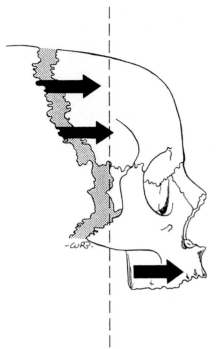

Figure 2–2. The cranial bones increase in size by sutural bone growth as the forehead becomes displaced anteriorly. The nasomaxillary complex is carried anteriorly as well. (Redrawn from Enlow DH: Handbook of Facial Growth, ed 3. Philadelphia: WB Saunders, 1990.)

Another finding is reported deviation in the orientation of the anterior nasal spine.[32,34,66,117,155]

The mandible in the CLA population has been reported to be smaller and the gonial angle larger, and both posterior and anterior facial heights are slightly reduced,[32,177] but overall these differences are minor.

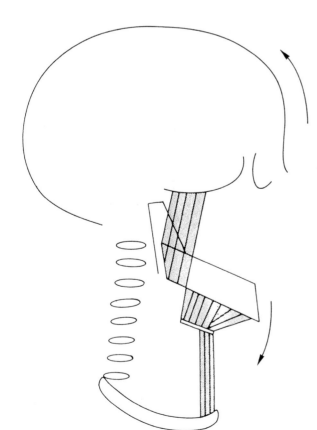

Figure 2–3. Hypothetical representation of growth disturbance associated with nasal obstruction; as the head tilts backward to reduce airway obstruction, the anterior mandible is subjected to a downward pull as the muscles and fascia between the mandible, hyoid, and shoulder are stretched. (Modified from Houston WJB: Mandibular growth rotations—Their mechanisms and importance. Eur J Orthod 1988; 10:369–373.)

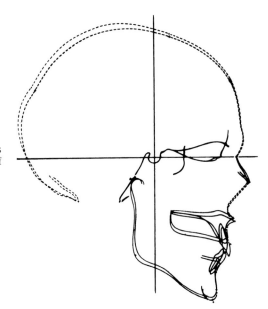

Figure 2–4. Average facial shape in adult patients with cleft lip/alveolus compared with a noncleft sample. (Courtesy of Dr. E. Dahl, University of Copenhagen.)

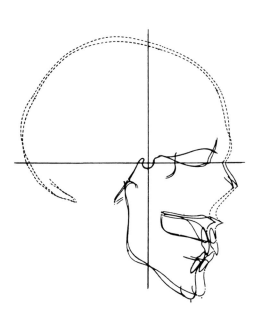

Figure 2–5. Average facial shape in adult patients with isolated cleft palate compared with a noncleft sample. (Courtesy of Dr. E. Dahl, University of Copenhagen.)

Figure 2–6. Average facial shape in adult patients with unilateral complete cleft lip and palate compared with a noncleft sample. (Courtesy of Dr. E. Dahl, University of Copenhagen.)

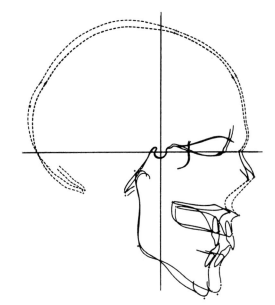

Cleft Palate Only

In contrast to subjects with primary palate clefting, interocular width in patients with clefts of the palate only (CPO) is not increased.[32, 34, 179] The cranial base angle is reported to be within the normal variation in most studies, but the upper face is characterized by a shorter and more retrusive maxilla relative to the cranial base.[17–19, 32, 93, 127, 145, 155, 172, 179, 192] As for the vertical dimensions, most authors have found a decrease in the posterior height,[32, 93, 172, 177, 179, 192] but there is disagreement about whether the anterior facial height is increased compared with that of the noncleft population. The width of the basal maxilla is found to be within normal variation or slightly reduced.[32, 179]

In CPO, the mandible is also smaller and retrusive with an obtuse gonial angle and a steep mandibular plane.[18, 32, 93, 172] In a longitudinal study of 52 Danish subjects with CPO observed from 5 to 21 years of age, Viteporn and coworkers[192] found anterior rotation of the mandible with a decrease in the gonial angle and mandibular inclination over time; they suggested that orthodontic treatment may have influenced the difference in mandibular growth pattern.

Because both the maxilla and the mandible are small and retrusive, the relationship between the jaws is usually satisfactory. Incisors in both jaws are retroclined and the dental arches slightly narrower and shorter,[4, 59] but an acceptable occlusion is usually obtained.

Where the extent of the palatal cleft has been considered, it appears that the above differences, at least for the maxillary dimensions, are more marked in association with larger clefts.[32, 69, 70, 85, 86, 93, 101, 179, 192] This was, however, not found in a study by Friede and coworkers.[59]

Complete Clefts of the Lip and Palate

The facial form of patients with repaired complete clefts differs to a greater extent than do the two other major cleft subtypes: cleft of the primary palate (CLA) and isolated cleft palate (CPO). There are, however, inconsistencies in reports concerning the cranial base angle. Some investigators find it to be increased,[32, 64, 146] others find no or just minor differences from the noncleft population,[25, 43, 75, 109, 145, 158, 162, 181, 188, 189] and Moss[111] and Harris[65] found it to be smaller. This disparity may be explained, at least in part, by the gender composition of samples. Semb[162] found the cranial base angle in unilateral cleft lip-palate (UCLP) to be consistently 3 degrees larger in females from age 5 years to 18 years. This gender difference was also found in studies by Ross,[145] Sandham and Cheng,[158] and Paulin and Thilander.[130]

In a study comparing a group of neonates with CLA to a group with complete CLP, the spheno-occipital synchondrosis was found to be broader and the distance from the superior part of the synchondrosis to the sella point shorter in the latter group.[119] The authors suggested that this may be related to a defect or a delay in maturity in the early development of the cartilaginous cranial base in children with major clefts.

As in the CLA group, the interocular width in patients with CLP is increased,[3, 32, 83, 84, 116, 117, 156, 162, 181] but the width of the face and the width of the basal maxilla do not differ from those of the noncleft population,[32, 181] and the upper dental arch is narrower with frequent posterior crossbites.[156] The width of the nasal septum in subjects with bilateral cleft lip-palate (BCLP) is found to be larger.[5] Asymmetry in the anterior part of the maxilla in subjects with UCLP is observed.[32, 34, 66, 116, 117, 156, 162]

The facial form in adult individuals with repaired UCLP and that with repaired BCLP are similar and, in comparison with the facial form of noncleft subjects, is characterized by a general retrusion of the profile relative to the cranial base involving the nasal bone, maxilla, and mandible. Both the maxilla and mandible are shorter and retrusive, and the incisors in both jaws are retroclined. There is severe reduction in posterior but only slight reduction in anterior maxillary height. An increased vertical length of the anterior maxilla has also been reported.[30, 123] The mandible has an increased gonial angle and a steeper mandibular plane, and there is an increase in lower facial height.[32, 42, 49, 116, 130, 146, 156, 162, 163, 177, 180, 181] The bony nasopharynx is smaller.[32, 159, 183, 189] There is a tendency for facial growth to be more severely affected in males.[130, 146, 162]

The *pattern of growth* is also different from that in noncleft individuals. Semb[162] found almost no increase between 5 and 18 years of age in the length of the maxilla measured to the anterior outline of the alveolar process (ss′-pm) in a mixed longitudinal study of 257 cases of complete UCLP. This dimension increased by only 1.4 mm for the UCLP sample while increasing by approximately 10 mm in the noncleft sample recorded in the templates of the Bolton standards.[27] There was a concomitant reduction in maxillary prominence at the dentoalveolar level, as seen in Figure 2–7. A marked reduction in mandibular prominence over time was also found. The excessive lower face angulation changed little over time in the UCLP sample (approximately 3° greater than the Bolton standards at age 5 years), whereas it was reduced by 5° in the noncleft sample.

The nose had a more backward and downward direction of growth than that which has been described for noncleft individuals,[132] and the relationship of the upper and lower lip outlines worsened steadily during growth as the upper lip receded in prominence. The soft tissue profile became steadily straighter, and especially so after the age of 15 years, as has previously been noted by Sadowsky and coworkers.[157]

These findings also concur with those of the longitudinal study reported by Enemark and coworkers.[42]

Figure 2–8 illustrates the development of the facial profile in a boy with UCLP.

In children with BCLP, the premaxilla is slowly molded back after lip repair, even when it is severely protruded at birth.

A mixed longitudinal study of 90 cases of complete BCLP[163] found the maxilla in BCLP to be relatively prominent in early childhood (4° more prominent at 5 years), but it steadily receded so that by 7 years it was similar to the value for noncleft subjects,[27] and by 18 years it was 6° less (see Fig. 2–7). Throughout the period of observation, the mandible was less prominent in subjects with BCLP—4° at 5 years —and remained so until the end of growth—6° less at 18 years. Vertically lower facial angulation remained higher in BCLP—2° at 5 years and 9° at 18 years.

This pattern of growth is similar in other studies, but some authors have reported a slower retrusion of the premaxilla so that by the end of growth, values were closer to those of noncleft subjects.[55, 68, 71, 121, 188]

The *growth pattern* was also different between UCLP and BCLP groups.[162, 163] In comparison with UCLP patients, subjects with BCLP displayed greater maxillary prominence in early childhood (s-n-ss was 5.3° larger at 5 years), but this difference was reduced with time so that by 18 years the maxilla was only slightly (1.4°) more prominent on average. In other respects facial growth patterns were similar in both conditions, although the gonial angle was somewhat greater (3°) in BCLP throughout the period of observation.

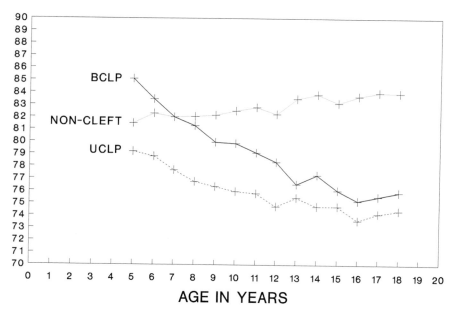

Figure 2–7. Changes in maxillary prominence (s-n-ss) for 257 patients with complete unilateral cleft lip and palate (UCLP) and 90 patients with complete bilateral cleft lip and palate (BCLP) compared with a noncleft sample (Bolton standards[27]).

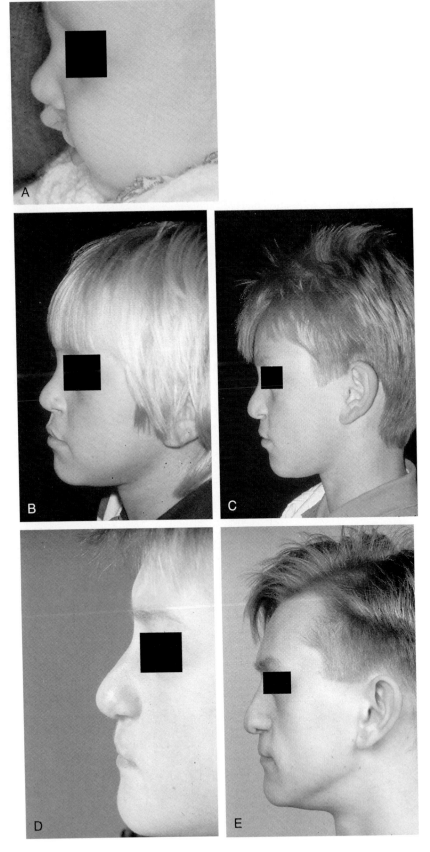

Figure 2-8. The development of the facial profile in a boy with unilateral cleft lip and palate: at 3 months of age, before lip closure (A), at 7 years of age (B), at 12 years of age (C), at 15 years of age (D), and at 21 years of age (E).

Figure 2–9 illustrates the development of the facial profile in a boy with BCLP. Presence of a soft tissue bridge in UCLP and BCLP, although reducing the need for secondary nasal corrections, had only minor influence on anteroposterior maxillary growth.[166]

Figure 2–9. The development of the facial profile in a boy with bilateral cleft lip and palate: at 3 months of age, before lip closure *(A)*, at 2 years of age *(B)*, at 5 years of age, before columellaplasty *(C)*, at 10 years of age *(D)*, at 15 years of age *(E)*, and at 21 years of age *(F)*.

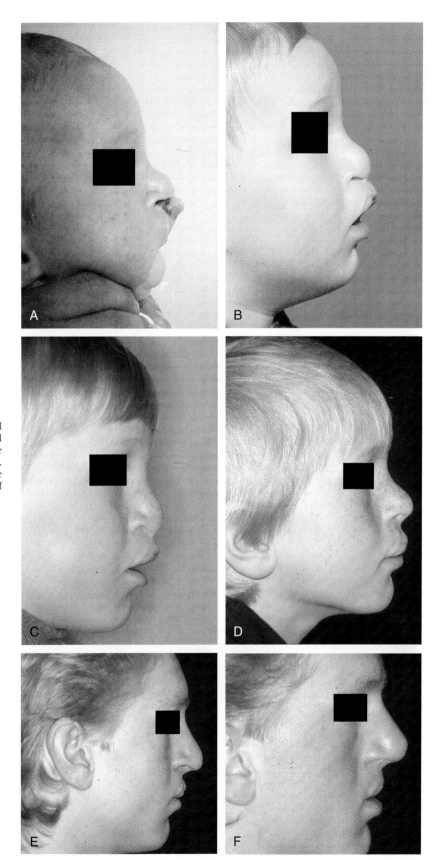

THE CAUSES OF GROWTH DISTURBANCES IN REPAIRED CLEFTS

Because the controlling forces in normal facial growth are obscure, the explanation of growth disturbance (or variation) associated with clefts and their repair must be somewhat speculative. Nonetheless, several factors are potential sources of interference with the normal growth pattern in individuals with clefts:

1. Congenital dysmorphology of the midface
2. Other variations intrinsically associated with the cleft
3. Functional adaptations
4. Surgical iatrogenesis

Congenital Dysmorphology of the Midface

The facial deformity present at birth represents a combination of the initial embryonic defect and subsequent changes occurring in utero. In complete unilateral clefting, features are asymmetry of the anterior maxilla, an upward tilt of the premaxillary region, and a distortion of the nasal septum, bulging laterally toward the cleft side. In bilateral clefts, the premaxilla, united by a cartilaginous joint to the vomer, occupies an extreme anterior position on the underside of the nasal septum, with the septopremaxillary ligament oriented upward rather than forward (Fig. 2–10). These anomalies are evident from the earliest stages after failure of union of the facial processes.[99, 100] However, the factors responsible remain unclear.[45] In addition to a more rapidly growing tongue, an increased growth rate of the fetal nasal septum has been demonstrated in CLP specimens, suggesting the possibility of an unrestrained primary overgrowth of the midline nasal capsule. The available data, however, do not preclude the possibility of a secondary response to extracapsular influences.[95]

The great variation observable in the eventual clinical presentation at birth suggests that there are possible secondary distortions during the fetal period. Differing patterns of intrauterine swallowing and tongue positioning, as well as variations in neuromuscular activity of the disrupted buccopharyngeal ring, may explain the diversity of segmental relationships seen in consecutive births (Fig. 2–11). In the absence of surgical repair, these dysmorphic features and relationships remain more or less constant throughout growth until adulthood (Fig. 2–12).

A variable degree of tissue deficiency is also likely to occur. Indeed, deficiency of mesoderm is considered to be an important factor in failure of embryonic union.[45] The measurement of deficient tissue is technically difficult, but cephalometric laminography has shown palatal shelf deficiency to occur within cleft subtypes involving a palatal cleft.[31] Huddart and coworkers,[81] in a comparative study on plaster models, found on average 13.7% tissue deficiency in the posterior palatal plane in UCLP and

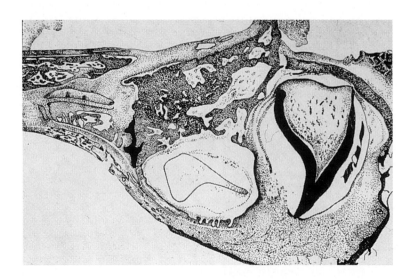

Figure 2–10. Sagittal section through premaxilla of a neonate with bilateral cleft lip and palate showing a prominent premaxilla united to the vomer by the premaxillary vomerine suture. Note the upward orientation of the anterior nasal spine. (Based on Latham RA: Development and structure of the premaxillary deformity in bilateral cleft lip and palate. Br J Plast Surg 1973; 26:1–11.)

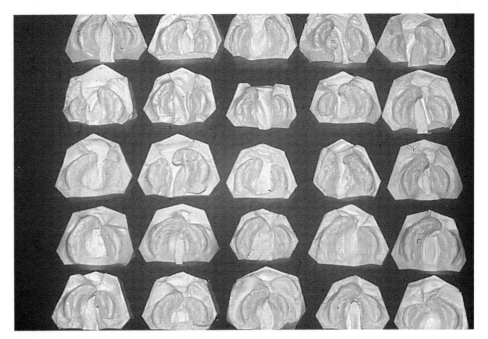

Figure 2–11. Neonatal study casts of 25 cases of consecutive UCLP.

significantly less in BCLP.[82] In contrast, Hotz and Gnoinski[78] and Hotz[76] could conclude that apart from a few cases of obvious hypoplasia, there is no tissue deficiency in the great majority of cleft cases. This is in accordance with the findings of Kuijpers-Jagtman.[98] The lack of landmarks makes it difficult to quantify deficiency of lip tissue, but the frequent absence of the lateral incisor and occasional absence of the central incisor in the alveolar process may indicate the occurrence of primary palate deficiency.[168] In some bilateral cases, the prolabium and the premaxilla are markedly reduced in size (Fig. 2–13).

Other Intrinsic Variations

It would be surprising if the catastrophic events leading to failed union of the facial processes were not associated with dysmorphology beyond the cleft site. Some indica-

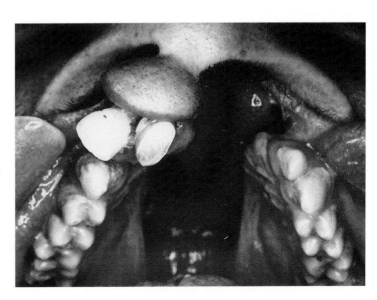

Figure 2–12. Arch form in an individual with unoperated BCLP. The segmental relationships may have changed little. (Courtesy of Hospital de Pesquisa e Reabilitacao de Lesoes Labio-Palatais, Bauru, Brazil.)

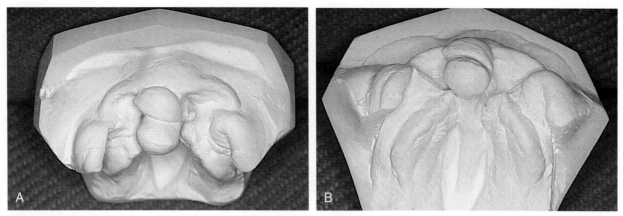

Figure 2–13. *A* and *B,* Study model of a patient with bilateral cleft lip and palate at 3 months with a very small prolabium and premaxilla.

tion of the extent to which the variations in facial form in CLP described above are intrinsic can be obtained by observations of patients with unrepaired clefts including neonates and twins.

Comparison of craniofacial dimensions of infants with clefts before surgery and of noncleft counterparts would indicate variations in form intrinsic to the clefting condition. Noncleft cephalograms are unavailable for ethical reasons, but Dahl and coworkers,[34, 35] using incomplete cleft lip as a near-normal reference group, found that CPO and BCLP were accompanied by a retrognathic maxilla, reduced posterior maxillary height, and a smaller, retruded mandible.

Studies of older individuals with unrepaired clefts provide further evidence of inherent differences in the face of individuals with clefts. In subjects with unrepaired clefts limited to the primary palate, increased interorbital width is the only major difference beyond the cleft region from subjects without clefting yet reported,[34] justifying their use as noncleft controls. Even in later years they display no difference in mandibular form.[20, 23] In subjects with unrepaired isolated clefts of the secondary palate, the bimaxillary retrusion and increased gonial angle noted at birth persist.[16, 32]

Additions to the literature of comparisons of older individuals with unrepaired complete clefts and their counterparts without clefting allow examination of the more generalized craniofacial configuration associated with clefting in the absence of surgery. On posteroanterior (PA) cephalograms, increased width of various facial parts in unoperated UCLP and BCLP has been found.[115] Capelozza and coworkers[29] compared a group of 13 males and 13 females (over 16 and 15 years of age, respectively) with unoperated unilateral complete CLP to a noncleft group matched for gender, age, and ethnicity. The maxilla in the UCLP group was smaller, but it was more protrusive at the alveolar level and at the level of the anterior nasal spine in the male subjects. The mandible was also smaller, the gonial angle was increased, the mandibular plane was steeper, and the lower incisors were retroclined in the UCLP group. There was a reduced posterior height and a tendency toward increased anterior lower facial height. These differences in mandibular shape were more marked in females. The nose was less protruded, but as a result of the maxillary protrusion, there was an increase in profile convexity.

These findings are largely in agreement with the results of a comparative study of 28 unoperated male subjects with UCLP from Sri Lanka over 13 years of age with a control group of Sri Lankan males without clefting,[106] except that the mandible in the Sri Lankan cleft group was retrusive as well as different in shape and smaller. There was also a tendency toward a larger cranial base angle in the Sri Lankan UCLP group, although this was not statistically significant.

These studies confirm the findings of previous studies of patients with unoperated complete clefts in which the samples were smaller and/or the age range greater.[20, 22, 23, 36, 110, 125, 126, 131]

One consistent finding is the *smaller* craniofacial dimensions (including size of the maxilla[29]) found in both unoperated and operated CLP subjects compared with noncleft subjects. This is often explained by the fact that the cleft population appears to be composed of smaller individuals overall.[32, 40, 88, 156] Thus caution is necessary in interpreting linear measurements.

Differences likely to be intrinsic in nature include abnormalities in the size and form of the cranial base (although the literature is contradictory on this point), and the increased interocular width in patients with CLP. The difference in size and shape of the mandible with small ramus height, increased gonial angle, and a steep mandibular plane that has been found in all clefts involving the secondary palate may also be inherited because it is associated with both repaired and unrepaired clefts,[16, 20, 23, 29, 30, 32, 106, 126] and is found in infants with CPO and BCLP.[34, 35] However, as discussed later, functional adaptations of the mandible secondary to hypoplasia of the nasal capsule cannot be ruled out.

Another indication of intrinsic difference between individuals with and without clefts is the consistent finding of smaller tooth size in patients with all cleft types.[47, 107, 108, 135]

Evidence that the prominence of the cleft maxilla is similar to that of the noncleft is a key issue in the debate concerning surgical iatrogenesis. Therefore it is noteworthy that the comparisons between persons without clefting and individuals with unoperated cleft have revealed that the anterior projection of the basal maxilla is the same in both groups,[29, 106] despite the finding (at least in the Capelozza and coworkers sample[29]) that the maxilla is smaller in subjects with unoperated clefts than in noncleft subjects, in keeping with the overall smaller size of patients with clefts. However, it requires adequate comparisons of cleft and noncleft neonates to rule out the possibility that the basal cleft maxilla has an initial retrusion (as the data of Dahl and coworkers[35] suggested) that is somehow overcome by excessive postnatal growth related to the presence of the unrepaired cleft.

The fairly rare occurrence of monozygotic twins discordant for CLP may also give some indication of inherited facial features of individuals with a predisposition to facial clefting. Research of this kind has seldom been reported. Interestingly, however, studies of 25 such pairs revealed nasal cavity width in 17 of the noncleft twins to be less than that for the normal population.[90, 91] This was considered to be a result of the reduced size of the embryonic medial nasal prominence.

Studies of the noncleft members of monozygotic twins discordant for CP suggest that they have an increased tongue size.[89, 96] Indeed, this may predispose the embryo to cleft palate by interfering with shelf elevation or by widening the midface so that the shelves are too far apart to make contact, even if they do elevate.

Functional Adaptations

The nasal airway is frequently impaired in individuals with CLP, nasal resistance being judged to be 20% to 30% higher than in the noncleft population. Nasal abnormalities such as deviated septum, vomerine spurs, alar constriction, turbinate hypertrophy, and thickened nasal mucosa tend to decrease nasal airway size and increase airway resistance.[2, 39, 46, 193, 194, 196] Impaired maxillary growth further constricts the nasal floor and reduces airway size and increases airway resistance. Ironically, surgical correction of the cleft nasal deformity may worsen the situation,[63, 194, 196] including surgical attempts to restore symmetry between the nostrils in unilateral clefts because surgery may lead to reduction in size of the unaffected nostril. Procedures to correct velopharyngeal inadequacy also significantly reduce the nasopharyngeal airspace and increase upper airway resistance[195, 197] and the prevalence of mouth breathing.[63, 193]

There is evidence that airway deficiency in individuals with UCLP is present in utero. Siegel and coworkers[173] observed that the fetal septum appeared to be enlarged and distorted and was flanked laterally by a reduced nasal airway passage at 17 weeks. They suggested that reduced nasal airway size may be a function of both nasal capsule deficiency and nasal septum hypertrophy. Reduced upper airway dimensions in CP infants were found by Dahl and coworkers.[35]

An impaired nasal airway and high airway resistance usually result in obligatory mouth breathing. Hairfield and coworkers[63] documented the unusually high prevalence of mouth breathing in individuals with clefts; about 68% of individuals with CLP breathe more in the oral mode than in the nasal mode. An unexpected finding was that the prevalence of mouth breathing in adults was the same as in children. Thus it appears that the improvement in nasal airway size with growth is not sufficient to induce a change in breathing mode. Another explanation is that obligatory mouth breathing is replaced by habitual mouth breathing rather than by nasal breathing. There is evidence in the literature that mouth breathing can be a learned behavior.[193]

Despite differences in nasal airway size among different cleft types, the prevalence of oral-nasal breathers is about the same in all groups because the open communication between the nose and mouth at birth prevents establishment of a normal nasal breathing pattern. Oral-nasal breathing also remains after surgical repair and may persist throughout life.[193]

Little doubt exists that nasal obstruction is a consistent finding in association with facial clefting. In keeping with the theories of mandibular adaptation to airway obstruction in noncleft individuals noted earlier, this may be responsible, at least in part, for the characteristic mandibular position and form in affected individuals. These adaptations need not necessarily be a consequence of surgical repair because, as noted earlier, there is evidence of airway deficiency in utero as a result of nasal capsule deficiency and septum hypertrophy.[173] It is possible, therefore, that airway insufficiency is the primary cause of the mandibular anomalies that are evident both in operated *and* in unoperated subjects and in newborns.

Because an oral mode of breathing is also associated with a lower tongue position, there is the possibility that narrowing of the maxillary arch may ensue. Thus, it is interesting that exactly this occurs, at least to some degree, in individuals with unoperated clefts of all types,[20, 23, 107, 108, 176, 186] despite excessive width in the posterior region at birth.[81, 82]

Surgical Iatrogenesis

From a clinical point of view, the impact of surgery on maxillary growth remains a central issue in the controversy surrounding the surgical management of orofacial clefts. Although attention was drawn to the dramatic effects of surgically induced growth impairment more than 50 years ago,[61, 62, 66, 73, 178] how much contemporary surgery interferes with growth and whether lip or palatal surgery is more harmful remain matters of dispute.[6, 30, 32, 106, 123, 146, 156] In addition, controversy remains about the importance of surgical technique, timing of surgery, and surgical skill.

Results of the comparison between noncleft and unoperated cleft subjects referred to earlier suggest that although the anterior dentoalveolar structures are flared anteriorly in the presence of an unrepaired cleft lip, and there are systematic differences in the structures adjacent to the maxilla, prominence of the basal maxilla in affected persons is remarkably similar to that in unaffected persons. The presence of an unrepaired cleft can hardly be considered normal, but these data suggest at least that the cleft maxilla has good potential for growth in the absence of surgery.

An indication of the extent of growth impairment induced by surgery may be obtained by comparing repaired and unrepaired samples. A series of Brazilian studies, including relatively large groups of the major cleft subtypes,[30, 123, 174] one study of Sri Lankan subjects with UCLP,[106] one Danish study,[32] and a Japanese study[200] permit some conclusions.

In isolated clefts of the primary palate, the effect of lip repair is to mold the distorted anterior dentoalveolar process into a normal configuration. The length, the prominence of the basal maxilla, the vertical maxillary relationships, and the mandible are all unaffected by lip closure.[30, 123, 175]

Similarly, in isolated cleft palate, repair of the cleft is not associated with alterations in the relationship of the maxilla or the mandible to each other or the craniofacial complex.[16, 30, 123, 174] This is largely in agreement with the findings of Dahl,[32] who found only minor differences in both jaws when comparing unoperated subjects with an operated group. However, the scar tissue in the palate may invariably influence the dentoalveolar structures.

Thus for these two cleft subtypes—isolated clefts of the primary (CLA) or the secondary palate (CPO)—surgery does not appear to adversely affect facial growth.

In contrast, in complete clefts of the lip and palate, surgery has a great impact on maxillary growth that becomes progressively apparent as patients reach maturity. It is especially in the anteroposterior dimension that growth is impaired, and subjects with repaired CLP demonstrate reduced prominence of the maxilla at the basal (anterior nasal spine) and dentoalveolar (A-point) level.[30, 106, 123] Vertically, maxillary growth is deficient in the posterior part, but is mostly unaffected anteriorly, with even increased vertical length of the anterior maxilla sometimes reported.[30, 123] The mandibular growth pattern is apparently unaffected by the surgical repair of complete clefts.[174]

In light of this evidence, there appears to be little doubt about the potential impairment for maxillary growth that surgery may induce in combined cleft lip and palate, and it is conceivable that cases with a significant deficiency of tissue are most at risk for postoperative maxillary distortion and restraint. However, the specific cause of growth disturbance remains unclear, with either lip surgery or palatal surgery being indicated as the major insult.[13, 30, 106, 123, 146–152, 156]

Lip and Palate Surgery and Growth Disturbance

Much has been written about the harmful effect of palatal scars that form on areas of the palate denuded during primary surgery.[62, 73, 97, 156] It has been postulated especially that scar tissue located in the region of the maxillary/palatine and palatine/pterygoid sutures acts to prevent the maxilla's normal downward and forward translation.[156] On the other hand, experimental animal studies have reported that increased pressure from the repaired cleft lip is the primary cause of maxillary growth restraint.[7–11] Lip pressure in infants with UCLP has been measured after lip repair and until 2 years of age and was found to be significantly higher than in a noncleft control group.[11]

Studies of partially operated human subjects with complete UCLP could conceivably shed light on this controversy by examining the effect of lip closure alone and the cumulative effect of surgery of both lip and palate.

Two studies have focused on this question on a relatively large sample of subjects with UCLP.[30, 106] Table 2–1 lists the findings from these studies. It seems that lip surgery alone has had a major influence on maxillary development. For example, the length of the maxilla (Ar-ANS) was reduced after lip surgery by 6.3 mm and 4.0 mm, respectively. Palatal surgery reduced this dimension by 1.0 mm in the Sri Lankan sample, and by 0.7 mm in the Brazilian sample. The same effect was seen in the prominence of the anterior alveolar process (SNA). Dahl[32] and Yoshida and co-workers[200] also found a substantial reduction in maxillary prominence in patients with UCLP who had undergone lip surgery only. However, because individuals with complete clefts who have undergone only palatal surgery are not available, this experiment cannot be considered complete. It is by no means certain that the effect of palatal repair alone would be limited to the values listed in the right hand column of Table 2–1 (i.e., which operation is undertaken first could have the major restraining effect).

Iatrogenic effects seem mainly limited to the maxillary base and arch. The anteroposterior growth impairment of the maxillary complex is the most obvious feature. The maxilla is shorter and is posteriorly displaced relative to the cranial base, although it also appears to be deficient in the posterior vertical dimension. The transverse dimension of the basal maxilla does not seem to be affected by surgery, but the dental arches are highly affected. Palatal closure often includes incisions along the dental arches, and the scars produced may induce an inward deflection of the dentoalveolar processes, resulting in anterior and transverse crossbites.[15, 32, 33, 42, 97, 156] It is therefore likely that different surgical techniques for closing the palate give rise to malocclusions of different extent without necessarily altering the neighboring structures.

Table 2–1. REDUCTION IN MAXILLARY PROMINENCE ASSOCIATED WITH LIP REPAIR ALONE OR LIP AND PALATE REPAIR OF UCLP

	UCLP Males, Sri Lankan; Changes After Lip Repair	UCLP Males, Brazilian; Changes After Palate Repair
Basal Maxilla (Ar-ANS)		
Effect of lip surgery	− 6.3 mm	− 4.0 mm
Additional effect of palatal repair	− 1.0 mm	− 0.7 mm
Alveolar Process (SNA)		
Effect of lip surgery	− 5.4°	− 6.1°
Additional effect of palatal repair	− 3.7°	− 1.2°

Surgical Skill, Technique, and Timing

The studies cited earlier demonstrate the vulnerability of the midface to surgical insult. Is it possible to determine whether some surgical approaches will be less harmful than others? A growing body of literature points to the desirability that surgery of all kinds be performed by high-volume operators,[38] and this has been recognized in relation to CLP surgery.[6, 130, 153, 154, 156, 169, 170] However, a confusing number of techniques has been recommended for the management of CLP,[79] and the literature is less helpful in regard to the choice of surgical protocol.[140]

Choices in Surgery in UCLP

The choice of technique for lip closure seems to be mostly a matter of personal preference for what the operator believes will give the best aesthetic and functional results. The choice ranges from lip adhesion, through various designs of nostril-lip reconstruction, to extensive undermining to effect primary lip and nose repair. The most popular time for lip closure seems to be when the patient is about 3 months of age,[79] when the nose and lip components have had a chance to increase in size along with the patient. However, a few centers practice definitive lip closure in newborns. If, as discussed earlier, lip surgery is more detrimental to growth than previously believed, this may possibly lead to greater growth impairment. It is not possible to study the effect of technique and timing of lip closure in isolation on maxillary growth in the Western world, because palatal surgery (soft and/or hard palate) is undertaken some months later. Studies of subsequent maxillary growth invariably show the cumulative effect of lip *and* palate closure.[33, 149, 164, 167]

The general finding for research on the long-term consequences of bone grafting in the neonatal period has been that maxillary growth is inhibited,[52, 92, 136, 137, 141] and the same is true for infant periosteoplasty.[71, 72] However, at least two centers have found growth after primary bone grafting to be satisfactory.[26, 122, 143, 144]

As for palatal closure, both technique and timing have been widely discussed, but their effect on maxillary growth is not resolved. The most controversial issue seems to be the timing of hard palate repair, in which two fundamentally different approaches may be contrasted—early closure of the complete cleft (before 1–1.5 years of age), and the delay of hard palate closure for several years, justified by a supposed avoidance of growth disturbance. The method of delayed hard palate closure was proposed by Gillies and Fry[60] and has become increasingly popular in the last two decades. In their review of the rationale and supporting evidence for this procedure, Witzel and coworkers[199] concluded that the beneficial effect on facial growth has not been proved (unless surgery is delayed until after 12 years of age). They pointed out that the deleterious effect on speech has not received proper attention.

Another area of disagreement is whether surgery to the alveolus at the time of lip repair will cause growth impairment. One theory is that interference with the vomero-premaxillary suture may cause growth disturbance.[48, 50, 53]

Different opinions exist regarding the disadvantages and benefits of the use of a single-layer vomer flap to close the hard palate.[28, 37, 42, 53, 54, 57, 94, 116, 162] Ross[148] stated that surgery to the alveolus impairs growth, especially in the vertical dimension. Most centers have discontinued primary bone grafting on the grounds that it impairs maxillary growth[54, 137] or that it does not give sufficient bone in the alveolar area for tooth migration so that a second bone grafting procedure is necessary.[26] Rosenstein and coworkers[144] nevertheless favored primary bone grafting.

The fourth issue of dispute has been whether push-back procedures, which supposedly give a longer soft palate but inevitably leave more scar tissue in the anterior palate, are more harmful to growth than other procedures (although there is still no evidence that the push-back procedure actually gives better speech[142]). Some authors have found a higher incidence of crossbites with the push-back procedure,[24, 33, 58, 128] whereas others have not.[21]

In a broad sense, some answers can be obtained from the results of multicenter comparisons. In one study, six European centers recalled consecutive 10-year-old patients with repaired complete UCLP and obtained an agreed-upon set of records including cephalometric radiographs, study casts, and photographs.[169] There was a wide variation in techniques and timing of lip and palate closure among the different centers. Statistical comparison of the six groups indicated that midfacial development was impaired at some centers more than at others, especially when soft tissue outline was considered.[118] A five-point ranking of anteroposterior dental arch relationship according to the Goslon yardstick[104] also showed that children at some centers had a considerably higher risk of midfacial retrusion that would call for surgical maxillary advancement.[105] This is illustrated in Figure 2–14.

It is impossible to say, however, which aspect of treatment was harmful because each team's protocol had several different elements. Common to the protocol of the two top-ranked centers was the fact that both closed the anterior cleft palate with a single-layer vomer flap at the time of lip closure, and neither used presurgical orthopedics. Perhaps more importantly, however, the top-ranked centers adhered to long-standing and strict protocol, with surgery carried out by high-volume operators, whereas the lowest ranked center had multiple operators and inconsistent protocols.

Maybe the most difficult problem for clinical researchers is fulfilling sample size requirements. Experience from the above intercenter study indicated that the sample of 30 patients with UCLP from each center appears to be too small to discern minor surgical effects. On the basis of the data gathered for the study, estimates of sample size required to discern different levels of outcome were attempted. It seems that roentgencephalometry, which is the most commonly used tool for evaluating craniofacial growth, is a very insensitive measure of outcome. For example, to detect a difference between a mean for two centers in maxillary prominence (s-n-ss) of 1.5° at 9 years of age, the required sample size is 117 for a two-center comparison.[171] These are sample sizes that most centers would have difficulty gathering. However, sample size requirements for this variable are likely to be reduced substantially with age,[140] with greater treatment effects being apparent at a later age because of the increasing divergence between cleft and noncleft growth curves (see Fig. 2–7). Evaluation of occlusion on study models (e.g., by the Goslon yardstick) appears to be more discriminating. For a systematic difference of 0.75 of a Goslon point to emerge between two centers, a sample size of 34 is needed to examine all pairwise differences.

With sample size considerations in mind, it is understandable that it has been difficult to draw concise conclusions on the differences in primary surgery management from the numerous retrospective reports in the literature, even when they have been intercenter comparative studies.[21, 26, 33, 58, 146–152, 171]

Table 2–2 summarizes the main features of several studies reporting a great variety of surgical technique and timing choices; in Tables 2–3 through 2–5, an attempt has been made to list equivalent values for individuals with UCLP.[1, 12, 26, 32, 42, 57, 71, 77, 116, 130, 144, 146, 162, 181–183] It must be noted, however, that these studies lack standardization of gender, cleft subtypes, and age range. There is a great variation in conventions adopted for allocation to age group. In cross-sectional reports, some authors have averaged age over ranges as high as 11 years. Several other reports have been excluded because the samples were small, the diagnostic groups were mixed, the age ranges were too wide, the subjects were not Caucasian, or dissimilar landmarks or forms of analysis had been used. Linear measurements have been excluded because of uncertainty about differences in magnification in the various reports.

The data in Tables 2–3 to 2–5 suggest that maxillary prominence (s-n-ss) and upper face angulation do not systematically differ between centers practicing early closure of the hard palate with a vomer flap (studies A, C, L, and O, as listed in Table 2–2), or by different one-stage palatoplasty, including push-back (B, D, E, F, G, H, and M),

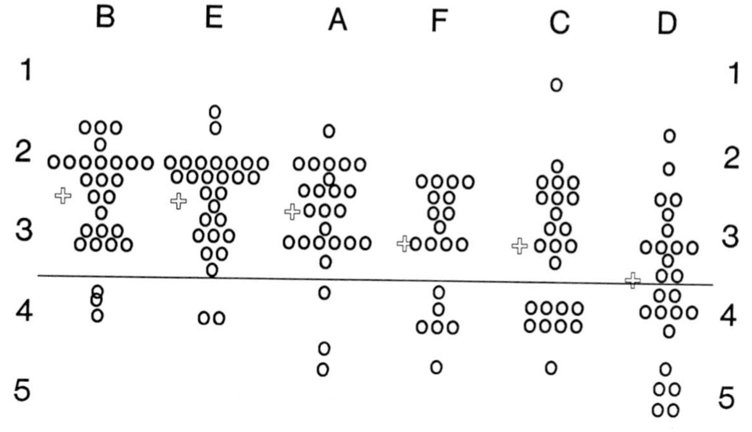

Figure 2–14. Ranking of mean Goslon score for individual patients from each center (B–D) where a score of 1 denotes a protrusive maxilla and a score of 5 a retrusive maxilla. A score below 3.5 would indicate a likely need for maxillary osteotomy to restore appearance and function. (From Shaw WC, Asher-McDade C, Brattström V, et al: Intercentre clinical audit for cleft lip and palate—A preliminary European investigation. *In* Jackson IT, Sommerlad BC [eds]: Recent Advances in Plastic Surgery, Number 4. Edinburgh: Churchill Livingstone, 1992.)

Table 2–2. REPORTS INCLUDED IN UCLP GROWTH STUDIES

	Sample Population			Soft Tissue Band	Data Type
	Total	Male	Female		
A. Semb (1991a)[162]	257	176	81	80	Mixed longitudinal
B. Aduss (1971)[1]	71	50	21	None	Mixed longitudinal
C. Enemark et al (1990)[42]	57	42	15	None	Longitudinal
D. Paulin and Thilander (1991)[130]	30	23	7	Not reported	Longitudinal
E. Hellquist et al (1983)[71]	19	13	6	Included	Longitudinal
F. Brattström (1991)[26]	18	12	6	3	Longitudinal
G. Toronto baseline: Ross (1987a)[146]	55	55	0	None	Mixed longitudinal
H. Rosenstein et al (1991)[144]	20	—*	—*	Not reported	Longitudinal
I. Hotz and Gnoinski (1976)[77]	18	18	0	Not reported	Cross-sectional
J. Smahel and Müllerova (1986)[182]	30	30	0	Not reported	Cross-sectional
K. Smahel and Müllerova (1994)[184]	32	32	0	Not reported	Cross-sectional
L. Mølsted (1987)[116]	31	19	12	10	Cross-sectional
M. Friede et al (1987)[57] (vomer flap group)	18	12	6	Included	Cross-sectional
N. Friede et al (1987)[57] (delayed closure group)	16	14	2	Included	Cross-sectional
O. Dahl (1970)[32]	78	78	0	Included	Cross-sectional
P. Smahel and Brejcha (1983)[181]	32	32	0	Included	Cross-sectional
Q. Marburg sample: Bardach et al (1984b)[12]	38	22	16	Not reported	Cross-sectional

* Not reported.

and those who delay hard palate closure until 4 to 8 years of age (I, J, K, N, and P). It is possible that eventual palatal surgery in the latter group may still have some adverse impact on late maxillary development,[80] but long-term follow-up results with delayed closure have not yet been reported. Furthermore, it is notable that the short-term results with delayed closure are not uniformly favorable. For example, samples A, B, C, D, E, and L, in which both the lip and hard and soft palate had been repaired, had less maxillary restraint at 5 to 6 years of age than sample J, in which only lip closure had been performed. In some cases, minimal periosteal flaps were placed at the base of the piriform fossa. Only for the exceptional delay of hard palate closure in the Marburg sample (Q) until mean age 13.2 years (range, 8 to 22 years) has a beneficial long-term effect on maxillary growth been reported,[12, 146] although the reported impairment of speech may outweigh this.[12] After the Marburg sample, group D had the highest mean for maxillary prominence at 18 years. These 30 patients had palatal closure at 1.9 years of age (in two stages for 7 patients, the hard palate being closed first) by a single surgeon.

The two groups M and N, in a preliminary report by Friede and coworkers,[57] were treated at the same center (one group before and the other after 1975), and the delayed group at 7 years showed some tendency for better maxillary growth than the vomer

Table 2–3. UCLP COMPARISON STUDY, MAXILLARY PROMINENCE (s-n-ss)

Age (Years)	Reference Study (see Table 2–2)																
	A	B	C	D	E	F	G	H	I	J	K	L	M	N	O	P	Q
5	79.6	79.2	79.7	80.4	79.8				79.8	76.9							
6	79.0	78.0				76.7						79.9					
7	77.9	78.4											78.8	80.3			
8	76.9	76.5	77.3	78.2	77.4												
9	76.6	76.4				75.3											
10	76.2	75.4									75.4						
11	75.9	76.5			76.0		75.7										
12	75.0	75.6	75.5														
13	75.6	75.1															
14	74.7	75.3			75.5			76.3									
15	74.8											74.0					
16	73.8		74.0	77.6		73.2	74.0										
17	74.1				75.1												
18	74.2		72.9	77.5											73.6	74.6	79.1

Table 2–4. UCLP COMPARISON STUDY, MAXILLO-MANDIBULAR RELATIONSHIP (ss-n-sm)

Age (Years)	A	B	C	D	E	F	G	H	I	J	K	L	M	N	O	P	Q
5	5.5		6.8	5.1	5.3				6.3	4.8							
6	4.7					2.9						5.6					
7	3.6												2.6	5.6			
8	2.6		4.6		2.8												
9	2.3					1.8											
10	1.7			2.4							2.2						
11	1.4				1.3		2.3										
12	0.4																
13	0.6																
14	0.4				0.3			2.4									
15	− 0.4											− 0.3					
16	− 1.7			0.6		− 1.9	0.0										
17	− 1.3				− 0.1												2.8
18	− 1.5		− 2.6												− 0.9	− 1.3	

flap group (though nonsignificantly for the values listed in Tables 2–3 to 2–5, except for the variable ss-n-sm). Unequivocal conclusions cannot be reached because the difference may reflect the small sample size, the short follow-up period, the disproportionate number of (larger) males in the delayed group, and the intrinsic shortcomings of historical control designs.[140]

With respect to dental arch relationship, a comparison of four groups in which timing of hard palate closure varied between 1.5 years to after 10 years of age did not reveal any difference among the groups.[124]

Choices in Surgery for BCLP

Fewer reports are available for BCLP (Table 2–6), and these suffer from the same shortcomings as the UCLP studies. Special attention has been given to the problems of the premaxilla, which may be extremely protruded at birth. After a successful lip repair, the premaxilla usually is molded back in the childhood years (see Fig. 2–9). However, if the lip is short or fastened high on the alveolus, it will not be able to mold back the alveolar process, and severe protrusion may persist. The lower lip will fall behind the premaxilla and the erupting teeth meet no resistance, and thus excessive eruption takes place (Fig. 2–15). In these cases, some centers advocate surgical set-back of the premaxilla, whereas others regard this as a procedure that involves too much risk of damaging maxillary growth and impairing the development of the teeth in the premaxilla. The results from studies of this surgery are controversial[13, 14, 51, 55, 67, 68] and more conservative approaches may be preferable (Fig. 2–16).

Table 2–5. UCLP COMPARISON STUDY, ANTERIOR FACE HEIGHT (NSL-ML)

Age (Years)	A	B	C	D	E	F	G	H	I	J	K	L	M	N	O	P	Q
5	36.1	38.3	37.6	36.2	38.2				35.2								
6	36.0	38.6				36.1						37.4					
7	35.7	38.9											35.1	38.7			
8	35.6	39.3	36.9		37.8												
9	35.3	39.2				37.3											
10	35.8	39.0		35.8								38.8					
11	35.5	38.6			37.3												
12	35.6	39.9	36.7														
13	35.7	38.1															
14	35.7	38.3			37.8			41.4									
15	35.9											37.4					
16	34.7		34.4	34.5		36.4											
17	34.8				37.6												
18	35.4		32.8	33.9											37.4	37.0	37.0

Table 2–6. REPORTS INCLUDED IN BCLP GROWTH STUDIES

	Sample Population			Soft Tissue Band	Data Type
	Total	Male	Female		
A. Semb (1991b)[163]	90	61	29	33	Mixed longitudinal
B. Hellquist and Svärdström (1990)[72] (periosteoplasty group)	35	23	12	Included	Mixed longitudinal
C. Hellquist and Svärdström (1990)[72] (no periosteoplasty group)	10	5	5	Included	Mixed longitudinal
D. Hellquist et al (1983)[71]	9	7	2	Included	Mixed longitudinal
E. Trotman and Ross (1993)[193]	30	30	0	Not reported	Longitudinal
F. Friede and Pruzansky (1972)[51]	17	—*	—*	None	Mixed longitudinal
G. Friede and Johanson (1977)[54]	13	12	1	Included	Mixed longitudinal
H. Friede and Pruzansky (1985)[55] (no set-back group)	14	9	5	Not reported	Cross-sectional
I. Friede and Pruzansky (1985)[55] (late set-back group)	7	3	4	Not reported	Cross-sectional
J. Bardach et al (1992)[14] (non-recession group)	11	8	3	Not reported	Cross-sectional
K. Bardach et al (1992)[14] (recession group)	17	15	2	Not reported	Cross-sectional
L. Heidbüchel et al (1994)[68]	21	14	7	Included	Mixed longitudinal
M. Rosenstein et al (1991)[144]	17	—*	—*	Not reported	Cross-sectional
N. Dahl (1970)[32]	49	49	0	Included	Cross-sectional
O. Smahel (1984b)[180]	26	26	0	Not reported	Cross-sectional

* Not reported.

Table 2–6 summarizes the main features of 13 studies of facial growth in BCLP in which a variety of different techniques have been used. A review of results follows. In Tables 2–7 to 2–9, an attempt has been made to list values for three variables that are directly equivalent.

In general, facial profile and other cephalometric variables were similar for all samples, except for two North American groups and one group from the Netherlands.[51, 55, 68, 188] The facial development in group A (90 subjects with BCLP treated by two-stage lip repair and a vomer flap to close the hard palate at 3 to 4 months of age, and subsequent posterior palatal closure by a modified von Langenbeck technique) was comparable with that found in three studies of adult males with BCLP.[32, 180, 190] In group N, consisting of 49 Danish subjects,[32] surgical history was undetermined in a sizable proportion, and some had not had palate repair. Approximately one third of the sample had vomer flaps at the time of lip repair. In the Czech group of 26 males (group O[180]) two-stage lip repair at 7 to 8 months and palatoplasty with push-back and primary pharyngeal flap at a mean age of 5.8 years were performed. Nine cases had premaxillary set-back surgery before palatoplasty. Vargervik's cross-sectional study[190]

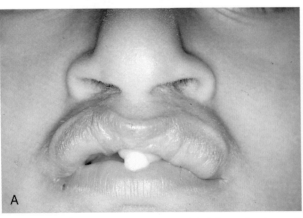
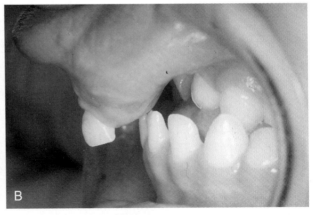

Figure 2–15. *A* and *B,* Closure of bilateral cleft lip and palate. After lip closure the lip is fastened high on the premaxilla, unable to influence its position.

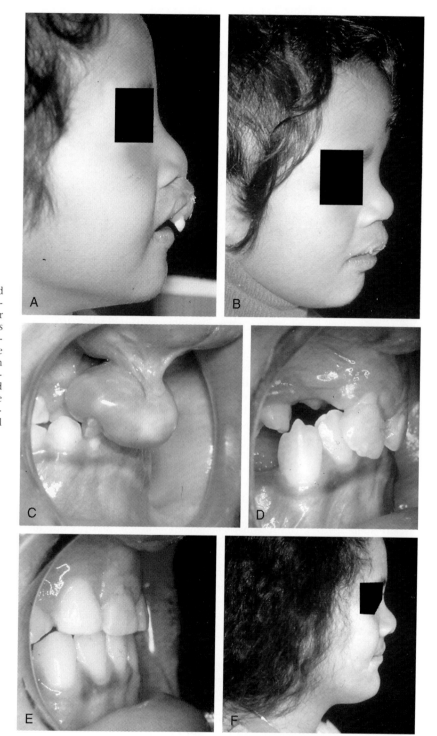

Figure 2–16. Patient with protruding and vertically displaced premaxilla after suboptimal lip closure: at 5 years of age *(A)*; four months after sulcusplasty, the profile is greatly improved as the lip covers the premaxilla *(B)*; one year after sulcusplasty, the premaxilla is molded back *(C)*; after derotation of permanent central incisors and bone grafting at age 11 years, the overjet is normalized but the overbite is still increased *(D)*; the overjet and overbite following routine orthodontic treatment for 22 months *(E)*; facial profile at age 18 years *(F)*.

of 51 males with BCLP treated with a variety of primary procedures (excluding premaxillary set-back procedures) also showed profiles similar to those in the Norwegian, Danish, and Czech samples; however, the variables listed were not compatible with those adopted for studies shown in Tables 2–7 to 2–9.

The BCLP patients in groups B, C, and D are from a Swedish center that performed periosteoplasty on some patients. All patients had lip closure without a vomer flap and push-back palatoplasty. Group B had periosteoplasty in infancy, group C had this procedure performed at a mean age of 6 years, and group D had never undergone periosteoplasty. Although the maxilla seems slightly more prominent with late perios-

Table 2–7. BCLP COMPARISON STUDY, MAXILLARY PROMINENCE (s-n-ss)

	Reference Study (see Table 2–6)														
Age (Years)	A	B	C	D	E	F	G	H	I	J	K	L	M	N	O
5	84.7	85.3	84.4	84.1											
6	83.5														
7	82.0				85.5	84.8	78.2								
8	81.3	81.5	83.7	81.4											
9	80.1														
10	79.9					82.2	78.8								
11	79.1	80.3	81.2	80.1											
12	78.7				82.9										
13	76.9														
14	77.5	78.3	79.7	79.5									77.9		
15	76.7														
16	75.2									77.7	75.5				
17	75.7	77.2	79.3	79.8	79.4			80.3	75.4						
18	75.6	74.7		77.6								79.3		75.5	74.4

teoplasty, the maxillomandibular relationship at the end of growth is not very different in these patients than in those from centers A, N, and O. Hellquist and Svärdström[72] also reported that infant periosteoplasty resulted in significant vertical growth inhibition of the anterior maxilla.

Friede and Johanson[54] reported facial growth in 13 Swedish children with BCLP (group G), five at age 7 and eight at age 10 years. The patients, who had lip adhesion and vomer flap (without premaxillary set-back procedures), final lip closure, and velar closure with push-back procedures, also have similar facial convexity to that reported in the above studies. Similar values were also obtained in group M, despite the fact that these subjects had received primary bone grafting.

As mentioned previously, the premaxillary set-back procedure in early childhood is a controversial issue, but the findings from two centers in which it has been practiced selectively indicate a tendency for more growth impairment in the set-back groups (H versus I, J versus K).[14,51,55] However, in a mixed longitudinal report of 21 patients in whom osteotomy of the premaxilla was performed on average at age 9 years showed favorable results (group L).[68]

Two studies from North American centers and the study from the Netherlands (Heidbüchel and coworkers[68]) demonstrate more favorable growth of the maxilla than the other reports. Trotman and Ross (group E),[188] in a longitudinal study on 30 male subjects with BCLP treated conventionally without surgical set-back procedures and vomerplasty, concluded that maxillary length reached normal values at age 16 and that the premaxilla probably attained a normal position in the mid-teens. Similarly, reports of 14 children observed to age 17 years (groups F and H) with no premaxillary

Table 2–8. BCLP COMPARISON STUDY, MAXILLOMANDIBULAR RELATIONSHIP (ss-n-sm)

	Reference Study (see Table 2–6)														
Age (Years)	A	B	C	D	E	F	G	H	I	J	K	L	M	N	O
5	10.9	9.5	8.9	10.1											
6	9.4				12.7										
7	7.6						6.1								
8	7.2	6.0	6.7	7.2											
9	5.7														
10	6.0						4.9								
11	4.8	5.2	4.8	5.2											
12	4.2				8.7										
13	2.8														
14	2.6	2.4	2.5	3.4									4.4		
15	1.7														
16	1.0									1.5	− 0.2				
17	0.8	0.5	− 0.3	1.8	4.2			6.4	− 0.2						
18	0.9	− 0.5	0.5											0.9	1.1

Table 2–9. BCLP COMPARISON STUDY, ANTERIOR FACE HEIGHT (NSL-ML)

Age (Years)	A	B	C	D	E	F	G	H	I	J	K	L	M	N	O
	Reference Study (see Table 2–6)														
5	36.3	37.2	37.7	36.5											
6	37.1				38.4										
7	35.8						37.1								
8	35.9	37.0	36.2	35.9											
9	36.3														
10	36.4						37.4								
11	36.5	36.9	36.4	35.8											
12	36.3				37.8										
13	37.5														
14	35.6	36.4	36.4	35.1											
15	34.9												43.1		
16	37.0									35.1	33.4				
17	34.8	34.7	35.0	34.6											
18	35.8	34.5	35.6		36.7							38.2		39.3	39.9

set-back procedures[55] show more favorable growth than the other studies mentioned. Unfortunately, it is not possible to determine which aspect of sample composition, surgical technique, or surgical skill is responsible.

Just as with UCLP, previously published series of treated cases cannot provide clear evidence of the efficacy of one surgical protocol over others. There seems to be little doubt that more rigorous research design is required to identify optimal models of delivering care and details of surgical technique that will maximize the potential for midfacial growth, while remaining consistent with other goals of management.

Secondary Procedures

Until growth is complete, secondary surgery also entails the possibility of growth impairment. The impact of pharyngeal flap and alveolar bone grafting has been formally studied.

Pharyngeal Flap Procedure

Presence of a pharyngeal flap may theoretically induce changes in facial growth by increasing airway resistance with resulting adaptation in the lower face, and by direct restraint of maxillary growth. Subtelny and Pineda Nieto[187] found the latter to occur after flap surgery, but their samples appear to have included an unmatched number of bilateral cleft subjects. This was also a feature of another report that found flap surgery to be associated with mandibular adaptation.[138] Long and McNamara[103] examined the effect of pharyngeal flap surgery on nine cases of CPO and eight of UCLP; they also found signs of increased vertical growth of the mandible. In contrast, Semb and Shaw,[165] in a matched comparison of 29 cases of UCLP, found similar postoperative growth increments in the flap group and in control groups (Table 2–10).

Alveolar Bone Grafting

Repair of the alveolar cleft with a bone graft may also impair maxillary growth. The effect of bone grafting on the mixed dentition has been studied. Enemark and co-workers[41] presented a follow-up of such grafting and reported no impairment of growth in the anterior dimension and only minor impairment of little clinical significance in the vertical dimension.

In a regression analysis of the 16-year-old cephalometric values of 58 subjects with UCLP, 28 of whom received bone grafts, Semb[161] found that early cephalometric form predicted later development and that bone grafting before the age of 12 years had no influence. This was confirmed in a study by Paulin and Thilander.[130]

Table 2–10. CONTROLLED COMPARISON OF AMOUNT OF CHANGE OCCURRING IN THE PHARYNGEAL FLAP GROUP BETWEEN PREOPERATIVE AND FOLLOW-UP REGISTRATION (29 MATCHED PAIRS)

	Flap Group (Mean Change)	Control Group (Mean Change)	Probability
Anteroposterior Relationships			
s-n-ss	− 3.86	− 3.43	0.568
s-n-pg	3.18	3.17	0.991
ss-n-sm	− 5.37	− 4.81	0.525
n-ss-pg	13.90	13.27	0.739
ss′-pm	0.88	1.13	0.747
Vertical Relationships			
NSL-NL	− 1.34	− 1.67	0.714
NSL-ML	− 1.63	− 1.81	0.873
NL-ML	− 0.29	− 0.14	0.912
n-ss′	9.89	9.02	0.100
ss′-gn	14.50	13.08	0.142
Cranial Base Angulation			
n-s-ba	− 1.51	− 1.08	0.592

Other Secondary Procedures

The impact of additional secondary procedures has not been studied, but it is possible that repeated attempts at fistula closure, lip revision, and radical nose revision entail some risk. Ironically, cases calling for multiple secondary procedures probably are the result of substandard primary surgery, and secondary operations will only compound the growth disturbance.

CONCLUSIONS

In review, we may conclude that the faces of children with repaired clefts will inevitably grow differently from those of their healthy counterparts. These differences are least with clefts confined to the primary palate and greatest for combined clefting of the lip and palate.

It is not justified to lay the blame for this at the door of the surgeon, since many aspects of facial dysmorphology associated with clefting are merely a continuation of initial embryonic distortion or intrinsic differences in growth pattern related perhaps to adaptation to an underdeveloped nasal capsule. Indeed, surgical repair of primary palate clefts and isolated cleft palate appears to have little or no influence on growth. There is, however, sufficient evidence that maxillary growth in combined cleft lip and palate is highly vulnerable to disruption by surgery, although the potential for good maxillary growth can be safeguarded if the surgery is performed atraumatically.

The search for ideal forms of surgery, at least as far as facial growth is concerned, is hindered by our lack of understanding of the very nature of facial growth. The primary controlling mechanisms are not known, and we are unable to say that any particular anatomic site is a ''growth center'' that must at all costs be preserved. All that can be said at present is that the quality of surgery will probably be maximized when it is performed by high-volume operators as part of a well-structured protocol.

Perhaps the breakthrough that is awaited will come from the biologic sciences if, for example, healing can be modulated in such a way to avoid scars. In the meantime, advances in surgical knowledge will come about only through rigorous multicenter studies, especially randomized trials.

The growth of our literature in this respect is at an embryonic stage.

References

1. Aduss H: Craniofacial growth in complete unilateral cleft lip and palate. Angle Orthod 1971; 41:202–213.
2. Aduss H, Pruzansky S: The nasal cavity in complete unilateral cleft lip and palate. Arch Otolaryngol 1967; 85:75–84.

3. Aduss H, Pruzansky S, Miller M: Interorbital distance in cleft lip and palate. Teratology 1971; 4:171–181.
4. Athanasiou AE, Mazaheri M, Zarrinnia K: Longitudinal study of the dental arch dimensions in hard and soft palate clefts. J Pedodontics 1987; 12:35–47.
5. Athanasiou AE, Tseng CY, Zarrinnia K, Mazaheri M: Frontal cephalometric study of dentofacial morphology in children with bilateral clefts of lip, alveolus and palate. J Craniomaxillofac Surg 1990; 18:49–54.
6. Bardach J: Cleft palate repair: Two-flap palatoplasty. Research, philosophy, technique, and results. *In* Bardach J, Morris HL (eds): Multidisciplinary Management of Cleft Lip and Palate. Philadelphia: WB Saunders, 1990, pp 352–365.
7. Bardach J, Eisbach KJ: The influence of primary unilateral cleft lip repair on facial growth. 1. Lip pressure. Cleft Palate J 1972; 14:88–97.
8. Bardach J, Mooney MP: The relationship between lip pressure following lip repair and craniofacial growth: An experimental study in beagles. Plast Reconstr Surg 1984; 73:544–555.
9. Bardach J, Kelly KM: The influence of lip repair with and without soft-tissue undermining on facial growth in beagles. Plast Reconstr Surg 1988; 82:747–755.
10. Bardach J, Mooney MP, Bakowska J: The influence of lip repair on facial growth: A comparative study in rabbits, beagles, and humans. *In* Williams HB (ed): Transactions of Seventh International Congress on Plastic Reconstructive Surgery. Canada: RBT Printing, 1983.
11. Bardach J, Bakowska J, McDermott-Murray J, et al: Lip pressure changes following lip repair in infants with unilateral clefts of the lip and palate. Plast Reconstr Surg 1984a; 74:476–479.
12. Bardach J, Morris HL, Olin WH: Late results of primary veloplasty: The Marburg project. Plast Reconstr Surg 1984b; 73:207–215.
13. Bardach J, Olin WH, Kelly K: Surgical-orthodontic correction of the protruded premaxilla. *In* Bardach J, Morris HL (eds): Multidisciplinary Management of Cleft Lip and Palate. Philadelphia: WB Saunders, 1990; pp 563–573.
14. Bardach J, Morris HL, Olin WH, et al: Result of a multidisciplinary management of bilateral cleft lip and palate at the Iowa Cleft Palate Center. Plast Reconstr Surg 1992; 89:419–432.
15. Bergland O, Sidhu SS: Occlusal changes from the deciduous to the early mixed dentition in unilateral complete clefts. Cleft Palate J 1974; 11:317–326.
16. Bishara SE: Cephalometric evaluation of facial growth in operated and non-operated individuals with isolated clefts of the palate. Cleft Palate J 1973; 10:239–246.
17. Bishara SE: Effects of the Wardill-Kilner (V/W-Y) palatoplasty on facial growth. Angle Orthod 1975; 45:55–64.
18. Bishara SE, Iversen WW: Cephalometric comparisons on the cranial base and face in individuals with isolated clefts of the palate. Cleft Palate J 1974; 11:162–175.
19. Bishara SE, Tharp RM: Effects of von Langenbeck palatoplasty on facial growth. Angle Orthod 1977; 47:34–41.
20. Bishara SE, Krause CJ, Olin WH, et al: Facial and dental relationships of individuals with unoperated clefts of the lip and/or palate. Cleft Palate J 1976a; 13:238–252.
21. Bishara SE, Enemark H, Tharp RF: Cephalometric comparisons of the results of the Wardill-Kilner and von Langenbeck palatoplasties. Cleft Palate J 1976b; 13:319–329.
22. Bishara SE, Arrendondo RSM de, Vales HP, Jakobsen JR: Dentofacial relationships in persons with unoperated clefts: Comparisons between three cleft types. Am J Orthod 1985; 87:481–507.
23. Bishara SE, Jakobsen JR, Krause JC, Sosa-Martinez R: Cephalometric comparisons of individuals from India and Mexico with unoperated cleft lip and palate. Cleft Palate J 1986; 23:116–125.
24. Blocksma R, Leuz CA, Mellerstig KE: A conservative program for managing cleft palates without the use of mucoperiosteal flaps. Plast Reconstr Surg 1975; 55:160–169.
25. Brader AC: A cephalometric appraisal of morphological variations in cranial base and associated pharyngeal structures. Angle Orthod 1957; 27:179–195.
26. Brattström V: Craniofacial development in cleft lip and palate children related to different treatment regimes [Thesis]. University of Stockholm, 1991.
27. Broadbent BH Sr, Broadbent BH Jr, Golden WH: Bolton Standards of Dentofacial Developmental Growth. St Louis: CV Mosby, 1975.
28. Bütow K-W, Steinhauser EW: Follow-up investigation of palatal closure by means of a one-layer cranially-based vomer-flap. Int J Oral Surg 1984; 13:396–400.
29. Capelozza L Jr, Taniguchi SM, da Silva OG Jr: Craniofacial morphology of adult unoperated complete unilateral cleft lip and palate patients. Cleft Palate Craniofac J 1993; 30:376–381.
30. Capelozza L Jr, Normando ADC, da Silva OG Jr: Isolated influence of lip and palate cleft repair on facial growth—a comparative study in adult males with complete unilateral cleft lip, alveolus and palate. Cleft Palate Craniofac J. In press.
31. Coupe TB, Subtelny JD: Cleft palate—deficiency or displacement of tissue? Plast Reconstr Surg 1960; 26:600–612.
32. Dahl E: Craniofacial morphology in congenital clefts of the lip and palate. An x-ray cephalometric study of young adult males [Dissertation]. Acta Odontol Scand 1970; 28[Suppl 57].
33. Dahl E, Hanusardottir B, Bergland O: A comparison of occlusions in two groups of children whose clefts were repaired by three different surgical procedures. Cleft Palate J 1981; 18:122–127.
34. Dahl E, Kreiborg S, Jensen BL, Fogh-Andersen P: Comparison of craniofacial morphology in infants with incomplete cleft lip and infants with isolated cleft palate. Cleft Palate J 1982; 19:258–266.
35. Dahl E, Kreiborg S, Jensen BL: Roentgencephalometric studies of infants with untreated cleft lip and palate. *In* Kriens O (ed): What Is a Cleft Lip and Palate? A Multidisciplinary Update. Stuttgart: Georg Thieme Verlag, 1989, pp 113–115.
36. DeJesus JA: Comparative cephalometric analysis of nonoperated cleft palate adults and normal adults. Am J Orthod 1959; 45:61–62.

37. Delaire J, Precious D: Avoidance of the use of vomerine mucosa in primary surgical management of velopalatine clefts. Oral Surg Oral Med Oral Pathol 1985; 60:589–597.
38. Devlin HB: Audit and the quality of clinical care. Ann R Coll Surg Engl 1990; 73[Suppl]:3–11.
39. Drettner B: The nasal airway and hearing in patients with cleft palate. Acta Otolaryngol 1960; 57:131–142.
40. Drillien CM, Ingram TTS, Wilkinson EM: The Causes and Natural History of Cleft Lip and Palate. Edinburgh: E & S Livingstone, 1966.
41. Enemark H, Sindet-Pedersen S, Bundgaard M: Long-term results after secondary bone grafting of alveolar clefts. J Oral Maxillofac Surg 1987; 45:913–918.
42. Enemark H, Bolund S, Jørgensen I: Evaluation of unilateral cleft lip and palate treatment: Long term results. Cleft Palate J 1990; 27:354–361.
43. Engman LT, Spriestersbach DC, Moll KL: Cranial base angle and nasopharyngeal depth. Cleft Palate J 1965; 2:32–39.
44. Enlow DH: Facial Growth, 3rd ed. Philadelphia: WB Saunders, 1990.
45. Ferguson MWJ: Craniofacial morphogenesis and prenatal growth. In Shaw WC (ed): Orthodontics and Occlusal Management. London: Heinemann, 1993, pp 1–25.
46. Foster TD: Maxillary deformities in repaired clefts of the lip and palate. Br J Plast Surg 1962; 15:182–190.
47. Foster TD, Lavelle CLB: The size of the dentition in complete cleft lip and palate. Cleft Palate J 1971; 8:307–313.
48. Friede H: A histological and enzyme-histochemical study of growth sites of the premaxilla in human foetuses and neonates. Arch Oral Biol 1975; 20:809–814.
49. Friede H: Studies on facial morphology and growth in bilateral cleft lip and palate [Thesis]. University of Gothenburg, 1977.
50. Friede H: The vomero-premaxillary suture—a neglected growth site in mid-facial development of unilateral cleft lip and palate patients. Cleft Palate J 1978; 15:398–404.
51. Friede H, Pruzansky S: Longitudinal study of growth in bilateral cleft lip and palate from infancy to adolescence. Plast Reconstr Surg 1972; 49:392–403.
52. Friede H, Johanson B: A follow-up study of cleft children treated with primary bone grafting. Scand J Plast Reconstr Surg 1974; 8:88–103.
53. Friede H, Morgan P: Growth of the vomero-premaxillary suture in children with bilateral cleft lip and palate. A histological and roentgencephalometric study. Scand J Plast Reconstr Surg 1976; 10:45–55.
54. Friede H, Johanson B: A follow-up study of cleft children treated with vomer flap as part of a three-stage soft tissue surgical procedure. Facial morphology and dental occlusion. Scand J Plast Reconstr Surg 1977; 11:45–57.
55. Friede H, Pruzansky S: Long-term effects of premaxillary setback on facial skeletal profile in complete bilateral cleft lip and palate. Cleft Palate J 1985; 22:97–105.
56. Friede H, Figueroa AA, Naegele ML, et al: Craniofacial growth data for cleft lip patients infancy to 6 years of age: Potential applications. Am J Orthod 1986; 90:388–409.
57. Friede H, Möller M, Lilja J, et al: Facial morphology and occlusion at the stage of early mixed dentition in cleft lip and palate patients treated with delayed closure of the hard palate. Scand J Plast Reconstr Surg 1987; 21:65–71.
58. Friede H, Enemark H, Semb G, et al: Craniofacial and occlusal characteristics in unilateral cleft lip and palate patients from four Scandinavian centers. Scand J Plast Reconstr Hand Surg 1991; 25:269–276.
59. Friede H, Persson EC, Lilja J, et al: Maxillary dental arch and occlusion in patients with repaired clefts of the secondary palate. Scand J Plast Reconstr Hand Surg 1993; 27:297–305.
60. Gillies HG, Fry WK: A new principle in the surgical treatment of "congenital cleft palate." Br Med J 1921; 1:335–338.
61. Graber TM: A cephalometric analysis of the developmental pattern and facial morphology in cleft palate. Angle Orthod 1949; 19:91–100.
62. Graber TM: The congenital cleft palate deformity. J Am Dent Assoc 1954; 48:375–395.
63. Hairfield MA, Warren DW, Seaton DL: Prevalence of mouth breathing in cleft lip and palate. Cleft Palate J 1988; 25:135–138.
64. Hama K: Morphological study of the craniofacial skeleton within a profile in cleft lip and palate. J Osaka Univ Dent School 1984; 4:41–67.
65. Harris EF: Size and form of the cranial base in isolated cleft lip and palate. Cleft Palate Craniofac J 1993; 30:170–174.
66. Harvold E: A roentgen study of the postnatal morphogenesis of the facial skeleton in cleft palate [Thesis]. University of Oslo, 1954.
67. Heidbüchel KLWM, Kuijpers-Jagtman AM, Freihofer HPM: An orthodontic and cephalometric study on the results of the combined surgical-orthodontic approach to the protruded premaxilla in bilateral clefts. J Craniomaxillofac Surg 1993; 21:60–66.
68. Heidbüchel KLWM, Kuijpers-Jagtman AM, Freihofer HPM: Facial growth in patients with bilateral cleft lip and palate: A cephalometric study. Cleft Palate Craniofac J 1994; 31:210–216.
69. Heliövaara A, Pere A, Ranta R: One-stage closure of isolated cleft palate with the Veau-Wardill-Kilner V to Y pushback procedure or the Cronin modification. Scand J Plast Reconstr Hand Surg 1994; 28:55–62.
70. Hellquist R, Ponten B, Skoog T: The influence of cleft length and palatoplasty on the dental arch and deciduous occlusion in cases of clefts and the secondary palate. Scand J Plast Reconstr Surg 1978; 12:45–54.
71. Hellquist R, Svärdström K, Ponten B: A longitudinal study of delayed periosteoplasty to the cleft alveolus. Cleft Palate J 1983; 20:277–288.
72. Hellquist R, Svärdström K: Craniofacial growth and dental occlusion in bilateral cleft lip and palate patients after infant periosteoplasty to the alveolar cleft—a longitudinal study to the age of 19 years. In Huddart AG, Ferguson MJW (eds): Cleft Lip and Palate. Long-Term Results and Future Prospects, Vol

1. The Presurgical Period, Initial Surgery, and Speech, Surgery, and Growth. Manchester: Manchester University Press, 1990, pp 166–178.

73. Herfert O: Experimenteller Beitrag zur Frage der Schädigung des Oberkiefer-Wachstums durch vorzeitige Gaumenspaltoperation. Dtsch Zahn-Mund-Kieferheilk 1954; 20:369–381.

74. Hirschfeld WJ, Aduss H: Interorbital distance in cleft lip and palate: Significant differences found by sign test. J Dent Res 1974; 53:947.

75. Horswell BB, Gallup BV: Cranial base morphology in cleft lip and palate. J Oral Maxillofac Surg 1992; 50:681–685.

76. Hotz M: Orofacial development under adverse conditions. Eur J Orthod 1983; 5:91–103.

77. Hotz M, Gnoinski W: Comprehensive care of cleft lip and palate children at Zurich University: A preliminary report. Am J Orthod 1976; 70:481–504.

78. Hotz M, Gnoinski W: Effects of early maxillary orthopaedics in coordination with delayed surgery for cleft lip and palate. J Maxillofac Surg 1979; 7:201–210.

79. Hotz M, Gnoinski W, Perko M, et al (eds): Early Treatment of Cleft Lip and Palate. Toronto: Hans Huber Publishers, 1986.

80. Huang CS, Hsu WY, Chen YR, Noordhoff MS: Dimensional Changes of Maxillary Dental Arch Following Anterior Palatoplasty [Abstract 29]. St. Louis: 47th annual meeting of the ACPA, 1990.

81. Huddart AG, MacCauley FJ, Davis MEH: Maxillary arch dimensions in normal and unilateral cleft palate subjects. Cleft Palate J 1969; 6:471–487.

82. Huddart AG: Maxillary arch dimensions in bilateral cleft lip and palate subjects. Cleft Palate J 1970; 7:139–155.

83. Ishiguro K, Krogman NM, Mazaheri M, Harding RL: A longitudinal study of morphological craniofacial patterns via P-A x-ray headfilms in cleft patients from birth to six years of age. Cleft Palate J 1976; 13:104–126.

84. Jain RB, Krogman WM: Craniofacial growth in clefting from one month to ten years as studied by P-A headfilms. Cleft Palate J 1983; 20:314–326.

85. Jakobsson OP, Hellquist R, Bergström R: Closure of the cleft palate in one or two stages: Maxillary alveolar-dental dimensions in 8 year old children born with isolated cleft palate. In Jakobsson OP: Repair of Isolated Cleft Palate. A Comparison of One- and Two-stage Surgery by Dental Arch Measurements, Cephalometry, and Speech Analysis [Dissertation]. Acta Universitatis Upsaliensis, Sweden, 1990a.

86. Jakobsson OP, Larson M, Hellquist R, Bergström R: Closure of the cleft palate in one or two stages: Cephalometric analysis of the maxilla and upper airway in 8 year old children born with isolated cleft palate. In Jakobsson OP: Repair of Isolated Cleft Palate. A Comparison of One- and Two-stage Surgery by Dental Arch Measurements, Cephalometry, and Speech Analysis [Dissertation]. Acta Universitatis Upsaliensis, Sweden, 1990b.

87. Jakobsson S: Cephalometric evaluation of treatment effect on Class II malocclusion. Am J Orthod 1967; 53:446–457.

88. Jensen BL, Dahl E, Kreiborg S: Longitudinal study of body height, radius length and skeletal maturity in Danish boys with cleft lip and palate. Scand J Dent Res 1983; 91:473–481.

89. Johnston MC: Animal models for human craniofacial malformations. In Bader JD (ed): Risk Assessment in Dentistry. Chapel Hill: University of North Carolina Dental Ecology, 1990.

90. Johnston MC, Hunter WS: Cephalometric analysis of monozygotic twins discordant for cleft lip/palate. J Dent Res 1989; 68:606.

91. Johnston MC, Hunter WS, Niswander JD: Facial morphology in monozygotic twins discordant for clefts of the lip and palate: A pilot study. In preparation.

92. Jolleys A, Robertson NRE: A study of the effects of early bone grafting in complete clefts of the lip and palate. Five year study. Br J Plast Surg 1972; 25:229–237.

93. Jonsson G, Thilander B: Occlusion, arch dimensions and craniofacial morphology after palatal surgery in a group of children with clefts in the secondary palate. Am J Orthod 1979; 76:243–255.

94. Jonsson G, Stenström S, Thilander B: The use of a vomer flap covered with an autogenous skin graft as part of the palatal repair in children with unilateral cleft lip and palate. Arch dimensions and occlusion up to the age of five. Scand J Plast Reconstr Surg 1980; 14:13–21.

95. Kimes KR, Siegel MI, Mooney MP, Todhunter J: Relative contributions of the nasal septum and airways to total nasal capsule volume in normal and cleft lip and palate fetal specimens. Cleft Palate J 1988; 25:282–287.

96. Kimes KR, Mooney MP, Siegel MI, Todhunter JS: Size and growth rate of the tongue in normals and cleft lip and palate human fetal specimens. Cleft Palate Craniofac J 1991; 28:212–216.

97. Kremenak CR: Physiological aspects of wound healing: contraction and growth. Otolaryngol Clin North Am 1984; 17:437–453.

98. Kuijpers-Jagtman AM: Maxillary arch dimensions from birth to 18 months in complete unilateral clefts. J Dent Res 1983; 62:461.

99. Latham RA: The pathogenesis of the skeletal deformity associate with unilateral cleft lip and palate. Cleft Palate J 1969; 6:404–414.

100. Latham RA: Development and structure of the premaxillary deformity in bilateral cleft lip and palate. Br J Plast Surg 1973; 26:1–11.

101. Levin HS: A radiographic cephalometric analysis of cleft palate patients displaying antero-posterior deficiencies in the middle one-third of the face [M.S. Thesis]. Chicago: Northwestern University, 1960.

102. Linder-Aronson S: Adenoids: their effect on mode of breathing and nasal airflow and their relationship to characteristics of the facial skeleton and their dentition. Acta Otolaryngol 1970; 265[Suppl]:1–132.

103. Long RE Jr, McNamara JA Jr: Facial growth following pharyngeal flap surgery: Skeletal assessment on serial lateral cephalometric radiographs. Am J Orthod 1985; 87:187–196.

104. Mars M, Plint DA, Houston WJB, et al: The Goslon Yardstick: A new system of assessing dental arch relationships in children with unilateral clefts of the lip and palate. Cleft Palate J 1987; 24:314–322.

105. Mars M, Asher-McDade C, Brattström V, et al: A six-center international study of treatment outcome

in patients with clefts of the lip and palate. Part 3. Dental arch relationships. Cleft alate Craniofac J 1992; 29:405–408.

106. Mars M, Houston WJB: A preliminary study of facial growth and morphology in unoperated male unilateral cleft lip and palate subjects over 13 years of age. Cleft Palate J 1990; 27:7–10.

107. McCance AM, Roberts-Harry D, Sherriff M, et al: A study model analysis of adult unoperated Sri Lankans with unilateral cleft lip and palate. Cleft Palate J 1990; 27:146–154.

108. McCance A, Roberts-Harry D, Sherriff M, et al: Sri Lankan cleft lip and palate study model analysis: Clefts of the secondary palate. Cleft Palate Craniofac J 1993; 30:227–230.

109. McNeill RW: A roentgen cephalometric study of nasopharyngeal and cranial base growth in cleft palate children. Int Assoc Dent Res 1962; 41:53.

110. Mestre JC, DeJesus J, Subtelny JD: Unoperated oral clefts at maturation. Angle Orthod 1960; 30:78–85.

111. Moss ML: Malformations of the skull base associated with cleft palate deformity. Plast Reconstr Surg 1956; 17:226–234.

112. Moss ML: The functional matrix. In Kraus BS, Riedel RA (eds): Vistas of Orthodontics. Philadelphia: Lea & Febiger, 1962.

113. Moss ML: The role of the nasal septal cartilage in midfacial growth. In McNamara J Jr (ed): Factors Affecting the Growth of the Midface. Craniofacial Growth Series. Ann Arbor, MI: Center for Human Growth and Development, 1976.

114. Moss ML, Bromberg BE, Song IC, Eisenman G: The passive role of nasal septal cartilage in mid-facial growth. Plast Reconstr Surg 1968; 41:536–542.

115. Motohashi N, Kuroda T, Capelozza L Jr, de Souza Freitas JA: P-A cephalometric analysis of nonoperated adult cleft lip and palate. Cleft Palate Craniofac J 1994; 31:193–200.

116. Mølsted K: Kraniofacial morfologi hos børn med komplet unilateral læbe-og ganespalte [Master Dissertation]. University of Copenhagen, 1987.

117. Mølsted K, Dahl E: Asymmetry of the maxilla in children with complete unilateral cleft lip and palate. Cleft Palate J 1990; 27:184–190.

118. Mølsted K, Asher-McDade C, Brattström V, et al: A six-center international study of treatment outcome in patients with clefts of the lip and palate. Part 2. Craniofacial form and soft tissue profile. Cleft Palate Craniofac J 1992; 29:398–404.

119. Mølsted K, Kjær I, Dahl E: Spheno-occipital synchondrosis in three-month-old children with clefts of the lip and palate: A radiographic study. Cleft Palate Craniofac J 1993; 30:569–573.

120. Nakamura S, Savara BS, Thomas DR: Facial growth in children with cleft lip and/or palate. Cleft Palate J 1972; 9:120–131.

121. Narula JK, Ross RB: Facial growth in children with complete bilateral cleft lip and palate. Cleft Palate J 1970; 7:239–248.

122. Nordin KE, Larson O, Nylen B, Eklund G: Early bone grafting in complete cleft lip and palate cases following maxillofacial orthopedics. I. The method and the skeletal development from seven to thirteen years of age. Scand J Plast Reconstr Surg 1983; 17:33–50.

123. Normando ADC, da Silva OG Jr, Capelozza L Jr: Influence of surgery on maxillary growth in cleft lip and/or palate patients. J Craniomaxillofac Surg 1992; 20:111–118.

124. Noverraz AEM, Kuijpers-Jagtman AM, Mars M, Van't Hof MA: Timing of hard palate closure and dental arch relationships in unilateral cleft lip and palate patients: A mixed longitudinal study. Cleft Palate Craniofac J 1993; 30:391–396.

125. Ortiz-Monasterio F, Rebeil AS, Valderrama M, Cruz R: Cephalometric measurements on adult patients with nonoperated cleft palates. Plast Reconstr Surg 1959; 24:53–61.

126. Ortiz-Monasterio F, Serrano AR, Barrera GP, et al: A study of untreated adult cleft palate patients. Plast Reconstr Surg 1966; 38:36–41.

127. Osborne HA: A serial cephalometric analysis of facial growth in adolescent cleft palate subjects. Angle Orthod 1966; 36:211–223.

128. Palmer CR, Hamlen M, Ross RB, Lindsay WK: Cleft palate repair: Comparison of the results of two surgical techniques. Can J Surg 1969; 12:32–39.

129. Paul JL, Nanda RS: Effect of mouth breathing on dental occlusion. Angle Orthod 1973; 43:201–206.

130. Paulin G, Thilander B: Dentofacial relations in young adults with unilateral complete cleft lip and palate. A follow-up study. Scand J Plast Reconstr Hand Surg 1991; 25:63–72.

131. Pitanguy I, Franco T: Nonoperated facial fissures in adults. Plast Reconstr Surg 1967; 39:569–577.

132. Posen JM: A longitudinal study of the growth of the nose. Am J Orthod 1967; 53:746–756.

133. Proffit WR: Contemporary Orthodontics. St. Louis: CV Mosby, 1986.

134. Quinn GW: Airway interference and its effect upon growth and development of the face, jaws, dentition and associated parts. NC Dent J 1978; 60:28–31.

135. Ranta R: A review of tooth formation in children with cleft lip/palate. Am J Orthod Dentofac Orthop 1986; 90:11–18.

136. Rehrmann AH: The effect of early bone grafting on the growth of the upper jaw in cleft lip and palate children. A computer evaluation. Minerva Chir 1971; 26:874–877.

137. Rehrmann AH, Koberg WR, Koch H: Long-term postoperative results of primary and secondary bone grafting in complete clefts of lip and palate. Cleft Palate J 1970; 7:206–221.

138. Ren Y-F, Isberg A, Henningson G: Interactive influence of a pharyngeal flap and an adenoid on maxillofacial growth in cleft lip and palate patients. Cleft Palate Craniofac J 1993; 30:144–149.

139. Ricketts RM: Respiratory obstruction syndrome. Am J Orthod 1968; 54:495–507.

140. Roberts CT, Semb G, Shaw WC: Strategies for the advancement of surgical methods in cleft lip and palate. Cleft Palate Craniofac J 1991; 28:141–149.

141. Robertson NRE, Jolleys A: Effects of early bone grafting in complete clefts of lip and palate. Preliminary report. Plast Reconstr Surg 1968; 42:414–421.

142. Rohrich RJ, Byrd HS: Optimal timing of cleft palate closure. Clin Plast Surg 1990; 17:27–36.

143. Rosenstein SW, Monroe CW, Kernahan DA, et al: The case for early bone grafting in cleft lip and cleft palate. Plast Reconstr Surg 1982; 70:297–307.
144. Rosenstein S, Dado DV, Kernahan D, et al: The case for early bone grafting in cleft lip and palate: A second report. Plast Reconstr Surg 1991; 87:644–654.
145. Ross RB: Cranial base in children with cleft lip and palate clefts. Cleft Palate J 1965; 2:157–166.
146. Ross RB: Treatment variables affecting facial growth in complete unilateral cleft lip and palate. Part 1: Treatment affecting growth. Cleft Palate J 1987a; 24:5–23.
147. Ross RB: Treatment variables affecting facial growth in complete unilateral cleft lip and palate. Part 2: Presurgical orthopaedic treatment. Cleft Palate J 1987b; 24:24–32.
148. Ross RB: Treatment variables affecting facial growth in complete unilateral cleft lip and palate. Part 3: Alveolus repair and bone grafting. Cleft Palate J 1987c; 24:33–44.
149. Ross RB: Treatment variables affecting facial growth in complete unilateral cleft lip and palate. Part 4: Repair of the cleft lip. Cleft Palate J 1987d; 24:45–53.
150. Ross RB: Treatment variables affecting facial growth in complete unilateral cleft lip and palate. Part 5: Timing of palatal repair. Cleft Palate J 1987e; 24:54–63.
151. Ross RB: Treatment variables affecting facial growth in complete unilateral cleft lip and palate. Part 6: Techniques of palate repair. Cleft Palate J 1987f; 24:64–70.
152. Ross RB: Treatment variables affecting facial growth in complete unilateral cleft lip and palate. Part 7: An overview of treatment and facial growth. Cleft Palate J 1987g; 24:71–77.
153. Ross RB: Facial growth in cleft lip and palate. In McCarthy JG (ed): Plastic Surgery, vol 4. Cleft Lip and Palate and Craniofacial Anomalies. Philadelphia: WB Saunders, 1990a, pp 2553–2580.
154. Ross RB: Prediction of craniofacial growth in cleft lip and palate. In Huddart AG, Ferguson MJW (eds): Cleft Lip and Palate. Long-term Results and Future Prospects. Volume 1. The Presurgical Period, Initial Surgery, and Speech, Surgery, and Growth. Manchester: Manchester University Press, 1990b, pp 475–491.
155. Ross RB, Coupe TB: Craniofacial morphology in six pairs of monozygotic twins discordant for cleft lip and palate. J Can Dent Assoc 1965; 31:149–157.
156. Ross RB, Johnston MC: Cleft Lip and Palate. Baltimore: Williams & Wilkins, 1972.
157. Sadowsky C, Aduss H, Pruzansky S: The soft tissue profile in unilateral clefts. Angle Orthod 1973; 43:233–246.
158. Sandham A, Cheng L: Cranial base and cleft lip and palate. Angle Orthod 1988; 58:163–168.
159. Scaf G, Capelozza L Jr, de Souza Freitas JA: Assessment of the nasopharyngeal area by cephalometry in cases of cleft lip and palate. J Nihon Univ Sch Dent 1991; 33:98–107.
160. Scott JH: The growth of the craniofacial skeleton. Ir J Med Sci 1962; 438:276–286.
161. Semb G: Effect of alveolar bone grafting on maxillary growth in unilateral cleft lip and palate patients. Cleft Palate J 1988; 25:288–295.
162. Semb G: A study of facial growth in patients with unilateral cleft lip and palate treated by the Oslo CLP Team. Cleft Palate Craniofac J 1991a; 28:1–21.
163. Semb G: A study of facial growth in patients with bilateral cleft lip and palate treated by the Oslo CLP Team. Cleft Palate Craniofac J 1991b; 28:22–39.
164. Semb G: Analysis of the Oslo cleft lip and palate archive. Long-term dentofacial development [Thesis]. University of Oslo, 1991c.
165. Semb G, Shaw WC: Pharyngeal flap and facial growth. Cleft Palate J 1990; 27:217–224.
166. Semb G, Shaw WC: Simonart's band and facial growth in unilateral clefts of the lip and palate. Cleft Palate Craniofac J 1991; 28:40–46.
167. Semb G, Roberts CT, Shaw WC: The scope and limitations of single center research in cleft lip and palate. In Vig KD, Vig PS (eds): Clinical Research as the Basis of Clinical Practice. Craniofacial Growth Series 25, Center for Human Growth and Development. Ann Arbor: The University of Michigan, 1991, pp 109–123.
168. Shaw WC: Early orthopaedic treatment of unilateral cleft lip and palate. Br J Orthod 1978; 5:119–132.
169. Shaw WC, Asher-McDade C, Brattström V, et al: A six-center international study of treatment outcome in patients with clefts of the lip and palate. Part 1. Principles and study design. Cleft Palate Craniofac J 1992a; 29:393–397.
170. Shaw WC, Dahl E, Asher-McDade C, Brattström V, et al: A six-center international study of treatment outcome in patients with clefts of the lip and palate. Part 5. General discussion and conclusions. Cleft Palate Craniofac J 1992b; 29:413–418.
171. Shaw WC, Asher-McDade C, Brattström V, et al: Intercentre clinical audit for cleft lip and palate—a preliminary European investigation. In Jackson IT, Sommerlad BC (eds): Recent Advances in Plastic Surgery, number 4. Edinburgh: Churchill Livingstone, 1992c.
172. Shibasaki Y, Ross RB: Facial growth in children with isolated cleft palate. Cleft Palate J 1969; 6:290–302.
173. Siegel MI, Mooney MP, Kimes KR, Todhunter JT: Analysis of size variability of the human normal and cleft palate fetus nasal capsule by means of three-dimensional computer reconstruction of histologic preparations. Cleft Palate J 1987; 24:190–199.
174. da Silva OG Jr, Normando ADC, Capelozza L Jr: Mandibular morphology and spatial position in patients with clefts: Intrinsic or iatrogenic? Cleft Palate Craniofac J 1992a; 29:369–375.
175. da Silva OG Jr, Ramos AL, Abdo RCC: Influence of surgery on maxillary growth in cleft lip and/or palate patients. J Craniomaxillofac Surg 1992b; 20:111–118.
176. da Silva OG Jr, Ramos AL, Abdo RCC: The influence of unilateral cleft lip and palate on maxillary dental arch morphology. Angle Orthod 1992c; 62:283–290.
177. da Silva OG Jr, Normando ADC, Capelozza Filho L: Mandibular growth in patients with cleft lip and/or palate—the influence of cleft type. Am J Orthod 1993; 104:269–275.
178. Slaughter WB, Brodie AG: Facial clefts and their surgical management in view of recent research. Plast Reconstr Surg 1949; 4:203–224.

179. Smahel Z: Variations in craniofacial morphology with severity of isolated cleft palate. Cleft Palate J 1984a; 21:140–158.
180. Smahel Z: Craniofacial morphology in adults with bilateral complete cleft lip and palate. Cleft Palate J 1984b; 21:159–169.
181. Smahel Z, Brejcha M: Differences in craniofacial morphology between complete and incomplete unilateral cleft lip and palate in adults. Cleft Palate J 1983; 20:113–127.
182. Smahel Z, Müllerova Z: Craniofacial morphology in unilateral cleft lip and palate prior to palatoplasty. Cleft Palate J 1986; 23:225–232.
183. Smahel Z, Müllerova Z: Nasopharyngeal characteristics in children with cleft lip and palate. Cleft Palate Craniofac J 1992; 29:282–286.
184. Smahel Z, Müllerova Z: Facial growth and development in unilateral cleft lip and palate during the period of puberty: Comparison of the development after periosteoplasty and after primary bone grafting. Cleft Palate Craniofac J 1994; 31:106–115.
185. Solow B, Tallgren A: Head posture and craniofacial morphology. Am J Phys Anthropol 1976; 44:417–436.
186. Spauwen PHM, Hardjowasito W, Boersma J, Latief BS: Dental cast study of adult patients with untreated unilateral cleft lip or cleft lip and palate in Indonesia compared with surgically treated patients in the Netherlands. Cleft Palate Craniofac J 1993; 30:313–319.
187. Subtelny JD, Pineda Nieto R: A longitudinal study of maxillary growth following pharyngeal-flap surgery. Cleft Palate J 1978; 15:118–131.
188. Trotman CA, Ross RB: Craniofacial growth in bilateral cleft lip and palate: Ages six years to adulthood. Cleft Palate Craniofac J 1993; 30:261–273.
189. Trotman CA, Collett AR, McNamara JA Jr, Cohen SR: Analyses of craniofacial and dental morphology in monozygotic twins discordant for cleft lip and unilateral cleft lip and palate. Angle Orthod 1993; 63:135–140.
190. Vargervik K: Growth characteristics of the premaxilla and orthodontic treatment principles in bilateral cleft lip and palate. Cleft Palate J 1983; 20:289–302.
191. Vig PS, Showfety KJ, Phillips C: Experimental manipulation of head posture. Am J Orthod 1980; 77:258–268.
192. Viteporn S, Enemark H, Melsen B: Postnatal craniofacial skeleton development following a pushback operation of patients with cleft palate. Cleft Palate Craniofac J 1991; 28:392–396.
193. Warren DW, Hairfield WM: The nasal airway in cleft palate. In Bardach J, Morris HL (eds): Multidisciplinary Management of Cleft Lip and Palate. Philadelphia: WB Saunders, 1990, pp 688–692.
194. Warren DW, Duany LF, Fischer ND: Nasal pathway resistance in normal and cleft lip and palate subjects. Cleft Palate J 1969; 6:134–140.
195. Warren DW, Trier WC, Bevin AG: Effect of restorative procedures on the nasopharyngeal airway in cleft palate. Cleft Palate J 1974; 11:367–373.
196. Warren DW, Hairfield WM, Seaton DL, et al: The relationship between size of the nasal airway and nasal-oral breathing. Am J Orthod 1988; 93:289–293.
197. Warren DW, Hairfield WM, Dalston ET: The relationship between nasal airway size and nasal-oral breathing in cleft lip and palate. Cleft Palate J 1990; 27:46–51.
198. Wieslander L: The effects of orthodontic treatment on the concurrent development of the craniofacial complex. Am J Orthod 1963; 49:15–27.
199. Witzel MA, Salyer KE, Ross BR: Delayed hard palate closure: The philosophy revisited. Cleft Palate J 1984; 21:263–269.
200. Yoshida H, Nakamura A, Michi K-I, et al: Cephalometric analysis of maxillofacial morphology in unoperated cleft palate patients. Cleft Palate Craniofac J 1992; 29:419–424.

3 | Syndrome Delineation and Growth in Orofacial Clefting and Craniosynostosis

Sven Kreiborg and M. Michael Cohen, Jr.

INTRODUCTION

Syndromology spans almost all fields of medicine. Approximately 1% of newborns have multiple anomalies or syndromes. Of these conditions, only 40% can be diagnosed as being recognized syndromes. The other 60% are unknown entities that need to be further delineated. Although many syndromes are individually rare, in the aggregate they make up a significant portion of medicine.[1]

HETEROGENEITY AND PLEIOTROPY

In syndromology, a decision must be made whether similar patients have an identical disorder with slightly different manifestations or etiologically separate disorders with somewhat similar manifestations. Two basic principles of genetic nosology are heterogeneity and pleiotropy (Fig. 3–1). *Heterogeneity* refers to multiple causes resulting in the same effect. *Pleiotropy* means multiple effects from a single cause. "Splitting" occurs with genetic heterogeneity, and "lumping" occurs with pleiotropy. Clinical, genetic, and molecular methods are used to recognize genetic heterogeneity. The process of syndrome delineation can lead to the establishment of separate etiologic entities that were once thought to constitute a single disorder. Such a fate has befallen "achondroplasia," "Seckel syndrome," "Robinow syndrome," and "CHARGE association." Syndromologists are "lumpers" to the extent that they pull together pleiotropic effects of a single genetic disorder. On occasion, different entities have been "lumped" together as a single entity because the process of syndrome delineation has later judged them to be the same. The Appelt-Gerken-Lenz syndrome, the SC-pseudothalidomide syndrome, and the Roberts syndrome are now known to represent the same syndrome. Similarly, Summitt syndrome, Goodman-type acrocephalopolysyndactyly, and Carpenter syndrome are now subsumed under the rubric of Carpenter syndrome.[2,3]

In the process of syndrome delineation, "splitting" occurs much more frequently than "lumping." Toriello[4] estimated that "new" syndromes are being described at the rate of one or more per week, and although some represent variable expression of previously recorded conditions, many actually represent newly recognized conditions. Tables 3–1 and 3–2 illustrate syndrome delineation through the years with respect to orofacial clefting[5–7] and craniosynostosis.[2]

ETIOLOGIC AND PATHOGENETIC HETEROGENEITY

Many clinicians prefer the spectrum thinking of classic medicine to the discontinuous thinking of medical geneticists. The former emphasizes relationships and similarities between various disorders; the latter emphasizes differences and discontinuities of the same disorders. These seemingly different perspectives are actually compatible. Disorders that are etiologically heterogeneous (discontinuous) may have similar or identical pathogenetic pathways. The etiology and the pathogenesis of a disorder should be considered separately. Figure 3–2 diagrams some possible relationships

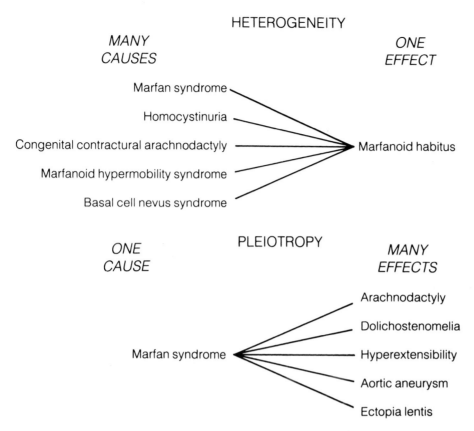

Figure 3–1. With genetic heterogeneity, etiologically separate disorders may have somewhat similar manifestations. With pleiotropy, different manifestations have a common cause. On the left side of the diagram, the causes are actually the various genes responsible for the disorders listed; the phenotype is listed simply for convenience. (From Cohen MM Jr: The Child with Multiple Birth Defects. New York: Raven Press, 1982.)

between etiology, pathogenesis, and the phenotype. Model I (top) shows etiologically heterogeneous disorders with a common pathogenetic mechanism that produces a single phenotype. Model II (middle) shows etiologically heterogeneous disorders with similar but not identical pathogenetic mechanisms and a single phenotype. Model III (bottom) shows etiologic and pathogenetic heterogeneity resulting in the same phenotype.[1]

Evidence to date suggests that many malformations are pathogenetically heterogeneous: that is, that several different mechanisms may be responsible for the same defect (see Fig. 3–2, model III). Consider holoprosencephaly, for example. The phenotype (P) (i.e., holoprosencephaly) is known to be etiologically heterogeneous (A, B, C) (e.g., may be caused in some cases by an autosomal recessive gene in the homozygous state, in other cases by trisomy 13, and in still other cases by the diabetic state of a pregnant woman). Etiologic heterogeneity suggests that the pathogenesis may also be heterogeneous (X, Y, Z) (e.g., may be based on an insult to the prechordal mesoderm in some instances, a slightly later insult to the neural plate in other

Table 3–1. SYNDROME DELINEATION INVOLVING OROFACIAL CLEFTING

Etiology	1971*	1978†	1990‡
Monogenic	39	79	193
Autosomal dominant	(17)	(35)	(69)
Autosomal recessive	(18)	(39)	(104)
X-linked	(4)	(5)	(20)
Environmentally induced	0	6	10
Chromosomal	15	29	49
Unknown cause§	18	40	90
Total	72	154	342

From Cohen MM Jr, Bankier A: Syndrome delineation involving orofacial clefting. Cleft Palate J 1991; 28:119–120.

* Based on Gorlin et al. (1971).[7]
† Based on Cohen (1978).[5]
‡ Based on POSSUM (1990).
§ Includes distinctive syndromes of unknown genesis and associations.

Table 3–2. SYNDROME DELINEATION INVOLVING CRANIOSYNOSTOSIS

Etiology	1975	1979	1986	1992
Chromosomal	0	11	14	16
Monogenic	12	26	31	40
Autosomal dominant	(5)	(12)	(13)	(15)
Autosomal recessive	(7)	(12)	(13)	(16)
X-linked	(0)	(2)	(2)	(3)
Inheritance pattern unclear	(0)	(0)	(3)	(6)
Environmentally induced	1	2	3	4
Unknown genesis	5	18	10	24
Miscellaneous	—	—	6	6
Total syndromes	18	57	64	90

Modified from Cohen MM Jr: Craniosynostosis: Diagnosis, Evaluation, and Management. New York: Raven Press, 1986.

instances, or an insult producing decreased cellular proliferation of all three germ layers simultaneously in still other instances). Although holoprosencephaly is known to be etiologically heterogeneous, in some cases the pathogenesis may be reduced to a common mechanism (X), as illustrated in model I, and in other cases may be reduced to a similar mechanism (X, X1), as illustrated in model II.[1] Figure 3–3 illustrates etiologic and pathogenetic heterogeneity with respect to the Robin sequence.

SYNDROME DELINEATION

The process of syndrome delineation can be divided into the following stages: (1) unknown-genesis syndromes, including provisionally unique-pattern syndromes and recurrent-pattern syndromes, and (2) known-genesis syndromes, including pedigree syndromes, chromosomal syndromes, biochemical-defect syndromes, and environmentally induced syndromes.[1]

In an unknown-genesis syndrome, the cause is simply not known. In a provisionally unique-pattern syndrome, several anomalies are observed in the same patient such that the clinician does not recognize the overall pattern of defects from his or her own experience, or from searching the literature, or from consultation with the most learned colleagues in the field. The patient illustrated in Figure 3–4 has a provisionally unique-pattern syndrome consisting of premature sutural fusion, cloverleaf skull, anomalies of the face, thumb duplication, micropenis, and bifid scrotum. The condition is known as COH syndrome. Most likely the anomalies have a common cause, though unknown, rather than having different causes acting independently. The probability that such anomalies occur in the same patient by chance becomes less likely the more anomalies the patient has and the rarer these anomalies are individually in the general population.[1,2]

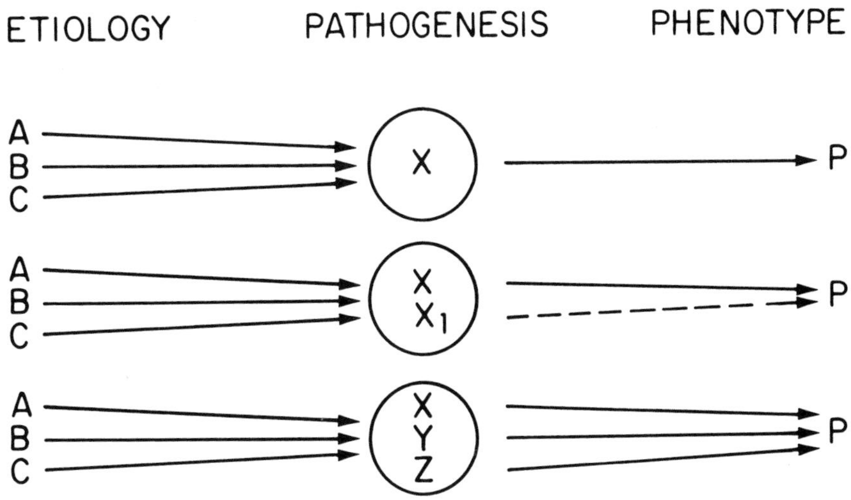

Figure 3–2. Possible relationships between etiology, pathogenesis, and the phenotype. See text. (From Cohen MM Jr: The Child with Multiple Birth Defects. New York: Raven Press, 1982.)

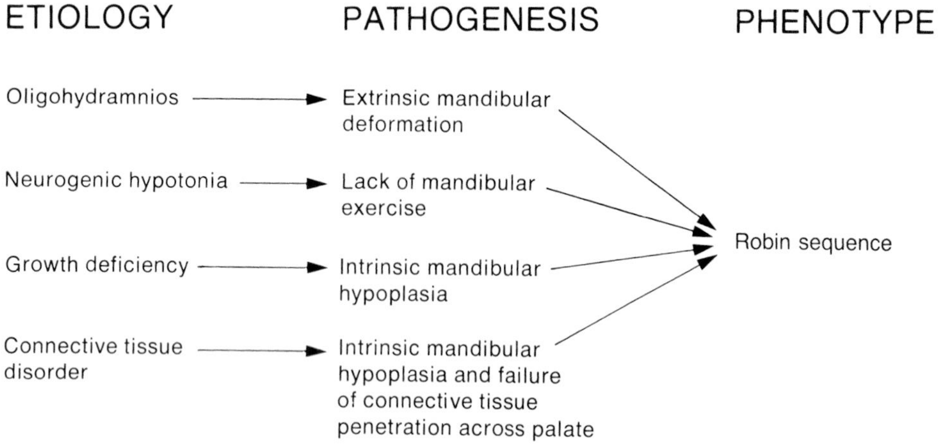

ETIOLOGY   PATHOGENESIS   PHENOTYPE

Oligohydramnios ──────▶ Extrinsic mandibular
                         deformation

Neurogenic hypotonia ──────▶ Lack of mandibular
                              exercise
                                                    Robin sequence

Growth deficiency ──────▶ Intrinsic mandibular
                           hypoplasia

Connective tissue ──────▶ Intrinsic mandibular
disorder   hypoplasia and failure
                          of connective tissue
                          penetration across palate

Figure 3–3. Etiologic heterogeneity suggests pathogenetic heterogeneity in the Robin sequence. The following pathogenetic possibilities should be considered. (1) Oligohydramnios results in decreased amnionic fluid, compressing the chin against the sternum and thus restricting mandibular growth. (2) If hypotonia restricts mouth opening during early fetal life prior to complete palatal closure, the Robin sequence might result from lack of mandibular exercise. (3) Growth deficiency, as observed in chromosomal syndromes such as dup(11q) syndrome, may produce the Robin sequence by intrinsic mandibular hypoplasia. (4) In a connective tissue disorder such as the Stickler syndrome, the Robin sequence may result from intrinsic hypoplasia and failure of connective tissue penetration across the palate. (From Cohen MM Jr: The Child with Multiple Birth Defects. New York: Raven Press, 1982.)

Obviously, if a second example comes to light, the condition is no longer unique. A provisionally unique-pattern syndrome is a one-of-a-kind syndrome to a particular observer at a particular point in time. There may be a 19th-century description of a similar instance that has been overlooked. There may also be some instances of the syndrome in different parts of the world that remain as yet unrecognized. Thus many syndromes appear to be unique at the time the initial patient is discovered but are no longer unique when two or more examples become known.[1]

A recurrent-pattern syndrome can be defined as similar or identical sets of anomalies in two or more unrelated patients. The three patients whose findings are summarized in Table 3–3 have a recurrent pattern syndrome known as Gomez-López-Hernández syndrome. Findings include mental deficiency, cerebellar ataxia, parietal alopecia, and a variety of craniofacial anomalies.[8] The same abnormalities in two or

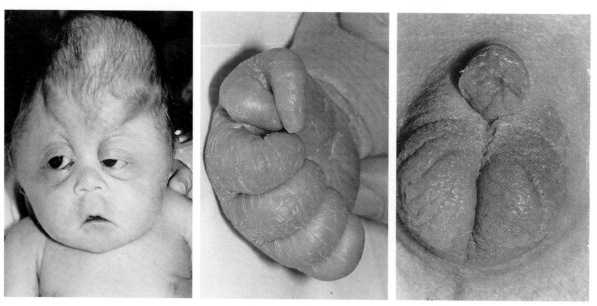

Figure 3–4. Provisionally unique pattern syndrome known as COH syndrome. Craniosynostosis, cloverleaf skull, facial anomalies, preaxial polydactyly, micropenis, and bifid scrotum. (From Cohen MM Jr: Craniosynostosis: Diagnosis, Evaluation, and Management. New York: Raven Press, 1986.)

Table 3-3. GOMEZ-LOPÉZ-HERNÁNDEZ SYNDROME

Findings	López-Hernández (1982)		Gomez (1979)
	Case 1	*Case 2*	*Case 3*
Sex	Female	Female	Female
Population	Mexico	Mexico	USA
Growth			
Short stature	+	+	?
Performance			
Mental deficiency	+	+	+
Central nervous system			
Pons-vermis fusion	+	+	?
Atresia of fourth ventricle	+	+	?
Cerebellar ataxia	+	+	+
Trigeminal anesthesia	+	+	+
Craniofacial			
Craniosynostosis	+	+	−
Parietal alopecia	+	+	+
Ocular hypertelorism	+	−	+
Corneal opacities	+	+	+
Midface deficiency	+	+	+
Low-set, posteriorly angulated ears	+	+	?
Limbs			
Clinodactyly	+	+	?
Genitalia			
Hypoplastic labia majora	+	+	?

From Cohen MM Jr: Craniosynostosis: Diagnosis, Evaluation, and Management. New York: Raven Press, 1986.

more patients suggest, but do not prove, that the pathogenesis in both cases may be the same. At the recurrent-pattern stage of syndrome delineation, the etiology is still unknown. In general, the validity of a recurrent-pattern syndrome increases with the more abnormalities found in the condition and the more patients recognized as having the syndrome.[1]

At the recurrent-pattern stage of syndrome delineation, the number of findings is usually expanded as the number of patients increases. However, because the etiology is unknown at this time, other examples of the syndrome tend to be selected because they most closely resemble the first case. This results in an artificial homogeneity of cases that emphasizes the most severe aspects of the syndrome. Thus we should be wary of estimated frequencies given in review articles and textbooks for anomalies that occur in a recurrent-pattern syndrome; they tend to be overestimates that can affect counseling on the prognostic risk for developing some features of the syndrome such as mental retardation.[1]

A known-genesis syndrome can be defined as several anomalies causally related on the basis of

1. Occurrence in the same family or, less conclusively, the same mode of inheritance in different families.
2. A chromosomal defect.
3. A defect in an enzyme or structural protein.
4. An environmental factor.[1]

Examples of known-genesis syndromes with orofacial clefting and craniosynostosis are shown in Tables 3-4 and 3-5. The term *pedigree syndrome* refers to known genesis on the basis of pedigree evidence alone; the basic defect remains undefined, although the condition is known to represent a monogenic disorder. An example is the autosomal recessive Carpenter syndrome, consisting of craniosynostosis and polysyndactyly. Most cases represent new mutations. The van der Woude syndrome, consisting of lip pits and cleft lip-palate, follows an autosomal dominant mode of inheritance with incomplete penetrance and variable expressivity. The gene is located on the long arm of chromosome 1 in the 1q23 region. A *chromosomal syndrome*, such as del(13q) syndrome, is cytogenetically defined. In a *biochemical-defect syndrome*, specific enzymatic defects are known in recessive syndromes. The term is also meant to include specific defects in structural proteins as these become known

Table 3–4. SOME TYPES OF KNOWN-GENESIS SYNDROMES WITH OROFACIAL CLEFTING

Type of Known-Genesis Syndrome	Syndrome Example	Striking Features	Orofacial Clefting	Etiology
Chromosomal	Trisomy 13 syndrome	Holoprosencephaly, seizures, apneic episodes, severe mental deficiency, early demise, ocular hypotelorism, flat nose, microphthalmia, iris coloboma, orofacial clefting, malformed ears, glabellar hemangioma, scalp defects, polydactyly, congenital heart defects, genital anomalies	Common	Trisomy 13
Pedigree (monogenic)	van der Woude syndrome	Lip pits and orofacial clefting	Common	Autosomal dominant, gene localized to 1q32
Teratogenic	Fetal alcohol syndrome	Growth deficiency, mental deficiency, microcephaly, narrow palpebral fissures, congenital heart defects, joint anomalies, other abnormalities	Uncommon	Chronic alcoholism during pregnancy

in some dominant disorders. The autosomal recessive mucopolysaccharidosis Hurler syndrome is characterized by α-L-iduronidase deficiency. Finally, an example of a condition caused by a teratogen is the fetal hydantoin syndrome, in which 6% have craniosynostosis.[2, 3]

Comments on Syndrome Delineation

The process of syndrome delineation is summarized in Figure 3–5. In general, a syndrome can be placed into one of the categories discussed. Occasionally, a syndrome may be delineated in a one-step delineation, thus bypassing several of the stages mentioned. For example, if a new chromosomal abnormality is discovered during the laboratory investigation of a patient clinically defined as having a provisionally unique-pattern syndrome, the patient represents a known-genesis syndrome of the chromosomal type in a one-step delineation. The variability of the clinical expression, however, must await the discovery of more patients. In other instances, such as a large dominant pedigree with many affected individuals, a known-genesis syndrome of the pedigree type and much of its phenotypic variability can be determined in one step.[1]

Table 3–5. SOME TYPES OF KNOWN-GENESIS SYNDROMES WITH CRANIOSYNOSTOSIS

Type of Known-Genesis Syndrome	Syndrome Example	Striking Features	Craniosynostosis	Etiology
Chromosomal	Deletion 13q	Lobar holoprosencephaly, mental retardation, microphthalmia, iris coloboma, retinoblastoma, malformed ears, micrognathia, hypoplastic thumbs, imperforate anus, hypospadias, cryptorchidism, congenital heart defects	Trigonocephaly with absent metopic suture in approximately 18% of cases	Deletion of long arm of chromosome 13
Pedigree (monogenic)	Carpenter	Preaxial polysyndactyly of the toes, brachydactyly and soft tissue syndactyly of the fingers, congenital heart defects, short stature, obesity	Multiple sutural synostosis with frequent asymmetric distortion	Autosomal recessive inheritance
Enzymatically defined	Hurler	Growth deficiency of postnatal onset, mental retardation, coarse facial appearance, corneal clouding, dysostosis multiplex	Premature fusion of metopic, sagittal, and lambdoidal sutures	α-L-Iduronidase deficiency (autosomal recessive)
Environmentally induced	Fetal hydantoin	Growth deficiency, mental retardation, hypoplastic nails, metopic ridging, ocular hypertelorism, other anomalies	Premature synostosis of sagittal or coronal suture in approximately 6% of cases	Diphenylhydantoin during pregnancy

From Cohen MM Jr: Craniosynostosis: Diagnosis, Evaluation, and Management. New York: Raven Press, 1986.

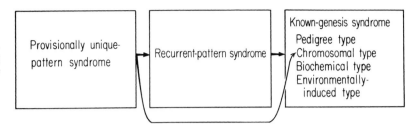

Figure 3–5. Diagrammatic summary of the process of syndrome delineation. (From Cohen MM Jr: The Child with Multiple Birth Defects. New York: Raven Press, 1982.)

In syndromes, anomalies are nonspecific. Each may occur as an isolated defect; each may occur as a component part of various syndromes. This is certainly true of orofacial clefting and craniosynostosis. Each may occur alone or together with various other abnormalities making up a large number of different syndromes. Because each may occur with various percentages in different syndromes, they are facultative rather than obligatory; that is, orofacial clefting or craniosynostosis may or may not be present in a given example of a condition in which either is known to be a feature.[1]

Significance of Syndrome Delineation

The significance of syndrome delineation cannot be overestimated. As an unknown-genesis syndrome becomes delineated, its phenotypic spectrum, its natural history, and its inheritance pattern or risk or recurrence become known, allowing for better patient care and family counseling.[1]

If the phenotypic spectrum is known, the clinician can search for suspected defects that may not be apparent but that may produce clinical problems later, such as a hemivertebra in Goldenhar syndrome. If a complication can occur in a given syndrome, such as Wilms tumor in the Beckwith-Wiedemann syndrome, the clinician is forewarned to monitor the patient for the possible development of neoplasia.[1]

Finally, if the recurrence risk is known, the parents can be counseled about future pregnancies. This is important if the risk is high and the disorder is handicapping or disfiguring, has mental deficiency as a component, or leads to a short life span. For example, cleft palate or Robin sequence is a common feature of the Stickler syndrome, an autosomal dominant disorder with a 50% risk of recurrence when one parent is affected. In this condition, retinal detachment occurs in 20% of reported cases and blindness occurs in 15%. Genetic counseling is important because the risk of developing serious ocular problems is high. This relatively common condition also illustrates the importance of syndrome delineation because the entity was unknown and unrecognized before 1965, although it had existed. Thus syndrome delineation fosters good patient care; the overall treatment program gains rationality. In contrast, with a provisionally unique-pattern syndrome, the treatment program and overall management frequently leave something to be desired.[1]

CRANIOFACIAL GROWTH

To exemplify the importance of syndrome delineation and the heterogeneity of orofacial clefting and craniosynostosis, a few striking examples of differences in craniofacial growth will be given. Some craniofacial disorders may resemble each other at one stage and differ markedly at another. Thus the importance of the time factor is essential for understanding growth, as previously pointed out by Pruzansky.[9] The implications for treatment will also be discussed.

Orofacial Clefting

Robin Sequence

The Robin sequence (Fig. 3–6) may have different etiologies and pathogeneses (see Fig. 3–3).

As part of a major study of cleft lip and palate in Denmark,[10] all new patients with clefts were examined clinically and roentgencephalometrically from 1976 to 1981.

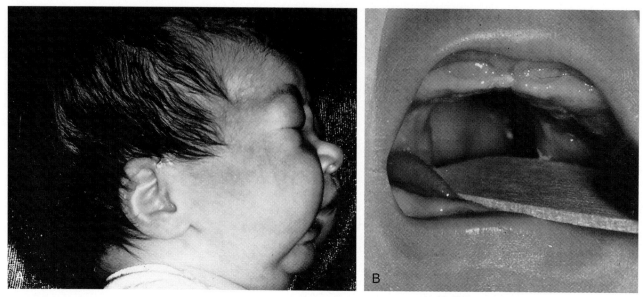

Figure 3–6. Robin sequence. *A,* Micrognathia. *B,* U-shaped cleft palate. (From Cohen MM Jr: The Child with Multiple Birth Defects. New York: Raven Press, 1982.)

During this period, nine patients with nonsyndromic Robin sequence were recorded. Eight were examined at 2 months and 22 months of age, before palatal closure.[11]

Facial growth in nonsyndromic Robin sequence was compared with facial growth in Danish children with isolated cleft palate examined during the same period, since Dahl and associates[12] observed that even infants with isolated cleft palate (without Robin sequence) have significantly smaller and more retrognathic mandibles than normal infants.

From 1976 to 1981, five cases of the Robin sequence occurring with syndromes, such as mandibulofacial dysostosis and Stickler syndrome, were recorded, and craniofacial growth in one girl with mandibulofacial dysostosis was monitored from infancy to age 9 years.

Similarities and differences in the phenotype between nonsyndromic and syndromic forms of the Robin sequence will be discussed with special reference to treatment strategies.

Isolated Robin Sequence

At 2 months of age, Robin sequence infants, on the average, had a significantly smaller cranial base angle (n-s-ba), shorter mandible (cd-pgn), and smaller depth of the bony nasopharynx than infants with isolated cleft palate (Fig. 3–7, Table 3–6). The mean difference in mandibular length was about 4 mm in comparison with the cleft palate group. However, when compared with cleft lip subjects, the difference was 8 mm. At 22 months of age, the mean mandibular length still differed significantly, now being 6 mm shorter in the Robin sequence group than in the cleft palate group (see Table 3–6; Fig. 3–8). At the same age, the mean increment in mandibular length was 24.5 mm for the Robin sequence group, in comparison with 26.8 mm for the isolated cleft palate group (Fig. 3–9*A,B*).[11]

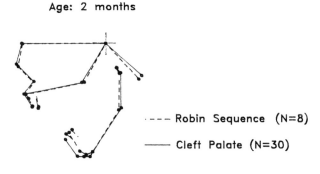

Age: 2 months

– – – **Robin Sequence (N=8)**

——— **Cleft Palate (N=30)**

Figure 3–7. Mean plots from lateral cephalograms of Robin sequence group (*n* = 8) and cleft palate group (*n* = 30) at 2 months of age. Superimposition on nasion-sella line, registered at sella. (Based on data from Kreiborg S, Jensen BL, Dahl E, Fogh-Andersen P: Pierre Robin syndrome. Early facial development. Fifth International Congress on Cleft Palate and Related Craniofacial Anomalies, Abstract 303. Monte Carlo, Monaco, 1985.)

Table 3–6. ROENTGENCEPHALOMETRIC VARIABLES SHOWING SIGNIFICANT
($p = 0.01**$) DIFFERENCES BETWEEN ROBIN SEQUENCE GROUP (RS)
AND ISOLATED CLEFT PALATE GROUP (CP$^+$)

Variable	Group	N	Age in Months	$\bar{x}$ (Degrees or mm)	Difference
n-s-ba	RS	8	2	133.6°	−4.8°**
	CP$^+$	30	2	138.4°	
	RS	8	22	130.8°	−2.2°
	CP	30	22	133.0°	
cd-pgn	RS	8	2	48.4 mm	−3.7 mm**
	CP$^+$	30	2	52.1 mm	
	RS	8	22	72.9 mm	−6.0 mm**
	CP	30	22	78.9 mm	
ML/RL	RS	8	2	146.9°	2.3°
	CP$^+$	30	2	144.6°	
	RS	8	22	145.6°	6.3°**
	CP	30	22	139.3°	

Abbreviations: n, nasion; s, sella; ba, basion; cd, condylion; pgn, prognathion; ML, mandibular line; RL, ramus line.

From Dahl E, Kreiborg S, Jensen BL, Fogh-Andersen P: Comparison of craniofacial morphology in infants with incomplete cleft lip and infants with isolated cleft palate. Cleft Palate J 1982; 19:258–266.

Age: 22 months

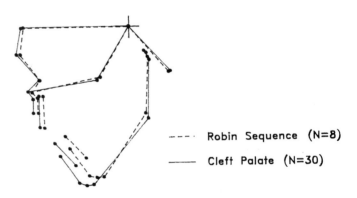

Figure 3–8. Mean plots from lateral cephalograms of Robin sequence group ($n = 8$) and cleft palate group ($n = 30$) at 22 months of age. Superimposition on nasion-sella line, registered at sella. (Based on data from Kreiborg S, Jensen BL, Dahl E, Fogh-Andersen P: Pierre Robin syndrome. Early facial development. Fifth International Congress on Cleft Palate and Related Craniofacial Anomalies, Abstract 303. Monte Carlo, Monaco, 1985.)

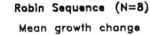

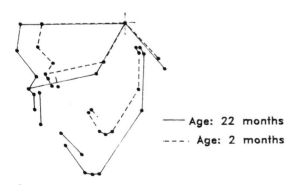

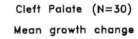

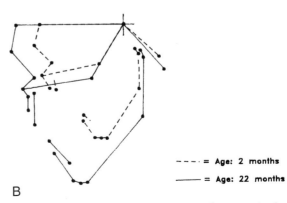

A   B

Figure 3–9. *A,* Mean growth pattern in the Robin sequence group from 2 to 22 months of age. *B,* Mean growth pattern in the cleft palate group from 2 to 22 months of age. (*A* and *B* based on data from Kreiborg S, Jensen BL, Dahl E, Fogh-Andersen P: Pierre Robin syndrome. Early facial development. Fifth International Congress on Cleft Palate and Related Craniofacial Anomalies, Abstract 303. Monte Carlo, Monaco, 1985.)

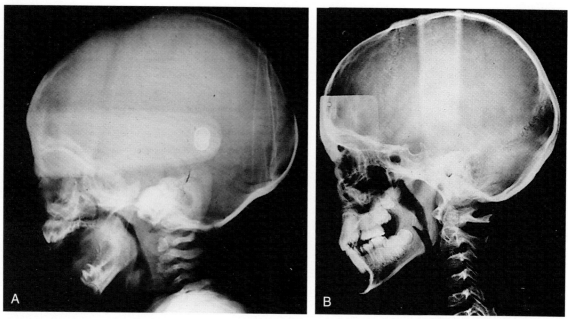

Figure 3–10. *A,* Robin sequence. Roentgencephalometric film at 2 months of age. Note short, retrognathic mandible and narrow airway. *B,* Robin sequence. Same child as in *A,* now 10 years of age. Note that facial morphology is within normal limits.

Two patients had fixation of the tongue; six were treated conservatively. At 22 months of age, before palatoplasty, glossoptosis had resolved in all Robin sequence patients as a result of downward and forward growth of the mandible. However, at this early age, it does not seem fully justified to term this "catch-up growth" because the mean increment in mandibular length was actually 2 mm less in the Robin sequence group than in the isolated cleft palate group. Furthermore, the mandible in the Robin sequence group had a significantly greater gonial angle than in the isolated cleft palate group (see Table 3–6).

Figure 3–10 illustrates facial development in one Robin sequence patient from 2 months to 10 years of age. Facial morphology at 10 years is within normal limits, but the mandible is still somewhat retrognathic, and the gonial angle is slightly larger than normal. Similar observations were made previously by Pruzansky[13] and Cohen.[1]

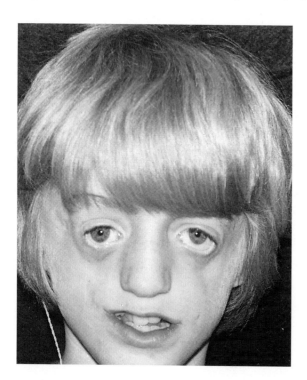

Figure 3–11. Mandibulofacial dysostosis. Downward-slanting palpebral fissures, malar deficiency; the child also wears a hearing aid. (From Cohen MM Jr: The Child with Multiple Birth Defects. New York: Raven Press, 1982.)

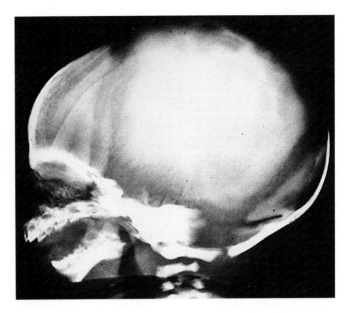

Figure 3–12. Mandibulofacial dysostosis. Lateral skull radiograph of a girl at 3 weeks of age. Note severe mandibular hypoplasia and obstruction of airway. (From Kreiborg S, Dahl E: The cranial base and the face in mandibulofacial dysostosis. Am J Med Genet 1993; 47:753–760.)

Syndromic Robin Sequence

Mandibulofacial dysostosis (Fig. 3–11) is a well-known autosomal dominant condition reviewed exhaustively elsewhere.[3, 14] The gene has been mapped to 5q31.3 → 5q33.3.[15] Cumulative evidence from the literature indicates that there are also 24 instances of affected sibs.[16] Although germinal mosaicism cannot be ruled out, it appears that mandibulofacial dysostosis is etiologically heterogeneous, with a less frequently occurring autosomal recessive type. The palate is cleft in about 35%, and many children with cleft palate have Robin sequence.

Mandibular growth is severely affected, thereby impinging on the oropharyngeal airway,[17, 18] and the cranial base angle becomes progressively more acute with time, thereby diminishing the nasopharyngeal airway.[19, 20] A case of severe mandibulofacial dysostosis is illustrated in Figures 3–12 and 3–13. At 3 weeks of age, severe respiratory and feeding difficulties were encountered (see Fig. 3–12), and antefixation of the tongue was carried out. After tongue release at 5 months, respiratory and feeding difficulties continued because of lack of downward and forward growth of the mandi-

Figure 3–13. Mandibulofacial dysostosis. Cephalometric growth tracing of the girl described in Figure 3–12 from 3 years to 8 years, 10 months of age. Superimposition on clivus, registered at mandibular condyle. Note downward and backward growth of mandible and bending of cranial base. (From Kreiborg S, Dahl E: The cranial base and the face in mandibulofacial dysostosis. Am J Med Genet 1993; 47:753–760.)

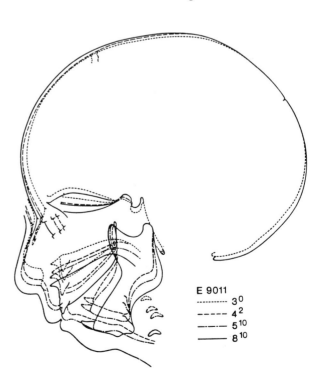

E 9011

---- 3⁰
---- 4²
---- 5¹⁰
—— 8¹⁰

ble. Tracheostomy was necessary and had to be maintained for several years even after palatal closure at 3 years. The growth pattern from age 3 to 8 years, 10 months is illustrated in Figure 13–13. The mandible grew downward and backward with minimal increase in height posteriorly. The cranial base angle became markedly more acute, and this phenomenon is discussed in detail elsewhere.[21]

Implications for Treatment

Isolated Robin sequence represents the lower end of the isolated cleft palate spectrum in terms of mandibular size, retrognathia, and perhaps the width of the cleft and basilar kyphosis. Isolated Robin sequence represents either a deformation sequence or a genetic predisposition for reduced mandibular size.[22]

In general, nonsyndromic Robin sequence infants usually can be treated by posture and by special care, including nasal intubation, about 66% of the time. The other 33% require fixation of the tongue or other forms of active treatment. Special care or treatment is usually required for only a relatively short period of time (3–6 months), since the downward and forward growth of the mandible is sufficient to help resolve the respiratory problem, even though the early mean increment in mandibular length is slightly less than in other cleft palate children.

In syndromic Robin sequence, treatment depends on accurate diagnosis of a specific syndrome and the type of Robin sequence.[23, 24] Infants with mandibulofacial dysostosis and the Robin sequence often have more severe and prolonged respiratory problems. Mandibular growth potential is poor, and respiratory function should be monitored carefully until the palatal cleft is closed and, most often, even after that. The Robin sequence in mandibulofacial dysostosis occurs on a malformational basis.

Craniosynostosis: Apert and Crouzon Syndromes

The syndromes of Apert and Crouzon (Figs. 3–14, 3–15) are characterized by severe developmental disturbances of nearly all the craniofacial regions, including the

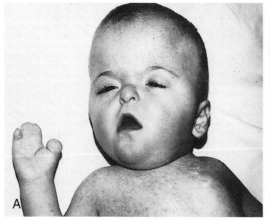
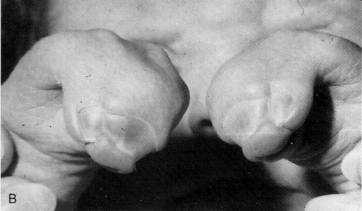
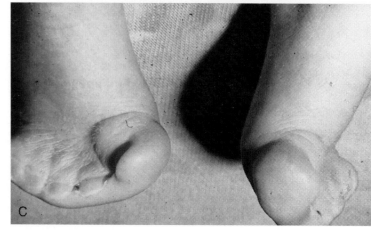
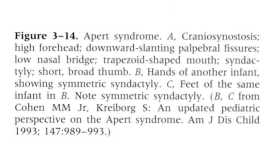

Figure 3–14. Apert syndrome. A, Craniosynostosis; high forehead; downward-slanting palpebral fissures; low nasal bridge; trapezoid-shaped mouth; syndactyly; short, broad thumb. B, Hands of another infant, showing symmetric syndactyly. C, Feet of the same infant in B. Note symmetric syndactyly. (B, C from Cohen MM Jr, Kreiborg S: An updated pediatric perspective on the Apert syndrome. Am J Dis Child 1993; 147:989–993.)

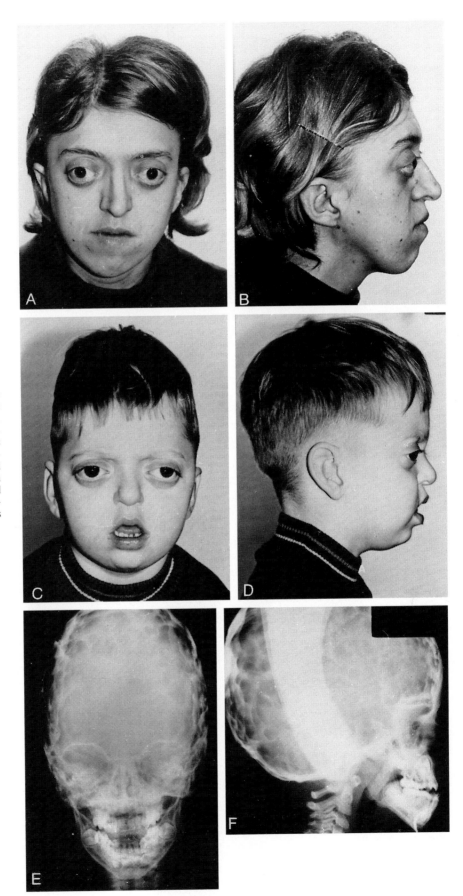

Figure 3–15. Crouzon syndrome in mother and son. *A* to *D*, Note brachycephaly, ocular proptosis, maxillary hypoplasia. *E, F,* Cephalometric roentgenograms of son. Note brachycephaly, increased digital markings, and maxillary hypoplasia. (From Cohen MM Jr: An etiologic and nosologic overview of craniosynostosis syndromes. Birth Defects 1975; 11(2):137–189.)

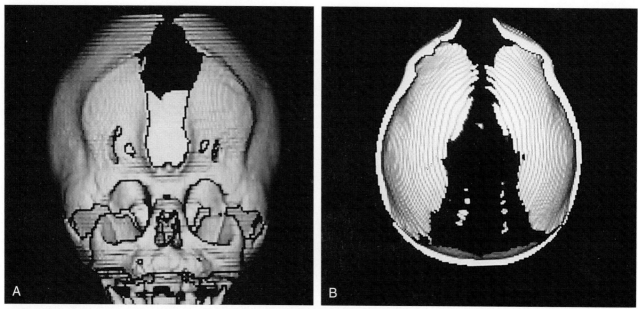

Figure 3–16. Apert syndrome. 1-month-old boy. Three-dimensional models from CT scans show extensive midline calvarial defect and unusually large anterolateral fontanelles. (From Kreiborg S, Marsh JL, Cohen MM Jr, et al: Comparative three-dimensional analysis of CT-scans of the calvaria and cranial base in Apert and Crouzon syndromes. J Craniomaxillofac Surg 1993; 21:181–188.) *B,* Apert syndrome. Same patient as in Figure 3–16*A.* Midline calvarial defect seen from inside of calvaria. (From Cohen MM Jr, Kreiborg S: An updated pediatric perspective on the Apert syndrome. Am J Dis Child 1993; 147:989–993.)

calvaria, cartilaginous cranial base, orbits, and maxillary complex.[25] Although it has been repeatedly stated that the cranial anomalies in the two syndromes are very similar, few comparative studies have been reported. The characteristics during infancy are markedly different.[26, 27]

In infancy a wide midline calvarial defect and patent sutures (except the coronal) and fontanelles characterize the Apert syndrome (Figs. 3–16, 3–17; Table 3–7); early closure of sutures and fontanelles characterizes the Crouzon syndrome (Fig. 3–18; see Table 3–7). In the cranial base, infants with Apert syndrome have a widened ethmoid and depressed cribriform plate. Progressive fusion of sutures and synchondroses is observed during the first few years of life in most cases (Table 3–8). Characteristic findings in infants with Crouzon syndrome include very early fusion of synchondroses and enlargement of the sella turcica (see Fig. 3–18, Table 3–8). The mean cranial

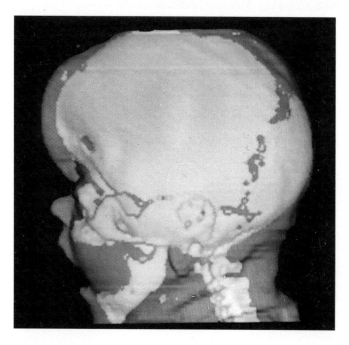

Figure 3–17. Apert syndrome. Same patient as shown in Figure 3–16. Note premature fusion of coronal suture area; all other sutures are patent. (From Kreiborg S, Cohen MM Jr: Characteristics of the infant Apert skull and its subsequent development. J Craniofac Genet Dev Biol 1990; 10:399–410.)

Table 3–7. ABNORMAL CALVARIAL FINDINGS

Findings	0–1 yr		1–4 yrs	
	Apert	*Crouzon*	*Apert*	*Crouzon*
Closure of sutures or suture areas*				
Coronal	+	+	+	+
Sagittal	–	+	+	+
Metopic	–	+	+	+
Squamosal	–	+	+	+
Lambdoid	–	+	–	+
Closure of fontanelles				
Anterior	–	+	+	+
Posterior	–	+	+	+
Anterolateral	–	+	+	+
Posterolateral	–	+	+	+
Midline calvarial defect	+	–	–†	–
Immature, thin calvaria	+	–	+	–
Increased digital markings	–	+	+	+

* In Apert syndrome, a widely patent midline calvarial defect extending from the glabella to the posterior fontanelle is observed in infancy.[26] We called this midline defect a suture area because no proper interdigitated suture formation ever took place. Rather, the midline defect was obliterated during the first 2 to 4 years of life by coalescence of bony islands that had formed in the defect. The term craniosynostosis may be misleading when applied to the metopic and sagittal areas of the Apert syndrome because no sutures form that then become prematurely synostosed. The lambdoid suture does form properly with interdigitations; we observed two instances with true Wormian bones.[26] From dry skull study, we think that proper suture formation may also occur in the squamosal area. Since the coronal suture area is fused at birth except in its most superior aspect, it is not known at present whether simple coalescence of bone takes place during intrauterine life or whether a "true pre-suture area" really develops.

† Midline calvarial defect in Apert syndrome closes by formation of bony islands that eventually coalesce.

From Kreiborg S, Marsh JL, Cohen MM Jr, et al: Comparative three-dimensional analysis of CT-scans of the calvaria and cranial base in Apert and Crouzon syndromes. J Craniomaxillofac Surg 1993; 21:181–188.

base angle (n-s-ba) tends toward platybasia in Apert syndrome ($\bar{x} = 134.4°$) and toward basilar kyphosis in Crouzon syndrome ($\bar{x} = 126.2°$).

In childhood and during adolescence, both syndromes are characterized by closure of all sutures in the calvaria, cranial base, orbits, and maxillary complex (Fig. 3–19) with progressive disharmony between the jaws, particularly in the sagittal plane[25] (Fig. 3–20).

In older children, adolescents, and adults, the two syndromes share a number of *qualitative* craniofacial traits in common: synostosis of nearly all sutures in the cal-

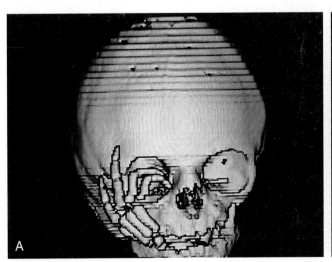 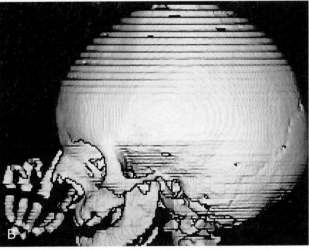

Figure 3–18. *A,* Crouzon syndrome. 11-month-old boy. Three-dimensional models from CT scans. Frontal view. Premature fusion of metopic, coronal, and sagittal sutures. Note absence of midline calvarial defect. (From Kreiborg S, Marsh JL, Cohen MM Jr, et al: Comparative three-dimensional analysis of CT-scans of the calvaria and cranial base in Apert and Crouzon syndromes. J Craniomaxillofac Surg 1993; 21:181–188.) *B,* Crouzon syndrome. Same patient as in Figure 3–18*A.* Lateral view. Premature fusion of all calvarial sutures except lambdoid suture. (From Kreiborg S, Marsh JL, Cohen MM Jr, et al: Comparative three dimensional analysis of CT-scans of the calvaria and cranial base in Apert and Crouzon syndromes. J Craniomaxillofac Surg 1993; 21:181–188.)

Table 3–8. ABNORMAL CRANIAL BASE FINDINGS*

Findings	0–1 yr		1–4 yrs		>4 yrs		Total	
	Apert	*Crouzon*	*Apert*	*Crouzon*	*Apert*	*Crouzon*	*Apert*	*Crouzon*
Fused synchondroses								
Spheno-occipital	0/6	2/3	0/3	3/5	3/3	10/11	3/12	15/19
Petro-occipital	0/6	2/2	2/3	3/3	3/3	10/11	5/12	15/18
Occipital	0/6	2/3	3/3	3/3	3/3	10/11	5/12	15/18
Asymmetry	2/6	0/3	1/3	0/5	1/3	1/11	4/12	1/19
V-shaped anterior cranial fossa	1/6	0/3	1/3	0/5	1/3	0/11	3/12	0/19
Enlarged sella turcica	0/6	3/3	3/3	5/5	3/3	11/11	6/12	19/19
Narrow floor of sella turcica	0/6	1/3	0/3	3/5	2/3	7/10	2/12	11/18
Widened ethmoid	6/6	0/3	2/3	1/5	3/3	2/11	11/12	3/19
Depressed cribriform plate	6/6	1/3	2/3	2/5	3/3	1/11	11/12	4/19
Thin clivus in midsagittal plane	0/6	1/3	0/3	2/4	0/3	7/11	10/11	0/12

* Tendency toward platybasia in Apert syndrome ($\bar{x}$ = 134.4°; range, 113°–153.5°) and basilar kyphosis in Crouzon syndrome ($\bar{x}$ = 126.2°; range, 113°–145.5°).

From Kreiborg S, Marsh JL, Cohen MM Jr, et al: Comparative three-dimensional analysis of CT-scans of the calvaria and cranial base in Apert and Crouzon syndromes. J Craniomaxillofac Surg 1993; 21:181–188.

varia, cranial base, orbit, and maxillary region; fusion of the synchondroses of the cranial base; and brachycephaly, hypertelorism, ocular proptosis, and maxillary hypoplasia. However, there are marked differences in *quantitative* craniofacial morphology, including marked cephalometric differences in the calvaria, cranial base, orbits, and maxilla.[28] Differences in oral, dental,[29] and cervical[30] characteristics have also been shown. In general, the craniofacial morphology is more abnormal in Apert syndrome than in Crouzon syndrome.[31] This is probably why the results of craniofacial surgery, most commonly carried out under the same principles in both syndromes, are generally less satisfactory in Apert than in Crouzon syndrome.

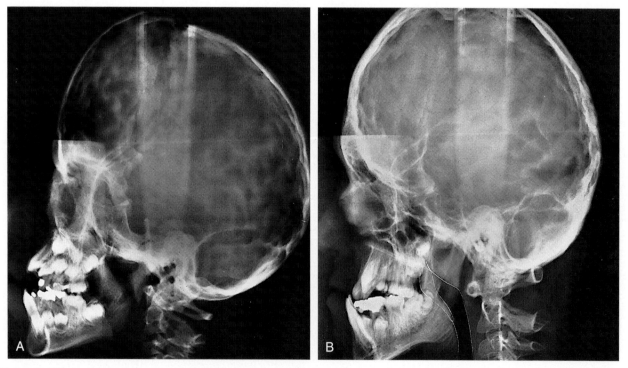

Figure 3–19. *A*, Apert syndrome. 8-year-old boy. Lateral cephalometric projection. Note closure of all sutures, increased digital markings, brachycephaly, enlarged sella turcica, maxillary hypoplasia, relative mandibular prognathism, and severe malocclusion. *B*, Crouzon syndrome. 8-year-old boy. Lateral cephalometric projection. Note closure of all sutures, increased digital markings, brachycephaly, enlarged sella turcica, maxillary hypoplasia, relative mandibular prognathism, and severe malocclusion. (From Kreiborg S, Aduss H, Cohen MM Jr: Apert's and Crouzon's syndromes contrasted: Qualitative craniofacial x-ray findings. *In* Marchac D [ed]: Proceedings of First International Congress on Craniofacial Surgery, pp 91–95. Berlin: Springer-Verlag, 1987.)

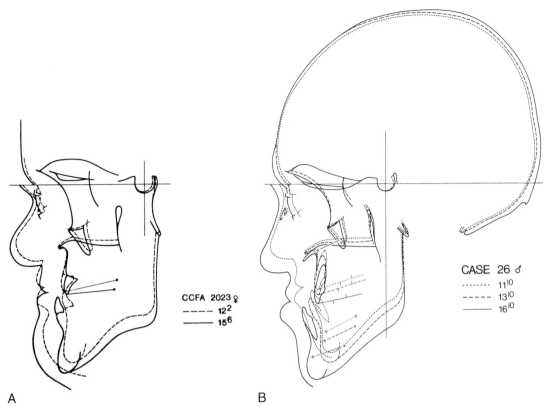

CCFA 2023 ♀
---- 12²
—— 15⁶

CASE 26 ♂
········ 11¹⁰
---- 13¹⁰
—— 16¹⁰

A   B

Figure 3–20. *A,* Apert syndrome. Cephalometric growth tracing of a girl observed from ages 12 years, 2 months to 15 years, 6 months. Note arrest of maxillary sutural growth and increasing sagittal disharmony between jaws. *B,* Crouzon syndrome. Cephalometric growth tracing of boy followed from 11 years, 10 months to 16 years, 10 months. Note arrest of maxillary sutural growth and increasing sagittal disharmony between jaws.

Primary Skull Defect

Because of cartilaginous abnormalities in the hands, feet,[2] cervical spine,[30] and trachea,[32] cartilage plays a primary role in the abnormal development of Apert syndrome very early during intrauterine life. This certainly includes craniofacial cartilage; the primary abnormality appears to involve the anterior cranial base, specifically the lesser wings of the sphenoid and the ethmoid with the cribriform plate and the crista galli.[27] The lesser wings of the sphenoid and crista galli are the three anterior points of dural attachment[33] and are much closer to each other in Apert syndrome than normally.[27] It seems likely that prenatal, altered, tensile forces in the dura result in dysmorphic brain growth and fusion of the coronal sutures.

The primary abnormality in Crouzon syndrome appears to be early fusion of the sutures and synchondroses. On the basis of the findings at birth and early infancy, it appears that sutural fusions generally occur relatively late in fetal life. The adult cranial form is explainable by the resultant dysmorphic and compensatory growth changes.[34, 35]

Implications for Treatment

In infants with Apert syndrome, the widely patent midline calvarial defect, together with open lambdoid and squamosal sutures, often permits adequate accommodation of the growing brain. Within the first year of life, it seems unlikely that increased intracranial pressure is a problem. However, the growth pattern may become very dysmorphic with hyperbrachycephaly and temporal bulging. We advocate early release (at 3–6 months) of the coronal sutures and advancement and reshaping of the frontal bone, not to prevent or treat increased intracranial pressure, but to reduce further dysmorphic and unwanted growth changes in the calvaria and cranial base.

In contrast, newborns with Crouzon syndrome have a high risk for developing increased intracranial pressure because of early multiple suture synostoses and fused synchondroses, forming a ''rigid box'' around the growing brain. Release of the fused sutures and frontal bone advancement are advocated as early as possible to prevent or treat increased intracranial pressure.

References

1. Cohen MM Jr: The Child with Multiple Birth Defects. New York: Raven Press, 1982.
2. Cohen MM Jr: Craniosynostosis: Diagnosis, Evaluation, and Management. New York: Raven Press, 1986.
3. Gorlin RJ, Cohen MM Jr, Levin LS: Syndromes of the Head and Neck. New York: Oxford University Press, 1990.
4. Toriello HV: New syndromes from old: The role of heterogeneity and variability in syndrome delineation. Am J Med Genet Suppl 1988; 1:50–70.
5. Cohen MM Jr: Syndromes with cleft lip and cleft palate. Cleft Palate J 1978; 15:306–328.
6. Cohen MM Jr, Bankier A: Syndrome delineation involving orofacial clefting. Cleft Palate J 1991; 28:119–120.
7. Gorlin RJ, Cervenka J, Pruzansky S: Facial clefting and its syndromes. Birth Defects 1971; 7(7):3–49.
8. Cohen MM Jr: Craniosynostosis update: 1986–1987. Am J Med Genet Suppl 1988; 4:99–148.
9. Pruzansky S: Time: The fourth dimension in syndrome analysis applied to craniofacial malformations. Birth Defects 1977; 13(3C): 3–38.
10. Jensen BL, Kreiborg S, Dahl E, Fogh-Andersen P: Cleft lip and palate in Denmark 1976–1981. Epidemiology, variability and early somatic development. Cleft Palate J 1988; 25:1–12.
11. Kreiborg S, Jensen BL, Dahl E, Fogh-Andersen P: Pierre Robin syndrome. Early facial development. Fifth International Congress on Cleft Palate and Related Craniofacial Anomalies, Abstract 303. Monte Carlo, Monaco, 1985.
12. Dahl E, Kreiborg S, Jensen BL, Fogh-Andersen P: Comparison of craniofacial morphology in infants with incomplete cleft lip and infants with isolated cleft palate. Cleft Palate J 1982; 19:258–266.
13. Pruzansky S: Not all dwarfed mandibles are alike. Birth Defects 1969; 5(2):120–129.
14. Dahl E, Kreiborg S, Björk A: A morphologic description of a dry skull with mandibulofacial dysostosis. Scand J Dent Res 1975; 83:257–266.
15. Jabs EW, Li X, Coss CA, et al: Mapping of the Treacher Collins syndrome locus to 5q31.3→5q33.3. Genomics 1991; 11:193–198.
16. Richieri-Costa A, Bortolozo MA, Lauris JRP, et al: Mandibulofacial dysostosis: Report on two Brazilian families suggesting autosomal recessive inheritance. Am J Med Genet 1993; 46:659–664.
17. Roberts F, Pruzansky S, Aduss H: An X-radiocephalometric study of mandibulofacial dysostosis in man. Arch Oral Biol 1975; 20:265–281.
18. Shprintzen RJ: Palatal and pharyngeal anomalies in craniofacial syndromes. Birth Defects 1982; 18(1):53–78.
19. Peterson-Falzone S, Figueroa AA: Longitudinal changes in cranial base angulation in mandibulofacial dysostosis. Cleft Palate J 1989; 26:31–35.
20. Arvystas M, Shprintzen RJ: Craniofacial morphology in Treacher Collins syndrome. Cleft Palate J 1991; 28:226–231.
21. Kreiborg S, Dahl E: The cranial base and the face in mandibulofacial dysostosis. Am J Med Genet 1993; 47:753–760.
22. Dahl E: Craniofacial morphology in congenital clefts of the lip and palate. Acta Odontol Scand 1970; 28(Suppl 57).
23. Shprintzen RJ: Pierre Robin, micrognathia, and airway obstruction: The dependency of treatment on accurate diagnosis. Int Anesthesiol Clin 1988; 26:84–91.
24. Shprintzen RJ: The implications of the diagnosis of Robin sequence. Cleft Palate J 1992; 29:205–209.
25. Kreiborg S: Postnatal growth and development of the craniofacial complex in patients with premature craniosynostosis. In Cohen MM Jr (ed): Craniosynostosis: Diagnosis, Evaluation and Management, pp 157–189. New York: Raven Press, 1986.
26. Kreiborg S, Cohen MM Jr: Characteristics of the infant Apert skull and its subsequent development. J Craniofac Genet Dev Biol 1990; 10:399–410.
27. Kreiborg S, Marsh JL, Cohen MM Jr, et al: Comparative three-dimensional analysis of CT-scans of the calvaria and cranial base in Apert and Crouzon syndromes. J Craniomaxillofac Surg 1993; 21:181–188.
28. Kreiborg S, Cohen MM Jr: A cephalometric study of the Apert syndrome in adults. J Craniofac Genet Dev Biol (submitted).
29. Kreiborg S, Cohen MM Jr: Oral manifestations of the Apert syndrome. J Craniofac Genet Dev Biol 1992; 12:41–48.
30. Kreiborg S, Barr M Jr, Cohen MM Jr: Cervical spine in the Apert syndrome. Am J Med Genet 1992; 43:704–708.
31. Kreiborg S, Cohen MM Jr: A clinical study of the craniofacial features in the Apert syndrome. Int J Oral Maxillofac Surg, in press.
32. Cohen MM Jr, Kreiborg S: Upper and lower airway compromise in the Apert syndrome. Am J Med Genet 1992; 44:90–93.
33. Moss M: The pathogenesis of premature cranial synostosis in man. Acta Anat 1959; 37:351–370.
34. Kreiborg S, Pruzansky S: Craniofacial growth in premature craniofacial synostosis. Scand J Plast Reconstr Surg 1981; 15:171–186.
35. Kreiborg S: Crouzon syndrome. A clinical and roentgencephalometric study. Scand J Plast Reconstr Surg [Suppl] 1981; 18:1–198.

36. Cohen MM Jr: An etiologic and nosologic overview of craniosynostosis syndromes. Birth Defects 1975; 11(2):137–189.

Genetic Considerations in Craniofacial Birth Defects

4

Arthur S. Aylsworth

INTRODUCTION

Most parents and many relatives of children with craniofacial malformations will be candidates for *genetic counseling* because they will have questions about issues such as primary cause, pathogenesis, and risk of recurrence. Therefore, each patient with a craniofacial malformation deserves to have an evaluation that is focused on *genetic considerations.* Such an evaluation should attempt to identify the genetic factors that were involved in the primary cause and/or pathogenesis of the patient's anomaly or syndrome. The purpose of this chapter is to outline how and why one should evaluate a patient with craniofacial anomalies with the goal of learning as much as possible about the cause and pathogenesis in order to gather information that will allow appropriate genetic counseling.

A committee of The American Society of Human Genetics has defined genetic counseling as follows:

A communication process which deals with the human problems associated with the occurrence, or the risk of occurrence, of a genetic disorder in a family. This process involves an attempt by one or more appropriately trained persons to help the individual or family to (1) comprehend the medical facts, including the diagnosis, probable course of the disorder, and the available management; (2) appreciate the way heredity contributes to the disorder, and the risk of recurrence in specified relatives; (3) understand the alternatives for dealing with the risk of recurrence; (4) choose the course of action which seems to them appropriate in view of their risk, their family goals, and their ethical and religious standards, and to act in accordance with that decision; and (5) to make the best possible adjustment to the disorder in an affected family member and/or to the risk of recurrence of that disorder.[1]

Even if families do not express an interest in genetic counseling, one should be alert to two situations that generally require more in-depth genetics evaluations. The first is when a craniofacial anomaly is *syndromic,* that is, it is associated with other birth defects. The other is when a craniofacial malformation is *familial,* that is, there is a family history of other similarly affected individuals. Families with either syndromic or familial craniofacial malformations usually will benefit from the information derived from such an evaluation, even though they may not actually understand the importance or significance of this approach beforehand.

The goal of the evaluation is to establish as correct a *genetic* diagnosis as possible and to understand what factors have led to the birth defect(s) observed. For a more extensive examination of diagnostic concepts, the reader is referred to several excellent references that deal with these topics. The books by Aase[2] and Cohen[3] and Cohen's more recent series of articles[4-14] provide an in-depth background about syndrome nosology and details of dysmorphic features, malformations, and syndromes. The updates by Jones[15] and Graham,[16] and the recent *Human Malformations and Related Anomalies,*[17] are excellent general references in which one can learn about causes and pathogenetic mechanisms of many craniofacial anomalies and syndromes encountered in clinical practice. The book by Gorlin et al[18] is a standard reference work on the genetics of craniofacial anomalies and syndromes. The article by Jones is specifically focused on facial clefting,[19] and the book edited by Cohen gives a comprehensive analysis of not only the causes of craniosynostosis, but also complications and management.[20]

METHODS

Accurate diagnosis depends on correct interpretation of data obtained through the patient history, family history, physical examination, and other studies. Medical records on the patient and other affected relatives usually need to be gathered in order to complete a thorough genetic evaluation.

In the *patient history,* it is important to document as precisely as possible the patient's anomalies and problems from conception onward. This should include a thorough gestational history to identify potential environmental teratogens. Childhood photographs are important to document the phenotype in an older patient. Growth records, radiographs, and other relevant laboratory reports may be helpful in establishing a good description of the original birth defects. The nature and extent of all anomalies should be documented and recorded.

The *family history* is used to identify relatives with similar malformations. Ask about relatives with the same or similar malformations, other congenital anomalies, mental retardation, miscarriages, or stillbirths and establish whether there may be parental consanguinity. A thorough evaluation will usually include examination of other, possibly affected, relatives, either in person or by photograph. A pedigree should be drawn to ensure completeness and to keep track of family history information. The process of taking a detailed family history and drawing the pedigree will frequently identify significant information that would not be obtained otherwise.

During the *physical examination,* structural variants and abnormal anatomic features are recorded. Photographs are useful for documenting significant findings. Measurements are made and interpreted by comparing to published standards.[15, 18, ,21–23]

Other studies depend on the patient's phenotype. Chromosome analysis should be done if the patient has multiple anomalies involving the craniofacies and any other organ system or region of the body when the pattern of anomalies does not fit a diagnosis that is etiologically well defined. Even if a patient has some features of a clear-cut diagnosis, it is also important to obtain a karyotype on anyone with atypical features or features of two or more distinct syndromes because of the chance that one might identify a chromosomal rearrangement that could be of diagnostic importance to other relatives and provide important information that can be used for mapping the gene(s) that are responsible for the phenotype. Karyotyping is also recommended for fetuses, stillbirths, and neonatal deaths in which there is only one obvious anomaly because of the possibility that there may be others found later at autopsy and because this will be the last chance to obtain an adequate sample of living tissue for chromosome analysis. Malformed fetuses, stillborn infants, and babies who die in the neonatal period should have thorough postmortem examinations to document all anomalies. Skeletal radiographs are obtained on any patient with dwarfism or skeletal anomalies. Special standardized radiographs may be useful for delineating anomalies of the craniofacies. DNA can be obtained and stored for future genetic studies from cultured fibroblasts and/or a blood sample for DNA extraction, or from a blood sample sent for lymphoblast transformation.

CLASSIFICATION

It should first be noted that all classification systems are arbitrary when viewed from another perspective. Anatomic systems of classification are commonly used by the surgical specialties. But a classification system based on embryologic development is much more appropriate in genetic diagnosis because of the importance of considering causative factors and pathogenetic mechanisms. Both types of classification systems, therefore, have an important role in the evaluation and management of patients with craniofacial anomalies.

While nomenclature in the field of dysmorphology continues to evolve, recommendations made in 1982[24] are still widely accepted and will be used here. In the *genetic approach,* one attempts to classify craniofacial anomalies into categories that have etiologic and pathogenetic implications by deciding whether each is a *deformation,* a *disruption,* a *malformation,* or associated with an underlying *dysplasia.*

Deformations

A *deformation* is "an abnormal form, shape, or position of a part of the body caused by mechanical forces."[24] Relatively common deformations seen in the newborn include craniofacial asymmetry, bowed legs, tibial torsion, clubfoot, dislocated hip, and arthrogryposis.[16] Some types of craniosynostosis have been attributed to intrauterine compression and, therefore, can be considered primary deformations.[25–27] Fetal crowding, especially in the third trimester, appears to cause many of the common deformations seen in newborns. Situations that are thought to contribute to fetal crowding include oligohydramnios, multiple fetuses, uterine malformation, and uterine fibroids. Many deformations associated with late intrauterine fetal crowding, such as plagiocephaly, will tend to show postnatal catch-up growth. When plagiocephaly worsens postnatally, one should evaluate the patient for an underlying craniosynostosis, usually involving the coronal or lambdoidal suture, in the region of restricted growth. Intrinsic fetal abnormalities that cause deficient fetal movement in utero, such as malformations or dysplasias of the central nervous system, peripheral nerves, or muscles, may cause a deformation phenotype of multiple congenital joint contracture deformities called *arthrogryposis.* Amniotic bands may also cause deformations of the skull, trunk, and extremities, as well as the disruptions discussed later. Counseling about deformations will depend on the likelihood of the same causative factors being present again in a future pregnancy.

Disruptions

A *disruption* is "a morphologic defect of an organ, part of an organ, or a larger region of the body resulting from the extrinsic breakdown of, or an interference with, an originally normal developmental process."[24] An example of such a mechanical disruption is the situation in which a fetus becomes entangled in strands of torn amnion. Such *amniotic bands* can cause tearing of tissues with ring constrictions around extremities, vascular compromise, and amputation.[15, 28–30] When a fetus swallows an amniotic band, a facial tear or *cleft* can result (Fig. 4–1). Atypical facial clefts (i.e., clefts that do not follow a pattern related to underlying embryonic development) may be disruptions due to amniotic bands, and one should look elsewhere for evidence of band formation (Fig. 4–2). This situation illustrates why it is important to use an etiologic approach to the patient evaluation in addition to the anatomic approach usually used when planning surgery and management. For genetic counseling purposes, it obviously would be inaccurate and inappropriate to lump an atypical facial cleft caused by amniotic bands (which are usually sporadic or nonfamilial, with low recurrence risk) along with the more common types of clefts that are primary malformations. As mentioned, amniotic bands may also cause deformation as well as disruption. Counseling about disruptions will depend on the likelihood of the same causative

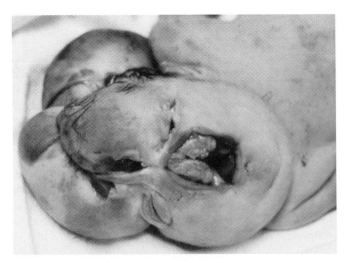

Figure 4–1. Severe craniofacial disruption caused by a swallowed amniotic band that wrapped around the calvaria.

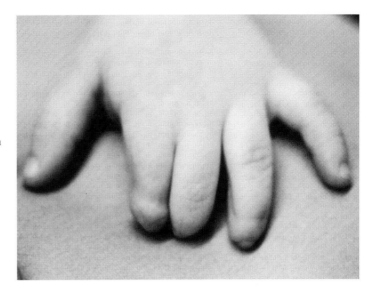

Figure 4–2. Mild degree of distal phalangeal amputation and subtle ring constriction caused by amniotic bands.

factors (such as a known teratogen or mechanical factor) being present again in a future pregnancy. The recurrence risk for amniotic band disruptions is usually low, probably less than 1% for most families.

Dysplasias

A *dysplasia* is "an abnormal organization of cells into tissue(s) and its morphologic result(s)." [24] The term is broadly applied to all "abnormalities of histogenesis" and tends to be tissue specific rather than organ specific. For example, patients with certain skeletal dysplasias may have an associated cleft palate. These include hypochondrogenesis, spondyloepiphyseal dysplasia congenita, Kniest syndrome, and Stickler syndrome. In each of these, cleft palate appears to be due to the underlying abnormalities of type II collagen that cause these bone dysplasias. [31–37] Counseling such patients and families about the cleft palate, therefore, must be based on knowledge about the underlying dysplasia rather than on empiric data collected on patients with other types of cleft palate. By the same token, investigators who study clefting should begin by separating study populations into causally related groups to improve the precision of their conclusions and the appropriateness of their recommendations. One must avoid giving patients with dysplasias erroneous diagnoses such as "Pierre Robin syndrome" (to be described) and inaccurate counseling that would be more appropriate for patients with nonsyndromic clefts.

Malformations

A *malformation* is "a morphologic defect of an organ, part of an organ, or larger region of the body resulting from an intrinsically abnormal developmental process." [24] This term is usually used to describe structural birth defects that result from intrinsic abnormalities in developing organs or morphogenetic processes; that is, they are thought of as inborn errors of morphogenesis. Most of the remainder of this discussion will focus on true malformations.

Major and Minor Anomalies

A *minor anomaly* is an unusual morphologic feature that is of no serious medical or cosmetic consequence to the patient. [15] A *major anomaly,* therefore, is one that is of medical or cosmetic significance. Minor anomalies include common structural variations such as frontal or parietal bossing, an unusually broad or narrow face, preauricular pits or tags, unusual external ear morphology, ocular hypertelorism or hypotelorism, upslanting or downslanting palpebral fissures, short columella, hypoplastic alae nasi, flat or broad nasal bridge, micrognathia or prognathism, macrostomia or microstomia, smooth philtrum (absence of the lateral philtral ridges), branchial arch remnants, branchial cleft cysts or pits, unusual scalp hair patterning, transverse palmar creases, and unusual dermal ridge patterns on the palm and fingertips.[2, 13, 15, 38] Many dysmorphic syndromes (for example, Down syndrome) are recognizable primarily because they have characteristic patterns of minor anomalies rather than by their major anomalies.

Minor anomalies are important to assess because they may provide clues about the cause or pathogenesis of major anomalies. While single malformations (i.e., those that are nonsyndromic or not associated with other anomalies) may be caused by a coincidental (i.e., accidental) combination of unknown genetic and/or environmental factors that would be unlikely to occur again, the finding of several other anomalies, even minor ones, suggests that there was a more widespread insult to or interference with early morphogenesis. Therefore, one's attempted explanation of underlying cause must take into account all minor as well as major anomalies.

Craniofacial Anomalies May Be Nonsyndromic or Syndromic

It is important to distinguish between syndromic and nonsyndromic patterns because each requires a different approach to evaluation and counseling. A malformation is *nonsyndromic* if it is the only anomaly present or if there are multiple anomalies that are all due to one pathogenetic sequence of events.

The term *sequence* has been used to describe "a pattern of multiple anomalies derived from a single known or presumed prior anomaly or mechanical factor."[24] Therefore, if several anomalies can be related back to one primary defect, factor, or event, this constitutes a pathogenetic *sequence.* For example, the patient with hydrocephalus, club feet, and a meningomyelocele does not have a "multiple congenital anomalies syndrome." Rather, this is a sequence related to a single, primary error of morphogenesis, the only primary malformation being the neural tube defect, with the hydrocephalus and club feet being secondary deformations. Similarly, oligohydramnios may cause multiple anomalies in a fetus, including pulmonary hypoplasia, craniofacial deformations, and contractures of the extremities. Note that the concept of a sequence implies a specific *pathogenetic* pathway that may have more than one underlying *cause* and produce more than one *anomaly* or phenotypic effect. Cleft lip with cleft palate can be thought of as a pathogenetic sequence, in which the palate defect is not a primary malformation but secondary to a cleft of the primary palate.

It should be noted that the so-called Pierre Robin syndrome is not a true multiple malformation syndrome at all. Rather, it is a collection of related anomalies in the same developmental region of the body that should be thought of as a single malformation or sequence. The term *Robin sequence* has been used to suggest that the combination of micrognathia, cleft palate, and glossoptosis is caused by a mechanism whereby the tongue remains up between the palatal shelves for an unusually long time so that when the shelves finally do come together, they are no longer capable of fusion. There are a number of possible underlying *causes,* including oligohydramnios causing external pressure on the mandible, neurogenic failure of the neck to extend, or primary growth deficiency in the mandible, all of which could act through this one *pathogenetic mechanism.* Also note that the Robin sequence, like other sequences, may be an isolated finding or part of a broader syndrome of malformation or dysplasia. The most common is Stickler syndrome, discussed elsewhere in this chapter. Cohen lists 33 of the more common and better delineated syndromes associated with the Robin sequence, but there are many more syndromes that have this anomaly as part of the phenotype.[18]

If more than one organ system, developmental field, or region of the body has been involved in dysmorphogenesis, the collection of anomalies is *syndromic.* Used in this way, the term does not necessarily imply that the phenotype constitutes a well-recognized syndrome. The word *syndrome* means "a running together," and it is used to refer to "a pattern of multiple anomalies thought to be pathogenetically related."[24] In clinical practice, this can be thought of as meaning anomalies in more than one organ system or region of the body. Surveys of craniofacial clinic populations suggest that as many as 40% to 65% of patients with clefts may have associated anomalies.[39-41] The

London Dysmorphology Database lists 110 noncytogenetic syndromes with non-midline cleft upper lip, 23 with midline cleft upper lip, 204 with cleft palate (including submucous cleft palate and absent, hypoplastic, or bifid uvula) without cleft lip, and 102 with craniosynostosis. For most malformation syndromes, *pathogenesis* is unknown, while *cause* may be known or unknown.

Causes of Malformations and Syndromes

Factors that affect morphogenesis can be thought of as falling into three major categories. First, *chromosome abnormalities* are structural rearrangements that usually involve many genes. These include deletions, duplications, inversions, translocations, etc. Second, *single gene mutations* are changes (base pair substitution, deletion, duplication) that occur within a single gene. These include all of the so-called Mendelian patterns of inheritance: autosomal dominant, autosomal recessive, and X-linked. Third, there are those conditions caused by a complex interaction of largely unknown genetic and/or environmental factors, referred to as *multifactorial.*

Associations and Syndromes of Unknown Cause

A recognizable pattern of birth defects may be called a syndrome even though there is no identifiable cause such as a visible chromosome abnormality, Mendelian inheritance pattern, or environmental teratogen. These have been called *unknown genesis syndromes* by Cohen.[3,7] Most of these phenotypes occur sporadically in families; that is, they tend to occur in only one individual and not to affect other relatives. Because only sporadic occurrences are observed, such phenotypes cannot be interpreted in Mendelian terms as possibly due to mutations in single genes. Some also have severe malformations and/or mental retardation, which causes affected individuals not to reproduce. In other words, they are *genetically lethal* conditions.

When diagnosing a patient with a syndrome of unknown genesis, one should keep in mind the possibility of causal heterogeneity; that is, some cases of the phenotype in question may be caused by one or more genetic mutations, while other cases might be due to one or more environmental teratogens. With the development of new laboratory techniques in genetics, and the observation of teratogenic effects of environmental agents on animal models, there has been a gradual accumulation of evidence that many of these phenotypes previously classified as ''unknown genesis syndromes'' are actually caused by identifiable genetic or environmental factors. Sporadic occurrence of a genetically lethal phenotype always raises the possibility of a new, dominantly expressed mutation in a single gene or a small chromosome deletion that is undetectable by routine standard cytogenetic banding techniques. For example, all of the syndromes mentioned later in the discussion of contiguous gene syndromes began as ''unknown genesis syndromes.''

The term *association* refers to a recurring complex of multiple malformations that has been observed in a number of patients for which the anomalies are not known to be related by common etiologic or pathogenetic mechanisms and the pattern occurs significantly more often than expected by chance. An association is a causally nonspecific category used to keep track of a heterogeneous group of undelineated syndromes and sequences. For example, the CHARGE association discussed later clearly is causally heterogeneous because some patients have chromosome 22q deletions, but most do not. Because the term *association* implies no knowledge of cause or pathogenesis, associations should not be used as final diagnoses. Rather, a patient with an association, that is, a recognized association of malformations, should be thought of as having undiagnosed syndromic anomalies that require a full evaluation, including thorough gestational and family history, examination, and karyotype to try to identify the underlying cause.

SYNDROMES

The known causes of *syndromes* are chromosomal abnormalities, including both cytogenetically detectable and submicroscopic abnormalities, single gene mutations, and environmental teratogens. Such genetic abnormalities cause syndromic birth defects, presumably because they interfere with multiple pathways during development. In a review of over 150 syndromes associated with facial clefting, Cohen found that approximately 20% were chromosomal, 50% Mendelian, a few teratogen-induced, and the rest (approximately 25%) of unknown cause.[42, 43] Recurrent, recognizable patterns of anomalies that are observed in unrelated patients, and for which there is no evident cause, have been called *unknown genesis syndromes,*[3] some of which are turning out to be submicroscopic rearrangements or *contiguous gene deletion syndromes* (to be discussed).

Single, *nonsyndromic* anomalies can be thought of as being caused by single genes or combinations of unknown environmental factors, unknown predisposing genes, and chance (i.e., multifactorial). Note that mutations in single genes may cause either syndromic or nonsyndromic malformations.

Chromosomal Abnormalities

Rearrangements of the genome large enough to see with the light microscope can be identified by cytogenetic techniques that are routinely available in numerous laboratories. In order for a rearrangement such as a deletion or translocation to be visible on routine karyotyping, at least several dozen genes are usually involved. Human autosomal abnormalities are characterized by prenatal and/or postnatal retardation of linear growth and/or brain growth, mental retardation, and multiple malformations resulting from a widespread disturbance of multiple morphogenetic pathways. Both major malformations and minor anomalies may be present. Sex chromosome abnormalities may be much more subtle in their manifestations than are autosomal abnormalities.

Because chromosome abnormalities typically cause multiple anomalies, patients with craniofacial malformations associated with birth defects involving any other region of the body should have a chromosome analysis unless the pattern of anomalies is typical of a well-defined syndrome that is known to be caused by something other than a chromosome abnormality. For example, one usually will not need to karyotype a patient with typical features of Treacher Collins syndrome, especially if the family history is positive and supports the diagnosis. In some situations where there is an apparent noncytogenetic diagnosis, however, karyotyping may be appropriate. This would be the case if a patient has features that are atypical for the apparent syndromic diagnosis, if the phenotype suggests the presence of a known cytogenetic syndrome as well as a noncytogenetic syndrome, or if the phenotype suggests the presence of more than one noncytogenetic syndrome. Features such as short stature, microcephaly, and/or mental retardation are indications for karyotyping if they are atypical for the syndrome. For example, a patient with features of Treacher Collins syndrome plus mental retardation, polydactyly, and congenital heart disease would obviously require a chromosome analysis for completeness. A diagnosis of a rare syndrome that is not well delineated, especially if short stature and/or mental retardation are present, can usually be made only after a chromosome abnormality has been ruled out.

A number of syndromes are now known to be caused by chromosomal deletions that involve several genes but are so small that only occasionally can they be seen with routine cytogenetic studies. Usually the deletions are submicroscopic, that is, not detectable by routine chromosome analysis. In such cases, molecular techniques such as fluorescence in situ hybridization (FISH) are required for detection of the genetic abnormality and establishment of a diagnosis. Syndromes caused by small, submicroscopic deletions are called *contiguous gene deletion syndromes* or *microdeletion syndromes.*[44] Like other chromosomal syndromes, they are characterized by multiple malformations, dysmorphic features, and mental retardation. Although frequently occurring sporadically, they may also be familial with variable expression in affected relatives.[45]

The syndrome of this type most relevant to craniofacial dysmorphology is the velo-cardio-facial syndrome (VCFS), characterized by cleft palate (including submucous cleft or velopharyngeal incompetence), conotruncal cardiac malformations, developmental delay with IQ usually in the low-normal to mildly retarded range, and dysmorphic facies characterized by a prominent, tubular-shaped nose, sometimes with narrow or notched alae nasi, short palpebral fissures, and slender, hyperextensible fingers.[46, 47] Many patients have been identified through craniofacial or cleft palate clinics. There is phenotypic overlap with the DiGeorge syndrome (DGS),[48–50] and patients with a nonrandom association of anomalies referred to as the CHARGE association (coloboma of the iris, heart malformation, choanal atresia, retarded growth and/or development, genital anomalies, and dysmorphic ears).[51,52] It is now clear that most patients with VCFS and DGS have either cytogenetically detectable or submicroscopic deletions in the proximal long arm of chromosome 22 at band 22q11, and a few patients with CHARGE anomalies also have deletions in that region.[50,53,54] The acronym CATCH 22 has been suggested to help one remember the major features that characterize this group of patients, namely cardiac defects, abnormal facies, thymic hypoplasia, cleft palate, hypocalcemia, and chromosome 22 deletion.[50,55]

Other examples of contiguous gene syndromes include previous ''unknown genesis'' syndromes such as the Prader-Willi and Angelman syndromes (deletion of 15q11-q13), Langer-Giedion syndrome (deletion of 8q24), Miller-Dieker syndrome (deletion of 17p13.3), and Williams syndrome (deletion of 7q11.23). It seems likely that in the future many other ''syndromes of unknown cause'' with apparently normal routine karyotypes will turn out to be caused by undetected, submicroscopic chromosomal deletions or duplications.

Single Gene Mutations

Craniofacial malformations and syndromes may be caused by mutations in single genes. To evaluate this possibility, one must carefully analyze the family history and examine close relatives. For example, it is important to examine first degree relatives of patients with facial clefts for evidence of hypernasal speech, submucous cleft palate, and lower lip pits, in addition to taking a careful family history looking for relatives with clefts or other anomalies. Similarly, in evaluating a patient with craniosynostosis, one should take a detailed family history and examine all available relatives for craniofacial asymmetry, microcephaly, digital anomalies, and other birth defects known to be associated with craniosynostosis.

Autosomal dominant inheritance is suggested by vertical transmission from generation to generation. Male-to-male transmission essentially rules out X-linked inheritance, leaving autosomal dominant inheritance strongly supported. Autosomal dominant syndromes may be characterized by interfamilial and/or intrafamilial variability of expression.

The Treacher Collins syndrome may manifest a wide variability of expression, even within families.[56] Mildly affected relatives may not be diagnosed until after the birth of a child with more severe and typical manifestations. The man whose mandible is shown in Figure 4–3 had no external features that strongly suggested the Treacher Collins syndrome, but he had a fully affected son. Because he did not have another affected ancestor, it was not possible to conclude definitely that he carried the same mutation that caused his son's anomalies, but his radiograph does raise that as a significant possibility. Variable expression of a single gene is one explanation for intrafamilial variability like that hypothesized for this family. Another is mosaicism; that is, a mildly affected parent might carry a Treacher Collins gene in only a fraction of his or her cells, thereby resulting in milder expression.

The phenotype of mandibulofacial dysostosis is causally heterogeneous. Some patients have other associated anomalies and other syndromic diagnoses, such as Nager syndrome with radial ray deficiencies.[57] When mandibulofacial dysostosis is not associated with other anomalies, it is usually diagnosed as Treacher Collins syndrome, but even in this group there is probably genetic heterogeneity. For example, while there is now good evidence that many families have Treacher Collins syndrome caused by mutations on the long arm of chromosome 5 in the region of q32-q33.2,[58] affected individuals have also been reported with chromosome deletions in other regions of the genome, including 4p15.32-p14[59] and 3p23-p24.12.[60]

Stickler syndrome, mentioned earlier in the discussion of dysplasias, is an example of an autosomal dominant cleft palate syndrome that may not be diagnosed because of mild expression and variable features. Associated problems include myopia with retinal detachment and osteoarthritis associated with a mild spondyloepiphyseal dysplasia and mild short stature. There are probably a number of patients with undiagnosed Stickler syndrome who are being treated in cleft palate clinics. Some may be diagnosed after individuals in two generations are affected. It is important to make the diagnosis early

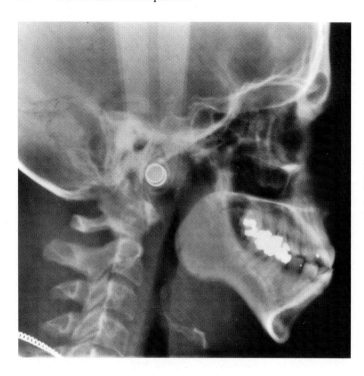

Figure 4–3. Lateral radiograph of mandible showing antegonial notching and down-curved configuration typical of Treacher Collins syndrome. Subject was the father of a fully affected boy but did not show any other obvious external features of the syndrome.

so that children can be followed closely by a pediatric ophthalmologist to prevent blindness caused by vitreoretinal degeneration and untreated retinal detachment, and so that appropriate genetic counseling can be provided to the family.

The clefting syndromes associated with lower lip pits constitute exceptions to the rule that cleft lip, with or without cleft palate [CL(P)], is causally and pathogenetically distinct from posterior cleft palate without cleft lip (CP). Familial clefting [either CL(P) or CP] associated with paramedian pits or mucous cysts of the lower lips (Fig. 4–4), usually occurs in an autosomal dominant pattern called van der Woude syndrome.[61] In van der Woude syndrome, CL(P) occurs approximately twice as frequently as CP, similar to the ratio in the general population. Other families have variant syndromes with lip pits, both CL(P) and CP, and associated malformations, including popliteal pterygia, jaw adhesions, eyelid adhesions, and genital anomalies. These syndromes are clearly different but may be either causally or pathogenetically related to more typical van der Woude syndrome. The gene that causes the van der Woude syndrome has been mapped to chromosome 1q32.[62,63] It should be noted that phenotypic expression in these families may be very subtle or even absent in some relatives who are obligate gene carriers.[61,64,65] An affected parent has approximately a 22% chance of having a child with some type of cleft, suggesting that penetrance for clefting is approximately 50%.[64] Therefore, genetic counseling for van der Woude

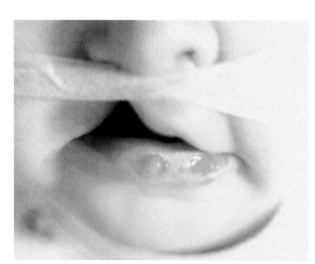

Figure 4–4. Mucous cysts/pits of the lower lip, typical of van der Woude syndrome.

syndrome is dramatically different from that for most other types of nonsyndromic clefting. This illustrates the importance of taking a careful family history and examining relatives to look for evidence of dominant inheritance and/or lower lip pits before counseling any patient with a cleft, either CL(P) or CP. So far studies in families with multiple cases of CL(P) or CP without lip pits have shown no evidence for linkage to the van der Woude gene locus on chromosome 1q.[66, 67]

Well over 100 craniosynostosis syndromes are known. Many are of unknown cause or due to rare chromosomal abnormalities or recessively expressed genes, but some of the better known and more commonly seen conditions are autosomal dominant. Crouzon syndrome, Apert syndrome, and Pfeiffer syndrome are relatively well known and have fairly distinctive and recognizable phenotypes. Saethre-Chotzen syndrome, on the other hand, demonstrates a broad and extremely varied pattern of expression, even within families.[68, 69] It is characterized by variable craniosynostosis that usually involves the coronal sutures and is asymmetric, causing facial asymmetry. Other features include eye abnormalities with hypertelorism and ptosis or blepharophimosis, low anterior hairline, beaked and/or deviated nose, prognathism, variable hand and foot anomalies, including brachydactyly and partial cutaneous syndactyly, and usually normal but occasionally delayed development. A variety of other anomalies are occasionally reported in the skeletal, cardiac, and genitourinary systems. When a syndrome appears to have findings as variable as seems to be the case for the Saethre-Chotzen syndrome, one should keep in mind the question of whether the broad phenotypic spectrum represents one condition with variable expression or a causally heterogeneous group of disorders with similar phenotypes. Final answers to this question will come as the responsible genes are identified in affected families. Evidence is accumulating that one or more genetic loci on the short arm of chromosome 7 cause the Saethre-Chotzen syndrome and other conditions associated with craniosynostosis.[70–75]

Isolated craniosynostosis frequently occurs sporadically. When it is familial, it usually follows a pattern compatible with and suggestive of autosomal dominant inheritance. While there is a great deal of current interest in craniosynostosis genes on 7p, over two dozen other regions of the human genome have been implicated as potential sites by observations of patients with craniosynostosis and chromosomal abnormalities.[18, 76, 77] Although most patients with chromosome abnormalities have multiple anomalies rather than isolated craniosynostosis, such observations are useful to help focus the search for single genes involved in the biology of cranial suture growth and fusion.

Autosomal recessive inheritance is suggested by the presence of parental consanguinity or affected siblings whose parents are unaffected. Keep in mind that the observation of multiple affected children of unaffected parents may also be compatible with other causes such as an environmental teratogen, autosomal dominant inheritance with incomplete penetrance, or parental gonadal mosaicism for a dominantly expressed mutation. In the evaluation of an individual patient with an unclassified malformation syndrome, parental consanguinity, no matter how distant, suggests an autosomal recessive etiology. The London Dysmorphology Database lists 104 autosomal recessive syndromes with either cleft lip/palate (44) or just posterior cleft palate (60) and 28 syndromes with craniosynostosis.

X-linked inheritance is characterized by multiple affected male relatives who are related through unaffected or less severely affected females. When carrier females are unaffected, the pattern is called *X-linked recessive.* But in some conditions, females may be as severely affected as males, a situation called *X-linked dominant inheritance.* As mentioned earlier, the presence of male-to-male transmission in a pedigree is strong evidence against X-linked inheritance because sons inherit a Y chromosome from their fathers. The London Dysmorphology Database lists 16 X-linked syndromes with either cleft lip/palate or just posterior cleft palate. At least one X-linked cleft palate gene has been mapped to the region Xq13-q21.31 in two large kindreds, one from Iceland and one from British Columbia.[78–80] In both families, ankyloglossia appears to be an associated feature in some individuals.

Teratogenic Syndromes

Environmental teratogens, including chemicals, drugs, physical agents, and maternal disease, may disrupt embryonic and fetal morphogenesis. While any environmental agent can be considered potentially teratogenic, the list of well-documented human teratogens is still relatively short.[15,18] Most human teratogens have been identified because they cause a recognizable pattern of anomalies. Different organ systems and tissues will have different susceptibilities in both time and exposure dose. Clinically important examples of human teratogens include alcohol and isotretinoin, both of which cause important craniofacial anomalies.[81–84] Isotretinoin causes an environmental phenocopy in the CATCH 22 phenotypic spectrum.[81] Teratogen-caused birth defects may be ''familial'' when relatives have similar exposures to environmental teratogenic agents for cultural or geographical reasons. For example, alcoholism may be familial, and children in more than one sibship in a family may show the effects of prenatal alcohol exposure.

Genetic Counseling for Syndromes

The possible causes of syndromic craniofacial malformations include chromosomal abnormalities, single gene mutations, and environmental teratogens. Counseling for syndromes of *known* cause, once a diagnosis has been made, is relatively straightforward compared to counseling for syndromes of unknown cause. For example, freestanding chromosomal trisomies have a relatively low empiric recurrence risk. Counseling for translocations and other rearrangements, however, must be based on the theoretical risk of transmission modified by observational data regarding the incidence of live-born babies with each particular abnormality.

Counseling about syndromes that demonstrate typical Mendelian inheritance patterns is based on the theoretical probability of transmission modified by knowledge about penetrance and expressivity of the condition. For dominantly expressed conditions, each gene carrier has a 50% chance of passing the mutation on to each child. But if expression is variable or penetrance is incomplete, the chance an affected child will have severe manifestations is less than 50%. The lower the penetrance, the less likely it is that a gene carrier will express the gene. Conversely, one can take into account the fact that the higher the penetrance, the less likely it is that an unaffected relative carries the gene with a risk of passing it on to children.[85]

Counseling families with Mendelian syndromes is difficult in the absence of good data about expressivity and penetrance, and accurate data are not available for many syndromes because more severely affected individuals tend to seek medical attention and are studied and reported first before less severely affected individuals are identified. It should be noted that information available in the literature about a syndrome may be inaccurate if relatives have not been personally examined.

Counseling about teratogenic syndromes is stressful because of parental guilt. Recurrence risks are based on the likelihood of teratogen exposure during subsequent pregnancies. It is assumed that genetic factors regulate maternal and fetal susceptibility to teratogenic insult, but these are largely unknown at present.

Counseling about syndromes of unknown cause and nonrandom associations is difficult because of the likelihood that there is etiologic or pathogenetic heterogeneity in any phenotypic category. Initially, sporadic occurrences tend to be reported. Then, familial cases are observed, and it becomes possible to separate out specific syndromes of known cause. A chromosome analysis is usually indicated for such patients, especially if they have short stature, microcephaly, or mental retardation, and the possibility of a submicroscopic deletion should be kept in mind.

NONSYNDROMIC ANOMALIES

Many patients with a single craniofacial malformation do not have other birth defects. These are *nonsyndromic* anomalies. Potential causes of single, nonsyndromic malformations include single gene mutations and presumed complex interactions of genetic factors, environmental factors, and chance.

The basic, underlying causes and pathogenetic mechanisms are not known for most nonsyndromic birth defects. Although some may occasionally be familial, pedigrees usually do not suggest an obvious pattern of Mendelian inheritance. If evidence for a single gene cause is not found in the family history, counseling is usually based on observed recurrence rates, which are commonly referred to as *empiric recurrence risks.*

As already suggested, it is sometimes necessary to examine relatives to avoid missing a positive family history. For example, it would be important for genetic counseling purposes to identify a submucous cleft in a relative of a child with a posterior cleft palate because a higher sib recurrence risk would be quoted than if no other relatives were affected. But a subtle submucous cleft in one parent or other relative might not be discovered if the affected individual is not examined.

Genetic Counseling for Nonsyndromic Anomalies

Malformations such as facial clefts and craniosynostosis that involve only one developmental region of the body or organ system may be caused by single genes or environmental factors, or a combination of both. Such nonsyndromic anomalies are usually not caused by chromosome abnormalities, which usually result in a more widespread interference with normal morphogenesis. Exceptions to this general rule would include isolated microcephaly and holoprosencephaly, both of which may appear to be the only major structural anomalies in children with small chromosomal deletions or duplications.

Genetic counseling for a nonsyndromic malformation usually relies on *observed recurrence rate* data to derive what is usually referred to as an *empiric recurrence risk*. It must be kept in mind that these so-called empiric risks are only crude guesses about risk based on average recurrence *rates* in populations that are probably very heterogeneous.

Counseling for isolated or nonsyndromic malformations should take into account whether the anomaly is familial or nonfamilial. Nonsyndromic birth defects are sometimes familial, but family pedigrees do not usually suggest a particular type of Mendelian inheritance pattern. Reports of the frequency of familial clefting from Denmark and South America range from 17% to 25% for CL(P) and from 3% to 12% for CP.[86, 87]

Frequently, however, the family history may indicate that a nonsyndromic malformation such as facial clefting appears to be familial, in which several distant relatives or only two close relatives are affected but in which the pattern does not follow or strongly suggest an obvious Mendelian inheritance pattern. Mathematical models have been constructed to explain these observed "non-Mendelian" patterns of familial recurrence. Models developed from the work of Falconer,[88] Edwards,[89] and Smith[90] assume that there is a continuous distribution of genetic "liability" or predisposition to malformation in the general population with a threshold point beyond which individuals are affected. A number of observations in human populations and experimental animals have been presented as being consistent with and, therefore, supporting such a model.[87, 91–98]

An alternative proposed to the polygenic/multifactorial model is that the underlying genetic "liability" or predisposition is determined by a single major gene with incomplete penetrance; that is, the gene is not always fully expressed in those who carry it. Studies based on complex segregation analysis have supported this model with evidence for both autosomal recessive and dominant or codominant major loci.[99–105] The relative merits of the polygenic/multifactorial and major single gene models have been and continue to be vigorously debated without clear resolution.[93–97, 99–102, 106–123]

Although much attention is now being paid to gene-environment interaction, another factor that is usually ignored when thinking about causation of abnormalities is chance. Kurnit and colleagues[124] have used computer modeling to show that the non-Mendelian familial clustering of anomalies usually attributed to concepts such as *reduced penetrance* and *multifactorial inheritance* may be accounted for by chance. In their computer model, multiple simulations of endocardial cushion closure using identical parameters resulted in widely varying outcomes, including complete (i.e., normal) closure, small ventricular or atrial septal defects, and wide open endocardial cushion defects. Numerous twin studies over the years have shown that concordance rates for "genetically caused" anomalies in monozygotic twins are frequently less than 100%. These observations support a model in which there is an underlying *predisposition* to malformation, and normal or abnormal morphogenesis is then a matter of chance. An important conclusion from these studies for health professionals who see patients with birth defects is that we should be thinking about the likelihood that there are many genes that do not always result in an abnormal phenotype but rather only *predispose* the embryo to abnormal morphogenesis. The complex processes of embryologic development are probably error prone, with some built-in margin of safety, and many genes probably exist that have small effects (which are, by themselves, "within normal limits") that subsequently, by chance, are amplified within a single morphogenetic pathway by the randomness that is inherent in all such complex systems, causing the embryo to swerve from its path of normal development.

If the factors that influence penetrance and expressivity include other genes as well as environmental factors and chance, it seems likely that that "liability" or predisposition to malformation will turn out to have many different potential genetic and environmental components, with possibly only one or a few being significant in any single patient or family. For this reason, the term *multifactorial* may eventually turn out to be satisfactory if one does not restrict it to imply an underlying "polygenic" predisposition but rather uses it to refer to the multiplicity of underlying causative factors that are potentially present.

Genomic imprinting is also a mechanism that could account for some of the non-Mendelian familial inheritance patterns that have been observed for birth defects and other conditions previously considered to be multifactorial or polygenic.[125] This refers to a phenomenon in which one or more genes are modified so that expression is determined by the sex of the parent from which the genes are inherited. In other words, some genes are expressed differently when inherited from the father than when inherited from the mother. It is clear that some, but certainly not all, portions of the human genome are imprinted in this fashion. For example, Figure 4–5 shows a pedigree in which two cousins have similar birth defects. If they had facial clefts, neural tube defects, congenital heart disease, or some other nonsyndromic malformation, the traditional way of interpreting the pedigree would be to say that this fits a *multifactorial* inheritance pattern. If, however, the anomaly is actually caused by a single gene that is only expressed when inherited from the father, then the risk of passing this birth defect on to a child would be 50% for the affected boy but negligible for the affected girl, quite different from the risk one might quote from empiric risk tables that are based on an assumption of an underlying polygenic or multifactorial causation. Furthermore, note that individuals IV-4, IV-6, and IV-9 could have as high as a 50% chance of having affected children if the gene is always expressed when inherited from the father (Fig. 4–6). Under the imprinting model, individuals I-2, II-2, II-3, III-1, and III-5 would be nonexpressing carriers of the gene responsible for the malformation, while those individuals labeled with a "?" are also potential carriers. In fact, it would be possible for any of the females in generation IV to have affected grandchildren if they were to pass the gene on to a son who then passed it on to a child (Fig. 4–7). Since this phenomenon can cause familial recurrence without following a traditional pattern of Mendelian inheritance, it is suggested that all such pedigrees, which are currently interpreted as multifactorial, be studied for evidence of genomic imprinting.

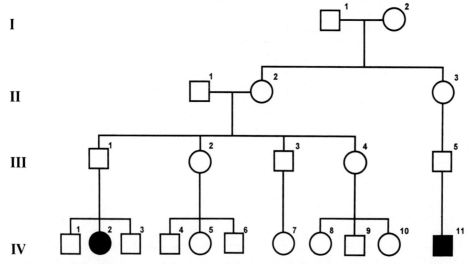

Figure 4–5. Pedigree where second cousins (fifth-degree relatives) have the same nonsyndromic craniofacial malformation. Health care professionals have been taught to interpret this situation as being of "polygenic" or "multifactorial" etiology. (Black symbols = affected)

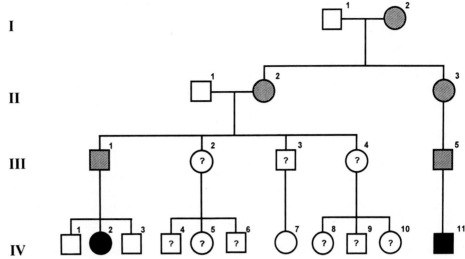

Figure 4–6. Imprinting model for pedigree shown in Fig. 4–5. A single, predisposing gene runs through the family, and is expressed only when inherited from the father. (Black symbols = affected. Shaded symbols = unaffected gene carriers. ? = possible gene carriers)

The mapping and identification of genes responsible for Mendelian craniofacial malformation syndromes by molecular techniques will allow more precise diagnoses for presymptomatic and nonexpressing gene carriers as well as for fetuses at risk. These techniques should also identify some of the major single genes that predispose embryos to develop nonsyndromic malformations. Both animal studies[126–130] and human studies[67, 117, 131–138] are underway. Genes of major interest have included those for transforming growth factor alpha and the retinoic acid receptor.

By this time it should be clear that any nonsyndromic craniofacial malformation has many different potential causes, including a random or coincidental combination of

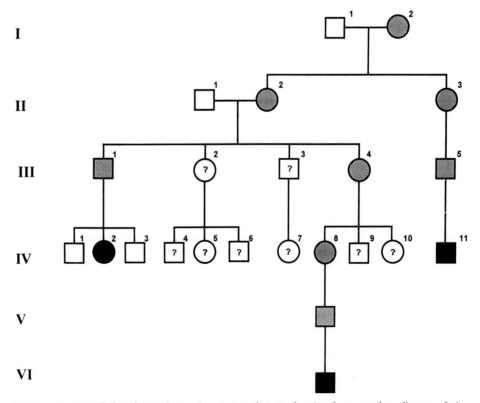

Figure 4–7. Extended pedigree from Figs. 4–5 and 4–6, showing how another distant relative could eventually be affected under the imprinting model. (Black symbols = affected. Shaded symbols = unaffected gene carriers. ? = possible gene carriers)

one or more genetic and/or environmental factors that predispose the embryo to dysmorphogenesis. Therefore, one must be very careful in interpreting the so-called empiric risk figures that are traditionally used. It is common practice to use an *empiric recurrence risk* (ERR) as an actual risk in counseling situations.[139–141] For example, when an unaffected couple has a child with CL(P), a 3% to 5% chance for recurrence in future children is frequently quoted because published recurrence rates range from 2% to 8%. But it is important to remember that an average 4% recurrence rate does not mean that everyone has a 4% risk. For example, it could represent a 25% risk for 16% of such couples and a negligible risk for 84%, if 16% of CL(P) is autosomal recessive and 84% is due to developmental accidents that are unlikely to occur again. On the other hand, an observed recurrence rate of 4% could represent a 25% risk for 12%, a 10% risk for 10% (if, for example, 10% is caused by a dominantly expressed gene with 20% penetrance), and a negligible risk for 78% of couples. Instead of telling such a couple that their risk *is* whatever "empiric risk" figure is found in the literature, one should be honest about what one knows and about the limitations of that knowledge. In view of our current knowledge about the many possible causes of birth defects, it is naive to base our counseling on an assumption of etiologic homogeneity. When the actual risk is unknown, this should be stated! The observed recurrence data should be presented as an *average* recurrence *rate* for individuals in a particular situation. The actual recurrence *risk* may be as high as 25% to 50% if there is a major single gene involved or negligible if the malformation is nonfamilial and was caused by a coincidental combination of factors (genetic, environmental, and chance) that would be very unlikely to occur again during future pregnancies. Counseling about uncertainty may be very difficult, but it is more appropriate to be honest than it is to try to appear omniscient.

Observed recurrence rates vary with the family history. When there are two first degree relatives affected (either siblings or parent and child), observed recurrence rates depend on the malformation but frequently are in the range of 5% to 15%. For more than two affected close relatives, recurrence rates are even higher, approaching 30%. The more affected relatives there are, the more one must consider the possibility that there is a major single gene running through the family predisposing gene carriers to malformation. The observation that apparent "risk" seems to change as more relatives are affected should cause one to be very humble about counseling based on this kind of empiric data, because it should be obvious that what has changed is not the actual risk but only our ability to estimate that risk. In other words, we should be very aware of the fact that families with the same past histories may actually have very different risks for the future.

Recent advances both increase our understanding of genetic causation and challenge long-standing concepts about the distinctness of some of the more common craniosynostosis syndromes. Mutations in two fibroblast growth factor receptor (FGFR) genes (FGFR1 and FGFR2) have been identified in patients with four craniosynostosis syndromes that were previously thought to be clinically and genetically different. (Mutation in another member of this family of tyrosine kinase receptors, FGFR3, has been identified as the cause of the autosomal dominant bone dysplasia, classic achondroplasia.) After linkage studies mapped both Crouzon and Jackson-Weiss syndromes to the same region on the long arm of chromosome 10 as FGFR2,[142] mutations in the same, highly conserved exon of FGFR2 were found both in patients with Crouzon syndrome and in the original family reported with Jackson-Weiss syndrome.[143, 144] Subsequently, a single missense mutation in a highly conserved codon of FGFR1 on chromosome 8p was reported to cause Pfeiffer syndrome in five unrelated families.[145] Cases of Pfeiffer syndrome caused by mutations in the same region of FGFR2 as the Crouzon and Jackson-Weiss mutations were then described; several of the Pfeiffer patients had mutations identical to those previously found in patients with Crouzon syndrome![146, 147] Finally, missense mutations involving two adjacent codons of FGFR2 have been identified as the cause of Apert syndrome in 40 unrelated patients.[148]

These findings illustrate the importance of good clinical phenotype definition and how it provides an essential basis for our ability to interpret and understand the significance of molecular genetic studies. The mechanisms by which identical or similar mutations produce different phenotypes in different individuals are unknown and constitute a fascinating biologic mystery. Readers interested in craniofacial development and the molecular mechanisms involved in gene expression are encouraged to read the references cited in the previous paragraph. A brief editorial review gives a good overview and summary.[149]

References

1. Epstein CJ, Childs B, Fraser FC, et al: Genetic counseling. Am J Hum Genet 1975; 27:240–242.
2. Aase JM: Diagnostic Dysmorphology. New York: Plenum Medical Book Company, 1990.
3. Cohen MM Jr: The Child with Multiple Birth Defects. New York: Raven Press, 1982.
4. Cohen MM Jr, Cole DEC: Origins of recognizable syndromes: Etiologic and pathogenetic mechanisms and the process of syndrome delineation. J Pediatr 1989; 115:161–164.
5. Cohen MM Jr: Syndromology: An updated conceptual overview. I. Syndrome concepts, designations, and population characteristics. Int J Oral Maxillofac Surg 1989; 18:216–222.
6. Cohen MM Jr: Syndromology: An updated conceptual overview. II. Syndrome classifications. Int J Oral Maxillofac Surg 1989; 18:223–228.
7. Cohen MM Jr: Syndromology: An updated conceptual overview. III. Syndrome delineation. Int J Oral Maxillofac Surg 1989; 18:281–285.
8. Cohen MM Jr: Syndromology: An updated conceptual overview. IV. Perspectives on malformation syndromes. Int J Oral Maxillofac Surg 1989; 18:286–290.
9. Cohen MM Jr: Syndromology: An updated conceptual overview. V. Aspects of aneuploidy. Int J Oral Maxillofac Surg 1989; 333–338.
10. Cohen MM Jr: Syndromology: An updated conceptual overview. VI. Molecular and biochemical aspects of dysmorphology. Int J Oral Maxillofac Surg 1989; 18:339–346.
11. Cohen MM Jr: Syndromology: An updated conceptual overview. VII. Aspects of teratogenesis. Int J Oral Maxillofac Surg 1990; 19:26–32.
12. Cohen MM Jr: Syndromology: An updated conceptual overview. VIII. Deformations and disruptions. Int J Oral Maxillofac Surg 1990; 19:33–37.
13. Cohen MM Jr: Syndromology: An updated conceptual overview. IX. Facial dysmorphology. Int J Oral Maxillofac Surg 1990; 19:81–88.
14. Cohen MM Jr: Syndromology: An updated conceptual overview. X. References. Int J Oral Maxillofac Surg 1990; 19:89–96.
15. Jones KL: Smith's Recognizable Patterns of Human Malformation. Philadelphia: WB Saunders, 1988.
16. Graham JM Jr: Smith's Recognizable Patterns of Human Deformation. Philadelphia: WB Saunders, 1988.
17. Stevenson RE, Hall JG, Goodman RM (eds): Human Malformations and Related Anomalies. New York: Oxford University Press, 1993.
18. Gorlin RJ, Cohen MM Jr, Levin LS: Syndromes of the Head and Neck. New York: Oxford University Press, 1990.
19. Jones MC: Facial clefting. Etiology and developmental pathogenesis. Clin Plast Surg 1993; 20:599–606.
20. Cohen MM Jr (ed): Craniosynostosis: Diagnosis, Evaluation, and Management. New York: Raven Press, 1986.
21. Saul RA, Stevenson RE, Rogers RC, et al: Growth References from Conception to Adulthood. Proc Greenwood Genet Ctr 1988; Suppl. #1.
22. Hall JG, Froster-Iskenius UG, Allanson JE: Handbook of Normal Physical Measurements. Oxford: Oxford Medical Publications, 1989.
23. Winter RM, Knowles SAS, Bieber FR, Baraitser M: The Malformed Fetus and Stillbirth. A Diagnostic Approach. Chichester: John Wiley & Sons, 1988.
24. Spranger J, Benirschke K, Hall JG, et al: Errors of morphogenesis: Concepts and terms. Recommendations of an international working group. J Pediatr 1982; 100:160–165.
25. Graham JM Jr, deSaxe M, Smith DW: Sagittal craniostenosis: Fetal head constraint as one possible cause. J Pediatr 1979; 95:747–750.
26. Graham JM Jr, Badura RJ, Smith DW: Coronal craniostenosis: Fetal head constraint as one possible cause. Pediatrics 1980; 65:995–999.
27. Graham JM Jr., Smith DW: Metopic craniostenosis as a consequence of fetal head constraint: Two interesting experiments of nature. Pediatrics 1980; 65:1000–1002.
28. Torpin R: Fetal Malformations Caused by Amnion Rupture During Gestation. Springfield, IL: Charles C. Thomas, 1968.
29. Jones KL, Smith DW, Hall BD, et al: A pattern of craniofacial and limb defects secondary to aberrant tissue bands. J Pediatr 1974; 84:90–95.
30. Higginbottom MC, Jones KL, Hall BD, Smith DW: The amniotic band disruption complex: Timing of amniotic rupture and variable spectra of consequent defects. J Pediatr 1979; 95:544–549.
31. Eyre DR, Upton MP, Shapiro FD, et al: Nonexpression of cartilage type II collagen in a case of Langer-Saldino achondrogenesis. Am J Hum Genet 1986; 39:52–67.
32. Francomano CA, Liberfarb RM, Hirose T, et al: The Stickler syndrome: Evidence for close linkage to the structural gene for type II collagen. Genomics 1987; 1:293–296.
33. Godfrey M, Hollister DW: Type II achondrogenesis-hypochondrogenesis: Identification of abnormal type II collagen. Am J Hum Genet 1988; 43:904–913.
34. Godfrey M, Keene DR, Blank E, et al: Type II achondrogenesis-hypochondrogenesis: Morphologic and immunohistopathologic studies. Am J Hum Genet 1988; 43:894–903.
35. Poole AR, Pidoux I, Reiner A, et al: Kniest dysplasia is characterized by an apparent abnormal processing of the C-propeptide of type II cartilage collagen resulting in imperfect fibril assembly. J Clin Invest 1988; 81:579–589.
36. Byers PH: Molecular heterogeneity in chondrodysplasias. Am J Hum Genet 1989; 45:1–4.
37. Murray LW, Bautista J, James PL, Rimoin DL: Type II collagen defects in the chondrodysplasias. I. Spondyloepiphyseal dysplasias. Am J Hum Genet 1989; 45:5–15.
38. Neuhauser G, Vogl J: Minor craniofacial anomalies in children. Eur J Pediatr 1980; 133:243–250.
39. Rollnick BR, Pruzansky S: Genetic services at a center for craniofacial anomalies. Cleft Palate J 1981; 18:304–313.
40. Shprintzen RJ, Siegel-Sadewitz VL, Amato J, Goldberg RB: Anomalies associated with cleft lip, cleft palate, or both. Am J Med Genet 1985; 20:585–595.

41. Hofstee Y, Kors N, Hennekam RC: Genetic survey of a group of children with clefting: Implications for genetic counseling. Cleft Palate Craniofac J 1993; 30:447–451.

42. Cohen MM Jr: Syndromes with cleft lip and cleft palate. Cleft Palate J 1978; 15:306–328.

43. Cohen MM Jr: Craniofacial disorders. In Emery AEH, Rimoin DL (eds): Principles and Practice of Medical Genetics, pp 576–621. Edinburgh: Churchill Livingstone, 1983.

44. Schmickel RD. Contiguous gene syndromes: A component of recognizable syndromes. J Pediatr 1986; 109:231–241.

45. Holder SE, Winter RM, Kamath S, Scambler PJ: Velocardiofacial syndrome in a mother and daughter: Variability of the clinical phenotype. J Med Genet 1993; 30:825–827.

46. Lipson AH, Yuille D, Angel M, et al: Velocardiofacial (Shprintzen) syndrome: An important syndrome for the dysmorphologist to recognise. J Med Genet 1991; 28:596–604.

47. Goldberg R, Motzkin B, Marion R, et al: Velo-cardio-facial syndrome: A review of 120 patients. Am J Med Genet 1993; 45:313–319.

48. Stevens CA, Carey JC, Shigeoka AO: DiGeorge anomaly and velocardiofacial syndrome. Pediatrics 1990; 85:526–530.

49. Greenberg F: DiGeorge syndrome: An historical review of clinical and cytogenetic features. J Med Genet 1993; 30:803–806.

50. Wilson DI, Burn J, Scambler P, Goodship J: DiGeorge syndrome: Part of CATCH 22. J Med Genet 1993; 30:852–856.

51. Beemer FA, de Nef JJ, Delleman JW, et al: Additional eye findings in a girl with the velo-cardio-facial syndrome. Am J Med Genet 1986; 24:541–542.

52. Pagon RA, Shprintzen RJ: Velo-cardio-facial syndrome vs. CHARGE "association" [letter to the editor]. Am J Med Genet 1987; 28:751–755.

53. Scambler PJ, Kelly D, Lindsay E, et al: Velo-cardio-facial syndrome associated with chromosome 22 deletions encompassing the DiGeorge locus. Lancet 1992; 339:1138–1139.

54. Driscoll DA, Salvin J, Sellinger B, et al: Prevalence of 22q11 microdeletions in DiGeorge and velocardiofacial syndromes: Implications for genetic counselling and prenatal diagnosis. J Med Genet 1993; 30:813–817.

55. Hall JG: CATCH 22. J Med Genet 1993; 30:801–802.

56. Rovin S, Dachi SF, Borenstein DB, Cotter WB: Mandibulofacial dysostosis, a familial study of five generations. J Pediatr 1964; 65:215–221.

57. Aylsworth AS, Lin AE, Friedman PA: Nager acrofacial dysostosis: Male-to-male transmission in 2 families. Am J Med Genet 1991; 41:83–88.

58. Dixon MJ, Dixon J, Houseal T, et al: Narrowing the position of the Treacher Collins syndrome locus to a small interval between three new microsatellite markers at 5q32-33.1. Am J Hum Genet 1993; 52:907–914.

59. Jabs EW, Coss CA, Hayflick SJ, et al: Chromosomal deletion 4p15.32-p14 in a Treacher Collins syndrome patient: Exclusion of the disease locus from and mapping of anonymous DNA sequences to this region. Genomics 1991; 11:188–192.

60. Arn PH, Mankinen C, Jabs EW: Mild mandibulofacial dysostosis in a child with a deletion of 3p. Am J Med Genet 1993; 46:534–536.

61. Burdick AB, Bixler D, Puckett CL: Genetic analysis in families with van der Woude syndrome. J Craniofac Genet Dev Biol 1985; 5:181–208.

62. Bocian M, Walker AP: Lip pits and deletion 1q32-41. Am J Med Genet 1987; 26:437–443.

63. Murray JC, Nishimura DY, Buetow KH, et al: Linkage of an autosomal dominant clefting syndrome (Van der Woude) to loci on chromosome 1q. Am J Hum Genet 1990; 46:486–491.

64. Burdick AB: Genetic epidemiology and control of genetic expression in van der Woude syndrome. J Craniofac Genet Dev Biol Suppl 1986; 2:99–105.

65. Menko FH, Koedijk PH, Baart JA, Kwee ML: Van der Woude syndrome—recognition of lesser expressions: Case report. Cleft Palate J 1988; 25:318–321.

66. Hecht JT, Wang Y, Blanton SH, Daiger SP: Van der Woude syndrome and nonsyndromic cleft lip and palate. Am J Hum Genet 1992; 51:442–444.

67. Vintiner GM, Lo KK, Holder SE, et al: Exclusion of candidate genes from a role in cleft lip with or without cleft palate: Linkage and association studies. J Med Genet 1993; 30:773–778.

68. Marini R, Temple K, Chitty L, et al: Pitfalls in counselling: The craniosynostoses. J Med Genet 1991; 28:117–121.

69. Niemann-Seyde SC, Eber SW, Zoll B: Saethre-Chotzen syndrome (ACS III) in four generations. Clin Genet 1991; 40:271–276.

70. Garcia-Esquivel L, Garcia-Cruz D, Rivera H, et al: De novo del(7)(pter-p21.2::p15.2-qter) and craniosynostosis. Implications for critical segment assignment in the 7p2 monosomy syndrome. Ann Genet 1986; 29:36–38.

71. Aughton DJ, Cassidy SB, Whiteman DA, et al: Chromosome 7p-syndrome: Craniosynostosis with preservation of region 7p2. Am J Med Genet 1991; 40:440–443.

72. Brueton LA, van Herwerden L, Chotai KA, Winter RM: The mapping of a gene for craniosynostosis: Evidence for linkage of the Saethre-Chotzen syndrome to distal chromosome 7p. J Med Genet 1992; 29:681–685.

73. Wang C, Maynard S, Glover TW, Biesecker LG: Mild phenotypic manifestation of a 7p15.3p21.2 deletion. J Med Genet 1993; 30:610–612.

74. Reardon W, McManus SP, Summers D, Winter RM: Cytogenetic evidence that the Saethre-Chotzen gene maps to 7p21.2. Am J Med Genet 1993; 47:633–636.

75. Reid CS, McMorrow LE, McDonald-McGinn DM, et al: Saethre-Chotzen syndrome with familial translocation at chromosome 7p22. Am J Med Genet 1993; 47:637–639.

76. Müller U, Warman ML, Mulliken JB, Weber JL: Assignment of a gene locus involved in craniosynostosis to chromosome 5qter. Hum Mol Genet 1993; 2:119–122.

77. Fryburg JS, Golden WL: Interstitial deletion of 8q13.3 → 22.1 associated with craniosynostosis. Am J Med Genet 1993; 45:638–641.
78. Moore GE, Williamson R, Jensson O, et al: Localization of a mutant gene for cleft palate and ankyloglossia in an X-linked Icelandic family. J Craniofac Genet Dev Biol 1991; 11:372–376.
79. Gorski SM, Adams KJ, Birch PH, et al: The gene responsible for X-linked cleft palate (CPX) in a British Columbia native kindred is localized between PGK1 and DXYS1. Am J Hum Genet 1992; 50:1129–1136.
80. Stanier P, Forbes SA, Arnason A, et al: The localization of a gene causing X-linked cleft palate and ankyloglossia (CPX) in an Icelandic kindred is between DXS326 and DXYS1X. Genomics 1993; 17:549–555.
81. Webster WS, Johnston MC, Lammer EJ, Sulik KK: Isotretinoin embryopathy and the cranial neural crest: An in vivo and in vitro study. J Craniofac Genet Dev Biol 1986; 6:211–222.
82. Sulik KK, Johnston MC, Daft PA, Russell WE, Dehart DB: Fetal alcohol syndrome and DiGeorge anomaly: Critical ethanol exposure periods for craniofacial malformations as illustrated in an animal model. Am J Med Genet Suppl 1986; 2:97–112.
83. Webster WS, Lipson AH, Sulik KK: Interference with gastrulation during the third week of pregnancy as a cause of some facial abnormalities and CNS defects. Am J Med Genet 1988; 31:505–512.
84. Sulik KK, Cook CS, Webster WS: Teratogens and craniofacial malformations: Relationships to cell death. Development 1988; 103:213–231.
85. Aylsworth AS, Kirkman HN: Genetic counseling for autosomal dominant disorders with incomplete penetrance. Birth Defects: Original Article Series 1979; XV(5C):25–38.
86. Bixler D: Genetics and clefting. Cleft Palate J 1981; 18:10–18.
87. Menegotto BG, Salzano FM: Clustering of malformations in the families of South American oral cleft neonates. J Med Genet 1991; 28:110–113.
88. Falconer DS: The inheritance of liability to certain diseases, estimated from the incidence among relatives. Ann Hum Genet 1965; 29:51–76.
89. Edwards JH: Familial predisposition in man. Br Med Bull 1969; 25:58–64.
90. Smith C: Heritability of liability and concordance in monozygous twins. Ann Hum Genet 1970; 34:85–91.
91. Carter CO: The inheritance of common congenital malformations. In Steinberg AG, Bearn AG (eds): Progress in Medical Genetics, pp 59–84. New York: Grune and Stratton, 1965.
92. Carter CO: Genetics of common disorders. Br Med Bull 1969; 25:52–57.
93. Carter CO: Genetics of common single malformations. Br Med Bull 1976; 32:21–26.
94. Fraser FC: The genetics of cleft lip and cleft palate. Am J Hum Genet 1970; 22:336–352.
95. Fraser FC: Evolution of a palatable multifactorial threshold model. Am J Hum Genet 1980; 32:796–813.
96. Smith DW, Aase JM: Polygenic inheritance of certain common malformations. Evidence and empiric recurrence risk data. J Pediatr 1970; 76:652–659.
97. Carter CO: Multifactorial genetic disease. In McKusick VA, Claiborne R (eds): Medical Genetics, pp 199–208. New York: HP Publishing, 1973.
98. Mitchell LE, Risch N: Mode of inheritance of nonsyndromic cleft lip with or without cleft palate: A reanalysis. Am J Hum Genet 1992; 51:323–332.
99. Melnick M, Bixler D, Fogh-Andersen P, Conneally PM: Cleft lip +/− cleft palate: An overview of the literature and an analysis of Danish cases born between 1941 and 1968. Am J Med Genet 1980; 6:83–97.
100. Marazita ML, Spence MA, Melnick M: Genetic analysis of cleft lip with or without cleft palate in Danish kindreds. Am J Med Genet 1984; 19:9–18.
101. Melnick M, Marazita ML, Hu DN: Genetic analysis of cleft lip with or without cleft palate in Chinese kindreds. Am J Med Genet Suppl 1986; 2:183–190.
102. Marazita ML, Spence MA, Melnick M: Major gene determination of liability to cleft lip with or without cleft palate: A multiracial view. J Craniofac Genet Dev Biol Suppl 1986; 2:89–97.
103. Nemana LJ, Marazita ML, Melnick M: Genetic analysis of cleft lip with or without cleft palate in Madras, India. Am J Med Genet 1992; 42:5–9.
104. Marazita ML, Hu DN, Spence MA, et al: Cleft lip with or without cleft palate in Shanghai, China: Evidence for an autosomal major locus. Am J Hum Genet 1992; 51:648–653.
105. Ray AK, Field LL, Marazita ML: Nonsyndromic cleft lip with or without cleft palate in West Bengal, India: Evidence for an autosomal major locus. Am J Hum Genet 1993; 52:1006–1011.
106. Fraser FC: The multifactorial/threshold concept—uses and misuses. Teratology 1976; 14:267–280.
107. Fraser FC: The genetics of common familial disorders—major genes or multifactorial? Can J Genet Cytol 1981; 23:1–8.
108. Melnick M, Shields ED, Bixler D: Studies of cleft lip and cleft palate in the population of Denmark. In Melnick M, Bixler D, Shields ED (eds): Etiology of Cleft Lip and Cleft Palate, pp 225–248. New York: Alan R. Liss, 1980.
109. Melnick M, Shields ED, Bixler D: Studies of cleft lip and cleft palate in the population of Denmark. Prog Clin Biol Res 1980; 46:225–248.
110. Mendell NR, Spence MA, Gladstien K, et al: Multifactorial/threshold models and their application to cleft lip and cleft palate. In Melnick M, Bixler D, Shields ED (eds): Etiology of Cleft Lip and Cleft Palate, pp 387–406. New York: Alan R. Liss, 1980.
111. Shields ED, Bixler D, Fogh-Andersen P: Facial clefts in Danish twins. Cleft Palate J 1979; 16:1–6.
112. Shields ED, Bixler D, Fogh-Andersen P: Cleft palate: A genetic and epidemiologic investigation. Clin Genet 1981; 20:13–24.
113. Liu SL, Erickson RP: Genetic differences among the A/JXC57BL/6J recombinant inbred mouse lines and their degree of association with glucocorticoid-induced cleft palate. Genetics 1986; 113:745–754.

114. Marazita ML, Goldstein AM, Smalley SL, Spence MA: Cleft lip with or without cleft palate: Reanalysis of a three-generation family study from England. Genet Epidemiol 1986; 3:335–342.

115. Biddle FG, Fraser FC: Major gene determination of liability to spontaneous cleft lip in the mouse. J Craniofac Genet Dev Biol Suppl 1986; 2:67–88.

116. Chung CS, Bixler D, Watanabe T, et al: Segregation analysis of cleft lip with or without cleft palate: A comparison of Danish and Japanese data. Am J Hum Genet 1986; 39:603–611.

117. Eiberg H, Bixler D, Nielsen LS, et al: Suggestion of linkage of a major locus for nonsyndromic orofacial cleft with F13A and tentative assignment to chromosome 6. Clin Genet 1987; 32:129–132.

118. Chung CS, Mi MP, Beechert AM: Genetic epidemiology of cleft lip with or without cleft palate in the population of Hawaii. Genet Epidemiol 1987; 4:415–423.

119. Juriloff DM, Harris MJ: Cleft palate: More genetic lessons from mice. J Craniofac Genet Dev Biol 1988; 8:127–134.

120. Farrall M, Holder S: Familial recurrence-pattern analysis of cleft lip with or without cleft palate. Am J Hum Genet 1992; 50:270–277.

121. Christensen K, Fogh-Andersen P: Cleft lip (+/− cleft palate) in Danish twins, 1970–1990. Am J Med Genet 1993; 47:910–916.

122. Hook EB: Genetic-counseling implications for cleft lip if an autosomal recessive major locus accounts for all cases. Am J Hum Genet 1993; 52:1270–1271.

123. Marazita ML, Spence MA, Melnick M: Genetic-counseling implications for cleft lip if an autosomal recessive major locus accounts for all cases. Reply. Am J Hum Genet 1993; 52:1271–1272.

124. Kurnit DM, Layton WM, Matthysse S: Genetics, chance, and morphogenesis. Am J Hum Genet 1987; 41:979–995.

125. Hall JG: Genomic imprinting: Review and relevance to human diseases. Am J Hum Genet 1990; 46:857–873.

126. Juriloff DM: Major genes that cause cleft lip in mice: Progress in the construction of a congenic strain and in linkage mapping. J Craniofac Genet Dev Biol Suppl 1986; 2:55–66.

127. Damm K, Heyman RA, Umesono K, Evans RM: Functional inhibition of retinoic acid response by dominant negative retinoic acid receptor mutants. Proc Natl Acad Sci USA 1993; 90:2989–2993.

128. Culiat CT, Stubbs L, Nicholls RD, et al: Concordance between isolated cleft palate in mice and alterations within a region including the gene encoding the α_3 subunit of the type A gamma-aminobutyric acid receptor. Proc Natl Acad Sci USA 1993; 90:5105–5109.

129. Karolyi J, Erickson RP: A region of the mouse genome homologous to human chromosome 1q21 affects facial clefting. J Craniofac Genet Dev Biol 1993; 13:1–5.

130. Juriloff DM: Current status of genetic linkage studies of a major gene that causes CL(P) in mice: Exclusion map. J Craniofac Genet Dev Biol 1993; 13:223–229.

131. Ardinger HH, Buetow KH, Bell GI, et al: Association of genetic variation of the transforming growth factor-alpha gene with cleft lip and palate. Am J Hum Genet 1989; 45:348–353.

132. Hecht JT, Wang YP, Blanton SH, et al: Cleft lip and palate: No evidence of linkage to transforming growth factor alpha. Am J Hum Genet 1991; 49:682–686.

133. Stoll C, Qian JF, Feingold J, et al: Genetic variation in transforming growth factor alpha: Possible association of BamHI polymorphism with bilateral sporadic cleft lip and palate. Am J Hum Genet 1992; 50:870–871.

134. Chenevix-Trench G, Jones K, Green AC, et al: Cleft lip with or without cleft palate: Associations with transforming growth factor alpha and retinoic acid receptor loci. Am J Hum Genet 1992; 51:1377–1385.

135. Stoll C, Qian JF, Feingold J, et al: Genetic variation in transforming growth factor alpha: Possible association of BamHI polymorphism with bilateral sporadic cleft lip and palate. Hum Genet 1993; 92:81–82.

136. Tenconi R, Clementi M, Turolla L: Theoretical recurrence risks for cleft lip derived from a population of consecutive newborns. J Med Genet 1988; 25:243–246.

137. Farrall M, Buetow KH, Murray JC: Resolving an apparent paradox concerning the role of TGFA in CL/P. Am J Hum Genet 1993; 52:434–437.

138. Hecht JT, Wang Y, Blanton SH, et al: Reply to letter: Resolving an apparent paradox concerning the role of TGFA in CL/P. Am J Hum Genet 1993; 52:436–437.

139. Carter CO: Recurrence risk of common congenital malformations. Practitioner 1974; 213:667–674.

140. Berini RY, Kahn E (eds): Clinical Genetics Handbook, pp 18, 294–309. Oradell, NJ: Medical Economics Books, 1987.

141. Harper PS: Practical Genetic Counseling. London: Butterworth, 1988.

142. Li X, Lewanda AF, Eluma F, et al: Two craniosynostotic syndrome loci, Crouzon and Jackson-Weiss, map to chromosome 10q23–q26. Genomics 1994; 22:418–424.

143. Reardon W, Winter RM, Rutland P, et al: Mutations in the fibroblast growth factor receptor 2 gene cause Crouzon syndrome. Nature Genet 1994; 8:98–103.

144. Jabs EW, Li X, Scott AF, et al: Jackson-Weiss and Crouzon syndromes are allelic with mutations in fibroblast growth factor receptor 2. Nature Genet 1994; 8:275–279.

145. Muenke M, Schell U, Hehr A, et al: A common mutation in the fibroblast growth factor receptor 1 gene in Pfeiffer syndrome. Nature Genet 1994; 8:269–274.

146. Lajeunie E, Ma HW, Bonaventure J, et al: FGFR2 mutations in Pfeiffer syndrome. Nature Genet 1995; 9:108.

147. Rutland P, Pulleyn LJ, Reardon W, et al: Identical mutations in the FGFR2 gene cause both Pfeiffer and Crouzon syndrome phenotypes. Nature Genet 1995; 9:173–176.

148. Wilkie AOM, Slaney SF, Oldridge M, et al: Apert syndrome results from localized mutations of FGFR2 and is allelic with Crouzon syndrome. Nature Genet 1995; 9:165–172.

149. Mulvihill JJ: Craniofacial syndromes: No such thing as a single-gene disease. Nature Genet 1995; 9:101–103.

5 | Facial Clefting Disorders and Craniofacial Synostoses: Skeletal Considerations

Stephen A. Schendel, Paul Tessier, and J.-F. Tulasne

The study of skeletal material provides a wealth of subjective and objective information for the anatomist and surgeon. This knowledge is invaluable in understanding the pathogenesis of craniofacial malformations and in planning their treatment. Unfortunately, skulls with craniofacial malformations are not common, and those known to exist are distributed among major museums, universities, and a few private collections. This makes it difficult for any individual to personally examine this material and have it available as a reference. Our purpose in this chapter is to provide the reader with a visual display of the bony pathology in a selection of craniofacial malformations. Nothing, however, will replace the intimate appreciation of a deformity, which is gained by handling and carefully examining the skull. We cover a series of simple craniosynostoses, finishing with Apert and Crouzon syndromes. Next, a series of skulls with facial clefts is presented, including the common cleft lip-palate case and the rare complete Treacher Collins skull. Unfortunately, many other types of craniofacial clefts are not found in the collections examined.

SUTURE OBLITERATION

Craniosynostosis results from obliteration of the involved suture or sutures by progressive fusion of the adjacent bones.[1] The resultant skull shape produced depends on which suture or sutures are involved. The diagnosis of craniosynostosis is based on the history of an unusual head shape at birth and on the physical examination. The particular head shape generally indicates the involved suture or sutures.[2] Dolichocephaly, or long skull, indicates sagittal suture involvement; scaphocephaly, a form of dolichocephaly, has more of a boat-shaped skull. Trigonocephaly, or a triangular shape, indicates involvement of the metopic suture and cranial base. Plagiocephaly, or oblique shape, is caused by unilateral closure of the coronal or lambdoidal sutures. Brachycephaly, or short skull, results from bilateral coronal suture involvement. Oxycephaly (sharp) and turricephaly (tower) result from the involvement of multiple sutures. Multiple suture closure is also associated with increased intracranial pressure that is frequently seen in radiographs by the so-called hammered silver appearance or in digital impressions. Multiple premature suture closure is typical of craniofacial dysostosis, or Crouzon syndrome, and acrocephalosyndactyly, or Apert syndrome. Many other syndromes involve various synostosed sutures and associated anomalies. Skeletal material for most of these syndromes is lacking, and we cover only the simple synostoses, Apert syndrome, and Crouzon syndrome in the following section.

Acknowledgments

The research and the study of abnormal skulls were conducted by Paul Tessier. We express our acknowledgments to the museums that have made possible this study: the Pathologisch-Anatomisches Bundesmuseum in Vienna (Prof. von Portele), the Royal College of Surgeons Museum in Edinburgh (Dr. Shivas), the Musée de l'Homme in Paris (Prof. Y. Coppens), the Institut für Pathologische Anatomie in Graz (Prof Ratzenhofer), Laboratory of Anatomy in Paris, and Anatomisch-Embryologisch Laboratorium in Amsterdam.

FACIAL CLEFTS

Craniofacial malformations associated with facial clefting were classified by Tessier into 15 locations, with the orbit as the primary reference[3,4] (Fig. 5–1). Many of these clefts were known under an older, sometimes misleading, nomenclature such as median facial dysraphia, cranium bifidum, frontonasal dysplasia, first and second branchial arch syndromes, and Treacher Collins or Franceschetti syndrome. Many of these clefts are rare, and we have no skeletal specimens; others, such as cleft lip and palate, are common.

Tessier outlined the principal concepts of these clefts. The term *hypoplasia* is useful in describing the bone surrounding the clefts but is not the same as clefting. *Clefting* is the interruption of either the soft tissue (hairline, eyebrows, eyelids, nostrils, lips, or ears) or the skeleton. Bone and soft tissues are, however, rarely involved to the same extent. Soft tissue defects are also more common and destructive from the midline to the infraorbital foramen; the ear is a notable exception. Conversely, defects of the bony structure are more severe lateral to the infraorbital foramen. Although this system does not refer to the embryology of the malformations classified, it is an excellent descriptive methodology for observing skeletal specimens. Unfortunately, examples of clefts between the central and lateral portions of the face have not been found in the museum and personal collections examined for this study. The next section anatomically describes the central and lateral facial clefting specimens found.

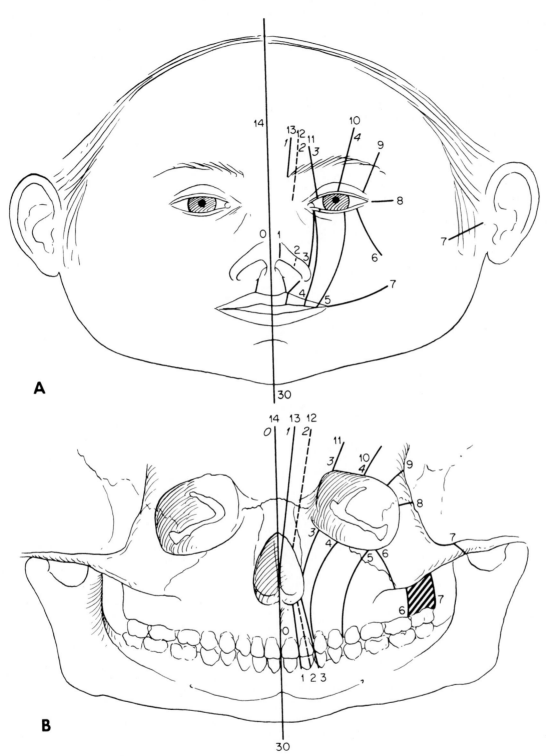

Figure 5–1. *A, B,* Tessier Craniofacial Cleft Classification.

SPECIMENS

Skull #343*

(Adult with Scaphocephaly)

Abnormal Findings

- Absence of the metopic and sagittal sutures (Figs. 5–2A, 5–3B)
- Reduced transverse dimension and increased anteroposterior (AP) skull dimensions (Figs. 5–2, 5–3)
- Bathmocephaly (Fig. 5–3A)

Normal Findings

- Symmetric facial and cranial bones
- Class I occlusion

---

* Pathologisch-Anatomisches Bundesmuseum, Vienna.

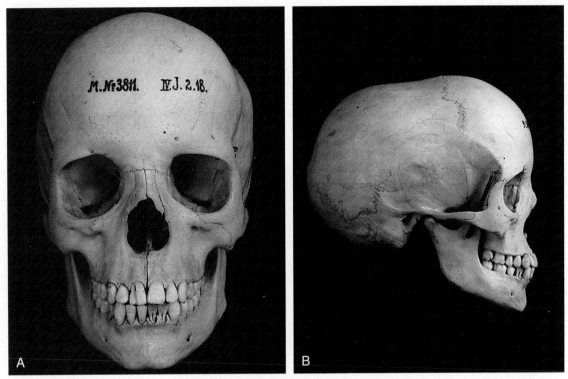

Figure 5–2. *A*, *B*, Skull #343 from Pathologisch-Anatomisches Bundesmuseum, Vienna.

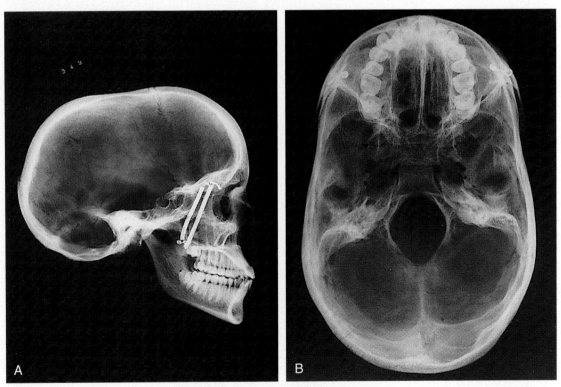

Figure 5–3. *A*, *B*, Radiographs of skull #343.

Skull #124*

(Adult with Scaphocephaly)

Abnormal Findings

- Absence of the metopic and sagittal sutures (Figs. 5–4*A,B*; 5–5*A*)
- Reduced transverse dimension and increased AP dimension of skull (Figs. 5–4*A,B,C,D*)

---

* Laboratory of Anatomy, Paris.

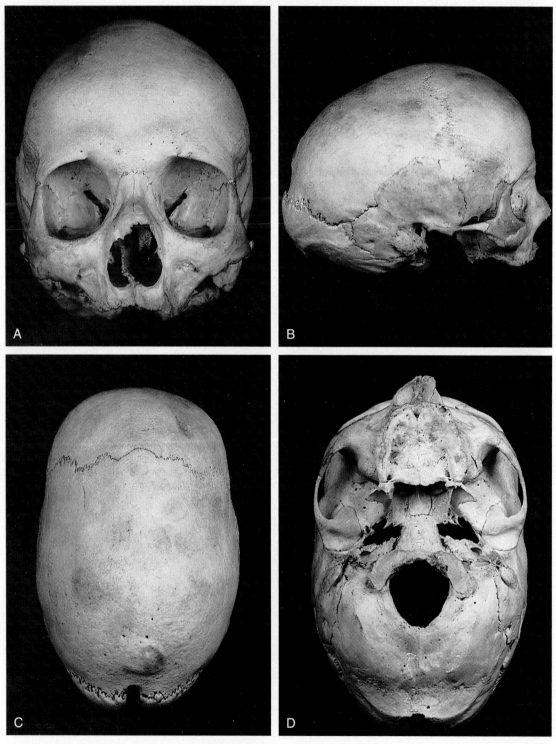

Figure 5–4. *A, B, C, D,* Skull #124 from the Laboratory of Anatomy, Paris.

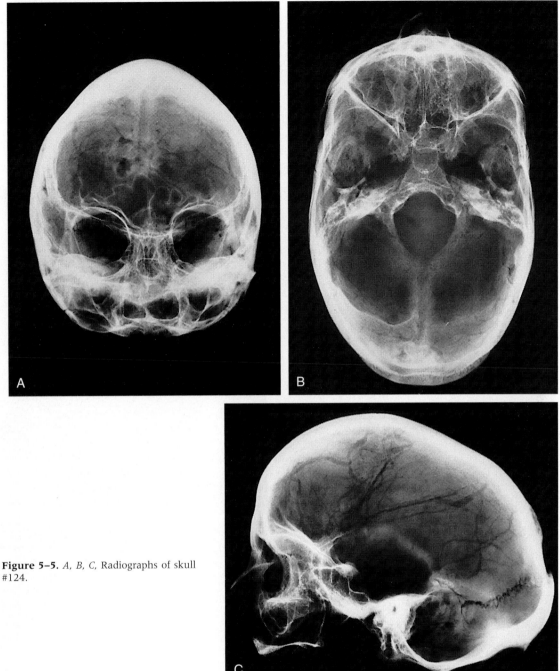

Figure 5–5. *A, B, C,* Radiographs of skull #124.

- Prominent vault (Figs. 5–4*A*, 5–5*A*)
- Bathmocephaly (Figs. 5–4*D*, 5–5*C*)
- Septal deviation and asymmetry of nasal bones (Fig. 5–4*A*)
- Narrow interorbital distance (Figs. 5–4*A*, 5–5*A*)

Normal Findings

- No orbital asymmetry
- Essentially normal maxillary position, although edentulous

Skull #121*

(Brachycephalic Skull)

Abnormal Findings

- Absence of right and left coronal sutures (Figs. 5–6*B,C*; 5–7*B*)
- Persistent, widened metopic suture (Figs. 5–6*A*, 5–7*A*)
- Increased transverse skull dimensions and shortened AP dimension (Figs. 5–6*A,B,C,D*; 5–7*A,B*)

---

* Laboratory of Anatomy, Paris.

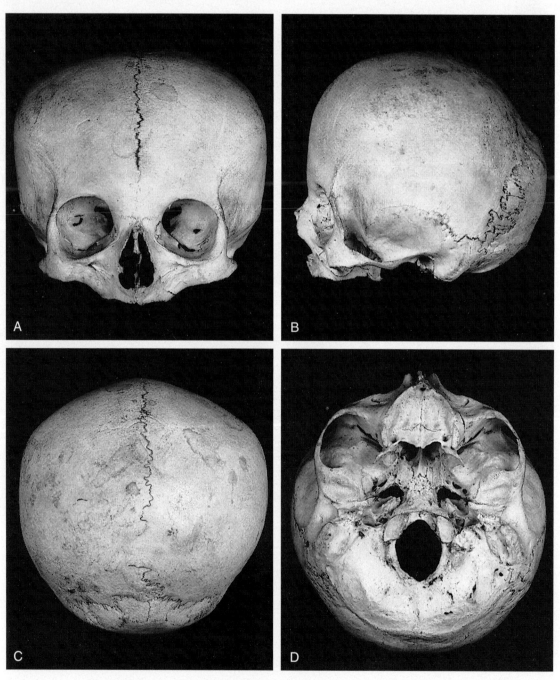

Figure 5–6. *A, B, C, D,* Skull #121 from the Laboratory of Anatomy, Paris.

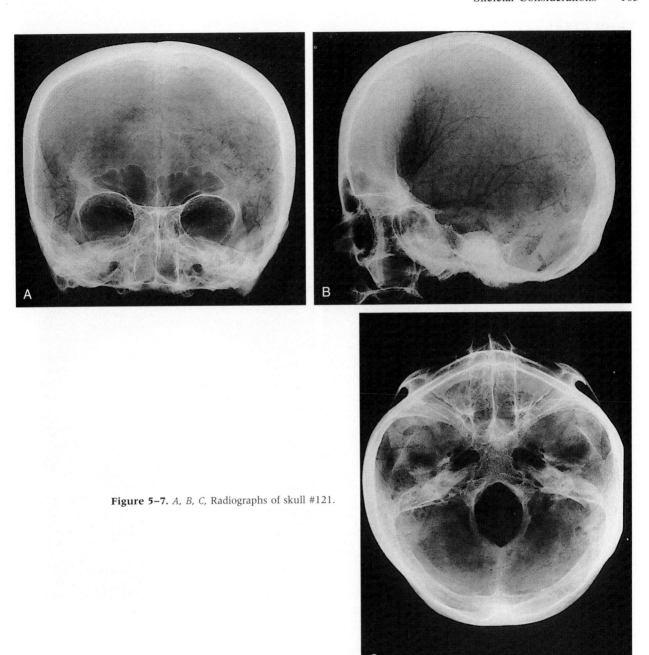

Figure 5–7. *A, B, C,* Radiographs of skull #121.

- Increased vertical dimension of the forehead and flatness, resulting in abnormal glabella (Figs. 5–6A,B; 5–7A,B)
- Wormian bones in occiput (Fig. 5–6C)
- Increased bowing of the zygomatic arches (Fig. 5–6D)
- Synostosis of sphenoid wings

Normal Findings

- Symmetric orbits and forehead (Fig. 5–6A)
- Normal foramen magnum (Figs. 5–6D, 5–7C)

Skull #156*

(Trigonocephalic Skull of a Young Child)

Abnormal Findings

- Absence of metopic suture with ridging (Figs. 5–8*A*, 5–9*A*)
- Pointed frontal bone, which slopes off laterally (Figs. 5–8*C*, 5–9*B*)
- Missing left zygomatic arch and complex, postmortem (Fig. 5–8*A*)
- Vertical orbital orientation, decreased interorbital distance (Figs. 5–8*A*, 5–9*A*)
- Vertically oriented frontal bone profile (Fig. 5–8*B*)

Normal Findings

- Asymmetry

* Anatomisch-Embryologisch Laboratorium, Amsterdam.

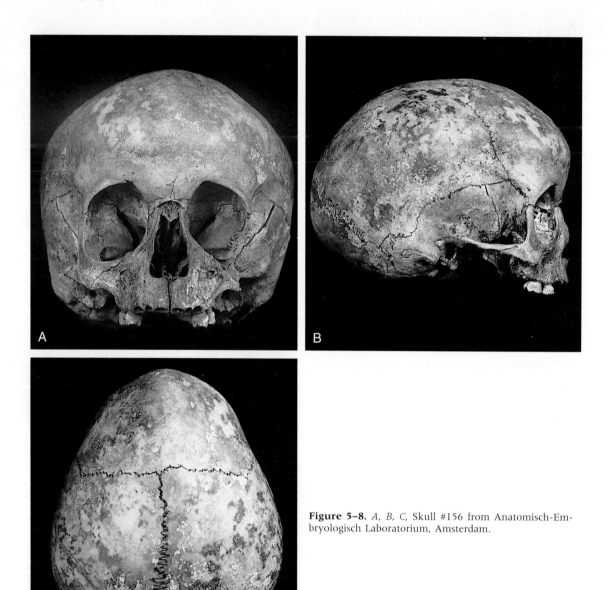

Figure 5–8. *A, B, C,* Skull #156 from Anatomisch-Embryologisch Laboratorium, Amsterdam.

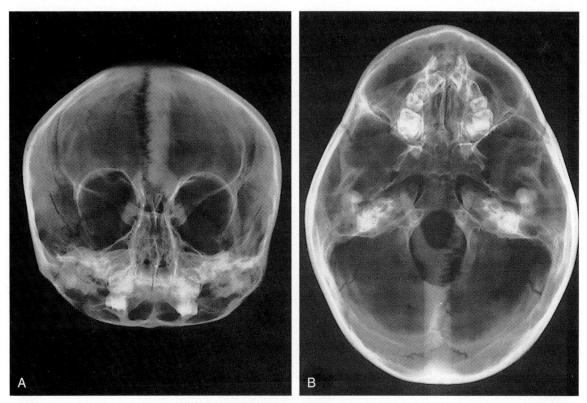

Figure 5–9. *A*, *B*, Radiographs of skull #156.

Skull #100*

(Skull with Plagiocephaly Caused by a Left Coronal Synostosis)

Abnormal Findings

- Absence of left coronal suture (Figs. 5–10*A*, 5–11*B,C*)
- Flattening of left frontal bone (Figs. 5–10*A*, 5–11*A*)
- Asymmetric orbits with elevation of lesser wing of sphenoid and malar eminences

---

* Collection Paul Tessier, Paris.

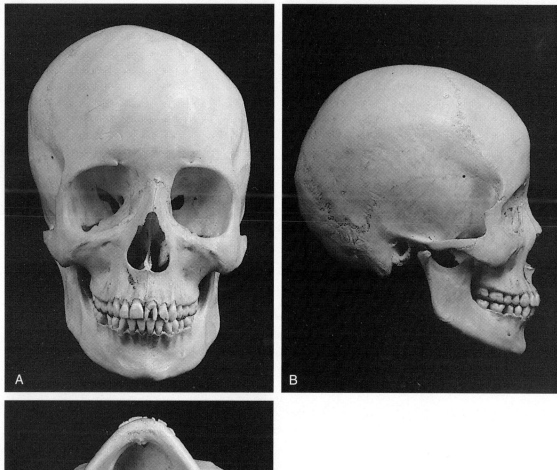

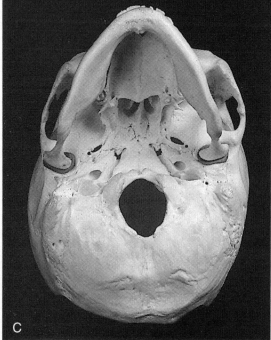

Figure 5–10. *A, B, C,* Skull #100 from Collection Paul Tessier, Paris.

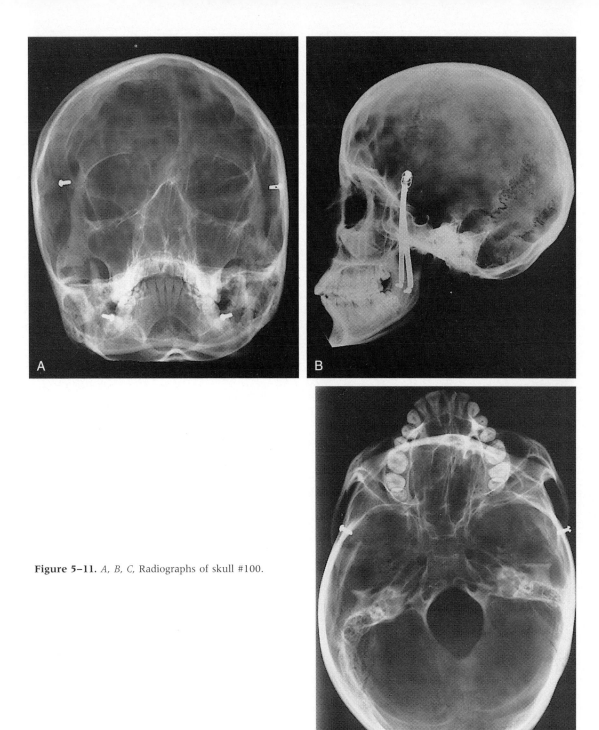

Figure 5–11. *A, B, C,* Radiographs of skull #100.

- Nasal root deviation to left (Figs. 5–10*A*, 5–11*A*)
- Asymmetric cranium, flattening right occipital area (Figs. 5–10*C*, 5–11*C*)
- S-shaped curve to skull midline
- Left petrous portion of temporal bone advanced, right portion retruded (Fig. 5–11*C*)
- Asymmetric glenoid fossae, maxilla, and mandible; left portions advanced (Figs. 5–10*C*, 5–11)
- Asymmetric foramen magnum
- Digital markings on anterior cranial vault (Fig. 5–11*A,B*)

Normal Findings

- Normal right lateral view (Fig. 5–10*B*)
- Class I occlusion

107

Skull #120*

(Skull with Plagiocephaly, Brachycephaly, and Hypertelorism)

Abnormal Findings

- Plagiocephaly and brachycephaly (Figs. 5–12, 5–13, 5–14)
- Absence of right coronal suture (Figs. 5–12C, 5–13C)
- Discrete temporal synostosis of left coronal suture (Figs. 5–14A,B)
- Midsagittal wormian bone (Fig. 5–12C)
- Flat, retruded right frontal bone (Figs. 5–12B,C; 5–14D)
- Hypertelorism and asymmetric orbits (Fig. 5–12A)
- Midsagittal suture deviation to right (Figs. 5–12C; 5–14A,B)
- Nasal root deviation to right, including vomer (Fig. 5–14A)
- Harlequin deformity of the right orbit and sphenoid wing (Figs. 5–12A; 5–13A,B)
- Hypoplastic, edentulous maxilla (Fig. 5–12A,B)
- Asymmetric zygomatic complexes and arches (Fig. 5–12B)
- Depression, anterior skull (Figs. 5–12A; 5–13A,B,C,D; 5–14C)
- Small frontal sinus; absence of maxillary sinuses (Fig. 5–14)
- Asymmetric petrous portions of the temporal bone and glenoid fossae: right portion advanced, left portion retruded (Figs. 5–12B, 5–14D)

---

* Laboratory of Anatomy, Paris.

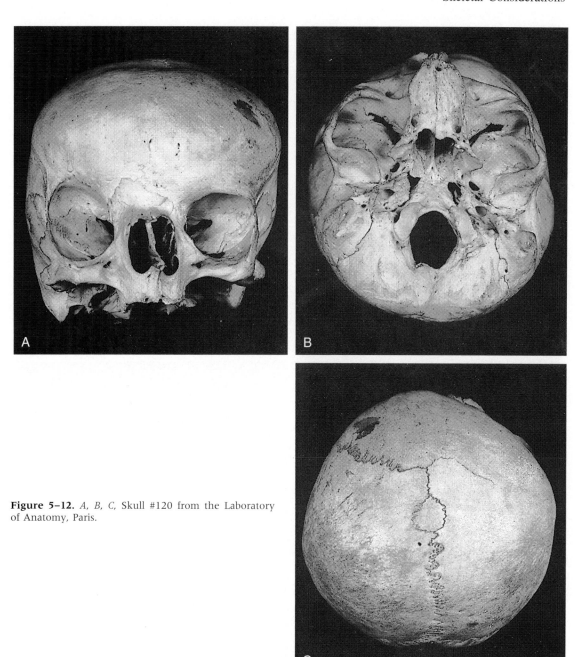

Figure 5–12. *A, B, C,* Skull #120 from the Laboratory of Anatomy, Paris.

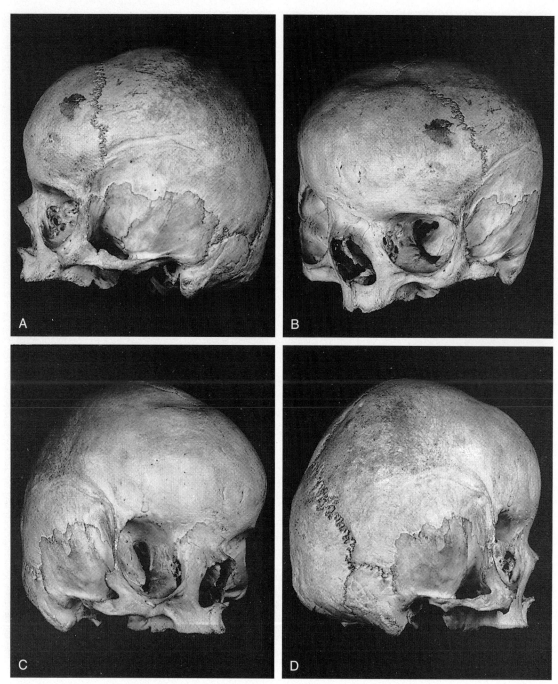

Figure 5–13. *A, B, C, D,* Lateral and oblique views of skull #120.

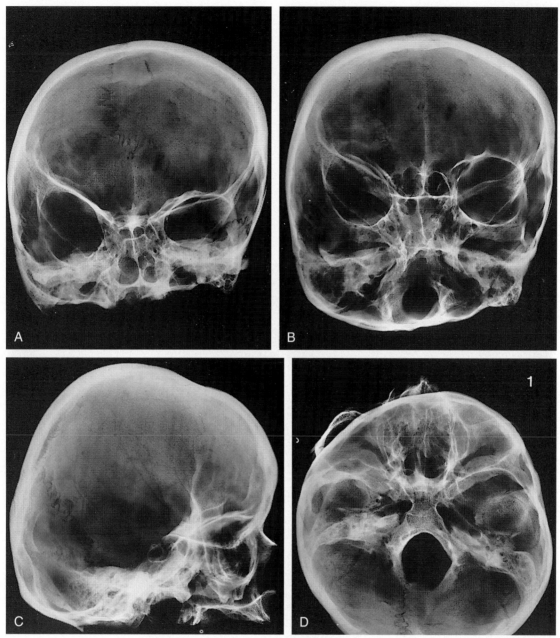

Figure 5–14. *A, B, C, D,* Radiographs of skull #120.

Skull #108*

(Skull of a Child with Apert Syndrome)

Abnormal Findings

- Brachycephaly (Figs. 5–15A,B,C)
- Inferior aspect (temporal) of closed coronal sutures (Figs. 5–15B, 5–16B)
- Widely open metopic suture (Figs. 5–15A,C; 5–16A)
- Hypertelorism (Figs. 5–15A; 5–16A)
- Rounded, protuberant frontal bone (Figs. 5–15B, 5–16B)
- Midface hypoplasia and retrusion (Figs. 5–15, 5–16)
- Small choanae (Figs. 5–15A, 5–16A)
- Abnormal cranial base and sella turcica (Fig. 5–16B)
- Hypoplastic maxilla (Figs. 5–15C, 5–16C)

---

* Musée de l'Homme, Paris.

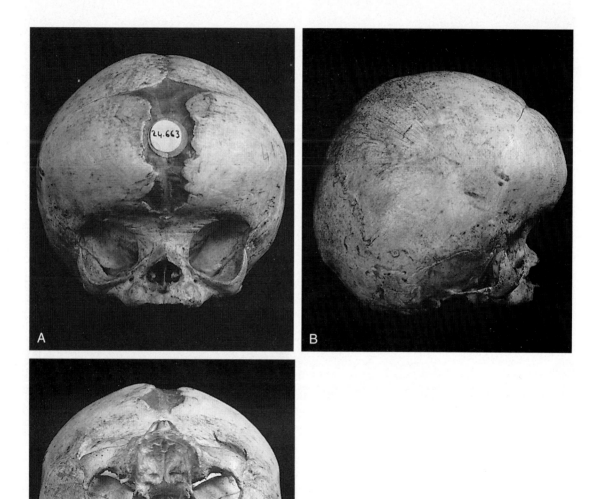

Figure 5–15. *A, B, C,* Skull #108 from the Musée de l'Homme, Paris.

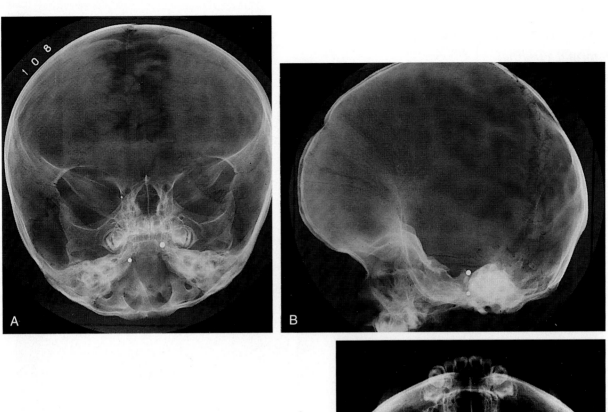

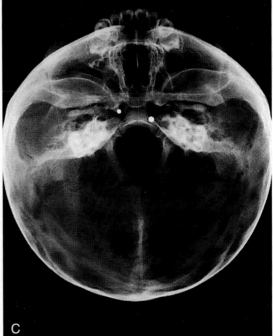

Figure 5–16. *A, B, C,* Radiographs of skull #108.

Skull #204*

(Skull of a One-Year-Old with Apert Syndrome)

Abnormal Findings

- Brachycephaly
- Closed coronal sutures, bilateral (Figs. 5–17*B,C*; 5–18*B*)
- Widely open metopic suture (Figs. 5–17*A*, 5–18*A*)
- Hypertelorism and abnormal orbital shape (Figs. 5–17*A,C*; 5–18*A*)
- Harlequin orbital deformity with sphenoid wing deformity (Figs. 5–17*A*, 5–18*A*)
- Small choanae

---

* Royal College of Surgeons Museum, Edinburgh.

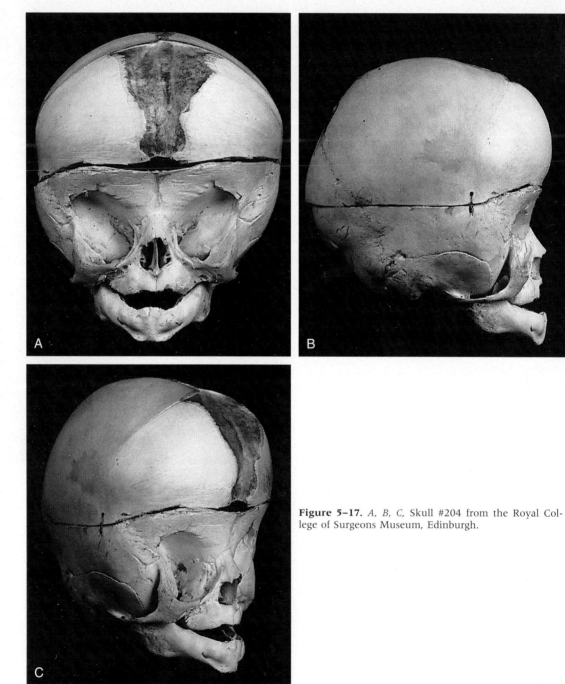

Figure 5–17. *A, B, C,* Skull #204 from the Royal College of Surgeons Museum, Edinburgh.

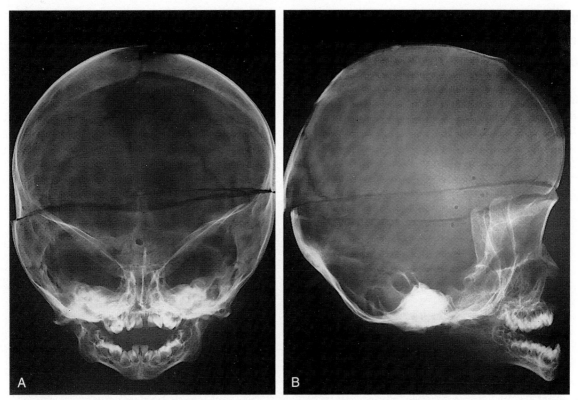

Figure 5–18. *A, B,* Radiographs of skull #204.

- Midface retrusion and hypoplastic maxilla (Figs. 5–17*A,B;* 5–18*A,B*)
- Cranial base deformity (Fig. 5–18*B*)
- Digital markings (Fig. 5–18)
- Mandibular deformity

Normal Findings

- Cranial and facial symmetry

Skull #430*

(Skull of an Adult with Crouzon Syndrome)

Abnormal Findings

- Absence of both coronal, metopic, lambdoid, and sagittal sutures (Figs. 5–19, 5–20)
- Frontal bone retrusion with midsagittal ridging and bossing
- Maxillary and midfacial retrusion and hypoplasia
- Temporal ballooning

* Reed Dingman Collection.

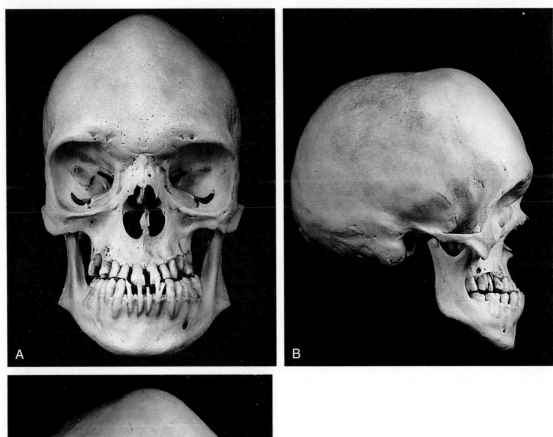

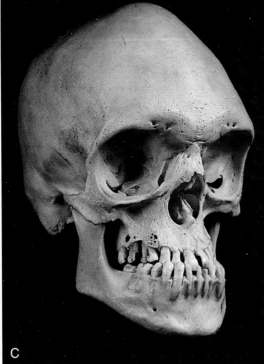

Figure 5–19. *A, B, C,* Skull #430 from Reed Dingman Collection.

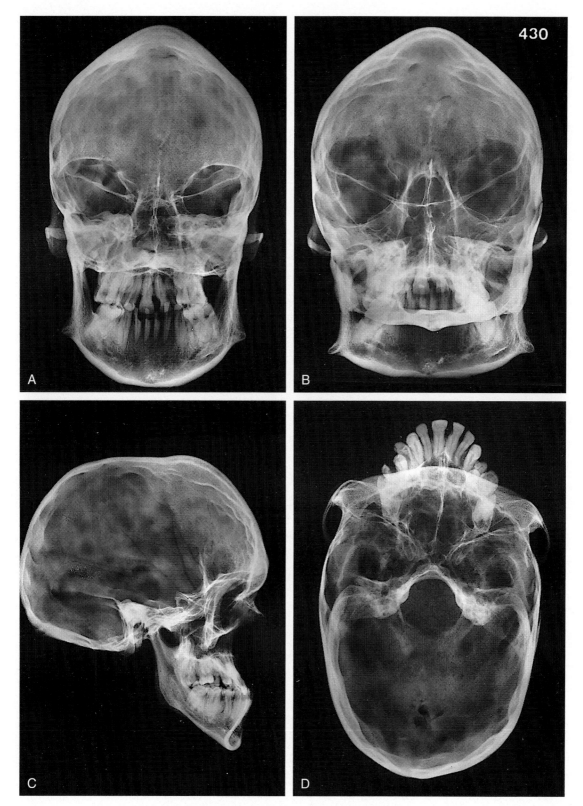

Figure 5–20. *A, B, C, D,* Radiographs of skull #430.

- Class III malocclusion, opening of mandibular gonial angle
- Short anterior cranial base
- Cranial base and sella turcica deformity (Fig. 5–20*C*)
- Digital markings (Fig. 5–20)
- Hypoplastic maxillary and frontal sinuses

Normal Findings

- Symmetric craniofacial structures
- Normal orbital cavity

Skull #161*

(Infant Skull with Holoprosencephaly, Tessier Cleft #0-14)

This cleft in the cranium appears as a lack of closure of the anterior neuropore. The cleft continues through the frontal bone (cranium bifidum, median encephalocele), midline nose, and columella and lip. The eyes may be widely separated (telorbitism), and midline structures such as the crista galli or septum may be duplicated. This cleft may also be associated with an absence of the premaxilla with arrhinencephaly, which predisposes the skull to cebocephaly, holoprosencephaly, or hypotelorism.

Abnormal Findings

- Extreme hypotelorism (Fig. 5–21A)
- Premaxillary agenesis, resulting in a midline cleft
- Absence of nasal cavity and nasal bones
- Orbital asymmetry
- Cranial asymmetry (Fig. 5–21B)
- Asymmetric, foreshortened anterior cranial base and sphenoid wing
- Trigonocephalic frontal bone with lateral sloping sides and midline ridge

Normal Findings

- Mandible

Skull #324†

(Infant Skull with Holoprosencephaly, Tessier Cleft #0-14)

Abnormal Findings

- Hypotelorism (Fig. 5–22A)
- Absence of nasal cavity and nasal bones
- Premaxillary agenesis, resulting in a midline cleft
- Trigonocephalic skull (Fig. 5–22B)
- Foreshortened anterior cranial base and sphenoid wing
- Absence of crista galli
- Foreshortened posterior cranial fossa with foramen magnum at posterior of skull

Normal Findings

- Orbital symmetry
- Mandible

---

* Anatomisch-Embryologisch Laboratorium, Amsterdam.
† Collection Rokitansky, Vienna.

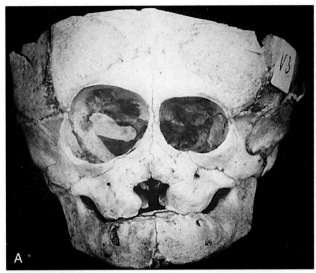

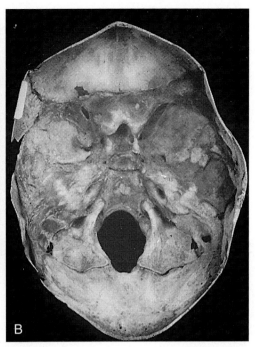

Figure 5–21. *A, B,* Skull #161 from Anatomisch-Embryologisch Laboratorium, Amsterdam.

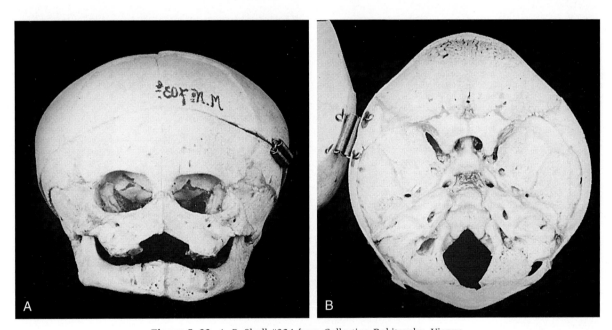

Figure 5–22. *A, B,* Skull #324 from Collection Rokitansky, Vienna.

Skull #352*

(Adult with Midline Maxillary and Palatal Clefts, Tessier Facial Cleft #0)

Abnormal Findings

- Midline maxillary cleft with agenesis of premaxillary segment (Fig. 5–23A)
- Absence of maxillary incisor teeth
- Palatal cleft (Figs. 5–23B, 5–24)
- Maxillary collapse
- Opened gonial angle of mandible (Fig. 5–23C)
- Class III malocclusion

---

* Institut für Pathologische Anatomie, Graz.

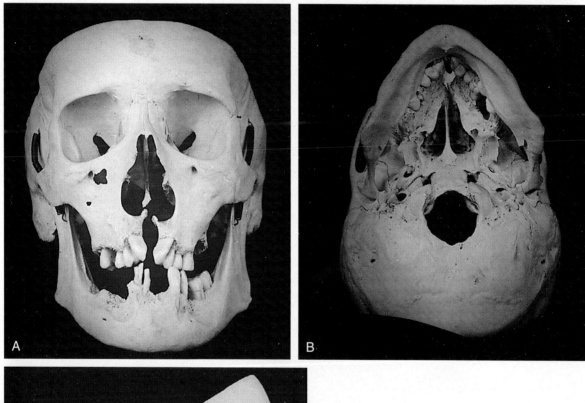

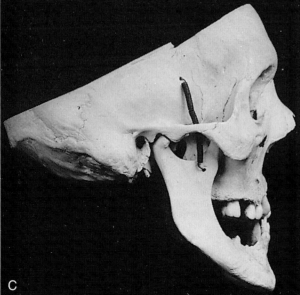

Figure 5–23. *A, B, C,* Skull #352 from Institut für Pathologische Anatomie, Graz.

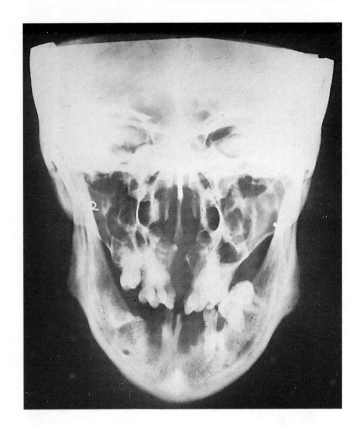

Figure 5–24. Radiograph of Skull #352.

- Maxillary retrusion
- Generalized periodontal bone loss

Normal Findings

- Interorbital distance
- Nasal cavity and septum
- Symmetry

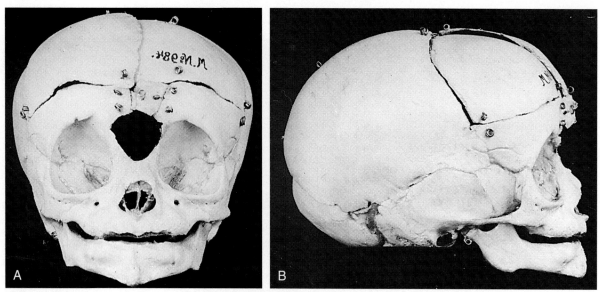

Figure 5–25. *A, B,* Skull #322 from Pathologisch-Anatomisches Bundesmuseum, Vienna.

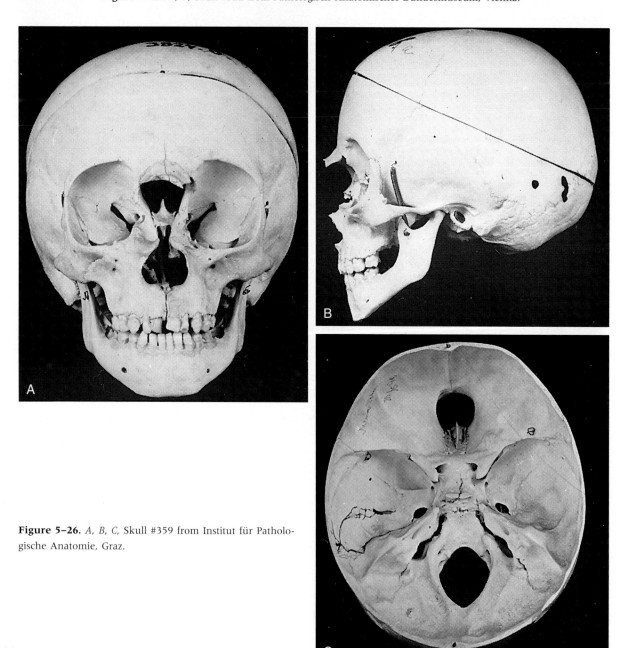

Figure 5–26. *A, B, C,* Skull #359 from Institut für Pathologische Anatomie, Graz.

Skull #322*

(Infant Skull with Encephalocele, Tessier Cleft #14)

Abnormal Findings

- Encephalocele defect in frontal bone displacing nasal cavity inferiorly (Fig. 5–25A,B)
- Oblique sphenoid, lesser wing
- Displaced nasal bones
- Abnormal orbital shape, increased vertical dimension
- Wide bifrontal dimension

Normal Findings

- Mandible

Skull #359†

(Child's Skull with Encephalocele Defect, Tessier Cleft 0-14)

Abnormal Findings

- Frontonasal encephalocele defects (Fig. 5–26A,B)
- Hourglass nasal cavity with nasal bones displaced superiorly
- Abnormal orbital shape with increased vertical dimension
- Vertical oblique orientation of lesser sphenoid wing
- Class I occlusion with crowding
- Anterior cranial base defect (Fig. 5–26C)
- Shortened cribriform plate and crista galli
- Shortened posterior fossa
- Posterior foramen magnum
- Digital markings (Fig. 5–27A,B)
- Depressed anterior cranial base and sella turcica
- Bathmocephaly

Normal Findings

- Mandible

* Pathologisch-Anatomisches Bundesmuseum, Vienna.
† Institut für Pathologische Anatomie, Graz.

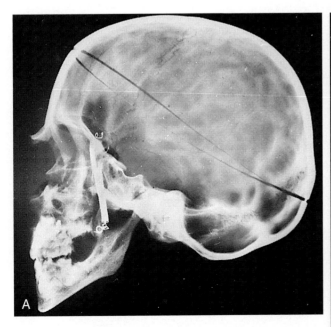
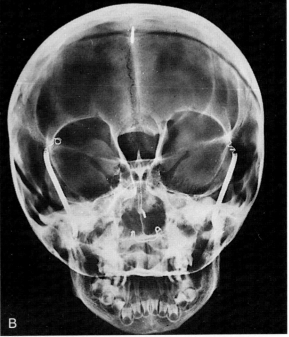

Figure 5–27. *A, B,* Radiographs of Skull #359.

Skull #312*

(Infant with Encephalocele and Bilateral Tessier Clefts #1, 13)

Paramedian craniofacial cleft extends through the frontal bone, through the olfactory groove of the cribriform plate, and between the nasal bone and the frontal process of the maxilla.

Abnormal Findings

- Paramedian encephalocele
- Defect between nasal bones and frontal process of maxilla splaying nasal bones (Fig. 5–28A,B)
- Small nasal cavity, displaced inferiorly
- Telorbitism
- Orbital cavities increased vertically
- Abnormally oriented sphenoid wings (Fig. 5–29A,B)
- Depressed sella turcica with more vertically oriented anterior cranial fossa

Normal Findings

- Mandible

Skull #160†

(Skull with Large Cleft Lip and Palate; Tessier Cleft #3 of the Hard Tissues)

Abnormal Findings

- Wide alveolar cleft (Fig. 5–30A,B)
- Cleft maxillary segment rotated in and up
- Noncleft maxillary segment rotated out and down anteriorly
- Vomer deviated to noncleft side
- Nasal bone on cleft side splaying
- Maxilla on cleft side posteriorly and laterally displaced, including pterygoid plates
- Noncleft maxillary segment rotated laterally, moving midline grossly to right

---

* Institut für Pathologische Anatomie, Graz.
† Anatomisch-Embryologisch Laboratorium, Amsterdam.

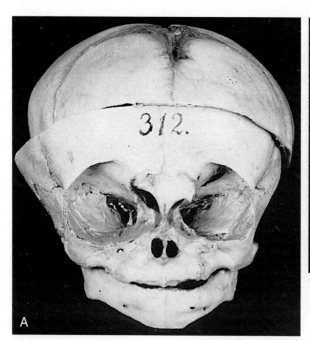

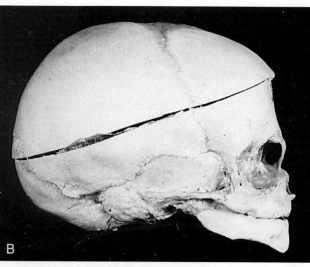

Figure 5–28. *A, B,* Skull #312 from Institut für Pathologische Anatomie, Graz.

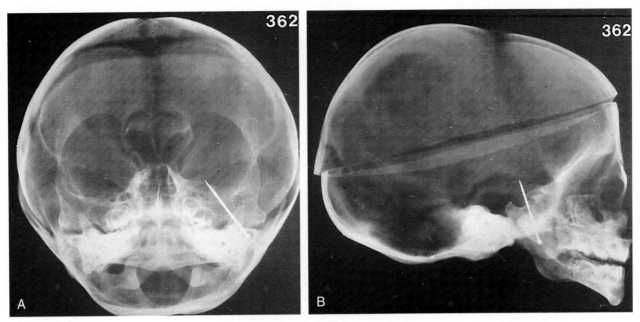

Figure 5–29. *A, B,* Radiographs of skull #312.

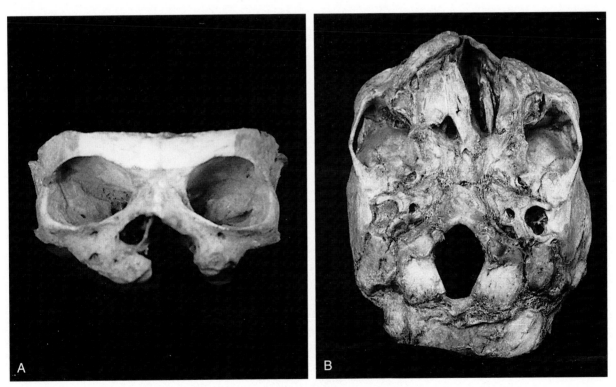

Figure 5–30. *A, B,* Skull #160 from Anatomisch-Embryologisch Laboratorium, Amsterdam.

Skull #0*

(Adult with Treacher Collins Syndrome (Franceschetti) Operated on with Zygomatic and Chin Implants[5])

Abnormal Findings

- Tessier clefts 6, 7, 8 (Fig. 5–31)
- Oblique downward-sloping orbital floors with lateral cleft, asymmetric
- Exostoses from previous zygomatic and chin implants
- Hypoplastic zygomatic processes rotated downward and in
- Asymmetric nasal cavity
- Hypoplastic (essentially absent) frontal bone component of the superior and lateral orbital rims
- Abnormal nasal bone structure and projection
- Absence of zygomatic arch and temporal processes
- Hypoplastic mandibular condyles, asymmetric
- Asymmetric projection of zygomatic processes
- Accentuated antegonial notch
- Microgenia
- Class III malocclusion
- Asymmetric projection of zygomatic processes

---

* Collection Paul Tessier, Paris.

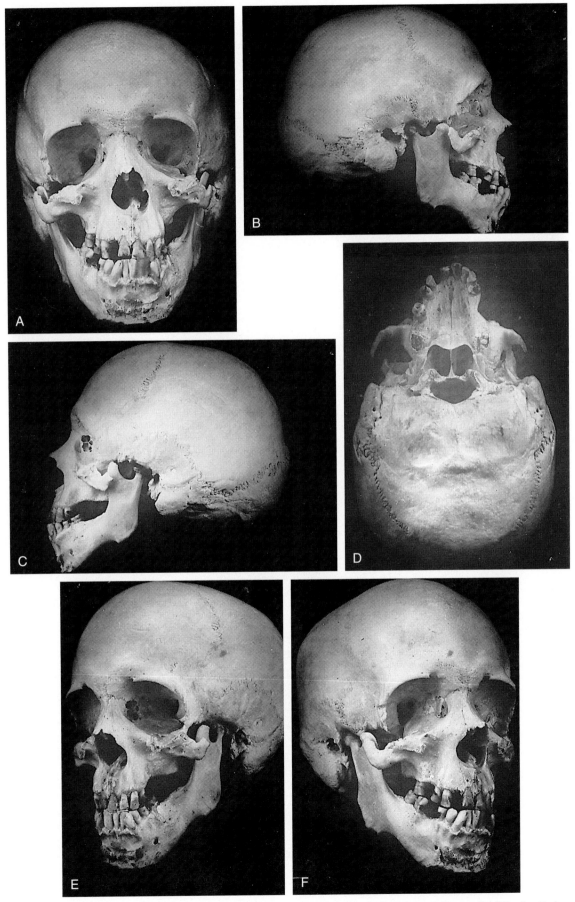

Figure 5–31. *A, B, C, D, E, F,* Treacher Collins Syndrome (Franceschetti) skull #0 from Collection Paul Tessier, Paris.

References

1. Pittman H: Diagnosis and management of craniosynostosis. Burrows Neurosurg Inst Q 1986; 2:28–40.
2. Tulasne JF, Tessier P: Analysis and late treatment of plagiocephaly: Unilateral coronal synostosis. Scand J Plast Reconstr Surg 1981; 15:257–263.
3. Tessier P: Fentes orbito-faciales verticales et obliques (colobomas) complètes et frustes. Ann Chir Plast 1969; 19:301–311.
4. Tessier P: Anatomical classification of facial, cranio-facial and laterofacial clefts. J Maxillofac Surg 1976; 4:69–92.
5. Schendel SA, Tessier P: Treacher Collins syndrome: Morphologic description of a skull with the complete form. *In* Caronni EP (ed): Craniofacial Surgery 3, pp. 394–396. Bologna: Monduzzi Editore, 1989.

II

Diagnosis and Treatment Planning

Comprehensive Team Management | 6

Ronald P. Strauss and James Henry Peter Ellis

Facial cleft and craniofacial care has often been described as optimally delivered by organized teams.[1] The advantages of such teams include their capacity to coordinate complex services, meet the psychological and social needs of families, and provide multifaceted evaluations.[2–4] As organizations, cleft/craniofacial teams have received little study as a health service. Typically cleft or craniofacial teams include medical, surgical, speech, psychosocial, and dental professionals, but large sample profiles of these organizations do not appear in the literature. Recent research on the attitudes and perspectives of team professionals[5] suggests that most teams function by consensus, even though each profession may view the needs of patients differently.

WHY TEAMWORK DEVELOPED

The literature that deals with teamwork in the delivery of health care suggests that there is little agreement on what a team is, or should be, who and what constitutes it, and what its goals and objectives are, yet there are more and more settings within which teamwork is being employed. Some studies address formal decision making and the authority structure of teams,[6] and team cost effectiveness in terms of personnel and other resources.[1]

Health care teams formed when a number of professionals and other health workers became involved in complex patient care demanding the insights and skills of various specialists. Teams, such as cleft palate or craniofacial teams, are a response to the elaboration of specialized knowledge and to the technological advances in modern medicine, which mandate that a variety of specialists become involved in the treatment of patients with facial birth defects. The availability of intensive care units and life support for newborns with craniofacial conditions has improved their survival and has resulted in increased and more specialized treatment demands on the cleft or craniofacial team.

The specialization and complexity of modern health professional practice may cause fragmentation of care, with dehumanizing implications.[7] To personalize and humanize care, health teams often include several psychosocial specialists, such as social workers, psychologists, therapists, and nurses. Commenting on the complex nature of craniofacial problems and the need for specialists to work together, Nackashi and Dixon-Wood[4] pointed out

> In chronic long-term conditions such as cleft lip and palate, the rehabilitative process is inclusive of medical, social, psychological, and vocational factors. Therefore a ''clinical team'' is required in order to provide the ''holistic'' approach to the patient or client. This is because no single discipline can provide all the needed curing and caring.

It is also increasingly realized that human problems tend to cluster[6] and need to be treated in a way that incorporates both medical and social intervention.[8] McKeganey and Bloor[9] argued that teamwork emerged particularly in those specialties in which social problems interpenetrated most strongly. Teamwork in health care delivery has evolved as a result of the recognition by health care professionals of the social and behavioral aspects of medical conditions.[10–14]

Teams have been built around the realization that all professionals, as well as patients or their agents, can make meaningful contributions to the treatment and management of craniofacial disorders or other complex health conditions. MacGregor[12] suggested that all team health care workers must demonstrate an awareness of the behavioral and social structural aspects of the sickness experience; this function cannot

130

be the exclusive concern of behavioral scientists. It has been critically important to involve family members, especially parents, in craniofacial team decision making and treatment planning.[1, 13–17] Craniofacial teams formed to efficiently meet the clinical and psychosocial needs of a complex patient population. The health outcomes of craniofacial team management have not as yet been established in the research literature, though clinicians and administrators report many advantages of team-based care over fragmented, community-based, multispecialty care.

TYPES OF TEAMS

Disagreement is evident about whether or not a health team is an identifiable social unit.[11, 18, 19] Most health teams are established and operated for particular and specialized purposes.[20–22] Specific organizational or institutional arrangements may also force some professionals to work together as a "team." [10, 18, 23]

Distinctions are drawn by some between intradisciplinary, multidisciplinary, and interdisciplinary teams.[1, 4, 11, 18, 19, 22, 24–27] The exact disciplinary composition of the team specialities may determine the categorization of a team. Furthermore, team categorization has to do with cohesiveness, level of cooperation between members, quality of relationships, and the maintenance of professional authority and autonomy.

An *intradisciplinary team* is composed of more or less similar specialists within a very narrow field of specialization, and is described as one in which ". . . each discipline is responsible for an initial independent assessment, but then information is shared and members are permitted to cross over one another's traditional role boundaries." [4] An intradisciplinary team operates with a narrow focus and ". . . is made up of people whose orientation is to one discipline, but who represent different aspects of that discipline, and differing educational levels, and who perform differing roles." [28]

Multidisciplinary teams may be specifically set up to enable a number of professionals to cooperate in a particular area while still maintaining autonomy from each other.[29, 30] Nackashi and Dixon-Wood[4] indicated that on multidisciplinary teams the members work independently because "Multidisciplinary teams . . . involve well-established, defined roles for the various professionals, with limited communication occurring among professionals on the team."

What some writers[18] refer to as multidisciplinary teams are work units in which a number of varied professionals are involved in a treatment situation. They form a loose collection of specialists treating various aspects of a patient's clustered problems without constructing mutually agreed-on plans. These are what Payne[29] preferred to call *work groups,* to be distinguished from a *collaborative team:* "A work group exists when people are brought into relationships with one another by virtue of the fact that they work together; but they do not share work tasks or responsibilities, and they do not use the fact that they work together to enhance the work they are doing." [29]

In proclaiming the virtues of *interdisciplinary teams* over multidisciplinary teams, Day[11] claimed that "A multidisciplinary approach can occur as a series of isolated evaluations by several disciplines and does not imply the merger of evaluative insights or the shared development of a treatment plan, hallmarks of a functional interdisciplinary team." An interdisciplinary team is therefore one in which a number of professionals from related, but not necessarily similar, disciplines are involved in conducting a joint evaluation and developing a treatment plan in which expertise is pooled and decision making is collective.[1, 11] Nackashi and Dixon-Wood[4] commented: "Interdisciplinary teams . . . meet often to plan assessment, . . . each professional performs assessment independent of those done by colleagues. This is followed by sharing of findings, recommendations for intervention, and the preparation of a single report incorporating all recommendations."

Such joint construction of a treatment plan may be actualized by an interdisciplinary team in which all members examine the patient, then representatives of the disciplines discuss findings and negotiate a plan of action based on interaction across professional lines. The team leader serves to facilitate and coordinate the treatment plan, and then he or she communicates this plan to the patient and the family.

TEAM STRUCTURE AND PROFESSIONAL AUTHORITY

The literature deals with team organizations by describing a dichotomy of "hierarchical" and "egalitarian" structures.[1,6] Authors such as Horwitz[26] distinguish between a "leader centered coordinated" team and a "fraternally oriented integrated" team. Others such as Logan and McKendry[22] compare "hierarchical" and "participative" teams. It would appear that teams may be divided into those that have a structured hierarchy of authority and power, and those that have shared authority with power allocated to the group. Hierarchical teams may be considered efficient because individual disciplines can maintain autonomy and conflicts are limited, whereas egalitarian teams allow for joint participation and decision making.[1] Webb and Hobdell[31] recognized the variable composition of health care teams and different skills involved, as they distinguished a "collegial team of coequal individualists," a "specialized collegial" team, an "apprenticeship" team (as in a training hospital), and a "complex" team.

There are important implications of team structure on team communication and cooperation. Multidisciplinary teams are often assumed to be hierarchical and interdisciplinary teams are assumed to be egalitarian in nature. Temkin-Greener[18] questioned the existence of egalitarian structured interdisciplinary teams, claiming that the structure of teams merely reflects traditional role and status arrangements in which physicians dominate. Bardach and associates[30] also regarded certain medical specialists as "cornerstones" of the team, whereas others are portrayed as contributing less central, but necessary, "support and treatment." The ability to communicate between disparate professions defines team function: "The ideal team interaction results in team members who not only learn about the other involved disciplines, but who can communicate comfortably in terms allowing for a unified frame of reference in regard to the patient/client."[4]

The role of the physician/surgeon is often critical to the function of health care teams. Some may expect that physicians will dominate on health care teams.[6] For instance, on a surgical operating team a hierarchy of professionals may be engaged, but ultimate authority and decision making is vested in the surgeon.[8] Medical interests are dominant on operating surgical teams, which are ". . . groups of people oriented to narrow and specific tasks, in which the doctor is the acknowledged expert, and they work under his direction. This is not to say that there are not occupational conflicts of various kinds but the ground tends to be undercut by the specificity of the work."[8]

It is suggested by some[8, 18, 26, 30, 31] that even on so-called egalitarian teams, medical professional interests will prevail. A contradiction often occurs between the stated ideals and the pragmatic implementation of a team program: ". . . sharing of power and a democratization of relationships among co-workers may be advocated, but if in a particular operating setting a convincing argument can be made that a hierarchical structure ensures more effective performance, that is the structure likeliest to be instituted. Authority may be shared to a degree, but the decision-making power commonly is more or less concentrated."[26]

The dominance of medical interests is usually accounted for by its traditional authority and its status as an archetype of modern professions.[6] The effects of medical training, the doctor-patient relationship, and the bureaucratic structure and technological nature of hospitals and medical schools reinforce status and power relationships on teams.[8, 18, 26] The fact that medical professionals have predominantly been males from higher socioeconomic backgrounds may play a role in maintaining this position.[8] In contrast, the assumed subservient and auxiliary roles of other professions are sometimes defined in limited terms on health care teams.[32–34] The interdisciplinary team may present a direct challenge to physician dominance as it emphasizes "role blurring" in teams as a ". . . recognition that each team member brings many individual attributes which may be determined more by personality and interests than by professional training."[27]

This does not mean that differences between the specialists are completely eliminated with respect to roles. The needs of legal and ethical accountability mandate the specificity of discipline roles and a clear division of labor with the identification of boundaries and common goals.[1,22] Ambiguity when role expectations are not clearly defined may lead to team conflict. The need for shared understanding and acceptance of role definitions is important to health care team function.[6, 19, 22, 26] A lack of such understanding can cause suspicion about other specialists and their methods.[36]

Some writers argue that group decisions are often made unilaterally by team leaders because of the hierarchical structure of teams.[6, 18, 30, 32] Others have found that joint decision making takes place where teams have more egalitarian and collegial structures and when there is sharing of common knowledge with colleagues and a willingness to learn about other disciplines.[1, 19, 22, 35] In order to achieve interdisciplinary function it is necessary that communicative openness and a shared vocabulary exists,[19, 36] as stated by Koepp-Baker: "The disquietude and restiveness often produced by specialistic jargon and vocabulary are reduced as the members of a team are required to simplify their language in order to affect the minds, actions, and feelings of specialists in a different field who are engaged in the same quest."[2] The same author also argued that the ". . . inescapable interdependence (in teamwork) demands/requires reductions and adjustments of individual and group dominances, and makes new subordinations necessary for a coordination of effort."[2] Where the formulation of a joint plan of action is the desired team goal, as is favored in interdisciplinary teams, it appears as if insistence on the dominance of one speciality can become counterproductive.

TEAM IDEOLOGY

Shared values relative to team operation and objectives are common on health care teams, providing guidelines for team members: "These norms are often unspoken and mandate appropriate behavior, regular attendance at team meetings and functions, contributions to the team, and use of team discussions for relevant material in a nonmonopolizing manner. In some cases insensitive team members may not be aware of these unspoken guidelines and the result is team interaction difficulties."[4]

Kane[27] found a strong shared ideology in 42% of 229 multidisciplinary teams studied in the United States. Team ideology may reflect the interests, values, and norms of dominant specialties or of particular individuals. It may also be the result of an interaction process that had incorporated the perspectives of the different disciplines, along with such values as egalitarianism, democracy, consensual decision making, mutual respect, and shared role definitions.[1, 11, 19, 21]

Team ideology may also reflect an emphasis on *process* or on *outcomes*. An emphasis on process involves a within-team focus on institutional demands, professional protocol, peer expectations, and team communication practices, while a focus on outcomes primarily considers how to best meet the needs and desires of patients/ clients. The latter thus constitutes a patient-centered ideology. When teams become process focused, they may become overly concerned with their internal relations and operations, resulting in inefficient operations that may not meet the needs of the patient. Webb and Hobdell[31] suggested two ways to ensure a patient-centered ideological orientation: (a) *"Consumer sovereignty"* helps to avoid the tendency to treat patients or clients as passive receivers of services or in isolation from their immediate social world. This is done through ". . . far greater attentiveness than is customary to the patient's or client's own definition of their needs, or the resources which they can muster . . . and to the patient's or client's satisfaction with the treatment received."[31] (b) *"Authority of relevance"* is the recognition that a variety of types of information are necessary for team decisions and that no single profession is so comprehensive in its scope that it can provide all the answers. If this orientation is part of team ideology, interaction is focused on the patient rather than on parochial professional interests.

When a number of members from different occupational groups have been cooperating in a limited way, teamwork may become a way to improve that cooperation.[29] Even highly formal teams, such as surgical operating teams, may develop informal patterns of cooperation, a sense that you "just know" that you have to cooperate with the rest of team in order to be able to meet your own responsibilities. Functional cooperation is therefore an essential element of team function: "At the heart of the concept of interdisciplinary teamwork is the joining of essentially dissimilar skills which colleagues in diverse occupations bring to bear upon different aspects of a common problem."[26]

It is generally argued that cooperation fosters a high level of solidarity or camaraderie in teams that interact frequently and informally.[26] Chief contributors are such interaction elements as common values, communication skills, openness, shared vocabulary, willingness to learn, consensual decision making, mutual respect for colleagues, informality, and humor.[11, 19, 21, 26, 36] Professional competence, as well as institutional support, are also important elements of cooperation in health care teamwork.

Team morale has been hypothesized as linked to patient satisfaction as an outcome measure of team function, but Kane[27] found no relationship between client and team member satisfaction. Merkel[37] also reported no significant relationship between actual patient satisfaction and physician perceptions of patient satisfaction, suggesting that measuring how satisfied patients are might not be a good index of team satisfaction and morale. The forces that bring cohesiveness to a team are as follows: "patient needs, institutional support, satisfaction with effective work, respect and friendship, and an understanding of the diagnostic process. Forces that tear a team apart include contradictory institutional practices, professional rivalries, misunderstanding the role of patient splitting, personal competitiveness and lack of understanding of the collaborative problem solving process."[21]

LEADERSHIP IN TEAMWORK

Leadership on health care teams can vary according to the nature of the team, the problem(s) dealt with, the institutional setup, personal leadership style, and personality. Some writers argue that these personal aspects are less important and that leadership should be viewed rather as a function than as a personal characteristic. Horwitz[26] viewed team leadership primarily as "facilitating the achievement of common goals." Margolis and Fiorelli[19] also viewed the leader as an "impartial facilitator" who ensures efficiency in the team's operation. Some authors[22] referred to a coordinator, rather than a leader, whose role should be clearly distinguished from the professional roles on the team, to avoid domination. Leadership can also be granted to the person who serves as the administrator of the team.

In some craniofacial team settings, team leadership is rotated between disciplines and their various members.[1, 26] This style of rotated leadership may reduce interprofessional barriers and assist in diminishing professional status hierarchies. The sharing of the position of team leader ensures that all disciplines experience centrality and are challenged by the necessity to develop interprofessional dialogue at the team conference.

Team leadership often implies the ability to resolve team conflict. Conflicts resulting from the structural constraints of a team organization can be dealt with by a team leader who can arbitrate conflicting positions[38]; however, conflicts that reflect larger interprofessional rivalries or "turf battles" may be more difficult to resolve on a local basis. On teams in which plastic surgeons, otolaryngologists, oral-maxillofacial surgeons, craniofacial surgeons, neurosurgeons, and ophthalmologists must negotiate their specific boundaries and responsibilities, conflicts may occur over the division of labor in patient care. The team leader must recognize such conflicts, but their resolution may actually depend upon the role definitions of the specific professionals involved and the "turf" definitions supported by their professional associations. Some hold that allowing autonomy to individual professions can avoid actual conflicts and avoid time consuming efforts to resolve conflicts.[30]

The team interaction approach to conflict resolution empowers the leader to facilitate team members in the settling of their differences, thus reducing role clashes, conflicting professional judgments, class, and gender differences.[1, 19, 21, 22] Conflict within the team and in team deliberations may be natural, inevitable, and productive. The expression of conflict may, if carefully managed, enhance the probability of choosing superior patient care plans and problem solutions.[19]

EVALUATING CLEFT PALATE AND CRANIOFACIAL TEAMS AS ORGANIZATIONS

Over the past 4 years an initiative has occurred to develop standards for types of teams to use in a team directory.[39] This effort has included a group of leading speech pathologists, orthodontists, general dentists, otolaryngologists, plastic surgeons, oral-maxillofacial surgeons, pediatric dentists, geneticist-pediatricians, psychologists, and nurses. Although at this moment the deliberations remain in draft form, two types of teams have been suggested for delineation. The two types of teams are the cleft palate team and the craniofacial team. In this chapter we review the basic kinds of measures that may be utilized in analyzing teams and examine whether there are basic features of effective cleft or craniofacial teams.

In evaluating a team, one would need to consider when the team formed. Teams that are in their first 5 years of evolution may remain in the formative stages of their development and cannot be evaluated with the same criteria as would more mature organizations. Another basic feature of a team relates to whether a craniofacial group or team operates as a separate organization from a given medical center's cleft palate group or team. When the two types of teams coexist or function in combined form, evaluation of how the organization responds to the needs of patients with complex craniofacial conditions may differ from evaluation of its approach to the needs of patients with a cleft lip or palate.

There are a variety of questions that might be asked about a given team's function that will provide basic data with which to understand its scope of care and patient load. Such questions include

1. The number of times the team meets face-to-face in a year
2. The number of new patients the team sees for evaluation in a year
3. The number of patients the team has in active treatment and/or routine follow-up
4. The number of initial surgical repairs of a cleft lip done by the team in a year
5. The number of initial surgical repairs of a cleft palate done by the team in a year
6. The number of maxillary/mandibular (orthognathic) osteotomy operations done by a team in a year
7. The number of intracranial operations done for patients with craniofacial conditions by the team in a year

In addition, one would want to examine structural aspects of quality assurance, such as

1. Whether the team systematically collects and stores clinical data on its patient population
2. Whether the team has a quality assurance program to measure treatment outcomes

Many professionals would suggest that, in general, the quality of care increases with the amount of experience the team has. The issue of whether numbers of procedures or patients equates to quality of team services is often debated. Most observers would conclude that a basic level of activity is necessary to ensure professional and team competence but that this is not a guarantee of quality. In considering team function, many professionals have argued that a baseline level of team and professional activity is required for effective care delivery; below that baseline it is unlikely that sufficient skill can be maintained. The actual numbers of *baseline* patients cared for or of procedures may be controversial, but the need for criteria has been generally accepted.

The Cleft Palate Team

The *cleft palate team* may be defined as a team of professionals who provide coordinated and interdisciplinary evaluation and treatment to patients with cleft lip and/or cleft palate. As a minimum a cleft palate team's professional group would include an actively involved surgeon, pediatric dentist or orthodontist, primary care physician (pediatrician, family physician, or general internist in the community or on the team), and speech-language pathologist. This core group of professionals would have education, training, and experience to have adequately prepared them for the performance of cleft palate care. Furthermore, the cleft palate team should support, encourage, or offer continuing education in cleft/craniofacial care for its members.

A cleft palate team should meet face to face for regularly scheduled meetings for treatment planning and case review, with a minimum of six meeting times per year. Such team meetings have been seen to benefit from professional input from at least four specialties, which are actually in attendance. The interaction between disciplinesis likely to result in improved treatment plans and more coordination between providers.

In considering the minimal range of professionals to develop a team treatment plan, one would expect that all patients evaluated by a cleft palate team would be seen by a surgeon, a primary care physician (pediatrician, family physician, or general internist in the community or on the team), a pediatric dentist or an orthodontist, and a speech-language pathologist. Additional professionals are often included on cleft palate teams or may be accessed by referral or through consultation. Cleft palate teams that evaluate at least 50 new or recall patients with cleft lip-palate in a year may be seen as generating sufficient experience to maintain professional skills and team function. For teams in rural areas, it may not be possible to see this number of patients, and careful attention will be required to ensure that patients in such settings receive comprehensive care and appropriate referral for procedures or evaluations that depend on specially honed skills.

Surgical skills are particularly difficult to maintain in the absence of activity, with some using the term *rusty hands* to describe surgeons who do not perform a basic number of procedures for a given population. Some would maintain that a surgeon on a cleft palate team should operate on 10 or more patients for primary repairs of a cleft lip and/or cleft palate in a year in order to remain at a high level of skill. Similarly, for patients requiring facial skeletal surgery, some have maintained that the cleft palate team should have, or should refer patients to, a surgeon whose education, training, and experience has adequately prepared him or her to provide facial skeletal surgery (bone graft, orthognathic surgery) and who does at least 10 orthognathic surgical procedures in a year. The cleft palate team also should have at least one surgeon who attends all the team meetings and who is adequately prepared for the diagnosis and treatment of patients with cleft lip-palate.

For patients requiring orthognathic treatment, the cleft palate team would have an orthodontist well prepared for the provision of orthognathic treatment. All orthognathic surgical treatments should be documented with preoperative and postoperative dental study models, facial and intraoral photographs, and cephalometric radiographs. In all cases of persons with cleft lip and palate, orthognathic surgical planning and outcomes should be routinely discussed at the cleft palate team meetings. Cleft palate teams depend on the presence of an orthodontist who attends all the team meetings and who is well qualified in the treatment of patients with cleft lip and palate. Such orthodontists would be likely to provide comprehensive orthodontic care for at least 10 patients with cleft lip-palate over the course of a year. Pediatric dentists and prosthodontists may serve to evaluate and treat dental conditions associated with the cleft.

Cleft palate teams should have a speech-language pathologist who attends team meetings and who is educated and equipped to diagnose and treat patients with cleft lip-palate. One speech-language pathologist on each team should optimally have provided speech therapy and/or a speech and language evaluation to a minimum of 10 patients with cleft lip-palate over the course of a year. On a cleft palate team, the speech-language pathologist routinely performs a structured speech assessment during team evaluations and uses clinical speech instrumentation (such as endoscopy, pressure flow, videofluoroscopy, etc.) to assess velopharyngeal function when indicated.

Evaluations with a cleft palate team routinely should include a screening hearing test. When a hearing loss is detected, patients should be referred to an otolaryngologist for examination, consultation, or treatment. Hearing evaluation routinely includes a test by an audiologist and an ear examination by an otolaryngologist before 1 year of age. The team *otolaryngologist* should have adequate preparation in the diagnosis and treatment of patients with cleft lip-palate.

The psychological and social issues related to facial clefting suggest that the team have a psychologist, clinical social worker, or other mental health professional who evaluates all patients on a regular basis. Furthermore, the team should routinely test or screen patients for learning disabilities and developmental, psychological, and language skills. Cleft palate teams benefit from routinely collecting school reports and other information relative to learning in school-age patients. The team should use a nurse or other trained professional who regularly provides supportive counseling and instruction (feeding, developmental) to interested parents of newborns. The team also should seek to sponsor or regularly make referrals to a parent support group or parent network in the community, as desired by families. The regular provision of supportive counseling and instruction to interested parents and patients preoperatively and postoperatively is a positive of effective cleft palate teams.

The involvement of primary care physicians on the team (pediatrician, family physician, or general internist) may be of great importance in detecting and responding to health problems of team patients. The regular attendance at team meetings of a primary care physician also assists in linking to community providers. On a cleft palate team, clinic and team reports are routinely sent to the patient's care providers in the community (schools, health department, local professionals) with the family's permission.

The cleft palate team should also provide formal genetic counseling or a clinical genetic evaluation for parents or patients who desire such evaluation.

All cleft palate teams should keep a central and shared file on each patient. The clinical files or records of the cleft palate team should routinely include

1. One or more diagnoses
2. A complete medical history
3. A treatment plan or goals that are reviewed periodically
4. A social and psychological history
5. Dental and orthodontic findings and history
6. Intraoral dental casts on patients, when indicated
7. Facial photographs on patients in treatment or evaluation
8. Lateral cephalometric radiographs (or the equivalent) on patients, when indicated

After a cleft palate team evaluation, the patient and family should routinely have an opportunity to ask questions and discuss the treatment plan with a team representative. Furthermore, the team routinely (for each evaluation) should write reports or summary letters, containing a treatment plan, to the family. The cleft palate team routinely provides case management (follow-up, referral, and coordination of care) and benefits advocacy/assistance (help families obtain financial or programmatic support), as needed. In order to function, it should have an office and coordinator or secretary.

The Craniofacial Team

The *craniofacial team* may be defined as a clinical group that provides coordinated and interdisciplinary evaluation and treatment for patients with a range of craniofacial anomalies or syndromes. In a very specific definition, craniofacial anomalies or syndromes may be defined as those conditions other than cleft lip-palate (unless cleft lip-palate is a feature of another condition) that are treated with craniofacial surgery. The American Cleft Palate-Craniofacial Association has developed a definition in consultation with other organizations that states that ''craniofacial surgery consists of the diagnosis, treatment planning, and surgical procedures in which the *intracranial approach to the midfacial segment* (including the orbit and/or supraorbital rim) is used.'' Given this limited definition of craniofacial procedures and thus craniofacial teams, it is important to consider characteristic elements needed for craniofacial team function. In most basic ways, the craniofacial team record and operation have characteristics of the cleft palate team, as discussed earlier.

On the craniofacial team, the operating surgeon, orthodontist, mental health professional, and speech-language pathologist would meet face to face at scheduled team meetings or conferences to evaluate patients with craniofacial anomalies or syndromes. Such meetings would optimally occur at least six times per year; meetings may coincide with cleft palate team meetings, although this is not always the case. Craniofacial teams generally see at least 20 patients with craniofacial anomalies or syndromes for evaluation over the course of a year. They always have a primary care physician (pediatrician, family physician, general internist) evaluate all patients before surgery. Craniofacial team facilities should have a pediatric intensive care unit.

Craniofacial teams fully document all craniofacial surgical treatments with preoperative and postoperative radiographs, facial photographs, and, where applicable, intraoral photographs. Craniofacial treatment plans and treatment outcomes (results) for all patients with craniofacial anomalies or syndromes are discussed at team meetings. The team surgeon attends all the team meetings and is educated, trained, and has experience in the diagnosis and treatment of patients requiring craniofacial surgery. The number of craniofacial surgical procedures required for a surgeon to maintain his or her skill level is unclear, but various professional organizations have suggested that at least one surgeon on the team provide craniofacial (as defined earlier) surgical treatment for a minimum of 10 to 20 patients with craniofacial anomalies or syndromes in a year.

The craniofacial team also has an orthodontist who attends all the team meetings and who is well qualified to treat patients with craniofacial anomalies or syndromes; indeed, at least one orthodontist should provide orthodontic evaluation or treatment for at least 10 patients with craniofacial anomalies or syndromes over a year.

In many regards, the craniofacial team possesses the baseline characteristics of the cleft palate team, with some additional expertise and focus. The speech-language pathologist should attend all the team meetings and similarly requires preparation in speech and language diagnosis and treatment of patients with craniofacial anomalies or syndromes. The craniofacial team also requires a mental health professional (psychologist, social worker, developmental pediatrician, psychiatrist) who attends all the team meetings. A nurse or other trained professional regularly provides supportive counseling and instruction (feeding, developmental) to interested parents of newborns.

In comparison with the cleft palate team, the craniofacial team must have a neurosurgeon adequately prepared for the neurosurgical diagnosis and treatment of patients with craniofacial anomalies or syndromes, and who can provide examination, treatment, and consultation for patients with craniofacial anomalies or syndromes. It also would have an otolaryngologist and ophthalmologist, who would be likewise qualified and involved. Routine hearing/ear and eye evaluations are part of the craniofacial team assessment. The team also uses a radiologist specialized in radiological evaluation of patients with craniofacial anomalies or syndromes and who has a facility with computed tomography capability and access to magnetic resonance imaging.

The craniofacial team generally also has a qualified and specifically trained pediatric dentist/general dentist/prosthodontist, audiologist, and geneticist. Craniofacial teams provide formal genetic counseling or a clinical genetic evaluation for parents or patients who desire such evaluation.

In addition to cleft palate and craniofacial teams, there are *evaluation and treatment review* teams that function solely as evaluation centers or treatment review/planning panels or boards, and in which members do not generally serve as the providers of clinical care or treatment. In low-population states or areas, teams may not easily fit into the typology previously reviewed. For example, in the United States such teams are generally found in the states with populations of less than 2 million persons and where there is a mean population density of less than 30 persons/square mile. These teams may use regional referral networks and sometimes are composed of fewer core professionals.

1991 SURVEY OF U.S. AND CANADIAN CLEFT/CRANIOFACIAL TEAMS

In 1991 a survey was done to examine cleft/craniofacial team organization, team services, and quality assurance. The survey was a comprehensive and national survey of cleft/craniofacial teams. Small sample or focused studies have been previously reported.[5, 40–46] A mailed self-administered questionnaire was sent to all 237 cleft/craniofacial teams that are listed in the Team Directory of the American Cleft Palate-Craniofacial Association. This directory is updated on an annual basis and is considered to include a complete listing of all U.S. and Canadian teams. The questionnaire was sent to team clinical directors or leaders. Of the 237 teams contacted, 224 responded with completed questionnaires, a response rate of 94.5%. One hundred ninety-four of the teams responding were in the United States. The questionnaire collected as yet unpublished data on (1) the team director and the team organization, (2) levels and scope of team services, (3) team membership, and (4) 31 quality parameters of cleft palate team organization of care.

The responding team clinical and team leaders were most commonly physicians (60.7%, N = 136), with plastic surgeons being the most highly represented specialty (N = 107). Team clinical directors were most commonly male (80.4%, N = 176) and generally were members of only one such team (80.6%, N = 179). Nearly half (49.1%, N = 108) of the directors spend 30% or more of their work effort in cleft/

craniofacial care. Relatively few team directors (10.9%, N = 24) spend less than 10% of their effort in cleft/craniofacial care.

It was noted that cleft/craniofacial teams fall into two main categories: most teams (83.5%) deliver direct clinical care to patients, while other teams (16.5%) serve only as review boards that plan care but do not provide clinical services. At most medical centers cleft and craniofacial care is delivered by one team (76.8%), although some centers have independent craniofacial teams. Teams were well distributed across the United States, one in five (20.1%) serve a predominantly rural population, and some (16%) are located in states or provinces with populations of less than 2,000,000.

The most common defining feature of teams was face-to-face group meetings, and the mean number of such meetings in a year was 20 meetings. The range of team meeting frequency is shown on Table 6–1, part A. More than two out of three teams meet over 10 times per year. The mean number of new patients per year was 63 patients. While few teams saw more than 100 new patients (13.7%) per year, there were nearly a third of teams (31.4%) with fewer than 20 new patients per year. The mean number of active and follow-up patients was 319 patients, as shown on Table 6–1, part C. A substantial range was noted, with some teams (10.4%) having 40 or less such patients and others (17.9%) having more than 450 such patients.

It was noted (Table 6–2, part A) that more than 95% of such teams evaluated and treated patients with cleft lip, cleft palate, and velopharyngeal incompetence in a year. Teams were less likely to treat handicapping malocclusions, hemifacial microsomia, and craniosynostosis disorders. Team surgical activity varied, but teams performed a mean of 20 to 25 procedures for initial cleft lip repair, initial cleft palate repair, and maxillary or mandibular osteotomies in a year. It should be noted that a minority of teams performed five or less such procedures in a year. A specific query relative to intracranial operations showed that most teams (59.8%) had not done this procedure in a year, whereas a small group of teams (13.4%) have done this 20 or more times (Table 6–2, part A). It is interesting to note that most of the teams studied label themselves as cleft palate teams (90.6%). One third of teams (N = 74) also considered themselves craniofacial teams. A small number (N = 13) of teams did not feel they fit any categories.

This survey provides a starting place for health services research relative to cleft/craniofacial teams. The sample used was large and the response rate was unusually

Table 6–1. ORGANIZATIONAL CHARACTERISTICS OF
CLEFT/CRANIOFACIAL TEAMS

	%	N
Part A: Face-to-face team meetings in a year		
10 or less	28.5%	64
11–20	40.6%	91
21–50	26.8%	60
>50	4.0%	9
Part B: New team patients in a year		
10 or less	12.3%	27
11–20	19.1%	42
21–50	37.7%	83
51–100	17.3%	38
101–200	10.5%	23
>200	3.2%	7
Part C: Total number of active and follow-up team patients		
40 or less	10.4%	22
41–100	20.3%	43
101–250	33.0%	70
251–450	18.4%	39
>450	17.9%	38
Part D: Attendance at team meetings: Team members attending ¾ or more of the team meetings		
0–2 members	6.5%	10
3–8 members	35.5%	55
9–20 members	51.6%	80
>20 members	6.5%	10

Table 6–2. SCOPE OF CARE AND SURGICAL ACTIVITY

Part A: Diagnosis of Patients Treated in a Year	Percent of Teams Evaluating and Treating in a Year
Cleft lip	96.0%
Cleft palate	96.4%
Cleft lip and palate	96.4%
Velopharyngeal incompetence	95.5%
Handicapped malocclusion	83.9%
Pierre Robin sequence	91.5%
Hemifacial microsomia	75.0%
Craniosynostosis disorders	58.0%

Part B: Team Surgical Activity in a Year	Mean Number of Procedures/Team	Percent of Teams With 5 or Fewer Procedures/Year
Initial cleft lip repair	21.5	17.1% (34)
Initial surgical palatal repair	25.0	13.6% (27)
Maxillary/mandibular osteotomy	21.1	34.9% (66)

Part C: Frequency of Intracranial Operations for Craniofacial Conditions in a Year	
Not performed in a year	59.8% (134)
Performed 1–19 times	26.8% (60)
Performed 20 or more times	13.4% (30)

high. Profiles of cleft and craniofacial teams allow individual teams to examine their characteristics in comparison with teams at other institutions.

FUTURE PERSPECTIVES ON TEAM CARE DELIVERY

As the U.S. health system changes, it is predictable that increasing attention will be directed toward the rationale and value of cleft and craniofacial teams. Health planners are likely to ask

1. How can cleft/craniofacial teams be most productive?
2. Are limitations on the numbers of cleft/craniofacial teams in a region effective in controlling cost and improving the quality of care?
3. Is team care more cost effective than fragmented care? Does it result in improved outcomes for patients?
4. What constitutes a minimal team? an excellent team?

The ability for teams to provide answers to such questions will define the future for the cleft and craniofacial team. The scientific study of cleft and craniofacial teams as organizations is an important, and largely undeveloped, field of inquiry. Decisions about funding of team-based care will be made based upon evidence that cost-conscious and comprehensive care can most effectively be provided through the cleft/craniofacial team.

Team-based health care delivery may have the capacity to further integrate patient and family concerns into health deliberations and decisions. At some cleft palate and craniofacial centers, parents and patients are included in the team conference as members of the team, directly articulating their perspectives to the group. This concept has been based on the perception that parents and patients have a right to hear all discussions that relate to their care and to directly observe clinical uncertainties and controversies. Some observers have noted that complex social, marital, and psychological issues may not be discussed with the parents or patient in the room. Others have felt that parents cannot engage in a meaningful discussion with numbers of professionals, rather they benefit from private, face-to-face opportunities to ask questions and discuss treatment plans with a designated team representative. In the future it is likely that teams will be further appreciated as a vehicle to improve consumer involvement in personal health care decisions.

Cleft and craniofacial teams are widely seen as an effective means to avoid fragmentation and dehumanization in the delivery of highly specialized health care. Comprehensive cleft and craniofacial team management presents an organizational model that may prove applicable to other areas of health service delivery in the future.

References

1. Strauss RP, Broder H: Interdisciplinary team care of cleft lip and palate: Social and psychological aspects. Clin Plast Surg 1985; 12:543.
2. Koepp-Baker H: The craniofacial team. *In* Bzoch KR (ed): Communicative Disorders Related to Cleft Lip and Palate, 2nd ed, pp 52–61. Boston: Little, Brown, 1979.
3. Morris HL, Jakobi P, Harrington D: Editorial. Objectives and criteria for the management of cleft lip and palate and the delivery of management services. Cleft Palate J 1978; 15:1.
4. Nackashi JA, Dixon-Wood VL: The craniofacial team: Medical supervision and coordination. *In* Bzoch KR (ed): Communicative Disorders Related to Cleft Lip and Palate, 3rd ed, pp 63–74. Boston: Little, Brown, 1989.
5. Noar JH: A questionnaire survey of attitudes and concerns of three professional groups involved in the cleft palate team. Cleft Palate Craniofac J 1992; 29:92.
6. Nagi SS: Teamwork in health care in the United States: A sociological perspective. Milbank Memorial Fund Quarterly, Health and Society 1975; 53:75.
7. Feinstein AR: Editorial: On the coordination of care. J Chronic Dis 1983; 36:813.
8. Dingwall R: Problems of teamwork in primary care. *In* Lonsdale S, Webb A, Briggs TL (eds): Teamwork in the Personal Social Services and Health Care, p 111. London: Croom Helm, 1980.
9. McKeganey NP, Bloor MJ: Teamwork, information control and therapeutic effectiveness: A tale of two therapeutic communities. Sociol Health Illness 1987; 9:154.
10. Cluff CB, Cluff LF: Informal support for disabled persons: A role for religious and community organizations. J Chron Dis 1983; 36:815.
11. Day DW: Perspectives on care: The interdisciplinary team approach. Otolaryngol Clin North Am 1981; 14:769.
12. MacGregor FC: Foreword. Social psychological considerations in plastic surgery. Past, present and future. Clin Plast Surg 1982; 9:283.
13. Brantley HT, Clifford E: Cognitive self-concept and body image measures of normal, cleft palate, and obese adolescents. Cleft Palate J 1979; 16:177.
14. Day DW: Genetics of congenital lip defects. Clin Plast Surg 1984; 11:693.
15. Hill MJ: An investigation of the attitudes and information possessed by parents of children with clefts of the lip and palate. Cleft Palate Bull 1956; 6:3.
16. MacDonald SK: Parental needs and professional responses: A parental perspective. Cleft Palate J 1979; 16:188.
17. Phillips J, Whitaker LA: The social effects of cranofacial deformity and its correction. Cleft Palate J 1979; 16:7.
18. Temkin-Greener H: Interprofessional perspectives on teamwork in health care: A case-study. Milbank Memorial Fund Quarterly 1983; 61:641.
19. Margolis H, Fiorelli JS: An applied approach to facilitating interdisciplinary teamwork. J Rehabil 1984; 50:13–17.
20. Campbell LS, Whitenack DC: An interdisciplinary approach for consultation on multiproblem patients. NC Med J 1983; 44:81.
21. Nason F: Diagnosing the hospital team. Social Work Health Care 1983; 9:25.
22. Logan RL, McKendry M: The multi-disciplinary team: A different approach to patient-management. N Z Med J 1982; 95:883–884.
23. Furnham A, Pendleton D, Manicom C: The perception of different occupations within the medical profession. Soc Sci Med 1981; 15E:289.
24. Briggs TL: Research on intra-professional social work teams in the United States of America. *In* Lonsdale S, Webb A, Briggs TL (eds): Teamwork in the Personal Social Services and Health Care, p 32. London: Croom Helm, 1980.
25. DeSpirito AP, Grebler J: Interdisciplinary approach to developmental pediatrics in a hospital-based child evaluation center. J Med Society NJ 1983; 80:906.
26. Horwitz JJ: Team Practice and the Specialist. An Introduction to Interdisciplinary Teamwork. Springfield, IL: Charles C Thomas, 1970.
27. Kane RA: Multi-disciplinary teamwork in the United States: Trends, issues and implications for the social worker. *In* Lonsdale S, Webb A, Briggs TL (eds): Teamwork in the Personal Social Services and Health Care, p 138. London: Croom Helm, 1980.
28. Brill NI. Teamwork: Working Together in the Human Services. Philadelphia: JB Lippincott, 1976.
29. Payne M: Working in Teams. London: The MacMillan Press, 1982.
30. Bardach J, Morris H, Olin W, et al: Late results of multidisciplinary management of unilateral cleft lip and palate. Ann Plast Surg 1984; 12:235.
31. Webb AL, Hobdell M: Coordination and teamwork in the health and personal social services. *In* Lonsdale S, Webb A, Briggs TL (eds): Teamwork in the Personal Social Services and Health Care, p 97. London: Croom Helm, 1980.
32. Mason RM, Riski JE: The team approach to orofacial management. Ann Plast Surg 1982; 8:71.
33. Walker S, Middelkamp JN: Letter. Management of cleft palate. J Fam Pract 1982; 15:611.
34. De Santis G: From teams to hierarchy: A short-lived innovation in a hospital for the elderly. Soc Sci Med 1983; 17:1613.
35. Ellis JHP: Psychosocial aspects in health care teamwork: The dynamics of interaction in an interdisciplinary cleft lip and palate team. Unpublished Master's Thesis, Department of Sociology, University of North Carolina at Chapel Hill, 1986.
36. Lillywhite H: Communication problems in the cleft palate rehabilitation team. Cleft Palate Bull 1957; 7:8.
37. Merkel WT: Physician perception of patient satisfaction: Do doctors know which patients are satisfied? Med Care 1984; 22:453.
38. Lonsdale S, Webb A, Briggs TL (eds): Teamwork in the Personal Social Services and Health Care. London: Croom Helm, 1980.

39. American Cleft Palate Association: ACPA Directory. Pittsburgh, PA: American Cleft Palate, 1990.
40. Will LA, Parsons RW: Characteristics of new patients at Illinois cleft palate teams. Cleft Palate Craniofac J 1991; 28:378.
41. Pannbacker M, Lass NJ, Scheurle JF, et al: Survey of services and practices of cleft palate-craniofacial teams. Cleft Palate Craniofac J 1992; 29:164.
42. Cohn ES, Knapp DM, McWilliams BJ: The team approach to cleft care in the Commonwealth of Pennsylvania. Pennsylvania Dent J 1984; May/June.
43. Scheurle J, Habal MB, Frans NP: Cleft palate teams and the craniofacial centers in Florida: A state network. Fla Lang Speech Hear Assoc J July, 1986.
44. Fox DR, Lynch JI, Brauer RO: Physicians referral to cleft palate teams in Texas. Tex Med 1986; 82:32–35.
45. Noar JH. Questionnaire survey of attitudes and concerns of patients with cleft lip and palate and their parents. Cleft Palate Craniofac J 1991; 28:279.
46. Smoot EC III, Kucan JO, Cope JS, et al: The craniofacial team and the Navajo patient. Cleft Palate J 1988; 25:395.

7 | Psychosocial Considerations in Habilitation of Patients with Facial Deformity: A Developmental Perspective

Hillary L. Broder

This chapter introduces a variety of pertinent psychosocial issues and interventions in treating patients with craniofacial anomalies (CFA) and their families. Craniofacial habilitation usually involves multiple evaluations and interventions; these are often staged. Scheduling surgical interventions is typically determined by the team's assessment of the patient's physical development and structural status, which may incorporate assessments from other health specialists. Despite extensive documentation regarding the potentially negative psychosocial impact of facial disfigurement on body image and adjustment,[1,2] many teams do not have mental health professionals. Thus the omission of routinely scheduled psychological assessment of patients with CFA by trained specialists throughout the habilitation process is a common occurrence.

If the ultimate goal of habilitation is to improve the patient's quality of life, success is dependent, in part, on the psychosocial condition of the patient and family.[4] It is important for teams to recognize that "improvement" of appearance may not correlate with patients' satisfaction and psychological adjustment.[5,6] Therefore, when treatment plans that involve surgical alteration of the face are developed, consideration of the relationship between physical and psychological development is critical.[7]

This chapter focuses on psychosocial issues associated with specific developmental stages and highlights the relevance of these issues in the habilitation process. Throughout this process, which usually terminates during early adulthood, ongoing evaluations of psychosocial issues are essential, if compliance and satisfaction with the various stages of treatment planning are to be successfully implemented.[8–10]

Each developmental period is illustrated by a case study to focus on relevant developmental issues that warrant consideration in treatment planning. The case presentations are followed by a section on psychological issues and their clinical implications, including a review of salient research findings. Conclusions are drawn from a psychological perspective to summarize the current status of craniofacial habilitation and implications for future research.

The framework for this chapter is "the developmental ladder," with components as follows:

Infancy: Getting off to a good start—family acceptance
Toddlerhood: Playing and learning—readiness skills for school
Latency: Fitting into a group—social self-concept and psychological adjustment
Young adolescence: Deciding to decide—patient and family expectations and decision making
Late adolescence: Being a looker—physical attractiveness and adolescence
Young adulthood: Pulling up roots—autonomy and adulthood

Acknowledgment

The case studies in this chapter replicate specific psychosocial scenarios but may not represent actual patients. I thank the members of the University of North Carolina Craniofacial Center for providing an extraordinary environment for this psychologist to be a viable team member, carry out clinical responsibilities, and conduct research. In addition, I appreciate having served our patients and their families. As I have provided services for them, they have enriched my life.

**INFANCY—GETTING OFF TO A GOOD START—
FAMILY ACCEPTANCE**

CASE OF A 3-MONTH-OLD WITH CLEFT LIP
AND PALATE

Mr. and Mrs. T had been anxiously awaiting a multidisciplinary evaluation of their 3-month-old son, JJ, at the craniofacial center. After the birth of JJ, Mr. and Mrs. T's first child, several hours had passed before the doctor informed the mother that there were "some problems." Only then was she permitted to see her newborn, who had a bilateral cleft lip and palate. Her initial reaction was shock. During the next few months, the infant had difficulty gaining weight. Feeding him was an unexpectedly time-consuming ordeal. Both the father, who had a brother with a cleft, and the mother, who was a practicing nutritionist, felt guilty and anxious about their child's birth defect and current health status. Furthermore, the parents had financial concerns. Mrs. T had taken a leave of absence from work, and her husband feared losing his job because of his employer's recent cutbacks. The mother was the only caretaker for the child; she did not permit anyone to babysit. After the child's birth, the parents became socially isolated and did not go out alone for an evening without the child. Initially, the parents were informed that the child would require several operations, yet they were uncertain about the nature and timing of the procedures.

Psychosocial Issues and Clinical Implications

Several issues of concern for the habilitation team must be considered. The parents had unresolved feelings (i.e., anger, sadness) about their initial shock. They were displeased about having had to wait before speaking with the obstetrician about their son's condition. In addition, the parents received minimal information to facilitate their understanding about the habilitation process. Like many parents having a child with a birth defect, they had to experience particular stages (i.e., anger, denial) before achieving acceptance of not having a "normal" child.[11] Because the father had a relative with a cleft, he felt guilty and blamed himself for the child's medical condition. Because the child had failure to thrive, the mother felt "like a failure." Questions regarding recurrence risks are particularly relevant in situations like this with a firstborn child. The parents are burdened with negative emotions. Thus communication with the habilitation team is indicated.

Parental acceptance is critical to the child's self-image,[5, 12, 13] and supportive counseling is necessary. Other interventions should include genetic counseling, psychotherapy (individual, couple, or family), relaxation therapy, desensitization treatment, support groups, educational programs, hospital entry programs, and preoperative and postoperative psychological consultations. These interventions facilitate parental acceptance and reduce anxiety.[14]

The quality of a family's support system is positively correlated with parental adaptation and adjustment to a child's medical condition.[15, 16] Therefore, enhancing the quality of the parents' support system is a goal in counseling. The parents' social isolation and the mother's perception that no one else can care for their child needs to be addressed. Such feelings are typical for parents of children with chronic conditions.[11] Allowing parents to confront their unresolved feelings of anger and grief after the birth of their newborns is another issue of clinical import.[17] Encouraging parents to develop a support system can help to alleviate their anxiety and stress.[16]

With regard to the infant's difficulty in gaining weight, instruction and demonstration of specific feeding methods (e.g., tube feeding and use of other feeding devices) can be introduced. By implementing behavior techniques (e.g., modeling, scheduling, and positive reinforcement), caretakers can learn to effectively feed their offspring. Parents report feeling more empowered as they perceive that they have more control.[18] Changes in the medical condition and the occurrence of complications may necessitate additional evaluations by specialists (e.g., in nutrition, neurology, and/or pediatric pulmonary medicine).

Issues related to the genetic implications and recurrence risks of the birth defect necessitate consultations with a geneticist and a genetic counselor. The parents' questions should be answered regarding the cause, prognosis, recurrence risks, and emotional responses (e.g., guilt) associated with the clinical malformation.[19] Following the team evaluation and interpretive conference, a summary letter, which is based on interview data, is sent to report the team's findings and recommendations.[20]

This child underwent a repair of his cleft lip and palate subsequent to this initial visit. Supportive counseling and genetics counseling were scheduled in coordination with the child's preoperative and postoperative visits with the surgeon. The entire team evaluated the child at 1 year of age. At that time, the child's developmental skills and the family's adaptation were evaluated by the team psychologist.

THE TODDLER—PLAYING AND LEARNING— READINESS SKILLS

CASE OF A 3-YEAR-OLD WITH CRANIOFACIAL DYSOSTOSIS

Ms. Z, a single parent, was extremely worried about her child's growth and development. She reported that her 3-year-old daughter, K, did not look very much like the other members of the family, and at times K did not seem to listen or hear. The mother also indicated that "K's head appeared to be changing shape and was bigger." Ms. Z noted that her daughter would tilt her head to one side when looking at picture books. Although Ms. Z had spoken with the pediatrician from the local health department about her child's growth and development, the physician discounted her concerns and asserted that "not all children develop at the same rate." Ms. Z further observed that the child's speech and language development was "different" from that of her other children, and she had difficulty understanding K's utterances. Consequently, Ms. Z allowed the child to communicate by pointing and rarely encouraged verbal interaction with her. Within the previous 6 months, Ms. Z reported that K fell often and complained of headaches. Ms. Z reported, "I am doing everything I can for this child." The mother also indicated that she could not do without the help from her 6-year-old daughter, who accompanied the mother to the evaluation.

Psychological Issues and Implications for Clinicians

The physical examination and computed tomography (CT) scan confirmed that K's head circumference was large, and brachycephaly was observed. The child had Crouzon syndrome and craniosynostosis for which surgery was recommended. Surgery included a craniectomy and pressure equalization (PE) tube insertion. To facilitate the mother's comprehension of the need for and ramifications of surgery, the surgeon utilized three-dimension imaging to illustrate the child's condition and explain anticipated results from treatment. Supplying this information reduced fear and can improve compliance with treatment and help create more realistic expectations.[10, 21] Results from the psychological evaluation of the child's intellectual status affirmed Ms. Z's perceptions that her daughter had cognitive deficits. Tests by the otorhinolaryngologist confirmed that conductive hearing losses were present. Ocular involvement was also significant. Before surgery, Ms. Z received a preadmission orientation and was given the opportunity to contact other parents who had children with Crouzon syndrome. Such programs are reportedly desired by parents[22] and are deemed successful in mitigating parental anxiety.[14]

After surgery, evaluations for supportive counseling, genetics, and ophthalmology were recommended. K was fitted with corrective lenses. The genetics evaluation revealed that Ms. Z's family, including Ms. Z, had a positive history of Crouzon syndrome. Counseling provided an avenue for Ms. Z to deal with emotional issues associated with acceptance (e.g., guilt) and provided her with an avenue to vent her feelings (e.g., separation anxiety). Through her participation in a parent support group, Ms. Z acquired information about the syndrome and learned strategies to enhance her coping skills. The importance of language stimulation was reviewed. Furthermore, sibling adaptation and rivalry and possible school phobia were evaluated, which is appropriate for families with children having chronic conditions.[24] Increasing parents' perceived control through knowledge and support is useful in working with parents of children with disabilities.[11, 23]

After the recuperative period, the 3-year-old was enrolled in the local child development center. By federal law, such centers were mandated in every state to provide educational, physical, and social stimulation for preschool children with developmental disabilities. Intellectual, speech and language, and general pediatric and specialist (otorhinolaryngologic) evaluations became routine to follow K's growth and development. Ms. Z reported relief and satisfaction that her observations were validated, her concerns were addressed, and specific interventions were implemented immediately.

LATENCY—FITTING INTO A GROUP— PSYCHOLOGICAL ADJUSTMENT

CASE OF AN 8-YEAR-OLD WITH APERT SYNDROME

Patient B was an 8-year-old boy with Apert syndrome. His family had recently moved, and he was attending a new school. According to the mother's report, B was experiencing difficulty with academic achievement and did not like his current school. While on the schoolbus, B was teased repeatedly about his appearance. He reported an incident in which, as he entered the bathroom at school, another student screamed at him "You monster!" and punched B in the bridge of his nose. After spending the evening in the emergency room with her son because of his injury from this bathroom incident, B's mother withdrew him from the school. According to independent interview data from B and his mother, it was revealed that B had no peer support system and spent his leisure time with imaginary friends or playing video games. Fearing that B would encounter further attacks, B's mother prohibited her son from going anywhere without her supervision. Ms. B reported feeling depressed and very anxious. Surgical interventions planned for the future included orthognathic surgery (a LeFort procedure) and possible orbital augmentation.

Psychological Issues and Implications for Clinicians

Although B had no history of cognitive problems, he had reduced school achievement. Psychological testing was undertaken to discern whether learning disabilities were present, because learning disabilities are often underdiagnosed and may be covert until the latency developmental period. In addition, children with cleft lip and palate are at increased risk for learning problems.[25] Test results from the cognitive assessment revealed normal intellectual function. However, test results from a standardized self-concept inventory and interview data indicated a low self-concept with high loadings on the popularity, physical appearance, and anxiety factors. B's elevated anxiety could be a reflection of his mother's sentiments[26]; parental attitudes are often expressed in their children's self-images.[27] Children with facial differences are at risk for negative psychosocial sequelae, such as diminished self-concept[28, 29] and social inhibition.[30, 31]

Because children respond to parental attitudes[5, 32] and B's mother reported specific psychological symptoms, counseling was recommended for her and her son. For the mother parental overprotection of her child[33] and codependency were relevant issues. Regarding the latter, Farris[34] wrote, "love is letting go of fear." Farris advocated parents' confronting their codependency.

Patient B was unable to accomplish age-appropriate psychosocial tasks, such as establishing a sense of achievement and peer acceptance,[35] and thus counseling and implementation of concrete tools to develop his coping skills were suggested to foster his self-esteem and validate his identity. Concrete tools to deal with bullying and to enhance his body image (e.g., enrollment in a Tae Kwon Do class) were encouraged. To improve his social skills, enrollment in noncompetitive group activities (e.g., group counseling and Boy Scouts) was suggested.

Because behavior problems increase during the latency period, the importance of evaluating psychosocial adjustment is underscored.[36] Fostering effective parenting skills is pertinent. Using consistent behavior management techniques can successfully develop children's social behaviors, such as self-reliance.[18] Increasing children's responsibilities (e.g., performing specified chores, scheduling homework time) further contributes to the child's development. Discussing the mother's perceived need to overprotect B and reviewing the impact of her expectations on the son's behavior and self-esteem were accomplished.[32] The relationship between parental expectations and a child's behavior is well-documented in the social impression and implicit personality theory.[37–39]

It has been shown that parents of children with CFA tend to perceive their children's behavior differently than do school teachers.[40] Thus, teacher evaluations may provide further insight into a child's psychological adjustment. Setting limits and establishing specific rules are critical in the child's moral and social skill development. Developing social independence and taking responsibility for the consequences of behavior are important in counseling a child who has been overprotected or spoiled, or who has difficulty with behavior boundaries.[41] Teaching the child to assume responsibility for behavior can be reinforced through a cooperative effort between parents and teachers.

ADOLESCENCE—DECIDING TO DECIDE— PHYSICAL ATTRACTIVENESS

CASE OF A HIGH SCHOOL JUNIOR WITH TREACHER COLLINS SYNDROME

Patient Y, an adolescent female with Treacher Collins syndrome, was entering her junior year in high school. She had moderate-to-severe facial disfigurement associated with her craniofacial anomaly. According to the patient report, Y had increased feelings of inadequacy, compulsive behaviors, and suicidal ideation during the previous 6 months. Socially, she was withdrawing from friends by disengaging in after-school and weekend activities. Her withdrawal represented a change from her prior behavior. The mother and stepfather expressed no specific concerns about their daughter's physical or psychological status. They simply reported that Y was "doing just fine."

Despite the team's previous recommendations for major reconstructive surgery when the girl reached late adolescence, the parents expressed no desire to obtain surgical treatment for their daughter. However, during the independent psychological interview with Y, she expressed concern about her significant facial asymmetry and eagerness to change her appearance. The patient was reluctant to express these feelings in the presence of her parents. During a joint interview with Y and her parents, Y meekly revealed that she was mildly unhappy with her face but was very fearful about future treatment. Although Y stated that she wanted to "look normal," the parents reported that their daughter was "beautiful" and did not need additional surgery. When querying the family further about the patient's desire "to look normal" as well as her social behaviors and ideation, patient Y became tearful. She stated that her friends were dating, whereas she was spending more time at home and was scared to go outside.

Psychological Issues and Implications for Clinicians

Because of psychological factors, surgical recommendations were postponed until the issues were further explored and resolved. The parents subsequently reported that the patient's grandmother had recently died, and the father was currently unemployed. These events can affect treatment planning.

This case highlights the importance of conducting independent interviews and assessments with the parents and patients. Discrepancies were found between reports of parents and Y on psychological adjustment and satisfaction with appearance.[42] Major psychological issues for this patient included her increased social isolation, obsessive-compulsive behaviors, and fear, as well as her inability to confront her parents regarding her unhappiness with her appearance and desire for change. She was not accomplishing her expected psychosocial tasks and felt socially inept.

It is noteworthy that significant changes in behavior are often the best indicators of psychic disturbance. Patient Y's current behaviors and concerns were incongruent with her history, which represented a clear indicator that she was in need of further psychological evaluation. She had an extraordinary fear of abandonment. She believed that if her mother and stepfather knew of her intrapsychic conflicts, she would be perceived as a burden. Furthermore, she revealed that her stepfather might leave her mother as her biological father had left, ''because of me.'' Psychological counseling was coordinated in conjunction with the patient's dental appointments at the center. After extensive individual psychotherapy, which included cognitive therapy, as well as relaxation and mental imagery, the family engaged in counseling. The parents discussed their denial of the patient's obvious desire for change, her unhappiness, and her social dependency. The mother confronted her fears about Y's hospitalization after the loss of her own mother, who died in the hospital, and the stepfather discussed his concerns about the financial burden associated with treatment. After individual and family therapy, surgical plans were initiated.

Treatment plans, including surgical recommendations, are effectively communicated in a safe, supportive environment with a one-on-one discussion between the patient (and parent, if appropriate) and the physician who will render the proposed treatment.[8,43] Preparing questions before the consultation with the physician is useful for patients and family in improving communication and increasing satisfaction between patients and physicians.[45] Such preparation can relieve patient anxiety and increase compliance with treatment.

Patient Y used relaxation techniques to cope with her anxiety. Surgery was scheduled and successfully completed. Patient and family adaptation after treatment were unremarkable.

LATE ADOLESCENCE—BEING A LOOKER— PHYSICAL ATTRACTIVENESS

CASE OF A 19-YEAR-OLD WITH MALOCCLUSION AND FACIAL DISFIGUREMENT

Patient X, a 19-year-old male, had a class III malocclusion and moderate disfigurement associated with his cleft lip and palate. Throughout high school, X excelled academically. Although he was accepted by the most competitive colleges in the country, he chose to attend the university in his home town. Residing at home was a financial relief to the parents; however, in this upper middle class family financial concerns were minimal. This young man had several friends, but he never dated in high school. He felt like a ''social failure.'' Although he had extensive orthodontic treatment, he postponed surgical treatment for 2 years. Later he underwent maxillary advancement during the summer of his junior year at the university. After surgery, X became reclusive and seemed depressed. Despite his continued academic achievements, X's parents reported that his disposition changed. He was described as ''noncompliant'' and ''sullen'' and his overall appearance (dress and hair) had become ''sloppy.'' The parents were professors at the university. They had chosen repeatedly to deny psychological emotional concerns and avoided psychological team evaluations. When X began sleeping in his room for extended periods, avoiding regular meals, and going out for long periods without telling his parents of his whereabouts, psychological counseling was sought.

Psychological Issues and Implications for Clinicians

Being attractive and experiencing an intimate relationship were unfulfilled developmental goals for X.[35,44] Psychological issues that warranted counseling involved autonomy, identity formation, and expectations with treatment. This young man had successfully compensated for his feelings of social inadequacy during adolescence by achieving academic recognition. Although this adjustment can be useful, X denied his feeling of inadequacy. As he became more aware of his need for intimacy, he unsuccessfully attempted to have a relationship with a female student in his class. Further exacerbating his feelings of inadequacy were uncertainties about his sexual identity, and he felt ashamed to discuss homosexual feelings. This young man had always tried to "fit in" but had some cognitive dissonance; that is, he had a conflict between his feelings and thoughts. This conflict manifested itself in depression and rebellious attitudes, which typically emerge during adolescence.[32] X had mildly delayed social skills, and thus his rebellious behaviors were displayed at a somewhat later age than usual. Typical developmental concerns about body image and appearance increased in this patient.[44] Adapting to changes in appearance resulting from surgery can heighten anxiety, especially in the absence of adequate support and guidance.[42, 46]

It is important that patients have the opportunity to be involved in decision making during adolescence and adulthood,[21] and exploring expectations associated with treatment is critical.[47] Furthermore, through routine screening of psychological issues in conjunction with team evaluations, early identification and/or psychological counseling can help alleviate intrapsychic conflicts and increase the likelihood of avoiding a crisis. Postoperative depression is commonplace, as is repeatedly cited in the literature, and perhaps occurs more frequently after a long-awaited change that is visible to the public. Therefore, postoperative consultations are recommended to examine adaptation to treatment.[48]

As occurs with many patients who are dissatisfied with treatment, X had unrealistic expectations about surgery, including his belief that he would become attractive to women. Because of his internalized fears, he dressed poorly to distract attention from the changes in his facial appearance. Another fear was that having undergone corrective surgery, he no longer had an excuse for not dating women. Counseling helped him address identity formation, expectations from treatment, and autonomy. He worked through his conflict about his sexual preferences and moved away from home, where he enjoys a satisfying, intimate relationship.

EARLY ADULTHOOD—PULLING UP ROOTS— AUTONOMY AND INDEPENDENCE

CASE OF A YOUNG ADULT WITH AN ILL-FITTING APPLIANCE

Ms. S, a recent graduate student who had just moved to the state, was first seen by the team because she was dissatisfied with her appliance. She had moderate disfigurement associated with her bilateral cleft lip and palate, as well as a poorly fitting appliance and hypernasal speech. Being a teaching assistant at the university, Ms. S was required to lecture to medical students and wanted to improve her voice quality. At the initial psychology team evaluation, she reported satisfaction with her prior treatment, which included multiple surgical interventions culminating in a lip and nose revision during the summer before her senior year in high school. The team recommended constructing a new appliance for her. In the course of the dentist's subsequent interactions with her, he suggested that she meet with the team psychologist to explore her feelings and anxiety about her recent move to the area and need for a support system. Ms. S acquiesced, although she vehemently told the dentist that she "did not need to talk."

Throughout the psychological interview, Ms. S avoided eye contact and became tearful in discussing her life history. Although Ms. S was defensive about the desire to pursue supportive counseling, she agreed to undergo a more thorough assessment with the hope of qualifying for financial support for dental services through the Department of Vocational Rehabilitation. According to interview data and results from the psychological evaluation, she qualified for financial support because of the emotionally handicapping effects of her craniofacial anomaly on her potential employment capabilities.

Psychosocial Issues and Implications for Clinicians

Ms. S had an adjustment disorder with mixed emotional disturbance. She had a long history of not discussing her cleft with anybody because she believed that within her family there was an unspoken shame associated with the cleft. Ms. S explained that when she was in the second grade, her mother betrayed her by going to the school officials to ''expose how I was teased about my face.'' She felt humiliated and was still angry that her mother told everyone how sensitive S was about her facial appearance. She further described her father as being depressed and ''the man I could never please.'' Consequently, S's adaptation involved following her doctors' and parents' concerns, never revealing her own needs and concerns. On her 16th birthday, the doctor told her that her lip and nose would ''finally be fixed.'' Patient S explained with great sadness that the surgical results were extremely disappointing. She despised her lip scar and the bulging tip on her nose that ''the doctor created.''

Because the last procedure was supposed to ''fix'' her appearance and the doctor never said that he did not like the results, she lived with anger and disappointment with the surgical results and people's inattention to her feelings and perceptions. For 10 years, she refused to express any dissatisfaction about her appearance. She attempted to ''pass as normal'' but never felt normal. After months of psychotherapy, she decided to speak with the surgeon to see whether any surgical alterations could be accomplished to address her specific concerns. After talking about her expectations and consulting further with the surgeon, S decided to undergo surgery.

Before surgery was undertaken, issues related to delayed socialization skills, assertiveness, and need for companionship were thoroughly examined. It was imperative for her to understand and accept that these social issues would not be resolved as a result of surgery, and that she would continue counseling about identity issues, fear of social situations, and negative self-defeating behaviors. She underwent two procedures to improve the appearance of her lip and nose, but waited until after surgery to discuss her feelings and hospitalizations with her parents. Having ''pulled up her roots'' and relocating to a new area provided her with the courage to face her feelings of inadequacy and unresolved feelings toward her parents. Slowly, she developed her social skills and confidence to successfully teach and pursue a career in academia.

CONCLUSIONS AND IMPLICATIONS FOR CLINICAL PRACTICE AND RESEARCH

Health psychologists purport that psychosocial factors such as motivation, expectations, and personality are critical to the body image and patient and family adaptation. Specific issues are critical in the child's psychosocial development. Table 7–1 outlines developmental stages and summarizes the important psychosocial factors associated with each stage. Although surgeons or team members assert that surgery should be carried out because of psychological factors in patients with craniofacial anomalies, these assertions are frequently based on clinical hunches in the absence of an evaluation from a trained mental health professional. Mental health specialists emphasize the importance of proactively evaluating and addressing the psychological factors in patients with CFA and their families as part of the habilitation process. Through these routine assessments, timely interventions can be implemented to address psychosocial

Table 7–1. OVERVIEW OF DEVELOPMENTAL STAGES AND ASSOCIATED PSYCHOSOCIAL ISSUES

Infancy (0 to 3 Years)	Toddler (3 to 6 Years)	Latency (6 to 12 Years)	Adolescence (12 to 18 Years)	Young Adulthood (Late Teens to Early 20s)
Parental acceptance	School readiness skills	School achievement	Future goals	Educational or vocational decisions
Genetic implications	Communication, social, motor, and language	Peer acceptance	Abstract reasoning	Acceptance about treatment results
Feeding, breathing, crying		Moral and social development	Decision making about treatment	Autonomy
Developmental skills	Discipline	Social competence	Independence	Life stress
Parent and child attachment	Overprotection and spoiling	Self-concept and body image	Dating	Genetic counseling
Family adaptation	Social independence		Concern about appearance	Acceptance of treatment results
Life stressors	Identity formation		School performance	
Support system	Sibling acceptance		Genetic counseling	
Separation anxiety	Family stress and adaptation			
Overprotectiveness	Separation anxiety			

issues (see Table 7–1). These interventions may include supportive counseling (individual or family), school placement, vocational rehabilitation, mental health or health department referrals, pre- and postsurgical counseling, relaxation or desensitization therapy, supports groups, and genetic counseling.

Although patients with CFA and their families may have negative psychosocial sequelae, no predictive models include psychosocial function. Each individual's life varies, and it is naive to believe that the degree of psychological distress reflects the degree of morphologic deviance. It is equally unrealistic to believe that surgical alteration of morphologic deviance will completely alter or "fix" patients' psychological status. In other words, movement of millimeters of tissue or bone cannot ensure or predict patient satisfaction with treatment or with self.

Despite the sophistication of technology and precision of skillful surgical teams, satisfaction with treatment and self is likely to be associated with psychological issues. No longitudinal data currently exist on patients with CFA regarding the impact of treatment interventions on self-satisfaction and psychological adjustment, decision making, or the optimal timing of treatment. Thus, if treatment planning and interventions are to improve quality of life, positive psychological outcomes are needed. Therefore, assessment of patient and family adaptation, social competence, and satisfaction with appearance must be made throughout the habilitation process.

References

1. Bull R, Ramsey N: The Social Psychology of Facial Appearance. New York: Springer-Verlag, 1988.
2. Alley TR, Hildebrandt KA: Determinants and consequences of facial aesthetics. *In* Alley TR (ed): Social and Applied Aspects of Perceiving Faces. Hillsdale, NJ: Erlbaum Assoc, 1988, pp 101–140.
3. Broder HL, Richman LC: An examination of mental health services offered by cleft craniofacial teams. Cleft Palate J 1987; 24:158.
4. Strauss RP, Broder H: Directions and issues in psychosocial research and methods as applied to cleft lip and palate and craniofacial anomalies. Cleft Palate Craniofacial J 1991; 28(2):150.
5. Macgregor FC: Transformation and Identity—The Face and Plastic Surgery. New York: Quadrangle/New York Times, 1974.
6. Fisher S: Development and Structure of the Body Image. Hillsdale, NJ: Erlbaum Assoc, 1986.
7. American Cleft Palate Association (ACPA): Parameters for Evaluation and Treatment of Patients with Cleft Lip/Palate or Other Craniofacial Anomalies. Pittsburgh: ACPA, 1993.
8. Waitzkin H: Information giving in medical care. J Health Soc Behav 1985; 26:81.
9. Schorr D, Rodin J: The role of perceived control in practitioner-patient relationships. *In* Wills T (ed): Basic Processes in Helping Relationships. New York: Academic Press, 1982.
10. Rodin J, Janis IL: The social power of health-care practitioners as agents of change. J Soc Issues 1979; 35(1):60.
11. Wright BA: Physical Disability: A Psychosocial Approach. New York: Harper & Row, 1983.
12. Spriesterbach DC: Psychological Aspects of the Cleft Palate Problem, vols 1, 2. Iowa City: University of Iowa Press, 1973.
13. Macgregor FC: Facial disfigurement: Problems and management of social interaction and implications for mental health. Aesthetic Plast Surg 1990; 14:249.
14. Petrillo M, Sanger S: Emotional Care of Hospitalized Children: An Environmental Approach, 2nd ed. Philadelphia: JB Lippincott, 1980.
15. Garrison WT, McQuestion S: Chronic illness during childhood and adolescence: Psychological aspects. Dev Clin Psych Psychiatr 1989; 19:19.
16. Cohen S, McKay G: Social support, stress and the buffering hypothesis. *In* Baum A, Taylor SE, Singer JE (eds): Handbook of Psychology and Health, vol 4. Hillsdale, NJ: Erlbaum Assoc, 1984, pp 253–276.
17. Affleck G, Allen D, Tennen H, et al: Causal and control cognitions in parents coping with a chronically ill child. J Soc Clin Psychol 1986; 3:369–379.
18. Berkson AG: Children with Handicaps: A Review of Behavioral Research. Hillsdale, NJ: Erlbaum Assoc, 1992.
19. Broder HL, Trier WC: The effectiveness of genetic counseling for families with craniofacial disorders. Cleft Palate J 1985; 157.
20. Broder HL: Should parents attend team meeting? Paper presented at the American Craniofacial Association, Pittsburgh, April, 1993.
21. Janis IL: Vigilance and decision-making in personal crisis. *In* Coelho GV, Hamburg DA, Adams JE (eds): Coping and Adaptation. New York: Basic Books, 1974, pp 139–175.
22. Pannbacker M, Scheurle J: Parents' attitudes toward family involvement in cleft palate treatment. Cleft Palate Craniofac J 1993; 30(1):87.
23. Partridge C, Johnston M: Perceived control of recovery: Measurement and prediction. Br J Clin Psychol 1989; 28:53.
24. LaVign E, Ryan M: Psychologic adjustment of children with chronic illness. Pediatrics 1979; 63:616.
25. Richman L, Eliason M: Type of reading disability related to cleft type and neuropsychological patterns. Cleft Palate J 1984; 21:1.
26. Dolgin MJ, Phipps S, Harow E: Parental management of fear in chronically ill and healthy children. J Pediatr Psychol 1990; 15(6):633.
27. Fishman CA, Fishman DB: Maternal correlates of self-esteem and overall adjustment in children with birth defects. Child Psychol Hum Dev 1971; 1(4):255.

28. Broder HL, Strauss RP: Self-concept of primary school age children with and without visible defects. Cleft Palate J 1991; 29:158.
29. Kapp-Simon K: Self-concept of primary school age children with cleft lip, cleft palate or both. Cleft Palate J 1986; 23:24.
30. Richman LC, Harper DC: Observable stigmata and perceived maternal behavior. Cleft Palate J 1978; 15:215.
31. Pertschuk MJ, Whitaker LA: Psychosocial outcome of craniofacial surgery in children. Plast Reconstr Surg 1988; 82:741.
32. Leach P: Your growing child—from baby through adolescents. New York: Knopf, 1991.
33. Tobiasen JM, Hiebert JM: Parents' tolerance for the conduct problems of cleft palate children. Cleft Palate J 1984; 21:82.
34. Farris JM: Parents Who Care Too Much. Minneapolis: Life Care Books, 1992.
35. Sullivan HS: The Interpersonal Theory of Psychiatry. New York: Norton, 1953.
36. Achenbach TM: The child behavior profile: I. J Consult Clin Psychol 1978; 46:478.
37. Tagiuri R: Person perception. In Lindzey G, Aronson E (eds): Handbook of Social Psychology. Reading, MA: Addison-Wesley, 1969.
38. Schneider DJ: Implicit personality theory: A review. Psychol Bull 1973; 79:294.
39. Schneiderman CR, Auer KE: The behavior of the child with cleft lip and palate as perceived by parents and teachers. Cleft Palate J 1984; 21:224.
40. Richman LC, Harper DC: The effects of facial disfigurement on teachers' perception of ability in cleft palate children. Cleft Palate J 1978; 15:155.
41. Brazelton TB: Touchpoints: Your Child's Emotional and Behavioral Development. Reading, MA: Addison-Wesley, 1992.
42. Broder HL, Smith F, Strauss RP: Habilitation of patients with clefts: Parent and child ratings of satisfaction with appearance and speech. Cleft Craniofac J 1992; 29:262.
43. Bertakis KD: The communication of information from physician to patient: A method of increasing patient retention and satisfaction. J Fam Pract 1977; 7:217.
44. Schonfeld WA: The body and body image in adolescents. In Caplan G, Lebovici S (eds): Adolescence: Psychological Perspectives. New York: Basic Books, 1969, pp 50–78.
45. Thompson SC, Nanni C: Patient oriented interventions to improve communication in a medical office visit. Health Psychol 1990; 9(4):390.
46. Stern MT: Children's encounters with illness. In Dixon SD, Stern MT (eds): Pediatric Behavior and Development. Chicago: Mosby Year Book, 1987, pp 367–374.
47. Kiyak HA, Vitaliano PP, Crinean J: Patients' expectations as predictors of orthognathic surgery outcome. Health Psychol 1988; 7(3):251.
48. Broder HL, Strauss RP: Psychosocial problems and referrals among oralfacial team patients. J Rehab 1991; 57:31.

8 | Nursing Considerations for Children with Craniofacial Anomalies

Mary Breen, Ginny Curtin, and Carol Ursich

INTRODUCTION

Children with craniofacial anomalies require complex interdisciplinary care. Nursing care is provided in the tertiary setting at birth, at the time of surgical interventions, and in the outpatient setting by a person who serves as service coordinator and as patient educator. Ideally, the nurse should be an interactive member of the multidisciplinary craniofacial team and be part of the decision-making process. This chapter focuses on the role of nursing services in the long-term management of craniofacial care. The roles of education, support, and coordination with the patient and family are discussed, followed by a description of the consultative and research roles of other health care and education professionals. The specific clinical care of the child with craniofacial anomalies such as cleft lip and palate, cranial suture synostosis, and other complex syndromes is outlined.

PATIENT FAMILY EDUCATION

Newborns

The family of an infant born with a craniofacial anomaly has many educational and emotional needs. The optimal time for the first contact with the family and evaluation of the child is within the tertiary setting at birth, with follow-up during the first few weeks of life.[1] Initial questions regarding the diagnosis, the etiology, and the proposed plan of initial management need to be addressed. In addition, the family needs to know about the basic care of the newborn, including airway management, positioning, nutritional needs, routine hygiene, and feeding techniques. The nurse may have the opportunity to support the mother's choice to breastfeed or to provide expressed breast milk. These decisions can positively influence the infant's health status. Presenting the criteria for adequate intake/weight gain as well as routine formula/expressed breast milk preparation and storage is also helpful. The nurse can introduce the new family to the concept of the multidisciplinary team approach to craniofacial care, describe the resources that will be available through team management, and arrange a referral to a craniofacial team and a local parent support group. Before the infant's discharge from the newborn nursery, the family should make an appointment or be given the resource numbers to call for a pediatric evaluation by the primary care provider and/or a visit by a public health nurse. When possible, this postdischarge visit should be scheduled within a week to determine that nutritional intake and weight gain are adequate.

During the initial consultation, parents generally find that instructions about newborn care and early management are helpful. However, they can become overwhelmed if the long-term care considerations, such as school entry, peer acceptance and teasing, and orthodontic management, extend to an older child. Those issues should be discussed at a later time. Sharing ''before and after'' pictures of other similar patients with family members may give them some hope and encouragement in what they often feel is a frightening and hopeless situation.

Written materials to supplement the orally communicated information, including feeding pamphlets, information about and publications by the American Cleft Palate Association (ACPA), and a team brochure should be available. The family can review these materials for answers and to pose further questions. Table 8–1 lists some helpful

Table 8–1. SELECTED PATIENT/FAMILY EDUCATIONAL RESOURCES

ACPA Literature
Various pamphlets and fact sheets on clefting and other craniofacial conditions
1218 Grandview Avenue
Pittsburgh, PA 15211

Looking Forward—A Guide for Parents of the Child with Cleft Lip and Palate
Mead Johnson Nutritionals
2404 Pennsylvania Avenue
Evansville, IN 47721-0001
Publication No. L-B68-10-88

Bright Promise: For Your Child with Cleft Lip and Cleft Palate
[Un Futuro Prometedor: Para Su Niño con Labio Hendido y Paladar Hendido]
National Easter Seals Society
Publications Department
70 East Lake Street
Chicago, IL 60601
Publication No. E-26 (English) or E-27 (Spanish)

Feeding Young Children with Cleft Lip and Palate
Minnesota Dietetic Association
1821 University Avenue West
Suite S 280
St. Paul, MN 55104

Nursing Your Baby With Cleft Lip and Palate
Childbirth Graphics
P.O. Box 20508
Rochester, NY 14602-0508

Orthognathic Surgery: Reshaping Your Face with Orthodontics and Corrective Jaw Surgery
Krames Communications
312 90th Street
Daly City, CA 94015-1898

Apert, Crouzon and Other Craniosynostosis Syndromes
About Face
99 Crowns Lane, 3rd Floor
Toronto, Ontario
Canada M5R 3P4

Treacher Collins Syndrome: An Overview
Treacher Collins Foundation
P.O. Box 683
Norwich, VT 05055

resources that are culturally appropriate and written at a level of understanding that is useful. Parental stress and exhaustion in the first days after the birth interfere with understanding the nature of the concepts, and repetition is usually welcomed.

Preoperative Preparation

A family whose child requires a surgical procedure benefits from preoperative preparation. This includes discussions of both medical and psychosocial aspects of the condition, and the family needs to prepare for the sequence of events that includes admission and consent routines, anesthesia preparation, usual length of surgery, and nursing and surgical pre- and postoperative care routines. A hospital tour through the usual areas of admission, operating room, and intensive care and nursing units, as well as supportive discussion, helps the child and family prepare for the actual experience. Although many parents like to have the surgical procedure outlined, the child generally is satisfied with a simple explanation of what will occur while he or she is taking a nap.

Studies by Wolfer and Visintainer[2] documented that age-appropriate preoperative programs for children that offer medical play serve as stress inoculation for both the child and the family. Significant differences were found between experimental and control children and parents on ratings of (1) upset behavior, (2) cooperation with procedures and induction, (3) time of first void, (4) posthospital adjustment, and

(5) parental anxiety and satisfaction with information and care; these ratings were found to increase when the child and the family received systematic psychological support and preparation. Positive coping strategies can be identified and used at the time of the stressful event. Unrestricted visiting and parental involvement in care are encouraged, and a child-life specialist can promote resolution of the stress and return to a normal routine.

Families who are able to articulate the rationale for the multidisciplinary services comply better with the multiple provider evaluations and therapies, including speech pathology, audiology, otolaryngology, dentistry, and orthodontics. These services require a long-term commitment by the patient and the family. Treatment goals are achieved over an extended period of time, in contrast to a surgical procedure that may produce an immediate and dramatic change and whose outcome may not depend on the patient's or the family's compliance.

Resources

Identification of the patient's and parents' needs for financial assistance, parent support groups, and other community resources is an integral task of the nursing assessment process. In concert with the team's social services provider, the pediatric nurse is in a position to identify these needs and provide appropriate referrals. Parents may experience shock, grief, guilt, and anxiety with regard to the financial impact when their infant is born with a craniofacial abnormality. In addition to the craniofacial centered care provided by the team, parents may benefit from additional services offered by state, county, and community agencies and national organizations. Their services may include financial support, parent support groups, respite services, school programs, and home visits by a public health nurse. These resources vary from region to region. Table 8–2 lists various organizations and agencies available.

Financial assistance may be available through private self-pay insurance or state-supported private insurance that provides insurance coverage for low-income families. Federal and state funding is available through Medicaid, Children's Special Health Services (formerly Crippled Children's Program), and the Civilian Health and Medical Program of the Uniformed Services (CHAMPUS). Medicaid is a program that covers costs of medical care for low-income families. Children's Special Health Services provides comprehensive medical care to children from birth to age 21 years with congenital conditions, if certain medical and financial criteria are met. Information is generally available through the state Department of Health. CHAMPUS is a federal program providing medical benefits to military dependents.

The Cleft Palate Foundation, About Face, and Let's Face It are national organizations that offer information and educational materials and provide opportunities for contact with local and national support groups. Clifford reported that parents gain encouragement and nurturance when they contact each other.[3] They are able to ask questions and express concerns in a safe and supportive atmosphere. Initially, some parents may be reluctant to seek contact with other families; however, they may welcome this support as they prepare for hospitalization and surgery. Anticipation of these events may be less frightening to the new parents if they can share their fears and gain understanding and comfort from a parent or patient who has experienced a similar situation. The nurse should encourage this interaction as well as facilitate the development of a local support group if one is not available.

Public health nurses can provide educational reinforcement and information on newborn care and assist the family in accessing needed services. These community-based nurses can assist the team in ensuring compliance with team recommendations as well as monitoring the infant's growth, development, and nutritional status.

Early childhood education and intervention for handicapped and developmentally disabled children is mandated by Public Law 94-142. The availability and types of these services vary from state to state. The state Department of Education can provide information regarding local sources. Head Start is an example of such a program. The child with a craniofacial anomaly may benefit from an early intervention that may help to diminish some educational disabilities.

Regional Centers for the Developmentally Disabled are an example of a federally mandated service that provides for developmentally disabled clients as well as infants and toddlers to 3 years of age who are identified as ''at risk'' for developmental delay.

Table 8–2. RESOURCES FOR PARENTS AND CHILDREN

Organization/Resource	Contact	Service Provided
About Face An international information and support organization for people with facial differences	About Face 99 Crown's Lane, 3rd Floor Toronto, Ontario Canada M5R 3P4 USA:1-800-225-FACE	Support group information Publications for families
Association for the Care of Children's Health (ACCH) An international organization for professionals and parents to improve medical settings and experiences for children	7910 Woodmont Ave. Bethesda, MD 20814 301-654-6549	Publications Resources Conferences
Civilian Health and Medical Program of the Uniformed Services (CHAMPUS) A program of medical benefits for military personnel	Health benefits administrator at local military base	Funding
Children's Special Health Services Provides comprehensive medical care for children under 21 years with congenital conditions	State Department of Health	Funding
Cleft Palate Foundation Educational and parental resource component of the American Cleft Palate Craniofacial Association	1218 Grandview Avenue Pittsburgh, PA 15211 412-481-1376	Cleft Hotline: 1-800-24-CLEFT Referrals to local teams and support groups Selected bibliography of available resources Printed booklets and fact sheets
Faces National Association for the Craniofacially Handicapped	Box 11082 Chattanooga, TN 34709 615-266-1632	Financial assistance for nonmedical costs Newsletter Publications
Hemifacial Microsomia Family Support Network Offers support and educational materials	6 Country Way Philadelphia, PA 19115 215-677-4787	Newsletter Educational publication
Let's Face It A network for people with facial differences	Box 711 Concord, MA 01742-004 508-371-3186	Resource catalog listing support groups and available publications
Medicaid Federal assistance program for low-income families	County Office for Human Resources or Welfare	Funding
National Information System and Clearinghouse Phone consultation providing comprehensive information and referrals for children 0 to 3 years old with disabilities	Center for Developmental Disabilities University of South Carolina Benson Building Columbia, SC 29208 1-800-922-9234	Referrals to services for children with special health care needs or who are developmentally disabled Educate family about legal rights
Public Health Nursing, Visiting Nurse Association State and county nursing services provided in the home	State or county Health Department	In-home evaluations Education Supportive counseling
Regional Centers for the Developmentally Disabled Federal- and state-supported programs for the developmentally disabled	State or county offices for regional centers; State Department of Education; State Department of Health and Social Services	Respite services Developmental evaluations Physical therapy/occupational therapy
Treacher Collins Foundation Family support network able to link families and provides educational material	P.O. Box 683 Norwich, VT 05055 802-649-3020	Family networking Newsletters Educational publication
Wide Smiles Private, nonmedical publication providing information and networking for parents	P.O. Box 5153 Stockton, CA 95205-0153 209-942-2812	Quarterly newsletter with articles, communication focusing primarily on clefts

Adapted from resource lists provided by About Face, Cleft Palate Foundation, and Let's Face It.

Information regarding this service is available through state Departments of Education, Departments of Mental Retardation and Developmental Disabilities, or local Health Departments. Cleft palate–craniofacial patients who have communication disorders, are hearing impaired, or medically fragile may be eligible. There is no financial eligibility requirement. Individualized assessment and treatment plans are designed for each client. Respite services are usually available through these centers. A designated number of hours per month of skilled care can be provided. Parents of infants and children with tracheostomies, assistive devices, and complex home medical care can find their experience emotionally, physically, and financially exhausting when there is no relief for the primary caretaker. The goal of respite services is to decrease stress on the family and enhance their ability to cope, thereby reducing the potential for neglect and abuse.[4]

COORDINATION/CASE MANAGEMENT

The craniofacial team is composed of a group of professionals with interest and expertise in caring for children with craniofacial anomalies. A large measure of the team's success may be due to the efforts directed at the coordination of the specialized care. Each professional makes recommendations for the child's care; however, the coordination of those recommendations into a management scheme is no small task. Children with craniofacial anomalies are served by a multiplicity of providers on the team in addition to their local source of primary care. The nurse on the craniofacial team often serves as a coordinator or case manager. Families benefit from coordinated care when their children have a clear, mutually agreeable treatment plan and goals. Oftentimes, appointments for evaluations and surgical procedures can be combined to save time and travel costs for the family. Coordination of care may also involve outside agencies such as home nursing services, developmental programs, and the school.

Case management involves coordination of the multidisciplinary care as well as assurance that evaluations are performed, procedures are completed, and goals are accomplished. Periodic reevaluation by the entire team is necessary at major decision-making junctures in the treatment process. The 1993 ACPA Parameters for Evaluation and Treatment document underscores the need for ongoing coordinated multidisciplinary care.[5]

CONSULTATION, EDUCATION, AND RESEARCH ROLES

One of the most important functions of the team nurse as a consultant is to provide outreach education and coordination with community hospitals, especially newborn nurseries or neonatal intensive care units, as well as with pediatricians and community health clinics. This is critical at the time of birth or when the diagnosis is made in order to provide health care providers with accurate information and specialty expertise.

Health care personnel, whose experience in providing care for such infants may be limited, may not feel competent to offer the information that the family needs. Parents often comment that they had received inadequate or incorrect information from hospital personnel concerning the defect and the care of their infant, which compounds their already high degree of stress and frustration.[6] Parents express gratitude and relief when early contact is made with a professional who has knowledge and experience in caring for patients with craniofacial defects.

Another aspect of the nurse's consultant role can be described as "patient and family advocate." In this role, the nurse serves as a liaison to nursing staff, craniofacial team members, primary care providers, and community agencies. For example, to the nursing staff in the pediatric unit, a mother may seem overly anxious and concerned about feeding her infant after surgery and the possibility of weight loss. Nurses and staff support personnel may be more empathetic if they understand the initial problems and frustrations that the mother experiences when feeding her newborn and how weight gain is an important milestone.

Additional educational responsibilities of the craniofacial nurse include ongoing staff education of hospital-based nursing personnel who care for these families, as well as of nursing students or other health care providers. This education may extend into public areas such as the school system, community organizations, or government agencies.

A comparatively new aspect of the nurse's role is in the area of research. In the past, nurses assisted in the management of medical research studies, but now more nurses are originating research projects that investigate questions related to feeding methods and weight gain, postoperative feeding techniques, and pain management, as well as a variety of psychosocial issues. As more medical and nursing research results are shared and incorporated into clinical practice, the nursing care and treatment of children with craniofacial defects and their families will continue to improve.

CLEFT LIP AND CLEFT PALATE

Habilitation of the infant with a cleft deformity involves evaluation and treatment by multiple specialists on the craniofacial team from birth through adolescence. The parents and, later, the child need appropriate information to understand the rationale and steps involved in this complex management.[5] Parents may have the misconception that once the lip and/or palate is surgically repaired, treatment is complete.

The stages of cleft management and the related educational needs may be divided according to developmental levels and surgical staging. Caretto identified certain stress periods for parents and patients with clefts, including the newborn period, the time surrounding hospitalizations, the onset of speech, school entry, and adolescence.[8] During infancy, the lip and palate are surgically repaired. Audiologic and otoscopic assessment should be made, and when necessary, treatment of eustachian tube dysfunction with insertion of pressure-equalization tubes should be performed by an otolaryngologist. Genetic evaluation, assessment of speech and language development, and an initial assessment by a pediatric dentist or an orthodontist as appropriate should be included in the first year's treatment plan.

Toddlers and preschool children require frequent speech and language evaluations and possible therapy; continued dental follow-up, with emphasis on promoting good oral hygiene and the prevention of baby bottle caries; continued audiologic monitoring; and possible lip and nose revisions by a plastic surgeon.

During school-age years, active orthodontia may begin in preparation for alveolar bone grafting. Continued speech and language evaluations and audiologic monitoring occur. If velopharyngeal insufficiency is identified, secondary palatal surgeries may be indicated. Revisions of the lip and nose may occur at this time.

The adolescent may require orthodontic treatment, lip revisions, and rhinoplasty. If there are problems with underdevelopment of the midface, orthognathic surgery may be indicated.

Neonatal Intervention

Parents' initial anxiety may be alleviated by immediate information regarding management, surgery, and feeding.[8] Providing this information can be viewed as emergent in nature.[9] Upon receiving the referral, the nurse immediately makes phone calls to the nursery and to the parents to provide general information about the craniofacial team and arranges for a visit with the parents as soon after discharge as possible. Scheduling time with the nurse before the complete team evaluation is beneficial. During this visit, the nurse provides education regarding the nature of the defect, the usual timing of surgeries, potential middle ear involvement, and the role of each discipline on the team. This gives the parents a basic understanding of their infant's condition and management before they are confronted with the entire team of specialists, which can be overwhelming. Written materials are provided, and parents are encouraged to review it at a later time and jot down questions as they arise, to discuss with the specific specialists during the team evaluation.

An excellent means for demonstrating the potential results of surgery are nonclinical photographs of children with repaired clefts.

Feeding and Nutrition

Feeding the infant with cleft lip and palate or isolated cleft palate can be a difficult and challenging experience for parents and health professionals. By understanding normal physiology and the altered anatomy in the newborn with a cleft, the nurse, using special techniques, can guide the parents and infant toward a successful feeding experience.

The normal process for nipple feeding involves two basic tasks: sucking and swallowing.[10] The infant's sucking motion causes the soft palate to rise, sealing off the nasopharynx from the oropharynx and creating a negative intraoral pressure which draws liquid into the mouth to be swallowed.[11] Infants with cleft palates are unable to isolate the oral and nasal cavities and create this negative pressure. They appear to make normal sucking movements, holding the nipple with their gums and pushing against any intact palatal surface.[10] Without the capacity to create negative intraoral pressure, however, the infants expend much energy but fail to obtain adequate nourishment.[12] Without intervention, feeding times are prolonged, nasal regurgitation occurs, intake is inadequate, and weight gain is poor.[13] These problems have been well documented: weight gains of less than 500 g per month, histories of feeding problems, and parental frustration have been reported.[12,14,15]

These problems can be alleviated with immediate intervention provided in the first days of life.[16] It has been demonstrated that with early counseling by experienced professionals, growth is improved and parental anxiety decreased.[13,15] In 1992, Brine and associates demonstrated with 31 patients that nutritional outcome can be positive with early and ongoing feeding intervention.[17] Making phone contact with the nursery with regard to feeding protocols or providing community nurseries with written instructions can be helpful. A clinic visit for feeding instructions or follow-up observation should be scheduled as soon as possible after discharge. In addition to prevention of infant weight loss, parents should be helped to become comfortable and competent in the care of a newborn with a cleft.

Infants with isolated cleft lip or cleft lip and alveolus usually do not have sucking problems and can be fed in the usual ways. Breastfeeding is also possible with some slight adjustments. Placing a finger over the cleft may assist the infant in obtaining a better seal around the nipple. If feeding problems persist, further assessment is needed to rule out cardiac, respiratory, or neurologic problems or the possibility of a submucous cleft palate.[9]

The goals of feeding are to provide optimal nutrition, to maximize suck reflex, and to use as normal a technique as possible while considering expense, availability, and parental acceptance.[9,10,13] A variety of nipples, feeding devices, and syringes are available. Some are expensive, not readily available, and unusual in appearance (e.g., Lamb's nipple). A device with an unusual appearance may reinforce the parents' fear that their infant is different and in some way not normal. Parents are often reluctant to use them.[12]

Two successful devices that are readily available and inexpensive include a standard bottle with enlarged (¼ inch) cross-cut regular nipple and the Mead Johnson Cleft Palate Nurser. These two methods have been studied, and no significant difference in outcomes was found.[18]

The following techniques are used during feeding:

1. Direct the nipple to any intact part of the palate with gentle downward pressure on the tongue.
2. Tilt the bottle up so that liquid is always in the nipple.
3. Position the infant upright at a 45° to 60° angle to decrease nasal regurgitation.
4. Apply gentle upward pressure with a finger placed under the jaw to encourage the sucking motion.[13]
5. Burp the infant after every ½ to 1 oz if necessary, because excessive air may be swallowed.
6. Limit feedings to 30 minutes; lengthy feedings are tiring and burn more calories.[13]

During the feeding process, the infant's cues should be observed. Widening of the eyes or choking and gulping may indicate too rapid a flow, and this will need to be adjusted.[11]

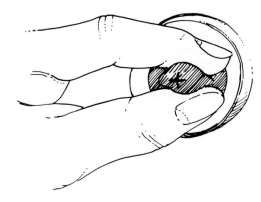

Figure 8–1. Enlarged illustration of a cross-cut nipple.

The first method involves a regular nipple with an enlarged cross-cut opening and a standard glass or plastic bottle. Enlarging the cut enables the infant to suck in greater quantities of formula in less time.[10] The cut opens when the infant squeezes the nipple, so that the infant is in control and able to prepare to swallow. This opening is preferable to merely a large hole, from which liquid pours out without the infant's control. The following procedure is used:

1. Using a No. 11 scalpel, art knife, or small pointed scissors, cut a cross ¼ inch in length into the existing minute cross-cut opening on a regular nipple (Fig. 8–1).
2. Use a 2- or 4-oz (plastic) bottle for initial feedings. (The smaller bottle is easier for a parent to hold and apply jaw pressure if needed.) As parent and infant become more experienced, any bottle can be used.
3. Assess for signs of too rapid flow or inadequate flow.
4. If flow is too rapid, feed with a smaller cross-cut opening; if too slow, enlarge the cut.

Premature-size nipples are not generally recommended for full-term infants with vigorous sucks as the nipple can collapse and increase air swallowing.[12]

The Mead-Johnson nurser, a compressible bottle with an elongated cross-cut nipple, is another option (Fig. 8–2). With this equipment, flow is increased by gently squeezing the bottle in rhythm with the infant's suck. Positioning of the baby and nipple is as described earlier. If feedings take longer than 30 to 45 minutes, attempt squeezing more during the suck phase. If the infant chokes or gags, squeeze more gently.[9] Care must be taken to squeeze gently because forcing can create aversive feeding behaviors or passive suck motions.

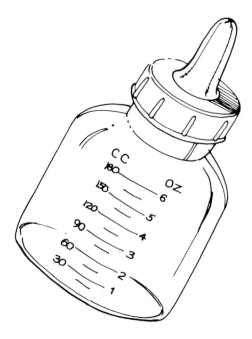

Figure 8–2. Illustration of a Mead Johnson cleft palate nurser.

Regardless of which method is used, consistency with the chosen technique for a minimum of 24 hours should be encouraged to allow both parent and infant time to adapt. Continuously switching nipples or methods causes the infant to become confused and will delay adaptation.

Breastfeeding the infant with cleft lip and palate or complete clefts of the palate is difficult and not usually successful. Infants with short, narrow clefts of the soft palate may be successful.[9] The problems are related to the inability to create negative intraoral pressure. Mothers who desire to breastfeed should be referred to a lactation consultant for additional assistance and support. Breastfeeding may be easier when the breast is full and the breast is massaged to stimulate letdown.[9,16] Applying pressure to the areola and holding it in the infant's mouth is also helpful.[16] While the infant is breastfed, biweekly weight checks and assessment of hydration status should be made until consistent weight gain has been achieved.

If direct breastfeeding is not successful, mothers may choose to feed expressed breast milk. It is essential that an electric pump be utilized at regular intervals to stimulate the usual infant feeding schedule in order to maintain an adequate milk supply. It must be considered that pumping and feeding expressed breast milk is time consuming and may not be practical, especially if there are preschoolers or toddlers in the home. The nurse can help counsel parents by exploring their feelings about breastfeeding. It is important that the mother understand that inability to breastfeed is not her failure but is caused by the infant's altered anatomy.

The use of feeding appliances varies across the country. They assist the infant in making a seal and creating negative intraoral pressure.[9] The ability of the parent to cope with removing and replacing it for cleaning, as well as the need for frequent visits to the dental specialist for evaluations and adjustments, should be considered before these appliances are used.[9] Appliances may be considered to assist with feeding, if other methods are not successful in the first week or two of life.

The parent holds the infant and provides the feeding, and the nurse acts as the coach or advisor. In addition to an explanation of the feeding technique, parents are provided with information regarding adequate intake requirements, frequency, and ideal duration of feedings and follow-up. Infants up to 6 months of age require 115 to 120 cal/kg of body weight (approximately 2½ to 3 oz/lb).[19,20] They are fed every 2 to 4 hours.[13,19] Maintaining a feeding record or diary gives the family a visual record of progress and assists the nurse in evaluating caloric intake in the first few weeks of life. Frequent phone follow-up by the nurse is encouraged in order to answer questions, identify problems, and provide support. Weekly follow-up weight checks are recommended until consistent weight gain is established. Normal gain is defined as ½ to 1 ounce per day.[13] Written instructions regarding the specific feeding program and follow-up is provided to alleviate confusion.

The methods described are appropriate for the infant with cleft palate but no other associated anomalies. If problems are encountered, possible cardiac, pulmonary, and neurologic deficits need to be assessed. Chewing, biting, or dysrhythmic sucking may be signs of neurologic deficits. Coughing or gagging may indicate swallowing problems.[10] Cyanosis, stridor, and retractions are indicative of cardiac or pulmonary disease. In these complicated situations, referral is made for further assessment. If oral feeding is not possible, nasogastric feedings may be used temporarily. This is not a long-term solution; possible complications include gagging, aspiration, decreased oral sensation, and oral aversive behaviors.[13] Gastrostomy tube placement must be considered if long-term problems are anticipated.[9,13] When these methods are used, an intensive oral stimulation or feeding program should be incorporated, usually guided by an occupational therapist.[10,13]

The timing of the introduction of solid foods and table foods is the same as for the infant without a cleft.[13] Pureed food is usually introduced at 4 to 6 months of age. Pureed food may be diluted slightly with formula or water and spoonfed, the food being placed posteriorly on the tongue. There may be some nasal regurgitation as the infant learns this new skill. Delaying the introduction of solid food and, subsequently, textured foods can create negative feeding behaviors.[13]

Clinical Management

Management of the cleft may include multiple surgeries throughout the treatment period. Preparing the parents and child for these events is one of the nurse's more important responsibilities. Parents and children experience powerlessness, anxiety, and confusion before and during hospitalization.[21] Parental concerns should be addressed and age-appropriate intervention for the child should be provided.[9]

The general postoperative management is similar to that given to any infant or child undergoing surgery. Fluids are usually provided parenterally until the patient is able to take maintenance fluids orally. Oral fluids begin with clear liquids and progress to full liquids as tolerated. The usual criteria for discharge are adequate fluid intake and the absence of any complications.

Pain management for infants and children is an integral part of postoperative nursing care. School-age children may be able to communicate their discomfort, but infants and toddlers cannot; therefore, these patients are at risk for inadequate pain management.[22] The team nurse can encourage the inpatient nursing staff to assess both verbal and nonverbal indications of discomfort (crying, facial expressions, restlessness, body posturing) at least every 4 hours. Medicating with either nonnarcotic or narcotic analgesics at least every 4 to 6 hours is recommended in the first 24 to 48 hours postoperatively unless contraindicated by an infant's or a child's behaviors. Patients who are experiencing pain may refuse oral feedings, thus delaying their discharge from the hospital. Before discharge, parents should be instructed in the home administration of pain medications.

Cleft Lip Repair

Primary repair of the lip is performed by 6 months of age. The infant's weight and overall physical condition are taken into consideration. Surgeons may use the "rule of 10" to determine timing: age 10 weeks, a weight of 10 lb, and a hemoglobin of 10 g. In selected patients, such as one with a wide unilateral complete cleft lip, the repair may be performed in two stages: lip adhesion in the first few weeks, followed by the definitive repair by 6 months of age.[5] Infants are usually hospitalized for 24 hours; however, increasing numbers of these operations are being performed on an outpatient basis. Because of decreasing lengths of stay, parental involvement and an understanding of and comfort with postoperative care are even more essential.

Postoperative management may vary according to the surgeon's preference. However, the goal of the postoperative nursing care is to protect the surgical site from manipulation by the infant and from infection. Feeding instructions may vary. In the past, syringes or cups were consistently used postoperatively. More recently, however, data regarding unrestricted postoperative feeding techniques have demonstrated that breast- or bottle-feeding postoperatively is safe and does not compromise suture line integrity.[23-25] Unrestricted feeding is more easily accepted by infants and parents. It has also been demonstrated that breast- or bottle-fed infants take maintenance fluids more rapidly and that their hospital stays are shorter in comparison with infants fed with a syringe or a cup.[23,25]

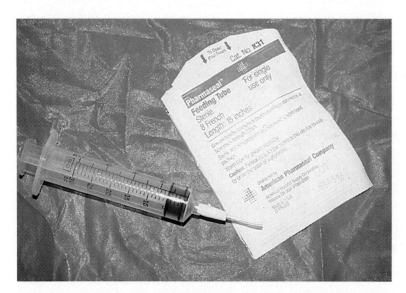

Figure 8–3. A 2-oz syringe with a feeding catheter tube cut to 1 inch may be used as an alternative method for postoperative feeding.

If restricted feedings are necessary (because of a surgeon's preference or an infant's refusal of a nipple), a 1- or 2-oz syringe with a feeding catheter tube cut to 1 inch and attached can be used (Fig. 8–3). The parent gently pushes the plunger while the tube is directed into the side of the mouth, allowing time for swallowing. This method may be easier to control than cup feeding. Pureed food may also be fed this way. The infant is offered water to rinse the mouth after feeding. Pacifiers and feeding utensils are eliminated for a specified postoperative period, and diet is limited to formula and pureed foods only.

The infant is placed in a supine position, on the side, or in an infant seat to prevent mechanical irritation of the surgical site.[26] Elbow restraints are applied to prevent flexion of the elbows so that the infant cannot place hands or objects on the lip or mouth. The restraints are removed every 4 hours for range-of-motion exercises and for assessing the skin for pressure areas. A tubular stockinette or a thin, long-sleeve tee shirt is worn against the skin to prevent rubbing. Some restraints may need to be pinned or taped to the infant's clothing to prevent accidental removal.

Normal saline solution may be used to cleanse the suture line three times a day, followed by application of an antibiotic ointment if indicated. This is best accomplished with sterile cotton-tipped applicators, rolling from the base of the nares downward. The suture site is observed for any signs of bleeding, swelling, or infection.

The length of time for feeding restrictions, for use of restraints, and for limitations on utensils and pacifiers is approximately 2 weeks.

Cleft Palate Repair

Primary palatoplasty is usually performed between 6 and 18 months of age; the timing depends on the infant's weight and physical condition and on the size of the cleft. The goal is to create a functional palate before speech development.[5] The length of hospital stay varies, but it is usually 48 to 72 hours.

In the postoperative period, close observation for airway compromise is necessary. Edema of the operative site, tongue swelling, and/or thickening of secretions may occur. Observation for increased respiratory rate, increased respiratory efforts, and adequate oxygenation is indicated.[21] High-humidity room air mist tents are often utilized if secretions thicken or edema occurs. Suctioning should be performed only if absolutely necessary and with care to avoid damage to the palate. Gentle oral insertion of the catheter is done in an emergency situation.

Swelling and discomfort during swallowing may create a reluctance in the infant to begin oral feedings. Fluids should be offered frequently and in small amounts. Oral feedings may be initiated when the infant is fully awake and responsive, beginning with clear liquids and progressing to full liquids when tolerated. A pureed diet is offered after 24 to 48 hours. Use of nipples may be restricted, and the cup or syringe method may be substituted as described previously. Unrestricted nipple feeding with cleft palate repairs without complication has been described.[24] However, no other objects may be placed inside the mouth, including pacifiers and feeding utensils. Pureed foods are fed by cup or syringe, followed by water to rinse the mouth after feeding. Elbow restraints are used as described previously.

Patients undergoing palatoplasty are older and more active than those undergoing lip repair and may have more difficulty adapting to restraints, physical limitations, and restricted feedings. They may be more irritable and difficult to console. Parents should be made aware of this possibility so that this behavioral change may be anticipated and managed with less anxiety.

Secondary Palate Management

School-age children with persistent nasality unresolved after speech therapy may be candidates for secondary palatal management with either pharyngoplasty or pharyngeal flap surgery. These surgeries are performed only after complete evaluations of the velopharyngeal mechanism, including such procedures as videofluoroscopy and videonasopharyngoscopy.[5]

Postoperative management involves the same principles as applied to the assessment and care after palatoplasty. The airway may be reduced in size and complicated by postoperative edema. Frequent observation for signs and symptoms of airway compromise is necessary. Restrictions include elimination of utensils and any other objects inside the mouth, blenderized diets by cup, and rinsing the mouth with water after feedings for approximately 2 weeks. The child needs to be included in the instructional process. It is helpful to have a dietitian consult with the parent and child regarding blenderized diet selections.

Alveolar Bone Grafting

The timing of bone grafting to the alveolar cleft is determined by the child's stage of dental development. It is usually placed before the permanent teeth erupt in the area of the cleft. Timing is decided in consultation with the orthodontist.[5] Bone is usually harvested from the iliac crest; however, costochondral or cranial sites may be used.

Careful observation of the graft and donor sites for bleeding and infection is necessary. The dietary restrictions are the same as those after secondary palate surgeries. The child stays on a blenderized diet for approximately 2 weeks and must have water rinses after every feeding. Avoidance of objects inside the mouth is stressed. Patients experience discomfort at the donor site as well as at the graft site. If iliac crest bone is harvested, ambulation may be difficult. Pain medication, offered 20 to 30 minutes before ambulation, may be helpful.

Additional Surgeries

Lip and nasal revisions may be performed before school entry to improve function or appearance as necessary. Care is similar to that provided after primary surgeries; all management is directed at preventing mechanical irritation and infection.

Rhinoplasty and nasal septal surgery are performed after completion of facial growth (at approximately 14 to 17 years of age).[5] The postoperative care should include iced compresses for the first 48 hours, as well as soft diets and fastidious oral hygiene.

Orthognathic surgery (i.e., maxillary advancement) is performed if the maxilla is underdeveloped and when orthodontic treatment to achieve proper occlusion has been unsuccessful. This is usually delayed until full growth is attained.[5] Postoperative management for these procedures is reviewed later in this chapter.

After all surgical procedures and before discharge from the hospital, instructions for home care are reviewed until the nurse feels assured that the parent or child is able to demonstrate any care required (i.e., applying restraints, syringe feedings, wound care). Written instructions are provided, and a postoperative visit with the surgeon should be scheduled.

PIERRE ROBIN SEQUENCE/STICKLER SYNDROME

Children with the Pierre Robin sequence have a classic triad of conditions: microretrognathia, glossoptosis, and a U-shaped cleft palate. This triad is termed a *sequence* because the initial malformation (microretrognathia) inhibits the tongue from assuming a natural in utero position on the floor of the mouth. The superior placement of the tongue subsequently prevents the palatal shelves from closing.[27] Figure 8–4 illustrates the altered anatomy.

Children with Stickler syndrome have the same findings as those with the Pierre Robin sequence; in addition, however, they have flat facies, myopia, skeletal changes such as arachnodactyly, and mild to moderate arthritis. The features of the Pierre Robin sequence may be part of other, less common syndromes; therefore, a comprehensive genetic evaluation is mandatory for all affected infants early in life. The child with Stickler syndrome also requires an early ophthalmologic assessment and symptomatic management of the arthritis.

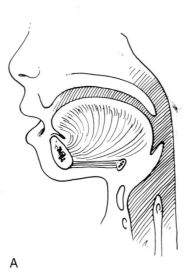
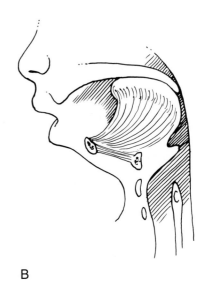

Figure 8–4. Anatomic features of upper airway. *A,* Normal. *B,* Mandibular microretrognathia found in infants with Pierre Robin sequence.

A   B

In addition to the aforementioned care for the child with cleft palate, nursing care for patients with the Pierre Robin sequence focuses on the airway management during the first year of life.

The mandible may appear to have some catch-up growth during this period of time.[28] In addition, it has been postulated that neurologic development improves oropharyngeal function and patency.[29]

Airway assessment for children with microretrognathia is aimed at detection of upper airway obstruction caused by decreased pharyngeal volume, which in turn produces increased airway resistance. Negative pressure is induced in the pharynx during the inspiratory phase, causing the tongue to be pulled into the pharyngeal airway. Symptoms of this upper airway obstruction include substernal, suprasternal, and intercostal retractions. Nasal flaring and noisy breathing may be present. Apnea/bradycardia monitors are not indicated for infants with obstructive apnea because thoracoabdominal movements continue during an obstructive event and bradycardia may occur only after a prolonged apneic event. Pulse oximetry likewise can reflect some severe events; however, it will not detect multiple short episodes of obstruction. Blood gas determinations can be helpful in detecting prolonged carbon dioxide retention and hypoxia by revealing the metabolic effects of elevated bicarbonate levels.[30] Additional diagnostic assessment of infants with any symptoms of upper airway obstruction secondary to microretrognathia often includes a polysomnographic (sleep) study, done over a period of 4 to 6 hours. The patient may be challenged by placement in different positions in order to determine the extent and frequency of obstructive events.[31]

Infants with upper airway obstruction also have symptoms of failure to thrive. This problem results from the airway compromise. Practitioners should take care not to attribute poor weight gain to the feeding method or to the presence of the cleft palate. This concept needs to be reinforced with families who may feel guilt and frustration with an unsuccessful feeding experience. Once the airway obstruction is relieved, the weight gain is expected to be adequate.[29] The parents may feed the child in an upright rather than a reclining position. During feeding, the tongue is generally thrust forward and inferiorly placed with pressure from the nipple. Care must be taken when the nipple is removed for burping because the tongue can easily slip back into the pharynx at this time and result in obstruction. Therefore, burping the infant in a seated position but leaning slightly forward will promote forward tongue position.

Prone positioning of the infant with mild microretrognathia is a management technique that requires careful instruction of the parents. The infant's ventilatory effort is more difficult to observe in this position. Prone positioning during travel is also a necessity and warrants consideration for discharge planning; an approved car bed, in which the infant is placed supine, is preferable to a traditional car seat. Infants who are discharged home with positioning as the primary treatment modality need careful follow-up observation. Parents need to be alert for increasing symptoms of obstruction, especially with the onset of the first infection of the upper respiratory tract. Home cardiorespiratory monitors are usually not indicated. Likewise, supplemental oxygen is not indicated. Follow-up appointments to assess airway status should be made with a physician experienced in this area of care.

Infants for whom prone positioning alone does not correct the upper airway obstruction require more aggressive methods of management. Temporary nasopharyngeal tube placement[30] or oral airway placement can be useful in relieving airway obstruction. The nasopharyngeal tube is longer and therefore may be easier to maintain in the correct position. Frequent suctioning and assessment of the tube patency is necessary. Taping to secure proper placement should be redone at least daily. Tubes need to be changed with care at frequent intervals if there is a build-up of secretions. Placement and changing of the tube are often easier if the infant is sitting up and leaning slightly forward. Feeding is accomplished via a nasogastric tube when the artificial airway is in place. Oral stimulation should continue at feeding times with a pacifier. The infant may remain with a nasopharyngeal airway in place for as long as 2 months with frequent reassessments for the growth of the pharyngeal airway and improved neuromuscular control. Some centers monitor progress by means of flexible fiberoptic nasopharyngoscopy,[29] whereas others perform follow-up polysomnography studies.

Infants who fail the management schemes just described are candidates for surgical treatment. One method is a glossopexy procedure, in which the tongue is moved anteriorly and attached to either the mandible or the lip.[29] Postoperatively, infants may have a nasopharyngeal airway in place for 48 hours, elbow restraints for 1 to 2 weeks, frequent suctioning, and eventual (after 5 to 7 days) reinstitution of oral feedings.[30]

In the absence of success with more conservative management protocols, a tracheostomy may be performed.[30] A tracheostomy requires complex nursing care and parent education. In general, infants who require tracheostomy have it in place until after the cleft palate is surgically repaired. Subsequently, they are assessed carefully for decannulation by bronchoscopy, polysomnographic study, and inpatient observation after decannulation.

Long-term care for patients with the Pierre Robin sequence and Stickler syndrome generally parallels the care required for all children with a cleft palate. However, children with Sticker syndrome may need regular ophthalmologic assessments and counseling to avoid impact sports, which may modify the risk of retinal detachment. There have been some reports of late childhood and adolescent deaths, presumably caused by sleep-state upper airway obstruction. History taking should include questions relating to the presence of sleep apnea. Some patients may be candidates for later genioplasty procedures to improve mandibular appearance and occlusion.

CRANIOSYNOSTOSIS

Craniosynostosis is the premature closure of one or more cranial sutures. It may manifest as an isolated occurrence, or it may be associated with other defects as part of a syndrome. The degree of skull and facial deformities may range from minimal, as in a mild metopic suture fusion, to severe, as in kleeblattschädel deformity, which involves multiple cranial sutures.[32]

The diagnosis of craniosynostosis and the referral to a craniofacial team may occur at different times. Severe deformities may be diagnosed at birth, and the initial contact occurs in the newborn period. Other patients may not be referred until later. Some families relate a history of always believing that their child's head looked ''different'' but being told by family, friends, or professionals that it would change. They may be angry or resentful when informed of the diagnosis. Others, especially parents of children with mild deformities, may have adjusted to the altered appearance and initially resist the diagnosis and suggestions for surgical correction. As the family attempts to gather more information and make a decision, the nurse's role may be to offer information, to clarify possible misconceptions, and to listen as the parents relate their fears and concerns. It is often helpful to be able to link a family whose child has a newly diagnosed condition to a support group or parent network.

Preoperative Preparation

The time and type of surgical procedure varies, depending on different factors, but the preoperative preparation has common elements.

Table 8-3. TOPICS COVERED BEFORE
CRANIAL SURGERY

ICU environment and routines
Monitors
Dressings, drains
Incision
Swelling
Pain relief
Nutriton
Behaviors to expect

Abbreviation: ICU, intensive care unit.

Because most initial surgeries for suture release are performed on infants or children less than 3 years of age, the parents undergo the preoperative preparation. Infants or children are not routinely admitted to the hospital preoperatively, and so the work-up and preparation are done on an outpatient basis. It is important to assess the family's level of understanding as it relates to the diagnosis, surgery, and hospitalization. The educational process may start at the clinic visit and continue until the surgery date through follow-up telephone calls and written information.

Instructions regarding the mechanics of the preoperative work-up are helpful. Explanations may include descriptions of x-rays, computed tomography (CT) scans, or other tests and their preparation. The infant or young child generally needs sedation in order to obtain an adequate CT or magnetic resonance imaging (MRI) study. The nursing care during this procedure includes monitoring for apnea/bradycardia and use of a pulse oximeter with careful attention to the presence of sleep-state upper airway obstruction during and after sedation.

The most important preparation involves an explanation of the anticipated postoperative course. Operative procedures vary, depending on the involved suture, the child's age, and the surgeon's preference; however, postoperative nursing care may be similar. When there are differences—for example, orbital swelling is not an anticipated event in a posterior procedure—then the information needs to be tailored to suit the procedure as well as the family's level of understanding. Table 8–3 summarizes the major points that need to be included in a discussion with the family. In addition, an opportunity to tour the intensive care unit (ICU) should be offered to the family.

Postoperative Care

Assessment of the patient in the initial postoperative period includes monitoring for increased intracranial pressure (ICP), blood loss, and possible syndrome of inappropriate secretion of antidiuretic hormone (SIADH). The infant usually has been extubated but may require supplemental oxygen via face mask or nasal cannula for a short period.

When the initial assessment has been completed, the parents should be allowed to visit as soon as possible. They are often very anxious to see for themselves that their child is alright and to observe the change in physical appearance. The countenance at this time before postoperative swelling begins is a good predictor of the patient's eventual appearance.

Giving explanations regarding the ICU routines, the child's monitoring equipment, and the anticipated course of treatment will reinforce the previous preoperative preparation. Parents should be allowed to participate in as much of their child's care as is possible.

Nursing care of the patient during the ICU stay includes several components. As mentioned, the infant usually has been extubated but may require supplemental oxygen via face mask or nasal cannula. Monitoring neurologic status includes assessing level of consciousness, pupil size, and reactivity. The head of the bed is elevated at a 30° angle. A closed wound drainage system may be used. A Foley catheter is used to assess accurate urine output, and intravenous fluids may be administered at less than maintenance requirement to prevent fluid overload. Clear liquids may be offered the first evening after surgery. The diet is advanced, depending on the child's tolerance.

Pain management is very important, and intravenous sedation with morphine sulfate is usually ordered for the first 24 hours.

The child is usually moved from the ICU to the acute care unit 24 hours postoperatively. The Foley catheter, arterial catheters, and drains are discontinued. Intravenous fluids are continued as necessary while the diet is being advanced. The child may also be weaned to oral narcotic or nonnarcotic analgesics.

After the removal of the head dressing, the incision should be cleansed and an antibiotic ointment applied if ordered. The nurse should be alert for signs of infection, including an increased temperature; redness, swelling, or drainage from the incision site; and drainage from the ear or nose, which could signify cerebrospinal fluid leakage.

Significant orbital edema, when present, is usually the symptom most distressing to both the patient and family. Swelling usually peaks 48 hours postoperatively. Restraints or distraction techniques may be necessary to prevent the child from rubbing the eyes. Toddlers especially may be distressed during this time and may have limited appetite and activity. The reassurance of the presence of familiar people and objects is helpful, and the parents also need to be reassured that this is a temporary state. An effective intervention is to use tape recordings of family members' voices or favorite music.

Discharge from the hospital is usually on the fourth or fifth postoperative day. Parents should be given instructions regarding suture care, safety precautions, pain management, signs and symptoms of infection or ICP, and follow-up care.

CRANIOFACIAL DYSOSTOSIS: CROUZON AND APERT SYNDROMES

Newborn Assessment and Management and Parent Education

Crouzon and Apert syndromes are the most common of the craniosynostosis syndromes. Patients with Crouzon syndrome have the characteristic features of craniosynostosis, exorbitism, and midface retrusion. Children with Apert syndrome in addition have syndactyly of the hands and feet.[33]

Patients with Crouzon syndrome may present to the craniofacial team at different ages. Severe cases may be recognized at birth, and immediate referral to a team is initiated, whereas subtle manifestations of Crouzon syndrome may not be diagnosed and referred until later. Apert syndrome, however, is usually diagnosed at birth as a result of the presence of syndactyly.

Parental acceptance of an infant and integration into the family are critical issues during the first year of life.[34] The birth and care of a newborn with Crouzon or Apert syndrome can be very stressful for a family. Parents who are trying to resolve negative feelings toward their infant may be embarrassed or reluctant to take the child out in public. This overprotection and/or alienation may create a negative impact on the child's psychological development.[34, 35] From the first interaction with the family, the nurse should be a role model of acceptance and nurturance.[5] The importance to the child in experiencing different environments and interactions with others should be discussed so that parents will not isolate the child. Discussing potential situations that families may experience in public may help prepare them for comments and questions both from strangers and from friends.

In addition to dealing with emotional stress, the family may have to deal with potential physical complications associated with the conditions. These may include respiratory difficulties, feeding problems, neurologic complications such as ICP or hydrocephalus, and the potential risk of development delay.[36]

If the infant experiences feeding difficulties, a thorough nursing assessment is necessary to determine the etiology. The two main causes for problems in this population include mechanical/structural defects, such as cleft or high arched palate, and respiratory defects, such as narrowing of the upper airway. Congenital maxillary retrusion may cause obstruction of the nasal airway and consequently interfere with the normal feeding process. Until the respiratory problem is resolved, oral feeding may be difficult.

In cases of severe midface retrusion and respiratory distress, a tracheostomy may be recommended. The nurse may then be involved in teaching the parents how to care for the tracheostomy at home and in arranging home health care for supplies and respite care is necessary. Even if an infant does not require a tracheostomy at birth, close monitoring for the development of chronic upper airway obstruction with resulting failure to thrive must continue throughout the first decade of life.

Children with craniofacial anomalies are also at a greater risk for obstructive sleep apnea. This may coincide with the expected enlargement of tonsillar and adenoid tissue in the preschool years. The diagnosis is usually established by a polysomnogram. The nurse should be familiar with the presenting symptoms, which can include snoring with apneic episodes, snorting or choking at night, restlessness during sleep, daytime hypersomnolence or hyperactivity, enuresis, failure to thrive, developmental delay, and behavioral problems.[37] A thorough nursing assessment may reveal some of these symptoms, which parents may have considered normal and neglected to report.

In Crouzon and Apert syndromes, synostosis or two or more cranial sutures is involved; therefore, there is a risk of increased intracranial pressure.[38] The nurse's responsibility may include ensuring consistent measurement and plotting of the infant's head circumference on the growth chart and assisting in monitoring for signs of ICP, such as irritability and vomiting. Delay in achievement of developmental milestones may also be an important indicator. Parents should be familiarized with signs of ICP and communicate with the pediatrician or neurosurgeon if there is concern.

Another potential complication is hydrocephalus. Although the incidence of hydrocephalus is lowest in single-suture synostosis, it is observed more frequently in patients with Crouzon and Apert syndrome.[39] If an infant requires a shunting procedure, the nurse's responsibility includes educating the family with regard to care of a child with a shunt and ensuring that appropriate antibiotic prophylactic measures are taken for invasive treatments.

Perhaps the area that raises the most emotional concern is the question of developmental delay. The reported incidence of mental retardation among patients with Crouzon syndrome is between 0% and 20%, whereas a higher incidence (approximately 20% to 30%) appears among patients with Apert syndrome.[33, 40] The nurse may be questioned by the family concerning these risks. Although it is important to not deny the possibility, it is essential that the child's individuality and the need for maximizing the child's potential and capabilities be emphasized. A referral to an infant simulation program may be appropriate.

Long-Term Care Considerations

Multidisciplinary long-term services for children with Apert and Crouzon syndromes should also include audiologic, speech, ophthalmologic, pediatric, dental, and orthodontic services. These children are at risk for conductive hearing loss and therefore should have frequent audiologic evaluations. Speech production may be altered because of the abnormal anatomic findings, such as an open bite deformity, byzantine-shaped or cleft palate, and decreased nasal air space. Consequently, frequent monitoring by a speech pathologist and therapy are often indicated. Ophthalmologic assessment is important because of the presence of exorbitism and the increased risk of eye muscle pathology. The nurse should assess for adequate corneal protection and instruct the parent in lubrication if necessary. Malocclusion is a universal finding; therefore, attention to dental and orthodontic services is critical.

Surgical Treatment

Treatment in infancy and early childhood is usually directed at the suture fusion, and nursing concerns and care are the same as those for children with craniosynostosis.

Surgical treatment of the midface deformity may be addressed during early school-age years, adolescence, or both, depending on the child's physical and emotional status and the philosophy of the craniofacial team.

Postoperative Care Following LeFort III Midface Advancement

After a midface advancement or LeFort III osteotomy, the child is transferred to the ICU for the first 24 to 48 hours. Factors influencing the length of ICU stay may include airway status and the presence of intermaxillary fixation (jaw wiring). However, the advent of microplates and screws for rigid internal fixation has reduced the use of intermaxillary fixation. This has resulted in easier postoperative airway access, increased patient comfort, and maintenance of optimal oral hygiene.[41] Management of the airway depends on various factors and may include extubation in the recovery room, a 24- to 48-hour use of nasal intubation, or, infrequently, a tracheostomy. Close assessment of the respiratory status is critical, especially in children with intermaxillary fixation.

After transfer to the pediatric unit, it is important to continue monitoring the airway status. If the jaws are wired, a wire cutter should be available at the bedside, and parents should be instructed in its use in an emergency. It is also appropriate to monitor the hemodynamic status after multiple osteotomies. Patients generally have significant postoperative edema. Local ice packs and elevation of head and the bed are recommended. Short-term steroids may be ordered to decrease the postoperative facial swelling.[42] Most patients require analgesics, initially narcotic and later nonnarcotic. Dietary modifications include blenderized food for approximately 1 month to allow bony and soft tissue healing. A consultation with a clinical nutritionist is appropriate. Oral hygiene needs to be meticulously performed.

Discharge criteria include a stable airway, stable hemodynamic status, and tolerance of blenderized diet. Discharge instruction on oral hygiene, incision care, activity limitations, and follow-up appointments should be presented.

Throughout the entire pre- and postoperative period, the child as well as the family must be actively involved in the planning and decision making to ensure compliance with recommendations. This includes both pre- and postoperative orthodontic management in addition to the immediate postoperative care restrictions.

TREACHER COLLINS SYNDROME

Children with Treacher Collins syndrome (mandibulofacial dysostosis) exhibit severe malar and mandibular hypoplasia. They have characteristic downward-slanting, palpebral fissures and colobomata of the lower lid. Severe external, middle, and inner ear malformations can occur with concomitant and conductive hearing loss. Approximately one third of patients have a cleft palate.[27]

Initial nursing management is similar to that provided for the patient with the Pierre Robin sequence with regard to airway and nutritional assessment and management. Children who have choanal atresia in addition to the mandibular hypoplasia are at particular respiratory risk in infancy, during which the patients are obligate nose breathers.

After the airway and nutritional needs are met, the child's audiologic status must be assessed. Middle ear anomalies are almost universal findings.[43] Experienced pediatric audiologists advocate early placement of hearing aids if warranted. The nurse can promote acceptance of this device and encourage compliance to afford the child maximal reception of auditory stimulation necessary for development.

Reconstruction of the malformed external ear may be performed when the ear has achieved nearly full growth (generally at about 5 to 6 years of age). Standard ear reconstruction techniques, employing costochondral grafting, are used.[44] A series of procedures may be necessary for reconstruction. The goal of postoperative care is to preserve the integrity of the reconstructed external ear with a well-padded head dressing that remains in place until the first postoperative visit. In addition, when a costochondral graft is harvested, the nurse needs to monitor for signs of pneumothorax and also promote good pulmonary hygiene to prevent pneumonia. Analgesia for localized discomfort is usually necessary.

Children with Treacher Collins syndrome may require bony reconstruction of the zygoma, zygomatic arch, anterior maxilla infraorbital rim, and orbital axis.[44] The reconstruction may be performed with calvarial vascularized bone graft or alloplastic material. Postoperative care for these patients includes meticulous attention to airway maintenance and to the hemodynamic status, particularly for patients with calvarial bone grafts. Symptomatic treatment for postoperative facial edema includes elevating the head of the bed and local application of ice packs.

Eyelid deformities may be corrected surgically, and the procedures generally can be performed on an outpatient basis unless there are airway problems. Postoperative care addresses the symptoms associated with periorbital edema.

Adolescents with Treacher Collins syndrome often require orthognathic surgery after a course of orthodontic management in the school-age years for a class II malocclusion and open bite deformity.[44] The postoperative nursing care for different orthognathic surgical procedures is similar to that previously described for the LeFort III midface advancement.

HEMIFACIAL MICROSOMIA/GOLDENHAR SYNDROME

Hemifacial microsomia comprises various defects in the development of the first and second branchial arches. It may be present in a mild form that involves mild facial asymmetry and microtia, or it may be present in a severe form that includes additional ocular, vertebral, cardiac, and renal malformations (also known as Goldenhar syndrome, or oculo-auriculovertebral dysplasia). The external ear, middle ear, mandible and maxilla, temporal bone, facial muscles, and muscles of mastication, tongue, and parotid gland may be underdeveloped. Affected children may have associated cleft lip-palate or macrostomia and also a branchial cleft sinus. Children who have a unilateral defect also have compensatory deformations of the unaffected side, especially in the mandible.[27,45] A minority of individuals exhibit a bilateral form of this condition.

Nursing care of infants with hemifacial microsomia or Goldenhar syndrome begins with airway assessment. Because the mandibular deficiency is most commonly unilateral, the incidence of upper airway obstruction is not as prevalent among these patients as among those with Treacher Collins syndrome and the Pierre Robin sequence. The infants may require some minor positioning adaptations for feeding because of the presence of an asymmetric mandible, macrostomia, or vertebral anomalies.

After airway and nutritional management, audiologic assessment and management similar to those in children with Treacher Collins syndrome is indicated.

Macrostomia and cleft lip and palate are repaired during infancy. Nursing care considerations have been previously described. Children with hemifacial microsomia may have epibulbar dermoids, microphthalmia, eyelid ptosis, coloboma of the upper eyelid, and strabismus.[33] As with Treacher Collins syndrome, the surgical management of these conditions is usually on an outpatient basis with symptomatic treatment postoperatively. The notable exception is in the use of an ocular prosthesis in increasing sizes for microphthalmia. Most children adjust to these prostheses well if the ocular care is initiated in infancy. Wearing glasses to protect the unaffected eye is also recommended for these children.

Children with hemifacial microsomia who have an atretic ear are candidates for external reconstruction, with the same care considerations outlined for patients with Treacher Collins syndrome. The timing of the procedure, however, is different in that it usually follows the reconstruction of the skeletal framework of the mandible and zygoma.

The most complex aspect of the treatment for patients with hemifacial microsomia and Goldenhar syndrome involves the management of the mandibular anomalies. The goals of the treatment include improved function (i.e., with mastication), optimal facial appearance, and symmetry upon achievement of full craniofacial growth.[45]

Children often require a combination of orthodontia with acrylic splints or activated appliances, in addition to surgical management.[45–47] These appliances necessitate vigilant oral hygiene practices, frequent appointments for adjustments, and strict compliance in maintaining proper placement in the mouth. This can be a challenge for the school-age child and the family.

Surgical management for the mandibular deficiency takes place at different ages, according to the degree of the problem and also to minimize interference with maxillary and midface growth. Depending on the extent of the deformity, children in their preschool and early school-age years may be candidates for orthognathic surgery. Additional surgical procedures may be needed in adolescence. Nursing care after surgical reconstruction is similar to postoperative care after midface advancement.

CONCLUSIONS

During the entire treatment program for any craniofacial anomaly, the nurse maintains contact with the family, continually reinforcing the treatment needs and coordinating care among the various specialists, community agencies, and the schools. At each interaction, the nurse assesses the child's and family's knowledge of the treatment program, the ability to cope with the multiple needs, and the ability to comply with treatment. If problems are identified, referrals to psychology and/or social services may be appropriate. It has been shown that increased information and involvement of the family in the health care program can decrease stress and improve outcomes.[48]

Advances in the prenatal diagnosis of craniofacial disorders will expand the role of the nurse as an educator and a consultant in the perinatal period.

References

1. MacDonald S: Parental needs and professional responses: A parental perspective. Cleft Palate J 1979; 16(2):188–192.
2. Wolfer JA, Visintainer MA: Prehospital psychological preparation for tonsillectomy patients: Effects on children's and parents' adjustment. Pediatrics 1979; 64(5):646–655.
3. Clifford E: Patients, parents and cleft palate teams. In Clifford E (ed): The Cleft Palate Experience: New Perspectives on Management, 1st ed, p 33. Springfield, IL: CC Thomas, 1987.
4. O'Connor P, Van der Plats S, Betz C: Respite care services to caretakers of chronically ill children in California. J Pediat Nurs 1992; 7(4):269.
5. American Cleft Palate–Craniofacial Association: Parameters for the Evaluation and Treatment of Patients with Cleft Lip/Palate or Other Craniofacial Anomalies. Cleft Palate–Craniofac J 1993; 30(Suppl 1).
6. Scheuerle J, Olsen S, Guildford AM: A survey of nursing care for parents and infants with cleft lip and palate. Cleft Palate J 1984; 21:110–114.
7. Rogers M, Barden RC, Kuczaj S: Psychosocial aspects of cleft lip and palate: The family. In Bardach J, Morris H (eds): Multidisciplinary Management of Cleft Lip and Palate. Philadelphia: WB Saunders, 1990.
8. Caretto V: Maternal responses to an infant with cleft lip and palate: A review of the literature. Matern Child Nurs J 1984; 10:197–205.
9. Curtin G: The infant with cleft lip or palate: More than a surgical problem. J Perinat Neonatal Nurs 1990; 3(3):80–89.
10. Clarren S, Anderson B, Wolf L: Feeding infants with cleft lip and palate. Cleft Palate J 1987; 24(3):244.
11. Richard M: Feeding the newborn with cleft lip and/or cleft palate: The enlargement, stimulate, swallow, rest (ESSR) method. J Pediat Nurs 1991; 6(5):317.
12. Pashayan H, McNab M: Simplified method of feeding infants born with cleft palate with or without cleft lip. Am J Dis Child 1979; 133:145.
13. Balluff M: Nutritional needs of an infant or child with a cleft lip or palate. Ear Nose Throat J 1986; 65:44.
14. Paradise J, McWilliams B, Elster B: Feeding infants with cleft palate [Letter]. Pediatrics 1985; 74:316.
15. Avedian LV, Ruberg RL: Impaired weight gain in cleft palate infants. Cleft Palate J 1980; 17:24–26.
16. Styer GW, Freeh K: Feeding infants with cleft lip and/or palate. J Obstet Gynecol Neonatal Nurs 1981; 10(5):329–331.
17. Brine E, Rickard K, Brady M, et al: Growth and Nutritional Outcome of Infants with Isolated Cleft Palate vs. Cleft Lip/Palate During the First 18 Months of Life. Presented at the 49th annual meeting of the American Cleft Palate–Craniofacial Association, Portland, OR, May 14, 1992.
18. Brine E, Rickard K, Brady M, et al: Efficacy of Two Feeding Methods in Improving Energy Intake and Growth of Infants with Cleft Palate. Presented at the 49th annual meeting of the American Cleft Palate–Craniofacial Association, Portland, OR, May 14, 1992.
19. Behrman RE, Klugman R: Nutrition and nutritional disorders. In Behrman RE (ed): Nelson Textbook of Pediatrics, 14th ed, pp 105, 124, 125. Philadelphia: WB Saunders, 1992.
20. Forbes MD, Woodruff C (eds): Pediatric Nutrition Handbook, 2nd ed, pp 19, 30. Elk Grove, IL: American Academy of Pediatrics, 1985.
21. McInerny T: Cleft palate repair: Surgical procedure and nursing care. AORN J 1985; 42(4):516–527.
22. Page G, Halvorson M: Pediatric nurses: The assessment and control of pain in preverbal infants. J Pediat Nurs 1991; 6(2):99–105.
23. Boekelheide A, Curtin G, Muraoka V, et al: Comparison of Postsurgical Feeding Techniques Following Cleft Lip Repair on Suture Line Integrity, Volume of Oral Fluid Intake and Length of Hospital Stay: A Multicenter Study. Presented at the 49th annual meeting of the American Cleft Palate–Craniofacial Association, Portland, OR, May 14, 1992.
24. Cohen M, Marschall M, Schafer M: Immediate unrestricted feeding of infants following cleft lip and palate repair. J Craniofac Surg 1992; 3(1):30–32.
25. Weatherly-White RCA, Kuelin DP, Mirrett P, et al: Early repair and breast feeding for infants with cleft lip. Plast Reconstr Surg 1987; 79(6):879–885.
26. Chase L, Starr D, Tvedte C, et al: Comprehensive nursing care of cleft patients. In Bardach J, Morris H (eds): Multidisciplinary Management of Cleft Lip and Palate, pp 840–847. Philadelphia: WB Saunders, 1990.

27. McPherson E: Genetic function in craniofacial syndromes. *In* Dufresne CR, Carson BS, Zinreich SJ (eds): Complex Craniofacial Problems: A Guide to Analysis and Treatment, pp 97–130. New York: Churchill Livingstone, 1992.

28. Figueroa AA, Glupker TJ, Fitz MG, et al: Mandible, tongue and airway in Pierre Robin sequence: A longitudinal cephalometric study. Cleft Palate–Craniofac J 1991; 28(4):425–434.

29. Sher AE: Mechanisms of airway obstruction in Robin sequence: Implications for treatment. Cleft Palate–Craniofac J 1992; 29(3):224–231.

30. Singer L, Sidoti EJ: Pediatric management of Robin sequence. Cleft Palate–Craniofacial J 1992; 29(3):220–223.

31. Freed G, Pearlman MA, Brown AS, et al: Polysomonographic indications for surgical intervention in Pierre Robin sequence: Acute airway management and follow-up studies after repair and take-down of tongue-lip adhesion. Cleft Palate J 1988; 25(2):151–155.

32. Dufresne CR: Classifications of craniofacial anomalies. *In* Dufresne CR, Carson BS, Zinreich SJ (eds): Complex Craniofacial Problems: A Guide to Analysis and Treatment, p 64. New York: Churchill Livingstone, 1992.

33. Jones KL: Smith's Recognizable Patterns of Human Malformation. Philadelphia: WB Saunders, 1988.

34. Campis LB: Children with Apert syndrome: Developmental and psychologic considerations. Clin Plast Surg 1991; 18(2):409.

35. Benson BA, Gross AM, Messer SC, et al: Social support networks among families of children with craniofacial anomalies. Health Psychol 1991; 10(4):252–258.

36. Kaplan LC: Management of Apert syndrome. Clin Plast Surg 1991; 18(2):217–225.

37. Volk MS, Arnold S, Brodsky L: Otolaryngology and audiology. *In* Brodsky L, Holt L, Ritter-Schmidt DH (eds): Craniofacial Anomalies: An Interdisciplinary Approach, p 173. St. Louis: Mosby Year Book, 1992.

38. Carson BS, Dufresne CR: Craniosynostosis and neurocranial asymmetry. *In* Dufresne CR, Carson BS, Zinreich SJ (eds): Complex Craniofacial Problems: A Guide to Analysis and Treatment, p 168. New York: Churchill Livingstone, 1992.

39. McCarthy JG: Plastic Surgery, vol 4: Cleft Lip and Palate and Craniofacial Anomalies. Philadelphia: WB Saunders, 1990.

40. Marsh JC, Vannier MW: Comprehensive Care for Craniofacial Deformities. St. Louis: CV Mosby, 1985.

41. Prein J, Hammer B: Stable internal fixation of midfacial fractures. Fac Plast Surg 1988; 5(3):221–229.

42. Schaberg SJ, Stuller CB, Edwards SM: Effect of methylprednisolone on swelling after orthognathic surgery. J Oral Maxillofac Surg 1984; 42:356–361.

43. Pron G, Galloway C, Armstrong D, et al: Ear malformation and hearing loss in patients with Treacher Collins syndrome. Cleft Palate–Craniofac J 1993; 30(1):97–103.

44. Dufresne CR: Treacher Collins syndrome. *In* Dufresne CR, Carson BS, Zinreich SJ (eds): Complex Craniofacial Problems: A Guide to Analysis and Treatment, pp 281–294. New York: Churchill Livingstone, 1992.

45. So IHS, Dufresne CR: Hemifacial microsomia. *In* Dufresne CR, Carson BS, Zinreich SJ (eds): Complex Craniofacial Problems: A Guide to Analysis and Treatment, pp 295–318. New York: Churchill Livingstone, 1992.

46. Munro IR: Hemifacial microsomia. *In* Marsh J (ed): Current Therapy in Plastic and Reconstructive Surgery of the Head and Neck, vol 1, pp 254–264. Toronto: BC Decker, 1989.

47. Vargervik K: Sequence and timing of treatment phases in hemifacial microsomia. *In* Harvold EP, Vargervik K, Chierici G (eds): Treatment of Hemifacial Microsomia, pp 133–137. New York: AR Liss, 1983.

48. Paynter E, Edmonson T, Jordan W: Accuracy of information reported by parents and children evaluated by a cleft palate team. Cleft Palate J 1991; 28(4):329–337.

Airway Management

Amelia F. Drake and James D. Sidman

INTRODUCTION

Airway management of patients with facial clefts or craniosynostosis is a challenging element of overall care. Just as in normals, airway obstruction in those with facial clefting might occur at different levels. The particular craniofacial anomaly, however, predisposes to certain types and degrees of involvement. Knowledge of the various causes of airway obstruction in the child with a cleft palate or craniofacial anomaly will better enable the pediatrician, otolaryngologist, and the rest of the craniofacial team to plan and direct the patient's care. Awareness of which types of obstruction improve with age will prevent needless and potentially ineffective treatment and/or surgery. Also, future investigation into appropriate methods of intervention is an essential aspect of the ongoing quest for optimal care of the craniofacial patient.

CAUSES OF UPPER AIRWAY OBSTRUCTION

Some of the conditions causing airway compromise in craniofacial patients are unique to the craniofacial population, while most types of airway compromise are found in those with or without craniofacial anomalies. Problems that are unique or found mostly in craniofacial patients include clefting of the midface (Tessier's classification) with nasopharyngeal stenosis or atresia secondary to midface hypoplasia, glossoptosis with oropharyngeal or hypopharyngeal obstruction, and laryngotracheo-esophageal clefting. Other causes of airway compromise, such as choanal atresia, laryngomalacia, pharyngeal hypotonia, and subglottic stenosis, are frequently found in children who do not have other craniofacial findings. It is not clear whether children with craniofacial abnormalities have these other abnormalities more often than the general population, and the authors are unaware of any epidemiologic studies to answer this question.

Anatomic Causes

An anatomic classification of site of obstruction is pragmatic, and the causes of upper airway obstruction are outlined in Table 9–1. Beginning with the nose, most sites of obstruction are not unique to the patient with a facial cleft or craniosynostosis. Examples are adenoid hypertrophy and allergic rhinitis, which cause nasal obstruction in much of the normal population. Children with repaired cleft palate have smaller nasal airways than unaffected normals of the same age. The nasal examination reveals significant nasal deformities and reduced nasal airway size in the presence of a repaired cleft palate.[1] Turbinate hypertrophy or septal spurs may be present and contribute to the problem. Growth improves the nasal airway size at the same rate as in normal controls, although the cleft nose remains significantly smaller than the noncleft nose through adulthood. The reduction in airway size is associated with an increase in the percent of oral breathing versus nasal breathing in the cleft population.[2]

The child is an obligatory nasal breather at birth, and 70% of newborn infants are unable to breathe orally on their own. Obligate nasal breathing lasts until 10 to 12 weeks of age, corrected to gestational age if the child is premature. This phenomenon is related to the anatomy of the food and air passageways. At birth, the soft palate reaches the level of the epiglottis (Fig. 9–1). This configuration permits the infant to breathe while nursing or feeding. The milk bolus travels laterally while air is inspired

Table 9–1. Causes of Airway Obstruction

Nasal/Nasopharyngeal

Nasal pyriform aperture stenosis
Choanal atresia
Advanced hypertrophy
Midfacial hypoplasia
  Apert syndrome
  Crouzon syndrome
  Pfeiffer syndrome

Oropharyngeal

Macroglossia
  Down syndrome
  Beckwith-Wiedemann syndrome
  Hemangioma/lymphangioma
Tonsillar hypertrophy
Mandibular hyperplasia
  Pierre Robin sequence
  Treacher Collins syndrome

Supraglottic/Glottic

Laryngomalacia
Atresia
Web
Laryngeal cleft
Saccular cysts
Vocal cord paralysis
Congenital subglottic stenosis

into the lungs. When normal nasal breathing is not possible, such as in situations of total or near-total nasal obstruction in the newborn, a problem arises. Posterior choanal atresia occurs in 1 in 8000 live births and can be unilateral or bilateral. Less commonly, it may be associated with other anomalies, such as in the case of the CHARGE syndrome (*c*oloboma, *h*eart defects, choanal *a*tresia, *r*etardation, *g*enitourinary anomalies, and *e*ar abnormalities).

Congenital obstruction at the anterior nose, known as congenital nasal pyriform aperture stenosis, has been described as a microform of holoprosencephaly, a midline developmental defect that sometimes includes a facial cleft.[3] A single maxillary incisor may be present on computed tomography scan, which is considered the diagnostic radiographic study (Fig. 9–2).

Figure 9–1. Proximate relationship of palate to larynx in infants.

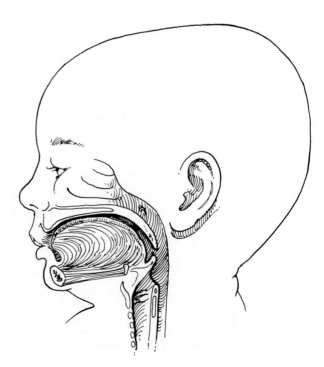

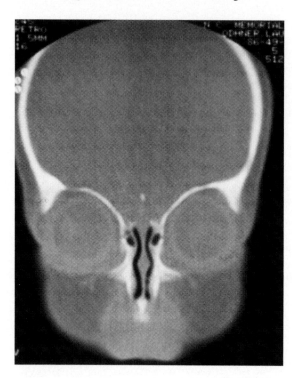

Figure 9–2. CT scan demonstrating congenital nasal pyriform aperture stenosis and single maxillary incisor.

At the level of the nasopharynx, midfacial hypoplasia often manifests as obstruction. Crouzon, Pfeiffer and Apert syndromes are all associated with midface hypoplasia. Because nasopharyngeal obstruction prevents normal nasal breathing, these patients may present during infancy with trouble breathing while feeding and, hence, with poor weight gain. Usually the diagnosis is obvious because of the suggestive facial features. Treatment is supportive, although tracheotomy may be helpful until nasal breathing is no longer necessary.

Similarly, obstruction at the oropharynx or hypopharynx may prevent normal respiration. Obstruction can be caused by glossoptosis or collapse of the tongue into the posterior pharyngeal airway. The cause of such collapse can be anatomic (a small mandible or large tongue). Infants with the Pierre Robin sequence (glossoptosis, cleft palate, micrognathia) will usually present with airway obstruction at birth if this is going to be a problem (Fig. 9–3). Many of these children will outgrow the problem by

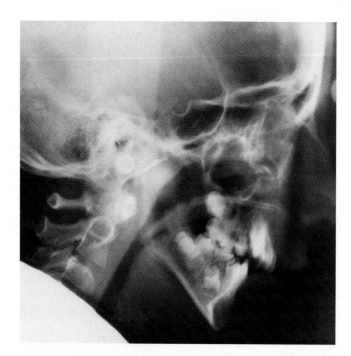

Figure 9–3. Lateral radiograph demonstrating hypoplastic mandible.

3 months of age. Manifestations of the obstruction include inspiratory stridor, moderate to severe sternal retractions, and poor feeding secondary to airway compromise. Diagnostic evaluation may reveal frequent episodes of oxygen desaturation, hypoxemia, hypercarbia, and acidosis. Commonly, the airway obstruction is exacerbated by the supine position (lying on the back) and is relieved by the prone position (lying on the abdomen). Some caregivers believe that the prone position gives a false sense of security because it simply covers up the retractions, but the airway obstruction persists.

Prone positioning helps relieve the degree of upper airway obstruction because the weight of the tongue is anterior, rather than posterior, to the airway. If a trial of positioning is initiated with a micrognathic child, monitoring with an oxygen saturation monitor should be done in the hospital before discharge. During sleep, the tone of the upper airway relaxes. The oxygen disassociation curve is important in determining at what level of O_2 saturation is acceptable. Below 90%, the oxygen-carrying capacity of the red blood cell drops off precipitously. Below this level, invasive treatment is generally accepted.

Prone positioning

↓

If O_2 saturation is 80% to 90%, consider oxygenation

↓

If $< 80\%$, consider intubation

↓

If chronic, consider tracheotomy

One advantage of tracheotomy in the micrognathic infant is that it allows for palatoplasty at an earlier age than would otherwise be possible in these children. Severe airway compromise is a common complication of palatoplasty in children with micrognathia when surgery is performed at the usual 10 to 14 months of age. Most surgeons agree that in children with the Robin sequence, even in the absence of airway problems, palatoplasty should be delayed until ages 15 to 18 months. If a tracheotomy is in place, then palatoplasty can be safely performed at 10 to 12 months.

The larynx is not involved in facial clefts or craniosynostosis per se. However, the subglottic larynx (the level of the cricoid cartilage) is the narrowest part of the upper airway in any infant or young child. For this reason, obstruction at this level becomes rapidly symptomatic. Laryngeal obstruction can be caused by laryngomalacia (literally "softening of the larynx" or collapse at the laryngeal inlet), which is the most frequent cause of stridor in the infant. This condition was formally called congenital laryngeal stridor. Although usually outgrown and no longer symptomatic, the obstruction associated with laryngomalacia can be exacerbated by gastroesophageal reflux or neurologic impairment.[4]

Laryngotracheoesophageal cleft, by contrast, is rare, unusually difficult to diagnose, and associated with life-threatening aspiration. Clefts of the posterior larynx are classified by severity (Fig. 9–4). They may extend down to the carina, a condition that is usually fatal due to massive aspiration. A cleft of the posterior larynx may occur as an isolated entity in an otherwise normal infant. It may also be associated with other anomalies, which may include cleft lip or palate. Patients with Opitz Frias syndrome can have clefts of the lip and palate as well as hypertelorism, hypogonadism, and laryngotracheoesophageal clefts. In these patients, the facial features (cleft lip/hypertelorism) might promote an evaluation for the more elusive laryngeal cleft. This diagnosis is made best with the rigid bronchoscope, at which time the posterior glottis can be palpated and its depth measured.[5] Surgical repair is the only long-term solution to such a defect.

Physiologic Causes of Upper Airway Obstruction

In some patients, the cleft palate is not obstructive in itself, but promotes behavior that may obstruct the upper airway. This is most commonly observed with abnormal oral motor development, in which the child persists in placing the tongue posteriorly in the oropharynx or superiorly in the nose, resulting in upper airway obstruction at one or two sites. This is seen in the Robin sequence and is probably a continuation of the tongue positioning that caused the in utero clefting in the first place. Some centers prescribe palatal obturators as a method to try to force the oral tongue forward, and

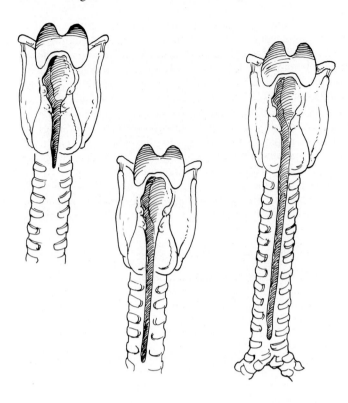

Figure 9–4. Illustrations of the three grades of laryngo-tracheoesophageal clefts.

tongue retention devices have also been tried. Neither of these techniques has been critically examined, and neither has gained widespread popularity.

Neurologic Causes

Neurologic impairment can affect the airway in a number of different ways. General hypotonia can manifest as airway obstruction secondary to pharyngeal and hypopharyngeal collapse, and may also be associated with cerebral palsy. It is often associated with global developmental delay. Syndromes associated with brainstem compression, such as Arnold-Chiari malformation or progressive fibroplasia, may present as acute airway obstruction secondary to bilateral vocal cord paralysis. Various degrees of holoprosencephaly can also manifest in cranial neuropathies. Möbius syndrome is rarely isolated to just the facial nerve but usually is a polyneuropathy and may present with airway obstruction or frequent aspiration. Glossopharyngeal, vagus, and hypoglossal neuropathies may present with aspiration and airway compromise. Neurogenic causes of upper airway obstruction usually portend a poor prognosis.

Obstructive Sleep Apnea

Obstructive sleep apnea (OSA) presents in adults with snoring or noisy respirations, nocturnal apnea, and daytime somnolence. In children, enuresis may also be a prominent feature. The most common cause of chronic upper airway obstruction in the child is adenotonsillar hypertrophy. Adenotonsillectomy is usually (>90%) curative in children. Diagnosis can usually be made by eliciting an accurate history from the parent or guardian. In adults or in patients with an uncertain history, a sleep study can be helpful. Indications for surgical intervention include (1) O_2 saturation dropping below 80%, (2) apnea index (number of apneas/hour) greater than 20, (3) significant daytime sleepiness, (4) heroic snoring, and (5) cardiac arrhythmia.[6] In the patient with a craniofacial syndrome or cleft palate, the management of OSA must be individualized. Adenoidectomy is not performed as a routine because of the possibility of resultant velopharyngeal incompetence.

EVALUATION

The initial evaluation of the patient with upper airway obstruction is the physical examination. This is helpful in determining both the site and severity of obstruction. Stridor may be present. Stridor, by definition, refers to noise originating from an obstructed airway. The type of noise can help localize the site of obstruction (see Table 9–1). Noise during inspiration originates from obstruction above the larynx, and expiratory noise (wheezes) originates from obstruction below the thoracic inlet. *Stertor* is another term for a snorting noise that results from nasal or nasopharyngeal obstruction. It should be noted that complete obstruction would not allow passage of air and would produce no sound. So the most complete obstruction (total obstruction) at any level has no associated noise and represents the most severe form of obstruction. (Such is the case with choanal atresia or laryngeal atresia.) Retraction of the intercostal or supraclavicular areas may indicate forcible effort during inspiration. Cyanosis may be present.

In addition to the physical examination, radiographic evaluation can be helpful in delineating the site and degree of upper airway obstruction. Plain anteroposterior and lateral films are perhaps the least costly and most useful in evaluating the patency of the upper airway. An air shadow should be traceable from the nose to the level of the larynx. Encroachment of hyperplastic adenoid or tonsillar tissue can be visualized. It should be recognized that the x-ray is only a two-dimensional representation of the overall picture.

Bronchoscopy, or upper airway endoscopy, permits total visualization of the upper airway. If the patient is experiencing obstruction, the location and cause of such obstruction should be discernible by locating the area of vibration that is causing the associated stridor.[7] Flexible bronchoscopy employs a flexible scope (Fig. 9–5). It is done with the patient breathing spontaneously, better simulating the normal dynamic situation. Rigid bronchoscopy generally requires general anesthesia but is more useful if active intervention is required.

INTERVENTION AND TREATMENT

Support of the airway might be required immediately in cases of acute airway obstruction or more long-term growth retardation or obstructive sleep apnea. In some instances, the patient's airway obstruction is lifelong and is related to the facial anomaly, such as midfacial or mandibular hypoplasia. In these situations, growth

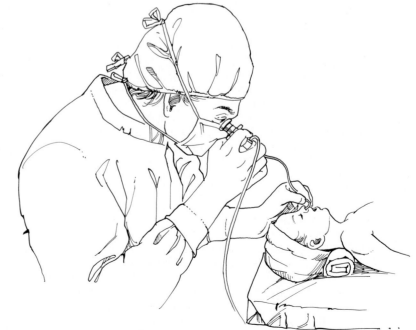

Figure 9–5. Technique of flexible bronchoscopy.

usually improves the amount of airway compromise. In other cases, a certain amount of airway obstruction can be the result of a surgical procedure, such as a posterior pharyngeal flap or closure of the cleft palate. In these surgeries, airway obstruction needs to be anticipated and circumvented as necessary.

Immediate Airway Intervention

In cases of immediate or sudden airway obstruction, endotracheal intubation may be necessary. This may be necessary shortly after birth if the infant is unable to breathe effectively on his or her own. An infant with the Pierre Robin sequence may be difficult to intubate as well, necessitating a more formal work-up with flexible intubation. The traditional and time-honored method of airway support for a child who is unable to breathe on his or her own is a tracheotomy. In some cases (e.g., laryngeal atresia) only an emergency tracheotomy can create an airway and save the life of the infant.

Tracheotomy

Tracheotomy is the surgical procedure of establishing an airway through the neck. The technique is usually performed over either an endotracheal tube or rigid broncho-scope. In a neonate or young child, the cricoid cartilage is palpated approximately two fingerbreadths above the sternal notch. A horizontal skin incision is made just below this, and then a vertical approach is made through the strap muscles in the midline raphe. A good practice is to use two stay sutures through the tracheal cartilage at the site of the tracheotomy. This allows rapid reinsertion of the tracheotomy tube in the event of accidental decannulation. Generally, the third tracheal ring is divided verti-cally and the tracheotomy tube is placed at this site. A tube is chosen, just as an endotracheal tube, not to be excessively large or small but to accommodate the inner dimensions of the trachea. Similarly, the length must be above the carina and is documented radiographically. The chief operative risks are hemorrhage, infection, and pneumothorax. The main long-term risk is mucus plugging of the tracheotomy tube, which can lead to death of the child.[8]

Perioperative Airway Management

The intraoperative or emergency management of the airway in children with micro-gnathia can be extremely difficult. This is often the case even in a micrognathic child who has not had airway problems. There is no reliable way to ascertain in advance which children will be difficult to intubate. Intubation with a laryngoscope can be difficult, or even impossible. In some cases, intubation over a flexible laryngoscope or bronchoscope is necessary. This should only be attempted by those with a depth of experience in fiberoptic endoscopy (an anesthesiologist, intensivist-pulmonologist, or otolaryngologist). In many instances, airway obstruction can be anticipated during the initial preoperative evaluation. Such is the case with patients with trismus or limited opening of the mouth due to any cause. A small mandible or large tongue are also indicators of potential difficulty with intubation. Most tertiary or children's hospitals have this capability but some community hospitals do not.

Decannulation

Once a child with the Pierre Robin sequence or other airway obstructing conditions has undergone tracheotomy, it is generally left in place until after the cleft palate repair (15 to 24 months of age). Delaying tracheotomy decannulation until after the craniofacial patient has undergone the majority of his or her early surgical reconstruc-tion procedures is recommended. This may mean that the tracheotomy is left in place until the child is 2 to 3 years old in the case of Apert or Crouzon syndrome patients. Downsizing the tracheotomy as a technique in decannulation is no longer employed in the younger child because it is neither physiologically sound nor safe. Before decannulation, flexible airway endoscopy is performed while the patient is both sedated and asleep. If the airway is adequate, then decannulation is performed and 48-hour hospitalization for observation and oxygen saturation monitoring is used. Removal of granulation tissue or other surgical intervention and decannulation are rarely combined in the same procedure.

Other Procedures

For infants in whom positioning alone does not provide an adequate airway, there are a variety of surgical interventions to be considered. A number of techniques to perform tongue-lip adhesion have been described.[9] Pulling the tongue forward and securing it with a pin through the base and anchoring it in the body of the mandible is another technique for improving the infant airway. All of these techniques are based on the principle that pulling the tongue anteriorly opens the site of obstruction at the tongue base. There are no studies with objective measurements that demonstrate benefit of these techniques, nor have the authors found them to be beneficial. Furthermore, it is commonly believed that these procedures may predispose children to an oral aversion and may, in fact, interfere with acquisition of speech.

In the authors' experience, the only reliable surgical intervention in the micrognathic infant with airway obstruction is tracheotomy. Although this procedure is distasteful to nearly all caregivers, it always circumvents the airway obstruction and resolves retractions, desaturation, and hypercarbia in tongue base obstruction. In children with pharyngeal and palatal collapse, tracheotomy is not the only therapy available. Nasal continuous positive airway pressure (CPAP) can often be beneficial. In the infant, CPAP can easily be delivered by nasal prongs, and in other age groups CPAP is administered by nasal mask. It is usually only necessary to use CPAP during sleep. Although it is difficult to accustom the child to the apparatus, persistence and encouragement on the part of the night-time nurses will help the child acclimate. If CPAP fails to resolve airway obstruction, then tonsillectomy with or without adenoidectomy can be considered. Partial uvulopalatopharyngoplasty (UPPP) or simple uvulectomy may sometimes suffice. It is important to be aware of potential speech complications to these procedures, especially in children with cleft palate.

In the UPPP procedure, the uvula and a narrow edge of the soft palate are resected and a tonsillectomy is performed if one has not been previously done.[10] Introduced into the United States by Fugita in 1981, the procedure is not uniformly effective. Therefore, its use tends to be individualized to patients who do not tolerate nasal CPAP. The supraglottoplasty or epiglottoplasty procedure for severe laryngomalacia has nearly completely superseded tracheotomy for this problem and can be successfully employed in craniofacial patients.[4] In this procedure, redundant tissue is trimmed from the epiglottic and arytenoid cartilages to prevent prolapse into the airway. At other times, procedures can be adapted to the craniofacial child. Such is the case with partial resection of the turbinates. In this procedure, tissue from the nasal turbinates is trimmed to establish an improved nasal airway.[11] Usually reserved for the patient with large turbinates from allergic causes, conservative application of this technique can be helpful in cases of midfacial hyperplasia in which the nasal airway is severely compromised.

CONCLUSIONS

It is critical for the members of the cleft/craniofacial team to be aware of the potential airway complications that are seen in a large number of craniofacial patients. If these problems remain unrecognized, many children will develop right-sided heart failure, failure to thrive, and other permanent sequelae of chronic airway obstruction.

In the modern practice of pulmonary medicine and otolaryngology, tracheotomy is no longer the only alternative for a child with a serious airway obstruction. Modern diagnostic techniques such as fiberoptic endoscopy will allow for exact localization of the obstruction, and then a rational treatment plan can be designed for the specific problem(s).

References

1. Warren DW, Hairfield WM, Dalston ET, Sidman JD, Pillsbury HC: Effects of cleft lip and palate on the nasal airway in children. Arch Otolaryngol Head Neck Surg 1988; 114:987–992.

2. Warren DW, Hairfield WM, Dalston ET: Effect of age on nasal cross-sectional area. Laryngoscope 1990; 100:89–93.

3. Arlis H, Ward RF: Congenital nasal pyriform aperture stenosis—isolated abnormality versus developmental field defect. Arch Otolaryngol Head Neck Surg 1992; 118:989–991.

4. Holinger LD, Konior RJ: Surgical management of severe laryngomalacia. Laryngoscope 1989; 99:136–142.

5. Pillsbury HC, Fischer ND: Laryngotracheoesophageal cleft: Diagnosis, management and presentation of a new diagnostic device. Arch Otolaryngol 1977; 103:735–737.

6. Simmons FB, Guilleminault C, Silvestin R: Snoring and some obstructive sleep apnea can be cured by oropharyngeal surgery: Palatopharyngoplasty. Arch Otolaryngol 1983; 109:503.

7. Wood RE: The diagnostic effectiveness of the flexible bronchoscope in children. Pediatr Pulmonol 1985; 1:188–192.

8. Fearon B, Cotton R: Surgical correction of subglottic stenosis of the larynx in infants and children. Ann Otol Rhinol Laryngol 1974; 83:428–491.

9. Douglas B: Treatment of micrognathia with obstruction by plastic procedure. Lyon Chir 1956; 52:420.

10. Fugita S, Conway W, Zorick F, Roth T: Surgical correction of anatomic abnormalities in obstructive sleep apnea syndrome: Uvulopalatopharyngoplasty. Otolaryngol Head Neck Surg 1981; 89:923.

11. Mabry RL: Surgery of the inferior turbinates: How much and when? Otolaryngol Head Neck Surg 1984; 92:571.

10 Ophthalmologic Considerations in Craniosynostosis, Hypertelorism, and Facial Clefts

*Marilyn T. Miller**

GENERAL PRINCIPLES AND THE EXAMINATION

Children with congenital malformations and syndromes involving craniofacial structures are at a significant risk for ocular anomalies. The number of syndromes and isolated malformations is great, and the spectrum of eye problems is vast. Therefore, the development of an approach to the dysmorphic child with craniofacial malformations is more productive than an attempt to memorize all ocular pathologic changes reported in the literature. One approach is to consider two categories:

1. Ocular complications secondary to abnormal size, shape, or position of bony and soft-tissue changes in orbital structures. These complications may occur during development or may be acquired after birth. The changes can be anticipated from the anatomic alterations in the surrounding tissues. They result from either a type of deformity or mechanical factors, and are not necessarily syndrome specific with the same anomaly present in multiple syndromes. The bony orbit is frequently affected in these patients, including changes in size, position, or symmetry between the two orbits, resulting in secondary, often serious, ocular problems. For example, in craniosynostosis the orbits are frequently shallow with abnormal configuration. This may predispose to corneal exposure or ulceration and motility disturbances. In cases with extensive cranial suture closure, the resultant increased intracranial pressure will result in papilledema and later optic atrophy.

2. Intrinsic ocular pathology. In this category malformations associated with craniofacial syndromes are primary. Examples are lid colobomas in mandibulofacial dysostosis and hemifacial microsomia, abnormalities in the ocular muscles frequently noted in craniosynostosis syndromes, Duane syndrome associated in some patients with Goldenhar syndrome, and less common malformations of the retina, optic disc, or anterior segment associated with many syndromes.

Most ocular findings are detected during a routine eye examination with a few modifications, for example, a more detailed search for milder forms of the "anticipated pathology," the documentation of negative or normal findings, and more detailed measurements of anatomic relationships. These extra measurements aid in the natural-history studies and evaluation of complications and effects of surgical intervention.

A careful history; careful examination of the eyelids, palpebral fissures, anterior segment, pupils, and fundus; cycloplegic refraction; and special attention to the optic disc are routine and mandatory. Motility evaluation should include measurements in the primary position and all fields of gaze, with particular attention to the presence or absence of A- or V-pattern deviations. Incomitant strabismus is frequently seen in these patients. Intraocular pressure measurements, visual field examination, exophthalmometry, corneal sensitivity tests, color vision tests, and tests of binocular vision should be performed when possible and desirable. In selected patients, less routine tests, such as fluorescein angiography or visualization of the lacrimal system by radiologic techniques, may be appropriate. When vision-threatening eye problems are suspected, a sedated examination or an examination under anesthesia may be necessary

* Supported in part by core grant EY 1792 from the National Eye Institute, Bethesda, Maryland.

if the patient cannot cooperate. However, before such a procedure is undertaken, consultation with other medical personnel should be conducted to anticipate anesthesia or sedation complications and, if possible, combined with other necessary tests such as computed tomography (CT) or magnetic resonance imaging (MRI). These patients are frequently at increased risk for airway complications and must be monitored closely.

Additional tests are important in patients with craniofacial anomalies. These include measurements and documentation of certain anatomic relationships: (1) inner and outer canthal distances, (2) interpupillary distance, (3) palpebral fissure size, (4) position of the lacrimal puncta, (5) obliquity of the palpebral fissure and asymmetry of orbits and orbital structures, and (6) degree of proptosis if present. These measurements prevent errors of recording false impressions, such as pseudohypertelorism due to soft-tissue changes in the canthal area, and provide useful data for the study of the syndrome characteristics and serve as a baseline if reconstructive surgery is performed. Normal values for these measurements for different ages and by sex may be found in many texts and articles.[1–9]

Interpupillary distance is an important observation in this group of patients. Most published values record the interpupillary distance obtained while the patient is fixating on a distant target. This may be difficult to accomplish in a child. If the measurement can be made only at the near position, this fact should be recorded, and the distance measurement can be estimated by adding approximately 3 cm. If an ocular deviation is present, the left eye is covered for fixation by the right eye, and the distance from the midpupil of the right eye to the midpoint over the nasal bridge is recorded. The right eye is then covered, and a similar measurement is made on the left side. The addition of the two values represents the interpupillary distance (usually for near). A more accurate and reproducible method of measuring orbital separation is the radiologic measurement of the bony intraorbital distance. Normal values for various age groups have been reported.[10,11] It is appropriate to calculate separately the anatomic distance for each half of the face, not only for interpupillary values but also for intercanthal values, as asymmetry is present in many clinical entities. The difference between the values obtained for each half of the face is an indication of the degree of asymmetry in the orbital region.

It is beyond the scope of this chapter to list all of the ocular findings reported in these patients, but because many ocular findings are not syndrome specific but are the result of an anatomic change that may occur in multiple syndromes, common or prototype syndromes have been selected. The ocular findings in this group are characteristic of many craniofacial syndromes or are associated with unusual or severe ocular malformations.

CRANIOSYNOSTOSIS

Common Causes of Visual Impairment

Visual loss is by far the most serious ophthalmologic problem in craniosynostosis patients. It may exist at birth, develop slowly, or progress rapidly during the growth of facial structures. Occasionally it may occur as a complication of reconstructive orbital surgery. Although visual loss can be unilateral or bilateral, the latter is obviously more devastating to the patient. The causes of visual disturbance are not unique to this group of patients, but the risk is significantly greater.

The most frequent causes of visual loss are acquired types of ocular pathology, such as optic atrophy and corneal damage occurring as a result of abnormalities in the surrounding structures or increased intracranial pressure. Amblyopia may be present due to strabismus or refractive differences between the two eyes.

Increased intracranial pressure can cause papilledema and, if not reversed, ultimately optic atrophy. In 1866, von Graefe[12] noted the association between an abnormal skull, increased intracranial pressure, and poor visual function. This association has been repeatedly observed in subsequent reports of craniosynostosis syndromes.[2,5,7,13–21] There is some disagreement as to whether the optic atrophy seen in craniosynostosis syndromes is always secondary to increased intracranial pressure or whether it may represent damage to the nerve from local changes in the optic canal.[13,21] Compression of the vascular supply to the optic nerve has been thought to occur in some situations from a sudden change in intracranial pressure.[22] Kinking of the optic nerve may also be a factor.[19, 23] Local causes of optic atrophy may explain why some patients demonstrate a marked difference in the degree of optic nerve involvement between the two eyes or lack a documented stage of papilledema. The latter situation could occur in a transient increase of pressures. Although we may not completely understand the relative importance of all the factors that might produce optic nerve damage, there appears to be no question that conditions that predispose to increased intracranial pressure are the most significant risk factors for subsequent nerve damage. Optic atrophy is infrequent in children if only the sagittal suture is involved or if suture closure is unilateral, as in plagiocephaly, and when present usually means multiple sutures are affected.

A mild chronic type of papilledema without retinal hemorrhages has also been described. This form of papilledema is difficult to differentiate from pseudopapilledema, a condition in which the optic disc gives the false appearance of papilledema. Papilledema may also disappear, leaving no residual signs. Some authors believe that the apparent increased frequency of tortuous vasculature in craniosynostosis represents evidence of previous papilledema (Fig. 10–1).[15] Medullated nerve fibers have also been noted in a significant number of patients with oxycephaly. It has been proposed that shallow orbits affect the myelinization process, leading to more medullated fibers.[24]

Although any child with premature closure of certain key sutures may show signs and symptoms of optic nerve damage, a very high frequency of optic nerve damage has been reported in Crouzon syndrome.[15] With the present earlier recognition of the presence of craniosynostosis, there seems to be a decreased incidence of papilledema and optic atrophy; however, these findings are still noted, and an initial ophthalmologic evaluation must always assess the status of the optic nerve. Ophthalmologic evidence of increased intracranial pressure frequently necessitates earlier neurosurgical intervention. Profound visual defects necessitate special schooling for the patient and counseling for the family. The common finding of optic atrophy in patients with Crouzon syndrome suggests periods of intracranial pressure at some phase of development, but the number of children with mental retardation is surprisingly quite low. Thus, the correlation among optic nerve damage, increased intracranial pressure, and mental retardation is somewhat unclear. In Apert syndrome, the percentage of mentally retarded patients is significantly higher, yet the frequency of optic nerve pathology is lower. Mental retardation may be a primary effect. CT and MRI are valuable tools to characterize the course of the optic nerve and to provide information on other anatomic factors that may cause or contribute to optic nerve damage.

Craniectomy prevents or alleviates some of the neurologic complications in these patients and also improves the shape of the developing skull. If increased intracranial

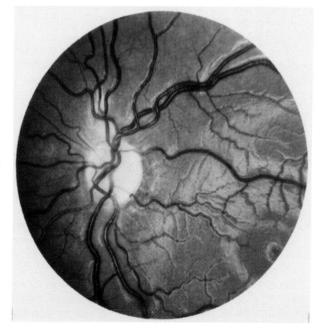

Figure 10–1. Fundus view of retina of patient with Crouzon disease. Note marked tortuosity of vessels. This may be related to some previous unrecognized episode of papilledema.

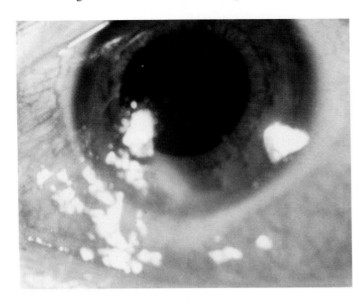

Figure 10–2. Exposure keratitis secondary to corneal ulcer in patient with Crouzon syndrome. This picture was taken postoperatively, after major reconstructive surgery. The corneal ulcer responded to therapy. Preoperatively, the patient also had recurrent mild keratitis.

pressure can be eliminated at a fairly early stage of papilledema, minimal visual impairment may ensue. It is important to realize that increased intracranial pressure in the presence of severe optic atrophy may not result in clinically noticeable disc changes. Therefore, the atrophic optic disc is not always a good indication of the status of cranial pressure.

The narrow or disturbed course of the optic canal that has been described in oxycephaly also may occur in other craniofacial syndromes. Radiologic evaluation of the canal is indicated for such patients and can be performed easily by CT scanning. Wood-Smith and coworkers[23] advocated surgical decompression for patients with progressive optic nerve change (often asymmetric) and radiologic evidence of diminished canal size.

The ophthalmologist is often the most experienced evaluator of the status of the optic nerve. This examination is crucial during infancy and early childhood because the damage is most severe when the brain is growing rapidly, and intracranial pressure in the untreated child may be elevated. However, increased intracranial pressure has been reported in older children and adults as well.[15]

Another acquired type of ocular pathology that may produce severe visual impairment is exposure keratitis. The cornea is vulnerable to the complication of exorbitism due to shallow orbits. The integrity of the cornea depends on the normal anatomy and function of the lids and the glandular structure in the lids. Defects or poor closure of the eyelid that leaves portions of the cornea unprotected cause exposure keratitis and, in some cases, infection and scarring of the cornea (Fig. 10–2). Corneal sensation may be diminished by repeated insults to the cornea or, on occasion, may represent a primary type of pathologic change. Reconstructive surgery around the orbit has been noted to result in a transient or permanent decrease in corneal sensitivity, with potential secondary corneal ulceration. Either situation intensifies the keratitis.

Proptosis and Corneal Complications

Proptosis (sometimes called exorbitism) caused by anatomic factors in the craniosynostosis syndromes is quantitatively different from exophthalmos secondary to tumors and pseudotumors in patients with normal orbits, and frequently shows a different rate of progression. However, the ophthalmic symptoms and complications are similar. The degree of proptosis varies dramatically, even in patients with the same craniosynostosis syndrome. Some cases show such severe corneal exposure that surgical intervention is required to save the cornea from ulceration and blindness. If the lids do not adequately protect the globe, the cornea is exposed to drying, causing punctate keratitis, pain, and conjunctival hyperemia (Fig. 10–3). If this is not adequately treated, perforation of the globe and further visual damage may result. Figures 10–3 and 10–4 show the variations in two patients with Crouzon syndrome. The patients in Figure 10–3 required immediate intervention and ultimately had fairly good visual

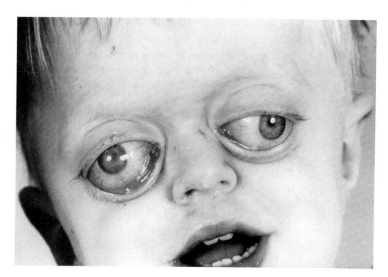

Figure 10–3. Crouzon patient with severe proptosis and secondary corneal exposure, which necessitated early reconstructive surgical intervention.

function without the long-term effects of the severe proptosis noted in infancy. The patient in Figure 10–4 had no corneal complications and required no special therapy for the proptosis. The small orbital volume causing proptosis in patients with cranio-synostosis differs significantly from more usual cases of proptosis caused by soft-tissue pathology (e.g., hyperthyroidism) and necessitates different surgical treatment. If conservative management is insufficient to prevent corneal damage, a tarsorrhaphy (usually lateral) may be indicated as a temporary or permanent measure, depending on the long-term management plan for the facial deformity in the patient. Eyelid surgery should be deferred if extensive reconstructive surgery is anticipated in the near future, unless the corneal integrity is severely threatened. Tarsorrhaphy may protect the cornea and diminish the proptotic appearance by narrowing the abnormally wide palpebral fissure, but the improvement may be short-lived, and recurrence results from constant mechanical force on the sutured lids. The definitive solution is reconstructive surgery involving the orbit. Standard decompression techniques that are useful in dealing with tumors or hyperthyroidism are not suitable for the severely reduced orbital volume that is characteristic of craniofacial synostosis.

Figure 10–4. Crouzon patient with mild proptosis and no symptoms, which necessitated no specific therapy.

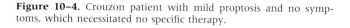

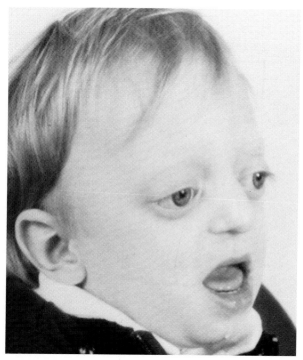

Occasionally during the examination of patients with marked exorbitism, slight retraction of the lid may cause luxation of the globe. Luxation may also occur spontaneously or with manipulation of the eyelids. This dramatic finding may be frightening to the examining ophthalmologist, especially if it occurs when the exophthalmos is measured with an instrument placed on the lateral orbit. Fortunately, the patients or their families usually know how to gently push the eye back by pulling the lid over it. If luxation is not reduced promptly, secondary conjunctival edema may ensue, making it more difficult to reduce the luxated globe. If edema is untreated, severe corneal exposure will follow, necessitating aggressive therapeutic intervention to prevent serious complications.

However, unlike many causes of exophthalmos, if proptosis is not severe at birth, it usually progresses slowly, and frequent monitoring of the cornea for warning symptoms will prevent serious complications in most cases. Such eyes respond to conservative treatment such as lubricating medication. If the cornea is exposed at night, ointment, taping, or other protective measures must be instituted to prevent extensive drying and exposure. Proptotic eyes are certainly more sensitive to the elements, and patients complain particularly about the irritating effects of the wind and sun. Such eyes also may be more vulnerable to any type of orbital trauma.

Refractive Errors, Ocular Motility Disturbances (Strabismus), and Amblyopia

Disturbances in ocular movement frequently occur in craniosynostosis syndromes, but accurate descriptions of the type and frequency of strabismus are often omitted in case reports. The associated defects in these patients are of such pronounced cosmetic or functional consequence that the treatment of strabismus is ignored or given low priority. As the number of patients undergoing reconstructive procedures for these severe bony defects increases, more detailed study will be made of all ocular problems, including variation in ocular motility. In this way, not only can treatment priority be logically determined, but also the relationship of bony, soft tissue, and central nervous system pathology to eye movement and oculomotor system functioning can be better understood.

In the early literature, authors attributed all cases of strabismus to poor visual acuity, but this was proven to be incorrect. Although decreased visual acuity may be an important factor in some patients, strabismus is often the result of anatomic and mechanical factors. The ocular deviation in the primary position is most frequently exotropia (Fig. 10–5) but also can be esotropia or straight eyes. A more consistent finding is the presence of an exotropia in the upgaze position with straight eyes or esotropia in downgaze, producing the V-pattern configuration.[9] Many patients also have associated overaction of the inferior oblique muscles. A subgroup of patients shows limitations in various fields of gaze. Although these findings may be attributed to mechanical effects of abnormally shaped and positioned orbits, there is increased evidence that a number of patients demonstrate abnormal insertion, structure, or orientation of the extraocular muscles.[25–28] Diamond and coworkers[27] reported extraocular muscle anomalies (primarily of the inferior and superior rectus muscles) in 42% of

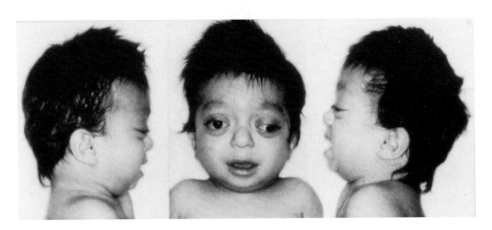

Figure 10–5. Patient with Crouzon disease, showing exotropia (outward deviation of the eye) in the straight-ahead position.

their patients with craniofacial dysostosis. Further information is being accumulated from CT findings. Orbital high-resolution CT scanning with small cuts (1 to 1.5 mm) will demonstrate changes in the location or size of extraocular muscles. Axial, coronal, and sagittal projections are useful in obtaining an accurate estimate of the degree of abnormality. For example, repositioning of the gantry to −15° provides good visualization of the course of the inferior rectus in the sagittal cut.[29] If sagittal cuts cannot be obtained, computer reformation may be used to acquire this information. Coronal sections may be direct or reformed. MRI can also be useful to study ocular muscles. Patients with gross limitation of movement are most likely to demonstrate CT or MRI abnormalities. Radiographic evaluation is indicated to plan appropriate surgical procedures in patients with severe limitation if ocular motility surgery is contemplated. It will allow preoperative alternative plans if the ocular muscles cannot be located. It is unclear whether this represents a pleiotropic effect of the gene or secondary changes in the position of the muscles of the globe due to local mechanical factors occurring during embryogenesis.

Most information about strabismus relates to patients with Crouzon and Apert syndromes, and there is some disagreement as to the timing of surgical intervention for strabismus. A few authors recommend early surgery,[30] but many prefer to defer surgery until after the reconstructive surgery.[9,31] Reconstructive surgery of the midface in craniosynostosis may not affect the degree or pattern of ocular motility, but in some cases a substantial effect does occur (in contrast to patients with hypertelorism and median facial cleft, in whom reconstructive surgery has been observed to significantly affect ocular motility).[32] Attainable goals of therapy in most patients are good vision in both eyes and a cosmetically acceptable position of the eyes in the primary position of gaze. Because of the potential anatomic abnormalities of the ocular muscle in addition to the disturbed anatomy of the orbits, it is often impossible to align the eyes in all fields of gaze, and so the surgery is more directed to a straight primary position.[9,31,33]

Although patients with craniosynostosis syndromes show an increased frequency of abnormalities such as astigmatism, paralytic deviations, and structural anomalies, the treatment modalities are modified only slightly from those used for the more routine strabismus of nonsyndromic patients. Correction of refractive errors, fundus evaluation, and amblyopia therapy remain the important modes of treatment and evaluation. Unless the patient has severe mental retardation or unusually limiting physical problems, correction of the refractive error and amblyopia therapy can be instituted concurrently with the evaluation and treatment of the patient's other problems.

Primary Malformations

The ocular problems described earlier occur secondary to increased intracranial pressure and/or pathology in surrounding structures and are the most visually debilitating and common. Intrinsic ocular pathology does occur in patients with the craniosynostosis syndrome but with low frequency. A few rare anomalies have been reported, such as iris coloboma, cataract, vitreous opacities, and medullated nerve fibers.

Margolis and associates[28] reported depigmentation of the hair, skin, and eyes in many patients with Apert syndrome. Iris transillumination and absent or diffuse foveal reflexes were also noted in these patients, but their visual acuity remained good, in contrast to more typical forms of albinism. Serum tyrosine and phenylalanine levels were found to be normal.

Bertelsen,[15] in his series of 40 patients with premature closure of cranial sutures, noted ptosis in two cases, a pathologic finding reported by other authors and noted in our patients also. Keratoconus was present in a few of our patients and also has been reported in the literature.[15]

The muscle changes noted in structure and location also may represent a primary anomaly. The frequency of these anomalies is difficult to ascertain unless the patient has an ocular muscle surgical procedure or unless an orbital CT scan is performed by a radiologist with knowledge of the normal size and location of ocular muscles. Nystagmus has been reported and is often secondary to very poor visual acuity, although it may occur, on occasion, as a primary abnormality.

In summary, many types of intrinsic ocular pathology may occur in craniosynostosis patients at a frequency significantly above that found in the general population but are

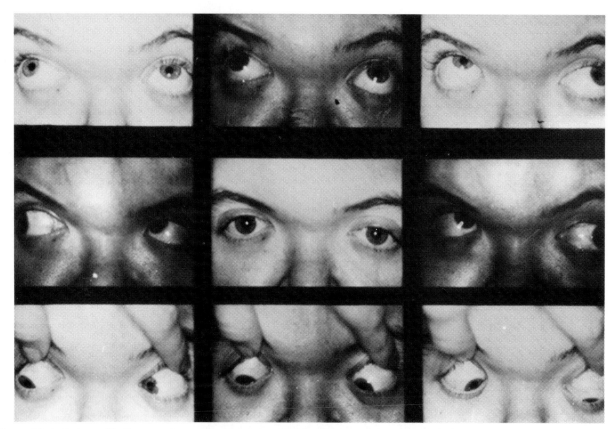

Figure 10–6. Patient with Crouzon disease showing a characteristic V-pattern, i.e., exotropia looking up and esotropia looking down, giving a V-formation. Also present are overacting inferior obliques, shown by elevation of the adducting eye.

still relatively rarely. The more serious types of pathology and those requiring early identification and intervention are almost always secondary complications.

Craniosynostosis Syndromes

Crouzon Syndrome

Ocular findings are frequent in this syndrome. Mild hypertelorism, downward slanting of palpebral fissures, and proptosis are commonly seen, along with a characteristic V-pattern strabismus (Fig. 10–6). Abnormal origins, size, or insertion of ocular muscles may be present. Infrequent findings include an albinotic appearance of the fundus, congenital glaucoma, and keratoconus.[5, 28]

Craniofacial findings in Crouzon syndrome are similar to those for Apert syndrome and other types of craniosynostosis, but the prevalence of various malformations and the family history are different, and there are no anomalies of the hands or feet. Crouzon syndrome has a clear autosomal dominant mode of inheritance, with about 67% of cases being familial.[34] The coronal suture is most frequently involved, but different combinations of sutures have been reported in 75% of cases.[35]

Proptosis occurs in most patients with Crouzon syndrome and may be severe, with vision-threatening corneal exposure necessitating earlier reconstructive surgery (see Fig. 10–3). Optic atrophy and blindness are also more frequent than in other types of craniosynostosis syndromes. Low-frequency anomalies reported include keratoconus, iris and corneal malformations, glaucoma, and ectopia lentis.[5] Abnormal location and position of ocular muscles have been reported frequently in both Crouzon and Apert syndromes.

Apert Syndrome

Apert syndrome is characterized by craniosynostosis midface hypoplasia and syndactyly of extremities (Fig. 10–7). Its transmission is believed to be autosomal domi-

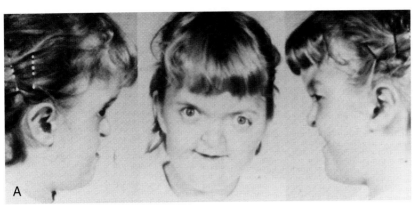
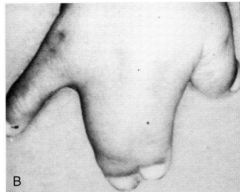

Figure 10–7. *A,* Frontal view of patient with Apert syndrome, characterized by midface hypoplasia, shallow orbits from premature closure of one or more sutures. *B,* Syndactyly of the hands, in this patient. There were also associated anomalies of the feet.

nant, but most cases are sporadic and are due to high neonatal mortality and reduced fitness of affected individuals.[34] Ocular findings are similar to those in Crouzon syndrome but there are fewer cases with severe proptosis.

Plagiocephaly

Plagiocephaly is defined as asymmetry of the skull caused by unilateral or asymmetric involvement of the cranial sutures or a deformation defect from compression in the uterus.[39] Figure 10–8*A* shows a patient with plagiocephaly. Frequently the asymmetry is best observed by looking down at a patient (Fig. 10–8*B*).

Plagiocephaly is sometimes divided into frontal or occipital types in the craniosynostosis group. The lamboidal suture is involved in the occipital type and the coronal suture in the frontal type. Unilateral coronal synostosis is estimated to occur in 1 per 10,000 births, 10 times more frequently than lamboidal synostosis.[40,41] Deformational plagiocephaly is more frequent, but many of these infants are not referred to craniofacial centers because of the natural history of improvement of this form of plagiocephaly. The following discussion concerns the frontal type of plagiocephaly, which is the most common type and the one of greatest concern to the ophthalmologist.

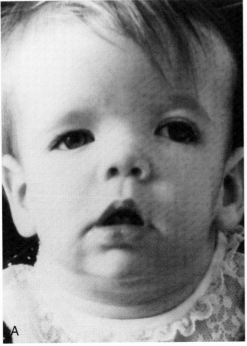
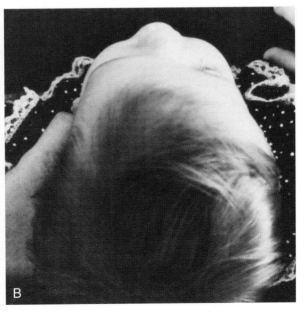

Figure 10–8. *A,* Frontal view of patient with plagiocephaly. *B,* Asymmetry is particularly obvious in the view from the top of the patient's head.

In the synostotic form the orbit is elevated on the affected side and the nasal root is also deviated on that side. Usually the ear is supraplaced, the forehead flattened, and the palpebral fissure more flattened on the involved side. The most reliable diagnostic tests are standard radiographs or CT scans. Primary radiographic findings may be unreliable in the first few months of life[40] and may need to be repeated if deformity remains or progresses, even when the initial early radiographic evaluation did not disclose any abnormality. Three-dimensional CT scans, although expensive, give more information on degree or orbital dysmorphology.[42]

Affected patients with plagiocephaly have a high incidence of vertical strabismus. The strabismus pattern depends on the type and degree of plagiocephaly. These children may show an abnormal head position with either the synostotic or deformation forms. With the deformation type the head tilt is often more to the affected side, while with the synostosed form the tilt is to the opposite side, often with a hypertropia secondary to a superior oblique palsy[43] on the side of the abnormal orbit as well as a classic upslanted overacting inferior oblique muscle. Surgery similar to that for a routine superior oblique palsy may be indicated. These patients should be examined carefully because they may exhibit other types of patterns or motility disturbances.

It is possible that other ocular symptoms or signs ascribed to craniosynostosis may exist that are limited to the affected side. However, because an adequate number of sutures are opened in most cases, there usually is no optic nerve damage or increased intraocular pressure.

Role of the Ophthalmologist

Changes in lid position may occur after midface surgery, necessitating secondary ptosis surgery. Because the levator muscle is often normal from a neuromuscular standpoint, resection may have a greater effect than one would predict if the ptosis were congenital.

Because lacrimal system dysfunction is common preoperatively and is related to an increased incidence of anatomic anomalies of the lacrimal excretory system or damage due to reconstructive surgery, the timing of lacrimal surgery depends on the severity of symptoms (recurrent infection) and the potential effect of future surgery on the anatomy. Preoperative tearing is best treated after reconstructive surgery unless there is recurrent severe dacryocystitis that cannot be medically treated. This issue must be discussed with the craniofacial medical team to arrive at an appropriate decision.[36, 37]

The ophthalmologist is an indispensable member of the craniofacial team for this group of patients. Initially, examination of the optic nerve status as an indicator of intracranial pressure is most crucial. This evaluation, along with determination of whether there is vision-threatening corneal exposure, will determine whether emergency surgical intervention by the craniofacial team is necessary. Subsequently, the identification and treatment of strabismus, amblyopia, refractive errors, dacryocystitis, and mild corneal exposure may require frequent ophthalmologic visits. Ophthalmologic input will be a factor in determining the time and extent of reconstructive craniofacial surgery.

Ocular complications following major reconstructive surgery are potentially serious. Direct or indirect damage to the neurologic pathways of the eye can result in permanent visual loss. Fortunately, blindness is a rare complication. In a combined report of 683 cases,[36] two patients sustained permanent visual loss; in another study of 75 cases,[37] only two patients had severe visual complications. Choy and associates[32] reported their complications in reconstructive surgery, and they and Diamond and associates[27] reported ocular alignment after surgery. The cause of serious complications was not uniform in the few reported cases, although postoperative hematoma and nerve decompression were reported in some cases. Monitoring of recorded evoked cortical potential at the time of surgery has been suggested.[38]

HYPERTELORISM

Hypertelorism is an anatomic description indicating an increased distance between the orbits (greater than 2 standard deviations from normal values). The most accurate diagnoses involve radiologic methods. The exact location for measuring the interorbital distance may vary among different investigators, but there are appropriate established norms for the various locations.[10, 44]

Soft-tissue variations, such as increased distance between the medial canthi (telecanthus), may result in a false diagnosis of hypertelorism. If the abnormality is confined to the soft tissue, the term *primary telecanthus* is sometimes used. Increased interorbital distance and proportional increased intercanthal distances is at times referred to as *secondary telecanthus*. A combination of telecanthus and lateral displacement of the lacrimal puncta occurs in Waardenburg syndrome and other syndromes.

Hypertelorism, a nonspecific finding in many dysmorphic individuals, is associated with a large, heterogeneous group of etiologies, such as craniofacial syndromes, teratogenic deformities, and disruption-type anomalies. It is a characteristic finding of a variety of chromosomal aberrations.[5] No one particular ocular abnormality is associated with the various types of hypertelorism, but dysfunction of the lacrimal excretory system due to disturbed midline anatomy exists in many patients without regard to the etiology of the hypertelorism. Lacrimal duct probings are not always successful because of these anatomic changes, necessitating more complex diagnostic evaluations of the lacrimal system.

Strabismus, usually exotropia, is frequently present if the hypertelorism is severe. If the bony orbits are abnormal more than in the horizontal position (e.g., craniosynostosis), other motility disturbances may also be present.

In median facial cleft syndrome, hypertelorism is the sine qua non. Other characteristic findings are bifidum occultum anterior cranium; midline clefting of nose, upper lip, premaxilla, and palate; and widow's peak (Fig. 10–9). There may also be notching of alae nasi. Intellectual development may be normal, but there is some increased incidence of mental retardation. Midbrain anomalies, including septo-optic dysplasia,[45] have been reported in addition to interhemispheric lipomas. Primary telecanthus superimposed on secondary telecanthus has been reported in some patients.

A few patients show some of the characteristics of Goldenhar syndrome (oculoauriculo-vertebral) with lid colobomas, epibulbar dermoids or lipodermoids, and vertebral anomalies.[46]

Exotropia occurs in many patients and seems related to the degree of hypertelorism. Uveal coloboma and microphthalmia have been noted in a few cases.[47–49] Optic atrophy is much rarer than in patients with craniosynostosis.

Routine ophthalmologic examination will reveal any low-incidence anomalies, but in most patients the strabismus, usually exotropia, becomes the main concern in addition to any ocular complications that may ensue after reconstructive surgery.

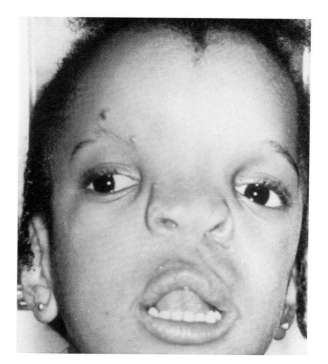

Figure 10–9. A median facial cleft that resulted in midline clefting of the nose and upper lip, widow's peak, and marked hypertelorism.

The exotropia appears to have a mechanical etiology due to the large separation of the orbits. Tessier[50] noted that the interorbital distance is much greater anteriorly than posteriorly. There may be a relative normal relationship horizontally between the optic canals. This related difference results in an increased angulation of the orbits. When the interorbital distance is reduced in reconstructive surgery, the degree of the exotropia frequently decreases or is eliminated. In a few patients esotropia with diplopia may actually occur postoperatively. This suggests that delaying possibly strabismus surgery until after reconstructive surgery may give better results.

MANDIBULOFACIAL DYSOSTOSIS

(MFD, Treacher Collins, Franceschetti-Zwahlen-Klein Syndromes)

This is a common syndrome that goes by many names depending on the medical specialty or the country of origin in the reports. Although this syndrome was first described in the literature in the 1800s by Berry,[51] Treacher Collins[52] and Franceschetti and colleagues[53] later published detailed descriptions of the major manifestations.

The disorder shows an unusually wide range of expressivity and involves structures primarily derived from the first branchial arch, groove, and pouch. The complete form is characterized by (1) coloboma or notching of the outer part of the lower eyelid; (2) lack of development of the malar bone and mandible; (3) antimongoloid slant of the palpebral fissures; (4) large mouth (macrostomia), abnormal (highly arched) palate, and anomalies of dentition; (5) malformations of the external and middle ear; (6) atypical hairline with projections toward the cheek; and (7) blind fistulas between the ears and angles of the mouth (Fig. 10–10). The condition is almost always bilateral. Incomplete and abortive cases are common.

The bilateral abnormalities are usually quite symmetric when compared with hemifacial microsomia. Intelligence in these patients is usually normal. A cleft palate exists in about 35% of patients with an additional 30% to 40% of patients showing more minor palatal anomalies.[5]

Although a variety of ocular abnormalities have been reported, vision is usually normal, and most of the ophthalmic defects are confined to the soft and hard tissues surrounding the globe. In the more severe cases there is a complete coloboma of the lower lid, which gives the lid a triangular shape. All structures of the lid may be affected at, and medial to, the site of the coloboma. In less severe cases only a notch of an S-shaped configuration of the lower lid exists, often with a decrease in the cilia of the lid medially. Significant astigmatism has been observed in a number of patients with off-axis cylinders, suggesting a possible relationship between the refraction and the defects in the surrounding soft and hard tissue.[54]

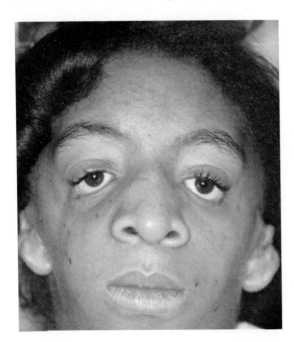

Figure 10–10. Mandibulofacial dysostosis, showing a downward slant of the palpebral fissure, abnormal ears, and coloboma of the outer third of the lower lid, with absent cilia nasal to coloboma.

The lacrimal puncta may also be involved or absent.[55,56] Wang and coworkers[57] examined 14 patients with mandibulofacial dysostosis and described in detail the changes observed in fissure length (decreased), shortening of the eyelid on forced closure, and the previously described punctal and lower lid anomalies. Low-incidence anomalies include upper eyelid colobomas, corneal guttata, and ptosis.[57,58]

Most of these patients require no ophthalmologic treatment other than routine management of strabismus, if it exists, and correction of the refractive error (although this may be somewhat difficult with eyeglasses because of the ear deformity). A few patients have tearing secondary to malformed positions of the palpebral fissures and other lacrimal anomalies requiring treatment.[55]

OCULO-AURICULO-VERTEBRAL SPECTRUM

(Hemifacial Microsomia, Goldenhar Syndrome, Facial Microsomia)

Hemifacial microsomia encompasses a heterogeneous spectrum of conditions characterized by malformations involving the ear and oral and mandibular structures. There are no absolute minimum criteria for diagnosis, and the incidence of this syndrome complex is unknown. Goldenhar syndrome is considered by many to be a variant in the group and is estimated to represent 10% of the total group.[59]

The designation of Goldenhar syndrome implies epibulbar or conjunctival lipodermoids with vertebral anomalies in addition to other characteristic findings. Ocular findings are thus more prevalent in this variant. Ocular and adnexal findings were reported by Hertle and colleagues[60] in 67% of cases in a facial microsomia series, with ptosis or a narrow palpebral fissure on the affected side in 10% of cases. Epibulbar dermoids and conjunctival lipodermoids occur frequently and most often inferotemporally.[61] Conjunctival lipodermoids also occur (Fig. 10–11). Upper lid colobomas are noted in about 20% of cases.[61] There appears to be a higher incidence of associated anophthalmia in cases with severe central nervous system anomalies.[5]

Hertle and colleagues[60] reviewed 49 cases of facial microsomia (5 bilateral and 44 unilateral). Visual loss was noted in 8% of cases, amblyopia in 16%, refractive errors in 27%, and strabismus in 22%. Strabismus is usually concomitant, but there is an increased occurrence of Duane syndrome[61,62] and other nonconcomitant types of strabismus.[63] Low-incidence anomalies include uveal colobomas,[61] corneal anesthesia,[64–66] iris coloboma,[67] optic nerve hypoplasia, and retinal abnormalities.[68]

Cosmetic and functional ocular malformations are common but extremely variable. In a few patients, the most important challenge may be cosmetic, with anophthalmia or microphthalmia. Many patients require routine treatment of refractive errors, ambly-

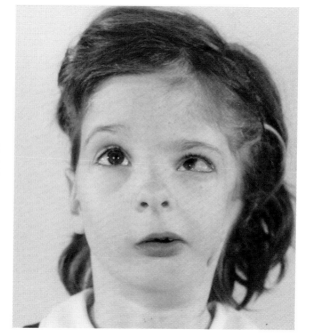

Figure 10–11. Goldenhar syndrome with large conjunctival lipodermoid and the typical manifestations of hemifacial microsomia. Lipodermoid extended far posteriorly, and only partial removal was possible.

opia, and strabismus. If corneal sensation is decreased, artificial tears may be indicated.

Epibulbar dermoids may result in astigmatism in the affected eye, and treatment will address amblyopia and the cosmetic appearance. Small, epibulbar dermoids and many conjunctival lipodermoids require only observation unless they increase in size. If surgical removal is necessary, care should be taken, as symblepharon formation may occur; removal is usually best limited to a readily visible section.[69] If the posterior aspect of a large lipodermoid is not visible, radiographic imaging may determine the extent of the lesion.

References

1. Aduss H, Pruzansky S, Miller M: Interorbital distance in cleft lip and palate. Teratology 1971; 4:171.
2. Cohen MM Jr: Malformation syndromes. *In* Bell WH, Proffit WR, White RD (eds): Surgical Correction of Dentofacial Deformities, pp 7–44. Philadelphia: WB Saunders, 1980.
3. Fox S: The palpebral fissure. Am J Ophthalmol 1966; 62:73.
4. Hall JG, Foster-Iskenius UG, Allanson JE (eds): Handbook of Normal Physical Measurements. New York: Oxford Medical Publication, 1989.
5. Gorlin RG, Cohen MM, Levin LS (eds): Syndromes of the Head and Neck, 3rd ed. New York: Oxford University Press, 1990.
6. Hoffman WY, McCarthy JG, Cutting CB, Zide BM: Computerized tomographic analysis of orbital hypertelorism repair: Spatial relationship of the globe and the bony orbit. Ann Plast Surg 1990; 25:124–131.
7. Jones KL (ed): Smith's Recognizable Pattern of Human Malformations, 4th ed. Philadelphia: WB Saunders, 1988.
8. Knudtzon K: On exophthalmometry. Acta Psychiatr Neurol 1949; 24:523.
9. Miller MT, Pruzansky S: Craniofacial anomalies. *In* Peyman GA, Sanders DR, Goldberg MF (eds): Principles and Practice of Ophthalmology, Vol 3, p 2354. Philadelphia: WB Saunders, 1980.
10. Hansman C: Growth of interorbital distance and skull thickness as observed in roentgenographic measurements. Radiology 1966; 86:87.
11. Morin JD, Hill J, Anderson J, et al: A study of growth in the interorbital region. Am J Ophthalmol 1963; 56:895.
12. von Graefe A: Graefe-Saemisch's Handbuch der gesamten Augenheilkunde, Vol 6, p 60. Leipzig: Engleman, 1880.
13. Anderson B, Woodhall B: Visual loss in primary skull deformities. Trans Acad Ophthalmol Otolaryngol 1953; 57:497–516.
14. Archer DB, Gordon DS, Maguire CJF, et al: Ophthalmic aspects of craniosynostosis. Trans Ophthalmol Soc UK 1974; 904:173.
15. Bertelson TI: The etiology of the premature synostosis of the cranial sutures. Acta Ophthalmol 1958; 36(Suppl 51):1–176.
16. Blodi FC: Developmental anomalies of the skull affecting the eye. Arch Ophthalmol 1957; 57:593–610.
17. Ingraham FD, Alexander E Jr, Matson DD: Clinical studies in craniosynostosis. Surgery 1948; 24:518–541.
18. McLaurin RL, Matson DD: Importance of early surgical treatment of craniosynostosis: Review of 36 cases treated during the first six months of life. Pediatrics 1951; 10:637–652.
19. Parks MM, Costenbader FD: Craniofacial dysostosis (Crouzon's disease). Am J Ophthalmol 1958; 33:782.
20. Pemberton JW, Freeman JM: Craniosynostosis. Am J Ophthalmol 1962; 54:641–650.
21. Friendenwald H: An optic nerve atrophy associated with cranial deformity. Arch Ophthalmol 1954; 30:405.
22. Lindenberg R, Walsh FP: Vascular compressions involving intracranial visual pathways. Trans Am Acad Ophthalmol Otolaryngol 1964; 68:677–694.
23. Wood-Smith D, Epstein F, Marello D: Transcranial decompression of the optic nerve in the osseous canal in Crouzon's disease. Clin Plast Surg 1976; 3:621–623.
24. Abeles M: Medullated optic nerve fibers accompanying oxycephaly and other cranial deformities. Arch Ophthalmol 1936; 16:188–196.
25. Weinstock FJS, Hardesty HH: Absence of superior recti in craniofacial dysostosis. Arch Ophthalmol 1965; 74:152–153.
26. Cuttone JM, Brazis PT, Miller MT, et al: Absence of the superior rectus muscle in Apert's syndrome. J Pediatr Ophthalmol Strabismus 1979; 16:349–354.
27. Diamond GR, Katowitz JA, Whitacker LA, et al: Variations in extraocular muscle number and structure in craniofacial dysostosis. Am J Ophthalmol 1980; 90:415–418.
28. Margolis S, Packter BR, Breinin GM: Structural alterations of extraocular muscle associated with Apert's syndrome. Br J Ophthalmol 1977; 61:683–689.
29. Mafee M, Miller M: Computed tomography: Scanning in the evaluation of ocular motility disorders. *In* Gonzales CF, Becker MH, Flanagan JC (eds): Diagnostic Imaging in Ophthalmology. New York: Springer-Verlag, 1986.
30. Nelson LB, Ingolia S, Breinin GM: Sensorimotor disturbances in craniostenosis. J Pediatr Ophthalmol Strabismus 1981; 18:32–41.
31. Bunsic JR: The ocular aspects of Apert syndrome. Clin Plast Surg 1991; 18:315–319.
32. Choy A, Margolis S, Breinin G, et al: Analysis of preoperative and postoperative extraocular muscle function in surgical translocation of bony orbits: A preliminary report. *In* Converse JM, McCarthy JG,

Wood-Smith D (eds): Symposium on Diagnosis and Treatment of Craniofacial Anomalies, pp 128–136. St. Louis, MO: CV Mosby, 1979.

33. Marsh JL, Galic M, Vannier MW: The surgical correction of craniofacial dysmorphology in Apert syndrome. Clin Plast Surg 1991; 18:251–275.

34. Cohen MM Jr (ed): Craniosynostosis: Diagnosis, Evaluation and Management. New York: Raven Press, 1986.

35. Kreiborg S: Craniofacial growth in premature craniofacial synostosis. Scand J Plast Reconstr Surg 1981; 15:171–184.

36. Whitacker LA, Munro IRF, Sayler KE, et al: Combined report and complications in 793 craniofacial operations. Plast Reconstr Surg 1979; 64:198–203.

37. David D, Poswillo D, Simpson D: The Craniosynostoses: Causes, Natural History and Management. New York: Springer-Verlag, 1982.

38. Handel N, Law J, Hoekn R, et al: Monitoring visual evoked responses during craniofacial surgery. Ann Plast Surg 1979; 2:257–258.

39. Clarren SK: Plagiocephaly and torticollis: Etiology, natural history, and helmet treatment. J Pediatr 1981; 98:92.

40. Bruneteau RJ, Mulliken JB: Frontal plagiocephaly: Synostotic, compensational, or deformational. Plast Reconstr Surg 1992; 89:21–31.

41. Friedrich DR, Mulliken JB, Robb RM: Ocular manifestation of deformational frontal plagiocephaly. J Pediatr Ophthalmol Strabismus 1993; 30:85–92.

42. Marsh JL, Vannier MA: Three dimensional surface imaging from CT scans for the study of craniofacial dysmorphology. J Craniofac Genet Dev Biol 1989; 6:61.

43. Robb RM, Boger WP III: Vertical strabismus associated with plagiocephaly. J Pediatr Ophthalmol Strabismus 1983; 20:58–63.

44. Becker MH, McCarthy JG, Chase N, et al: Computerized axial tomography of craniofacial malformations. Am J Dis Child 1976; 130:17.

45. François J, Eggermont E, Evens L, et al: Agenesis of the corpus callosum in the median facial cleft syndrome and associated ocular malformations. Am J Ophthalmol 1973; 76:241–245.

46. Naidich TP, Osborn RE, Bauer B, et al: Median cleft face syndrome: MR and CT data from 11 children. J Comp Assist Tomogr 1988; 12:57–64.

47. Baraitser M, Winter RM: Iris coloboma, ptosis, hypertelorism and mental retardation. J Med Genet 1988; 25:41–43.

48. Betharia SM, Kumar S: Facial cleft syndrome: A case report. Indian J Ophthalmol 1990; 38:198–199.

49. Pallotta R: Iris coloboma, ptosis, hypertelorism, and mental retardation: A new syndrome possibly localised on chromosome 2. J Med Genet 1991; 28:342–344.

50. Tessier P: Orbital hypertelorism. Scand J Plast Reconstr Surg 1972; 6:135.

51. Berry GA: Note on a congenital defect (? coloboma) of the lower lid. Ophthalmol Hosp Rep Lond 1888–1889; 12:255–257.

52. Treacher Collins E: Case with symmetrical congenital notches in the outer part of each lower lid and defective development of the malar bone. Trans Ophthalmol Soc UK 1960; 20:190–192.

53. Franceschetti A, Brocher JEW, Klein D: Dysostose mandibulo-faciale unilaterale avec déformations multiples du squelette (processus parastoïde, synostose des vertêbres, sacralisation, etc.) et torticolis clonique. Ophthalmologica 1949; 118:796–814.

54. Miller MT, Folk ER: Strabismus associated with craniofacial anomalies. Am Orthop J 1975; 25:27–36.

55. Bartley GB: Lacrimal drainage anomalies in mandibulofacial dysostosis. Am J Ophthalmol 1990; 109:571–574.

56. Franceschetti A, Klein D: The mandibulo-facial dysostosis. A new hereditary syndrome. Acta Ophthalmol 1949; 27:143–224.

57. Wang FM, Millman AL, Sidoti PA, et al: Ocular findings in Treacher Collins syndrome. Am J Ophthalmol 1990; 110:280–286.

58. Nucci P, Brancato R, Carones F, et al: Mandibulofacial dysostosis and cornea guttata. Am J Ophthalmol 1989; 109:204.

59. Rollnick BR, Kaye CI: Hemifacial microsomia and variants: Pedigree data. Am J Med Genet 1983; 15:233–253.

60. Hertle RW, Quinn GE, Katowitz JA: Ocular and adnexal findings in patients with facial microsomias. Ophthalmology 1992; 99:114–119.

61. Baum JL, Feingold M: Ocular aspects of Goldenhar's syndrome. Am J Ophthalmol 1973; 75:250–257.

62. Miller MT: Association of Duane retraction syndrome with craniofacial malformations. J Craniofac Genet Dev Biol Suppl 1985; 1:273–282.

63. Aleksic S, Budzilovich G, Choy A, et al: Congenital ophthalmoplegia in oculoauriculovertebral dysplasia: Hemifacial microsomia (Goldenhar-Gorlin syndrome). Neurology 1979; 26:638–644.

64. von Bijsterveld OP: Unilateral corneal anesthesia in oculoauriculovertebral dysplasia. Arch Ophthalmol 1969; 82:189–190.

65. Mohandessan MM, Romano PE: Neuroparalytic keratitis in Goldenhar-Gorlin syndrome. Am J Ophthalmol 1978; 85:111–113.

66. Snyder DA, Swartz M, Goldberg MF: Corneal ulcers associated with Goldenhar syndrome. J Pediatr Ophthalmol 1977; 14:286–290.

67. Feingold M, Gellis SS: Ocular abnormalities associated with the first and second arch syndromes. Surv Ophthalmol 1969; 14:30–42.

68. Margolis S, Aleksic J, Charles N, et al: Retinal and optic nerve findings in Goldenhar-Gorlin syndrome. Ophthalmology 1984; 91:1327–1333.

69. McNab AA, Wright JE, Caswell AG: Clinical features and surgical management of dermolipomas. Aust NZ J Ophthalmol 1990; 18:159–162.

Speech and Hearing Considerations in Facial Clefting and Craniosynostosis

11

Rodger M. Dalston and Donald W. Warren

INTRODUCTION

The principal focus of this chapter is to present information concerning those factors affecting the speech and language skills of persons born with facial clefts and those presenting with craniosynostosis in the context of Apert or Crouzon syndrome. Craniosynostoses without additional stigmata are not included because such patients typically do not present with communicative disorders.

The initial impact of giving birth to a child with a craniofacial anomaly, the subsequent adjustment of the affected individual and family, as well as the nature of the child's acceptance in society have important implications for speech and language performance among these patients. However, these issues are addressed elsewhere in this book. In addition, the interested reader is referred to several reviews of these topics.[1-4]

DEVELOPMENT OF SPEECH AND LANGUAGE SKILLS IN PATIENTS WITH FACIAL CLEFTING AND CRANIOSYNOSTOSIS

Prelinguistic Vocalizations

There is a growing body of information in the literature indicating that among normally developing children, the variety of babbling sounds produced during the second 6 months of life is highly predictive of the sound repertoire that will be present in early meaningful speech.[5-9] Moreover, there is evidence suggesting that children whose speech sound repertoire is reduced at 1 year of age will tend to have more articulation errors at age three.[10] In other words, a reduction in prespeech sound repertoire at 6 to 9 months of age may presage a reduction in consonant types at 1 year, and this, in turn, may foretell an increased frequency of speech sound errors at age three.

The apparent cascade described earlier has by no means been universally observed among patients at risk for developing communication problems. For example, Landahl and colleagues[11] conducted a longitudinal comparison of four children with Apert syndrome and four unaffected youngsters and found that children in the former group actually manifested a wider variety of babbling sounds than their unaffected peers during the period between 16 and 70 weeks of age. However, this precocious behavior had no apparent impact upon later speech sound development. The authors suggested that this may have been due to physical constraints within the oral cavity that adversely affected the ability to assume oral cavity configurations necessary for the production of acceptable English speech sounds.

The findings of Landahl and associates are in agreement with those of Smith and Oller,[12, 13] who studied another group of children who were at high risk for developing speech and language problems. To determine whether the early vocalizations of patients with Down syndrome could be differentiated from those of their normal peers, Smith and Oller[12] studied 9 normal and 10 Down syndrome infants at 3-month intervals beginning at 3 months of age. On the basis of parental reports and longitudinal phonetic transcriptions of tape-recorded utterances, they found that the onset of reduplicative babbling and the general sequence of consonant development in these two groups were similar throughout the first 15 months of life. Similar findings were obtained when Smith analyzed the phonologic development of 15 moderately to profoundly hearing-impaired infants.[13]

The findings reported earlier tend to suggest that among infants who do not manifest a palatal cleft, it may not be possible to predict phonologic development from phonetic analyses of prelinguistic vocalizations. In fact, Smith[14] stated that the variability generally associated with speech and language development may severely limit the ability to foresee eventual communicative disorders on the basis of vocal behavior manifested during infancy.

On the other hand, several recent studies have revealed that the early sound repertoire of children with unrepaired, or recently repaired, palatal clefts *is* qualitatively different from that of children without clefts.[15–18] Given the hypothesized sequence of speech sound development described earlier, the presence of these early qualitative differences may help explain the fact that youngsters with palatal clefts typically manifest numerous articulation problems in early childhood. For example, Dalston[19] reported that 74% of 4- to 5-year-old children seen for evaluation at the University of North Carolina Craniofacial Center (UNCCC) manifested articulation errors that were not considered to be normal for children of that age. By comparison, only 3.5% of the general preschool population manifest such errors.[20]

However, it should be emphasized that not all misarticulations exhibited by children with palatal clefts are the direct consequence of past or present velopharyngeal dysfunction. As a result, closure of the cleft cannot be expected to preclude the emergence of all articulation errors. Those errors that are considered to be related causally to velopharyngeal inadequacy are called *compensatory articulation errors.* This term is used because such misarticulations presumably arise from attempts to compensate for the inability to generate sufficient intraoral force for the production of pressure consonants. These compensatory errors include glottal stops, pharyngeal stops, pharyngeal fricatives, and posterior nasal fricatives. Many clinicians feel that mid-dorsum palatal stops, originally described by Trost,[21] also belong in this group. However, it is potentially significant to note that these errors occasionally are found in the consonant repertoire of individuals who do not manifest velopharyngeal impairment.[22] More information concerning the articulation performance of patients with oral-facial clefts and craniosynostosis will be provided later in this chapter.

Early Language Development

We have been unable to find any references in the literature concerning the early language competencies of patients with Apert, Crouzon, or Treacher Collins syndrome, although language delays would be expected among those individuals manifesting cognitive skill deficits. A computerized review of clinical records on syndromic craniosynostosis patients followed at the UNCCC indicated that 6 of 27 (22%) such patients manifested receptive and expressive language impairments at the time of their latest clinic visit. However, in all cases their language performance was commensurate with their overall level of intellectual functioning.

Currently available research suggests that the language abilities of individuals with oral-facial clefts are also somewhat impaired with respect to their noncleft peers,[23–31] although the differences tend to be small. In addition, there appears to be some evidence suggesting that these differences are present during early childhood. Fox and associates[32] compared 20 children with cleft lip and palate and four with cleft palate only to a matched group of 24 noncleft youngsters. These children ranged in age from 2 to 33 months. The mean age of the subjects with an oral-facial cleft was 17.7 months, and the mean age of the control group was 18.5 months. Administration of the Denver Developmental Screening Scale (DDS), the Receptive Expressive Emergent Language Scale (REEL), and the experimental version of the Birth-3 Scale (B-3S) indicated that the performance of the cleft palate youngsters generally fell 1 to 3 months below that of the control group. Statistically significant differences were evident on both REEL subtests and on the Language Expression, Personal/Social, and Motor subtests of the B-3S.

In an attempt to ascertain whether the language differences reported for older children[25] and adults are demonstrable in very young children, Long and Dalston[33-35] compared the preverbal communicative skills of 10 cleft lip and palate infants with those of 10 noncleft infants matched on the basis of age, sex, socioeconomic status, and dialect. Data were obtained from these 12-month-old subjects while they interacted with their mothers in a quasi-structured play situation. Analysis of the data, utilizing a protocol derived from the work of Bates and associates,[36] suggested that the children could not be differentiated on the basis of their comprehension, gestural, or paired gestural plus vocal expressive behaviors.

Whether the language skills of individual patients manifesting oral-facial clefts or craniosynostoses are truly different from those of their unaffected peers undoubtedly will depend upon a large number of variables. These variables include, but almost certainly are not limited to, intellectual capacity, auditory acuity, and articulatory proficiency.

Intellectual Skill Development

Richman and Eliason[37] provide an extensive review of information in the literature concerning the intellectual skills of cleft palate individuals. While the evidence reviewed by them was somewhat contradictory, they concluded that mean IQ scores for cleft palate subjects who have no other congenital anomalies tend to be somewhat depressed but within the normal range. McWilliams and colleagues[38] also provided a review of the literature concerning intellectual development among individuals with oral-facial clefts. The interested reader is directed to these two sources for additional information regarding this issue.

Impaired intellectual skill development is cited as a fairly common occurrence among patients with Apert syndrome,[39] although normal intelligence has been observed.[40,41] Mental retardation is less often observed among patients with Crouzon syndrome and is only occasionally observed among patients presenting with Treacher Collins syndrome. Among the 13 patients with Treacher Collins who are being followed longitudinally at the UNCCC, one (7.6%) has mild mental retardation. This agrees well with the findings of Stovin and coworkers,[42] who found four patients with mental deficiency among their group of 63 patients (6.3%).

Hearing Loss

Conductive hearing loss has been well documented as a frequent finding among children with Apert, Crouzon, and Treacher Collins syndromes.[38,43-50] The conductive nature of hearing loss observed in all three groups appears to be due to ossicular malformations and/or improper aeration of the middle ear due to structural crowding in the nasopharynx. Hearing loss among these patients tends to persist into adulthood.[47,51]

It is generally accepted that virtually all children born with a palatal cleft manifest conductive hearing losses that are the result of middle ear effusions at birth. While there is some evidence to the contrary,[52] most studies seem to substantiate this general impression.[53-55] Such effusions may be related to improper middle ear aeration resulting from abnormal auditory tube function.

The presence of substantial middle ear effusion necessarily causes a reduction in the efficiency with which the middle ear transmits airborne sound waves to the cochlea, thereby resulting in a conductive hearing loss. For this reason, it is generally assumed that children born with palatal clefts are at high risk for manifesting such hearing losses. This assumption clearly is borne out by numerous clinical investigations that indicate an inordinately high prevalence of conductive losses in these youngsters.[53,56-58] Moreover, Caldarelli and associates[50] and Heller and colleagues[60] suggested that middle ear disease also occurs frequently in patients with "congenital palatal incompetence" without signs of overt clefting.

There is no doubt that *pronounced* hearing loss can have a deleterious effect upon the development and maintenance of verbal communication skills.[61-69] However, conclusive evidence concerning the impact of a mild, conductive hearing loss on the development of these skills remains elusive.[70]

Despite the lack of definitive evidence linking mild conductive hearing loss and impaired communication skill development, it seems safe to say that the otologic management philosophy espoused by Paradise[55] has been adopted by many clinicians. He favored the placement of pressure-equalization (PE) tubes as early as possible in cleft palate infants in the hope of preventing otic and auditory handicaps as well as deficits in language and intellectual development. Unfortunately, no study has been reported that provides clear evidence that early otologic management actually does facilitate the development of normal speech and language skills. In fact, Potsic and coworkers[71] were not even able to demonstrate that hearing itself was improved in patients in whom PE tubes had been inserted. Moreover, Moller[72] cautioned against routine placement of tubes because of the possibility of provoking tympanosclerotic changes. Crysdale[73] and Paradise[55] also discussed the possibility of significant complications that can occur as a result of tube placement.

Comparably depressing conclusions were reached by Freeland and Evans[74] in their study of the prevalence of middle ear effusions among 27 children who received routine otologic surveillance and treatment, and 41 children who did not. They reported that vigorous screening and treatment of their cleft palate patients during the first 4 years of life resulted in only a modest 13% reduction in the prevalence of persistent middle ear effusions at 4 years of age. On the other hand, they did report that such treatment seemed to prevent tympanic perforations and attic retractions.

Regardless of the nature and timing of otologic treatment provided youngsters with palatal clefts, and perhaps in spite of such treatment,[74] it appears that auditory function does improve with age.[72, 75] Nevertheless, as is the case with craniosynostosis patients, impaired auditory tube function and conductive hearing loss seem to persist into adolescence and adulthood.[54, 76–78]

Articulation Errors Among Cleft Palate Speakers

As a basis for understanding the nature of many of the speech production errors made by persons with cleft palate with or without cleft lip, it is useful to dichotomize primary and secondary consequences of velopharyngeal impairment. A patient who cannot effectively close the velopharyngeal port can be expected to manifest hypernasal resonance on vowels and nasal emission of air on pressure consonants as a primary consequence of this inability. In cases of marked impairment, stop consonants would be expected to be replaced by homorganic nasals. However, these primary effects do not adequately describe the speech of a patient with velopharyngeal inadequacy. Many of the speech characteristics of such individuals are the result of compensatory adaptations made in an attempt to adjust to the velopharyngeal deficit.

Glottal stops and pharyngeal fricatives undoubtedly are the best-known forms of compensatory articulation manifested by speakers with impaired velopharyngeal function. Trost[21] described three additional types of compensatory articulation patterns that are useful in identifying the phonetic repertoire of individuals with cleft palate. The first of these, the pharyngeal stop, typically is substituted for /k/ or /g/. It involves approximation of the back of the tongue and the posterior pharyngeal wall. The second type, the mid-dorsum palatal stop, is produced by effecting broad lingual dorsum contact with the palatal vault, resulting in a stop sound that is perceptually ambiguous: neither /t/ nor /k/; neither /d/ nor /g/. It may be that these compensatory patterns are a reflection of the observation that cleft palate children tend to produce a preponderance of retracted lingual placements among their articulation errors.[79, 80]

The third articulatory behavior described by Trost is what she called a posterior nasal fricative. The distinguishing characteristic of this articulation is that audible turbulence is created at the velopharyngeal port. McWilliams and colleagues[38] and Terashima[81] described what appear to be similar compensatory patterns.

In addition to compensatory articulation errors, patients with oral-facial clefts also manifest a high frequency of sibilant articulation errors in their speech. Because the prevalence of dental abnormalities is quite high in the cleft lip and palate population,[82–84] it seems reasonable to suggest that the presence of these articulation errors is related causally to the patient's occlusal status. However, Bishara and colleagues[85] were unable to establish any consistent trends between dentofacial morphology and articulatory proficiency in the group of 72 cleft palate females they studied.

If there is a causal relationship between dentofacial morphology and speech proficiency, it would be reasonable to assume that articulation should be affected by the magnitude of structural change to the oral cavity resulting from orthognathic surgery. However, the current evidence is somewhat contradictory. Turvey and coworkers[86] found that surgical correction of anterior open bites in nine noncleft patients resulted in "significant improvement in self-correction" of interdental lisps. Vallino[87] obtained similar results in her study of 34 noncleft patients who underwent a LeFort I maxillary osteotomy, a bilateral sagittal split osteotomy, or a combination of the two. Conversely, Schwarz and Gruner[88] studied 31 cleft palate patients and found that a "slight" degradation in articulation ability occurred following maxillary advancement. Other authors have provided evidence suggesting that maxillary surgery has no perceptually discernible long-term effect upon articulation.[89–92]

Even if orthognathic surgery does not result in perceptually significant alterations to speech, there is no justification for concluding that such surgery has no impact upon the motor control processes underlying speech. Indeed, quite the opposite may be true. Orthognathic surgery necessarily changes the biomechanical properties of the speech mechanism, thereby necessitating a change in motor programming if preoperative speech performance is to be maintained.[93] The extent to which dentofacial abnormalities associated with orofacial clefting may have an impact upon the development of motor programming for speech is still not fully understood.

Articulation Errors Among Patients with Craniosynostosis

Patients with Apert and Crouzon syndromes all manifest certain structural hazards that predispose these individuals to produce certain types of speech sound errors. Although variable expressivity affects the extent to which certain morphologic differences are present in a given patient, the structural impediments to normal articulation are apparent in most affected individuals. Of primary significance is the fact that these patients present with midface hypoplasia that causes the tongue to assume a protrusive posture with respect to the upper dental arch. As a consequence, these individuals typically manifest distortions of sibilants and affricates.

Midface hypoplasia and an abnormally acute cranial base angle[94, 95] both contribute to a reduction in the velopharyngeal port area. So also does the fact that patients with syndromic craniosynostosis usually present with an inordinately high nasal cavity resistance. As a consequence, these individuals usually have difficulty producing nasal consonants and have speech that is characterized by hyponasality. These structural differences also predispose them to obstructive sleep apnea and obligatory mouth breathing. Assessment of upper airway resistance and its impact upon breathing and speech are discussed in the next section of this chapter.

UPPER AIRWAY PROBLEMS IN PATIENTS WITH FACIAL CLEFTING AND CRANIOSYNOSTOSIS

There is a high prevalence of breathing problems associated with facial clefts and craniosynostosis. Clefts of the lip and palate frequently produce significant nasal deformities, such as deviated septum, vomerine spurs, and atresia of the nostrils, as well as maxillary growth deficits that alter the nasal floor.[96–98] These abnormalities tend to reduce the size of the nasal airway, resulting in nasal resistance values that are about 20% to 30% higher than in the normal population.[97, 98]

There is evidence that airway deficiency in unilateral cleft lip/palate is present in utero. Siegel and associates[99] observed that the fetal septum appeared enlarged and distorted, and was flanked laterally by reduced nasal airway passages at 17 weeks of gestation. They suggested that reduced nasal size may be a function of both nasal capsule deficiency and nasal septum hypertrophy. In addition, histochemical abnormalities in the facial muscles of unrepaired clefts, including mitochondrial abnormalities and muscle fiber hypoplasia, suggesting a myopathy or delayed maturation, have also been demonstrated.[100] These abnormalities may affect the nasal musculature as well. In repaired clefts, abnormal muscle bundles and connective tissue have also been identified at some distance from the cleft margin.[101] Their appearance is consistent with surgical denervation of VII nerve muscle groups in the perialar region.

The nasal airway of an adult with a repaired cleft lip and/or palate generally is about 25% smaller than that of a normal adult.[98] The normal adult nose is about 0.62 cm² in the smallest cross-sectional area, whereas the nose of an adult subject with cleft is about 0.43 cm².[97, 98, 102, 103] Evidence that the cleft airway is narrow implies that the airway is impaired and mouthbreathing is common. Indeed, a study by Hairfield and coworkers[104] confirmed this. Approximately 70% of the subjects with cleft lip/palate evaluated were either oral, predominantly oral, or mixed oral-nasal breathers. Published data on the prevalence of mouthbreathing in the normal population indicate that the proportion is approximately 15%.[105–107]

Children

For children, the type of cleft appears to affect nasal airway size but not necessarily breathing mode.[108] Table 11–1 presents data on nasal airway size during inspiration and expiration according to the type of cleft. Normative data also are shown for comparison. The differences among cleft types are readily apparent. The group with bilateral cleft lip and palate and the group with unilateral cleft lip demonstrate nasal cross-sectional areas that are significantly larger than the other cleft types. Indeed, the group with bilateral cleft lip and palate has an area slightly larger than the normal group.

Usually the nasal valve is the site of the smallest cross-section of the nose and the region of greatest flow resistance.[109–111] However, in the cleft population other areas may be involved as well. Septal deformities occur most frequently, but stenosed nasal apertures, thickened nasal mucosa, and hypertrophied turbinates are also observed. Similarly, the collapsed nasal ala associated with the typical cleft lip-nasal deformity is frequently present, especially in the group with unilateral cleft lip and palate. There is evidence that conditions or procedures that alter the shape or function of the nasal valve also affect the nasal cross-sectional area. As noted earlier, histologic abnormalities in the perialar musculature suggestive of surgical denervation/reinnervation have been demonstrated and undoubtedly adversely affect the nasal valve upon which they insert.[101] Turvey and colleagues[112] and Guenthner and associates[113] demonstrated that superior repositioning of the maxilla increases nasal area, presumably by changing the shape of the nasal valve. Cosmetic procedures that inappropriately scar or cause collapse of upper lateral cartilage also narrow the airway.[114] In fact, any morphologic changes within the critical nasal valve region may influence the mode of breathing. Individuals with bilateral cleft lip and palate usually undergo surgery that lengthens the columella. Presumably, this procedure would have a positive effect on ala shape and widen or stent the nasal valve. It is quite possible that the difference in airway size between the group with bilateral cleft lip and palate and the group with unilateral cleft lip and palate stems from this surgery.

Another factor that affects nasal airway size is age. Figure 11–1 demonstrates that nasal cross-sectional area increases with age in the cleft as well as the noncleft populations. However, the 25% to 30% difference in airway size apparently remains over time. This difference is also reflected in the extent to which the cleft group tends to maintain a more oral pattern of breathing (Fig. 11–2). These findings pose interesting clinical questions. Specifically, all palate-involved groups, including the group with

Table 11–1. NASAL AIRWAY SIZE BY TYPE OF CLEFT IN CHILDREN

| | Nasal Airway Size, cm² (Mean ± Standard Deviation) | | | | | |
	UCL	UCLP	BCLP	CHP	CSP	Normal
Inspiration	0.37 ± 0.22	0.21 ± 0.13	0.40 ± 0.15	0.26 ± 0.14	0.26 ± 0.05	0.36 ± 0.18
Expiration	0.36 ± 0.20	0.22 ± 0.12	0.41 ± 0.14	0.27 ± 0.15	0.23 ± 0.05	0.34 ± 0.17

Abbreviations: UCL, unilateral cleft lip; UCLP, unilateral cleft lip/palate; BCLP, bilateral cleft lip/palate; CHP, cleft of hard palate; CSP, cleft of soft palate.

From Warren DW, Drake AF, Davis JU: Nasal airway in breathing and speech. Cleft Palate J 1992; 29:511–519.

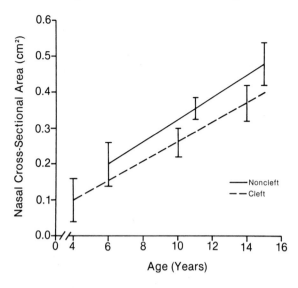

Figure 11-1. The relationship between age and nasal cross-sectional area in patients with ("cleft") and without ("noncleft") cleft lip and palate. (From Warren DW, Drake AF, Davis JU: Nasal airway in breathing and speech. Cleft Palate J 29:511–519, 1992.)

bilateral cleft lip and palate, were more oral than nasal breathers. The group with bilateral cleft lip and palate should have had a higher mean percent of nasal breathing based on airway size. In fact, a percent of nasal breathing similar to that observed in the group with unilateral cleft lip would be expected. Although it is only conjecture, we suggest that distortion of the nasal valve and alar collapse, so frequently associated with bilateral cleft lip and palate prior to initial repair and columellar lengthening, resulted in high nasal resistance.

Since there is open communication between the nose and mouth at birth, a normal nasal breathing pattern is not established. In addition, endoscopic studies of some of our bilateral cleft lip and palate patients indicate that the tongue is often placed in the nose during breathing prior to palatal repair. Such conditions may produce a persistent pattern of mouthbreathing that remains even after surgical repair.

Adults

Type of cleft does not appear to have the same effect in adults. As Table 11–2 indicates, there is no difference in nasal cross-sectional area between the unilateral cleft lip/palate and the bilateral cleft lip/palate. Obviously, secondary surgical procedures to correct septal and other defects are partially responsible for this change with age. Some dramatic differences are apparent, however. Whereas the mean unilateral cleft lip/palate nasal area almost doubled (i.e., 0.22 cm^2 in children at a mean age of 9.7 years vs. 0.41 cm^2 in adults), less change occurred with age in the bilateral cleft lip/palate group. In fact, during inspiration, the bilateral cleft lip/palate nose tends to

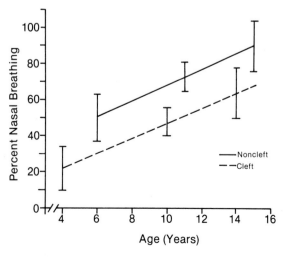

Figure 11-2. The relationship between age and percentage of nasal breathing by patients with ("cleft") and without ("noncleft") cleft lip and palate. (From Warren DW, Drake AF, Davis JU: Nasal airway in breathing and speech. Cleft Palate J 29:511–519, 1992.)

Table 11–2. NASAL AIRWAY SIZE BY TYPE OF CLEFT IN ADULTS

Group	Inspiratory (cm² ± SD)	Expiratory (cm² ± SD)	Nasal Area < 0.40 cm² (%)
N	0.63 ± 0.17	0.56 ± 0.14	20%
UCLP	0.41 ± 0.14	0.41 ± 0.13	45%
BCLP	0.34 ± 0.23	0.45 ± 0.29	67%
CP	0.35 ± 0.17	0.32 ± 0.16	67%
U/BCL	0.40 ± 0.16	0.44 ± 0.13	60%

See Table 11–1 for abbreviations.
From Warren DW, Drake AF, Davis JU: Nasal airway in breathing and speech. Cleft Palate J 1992; 29:511–519.

collapse with the negative inspiratory pressures. This apparent lack of growth in the bilateral cleft lip/palate group is a concern. The columellar lengthening procedure apparently provides an adequate nasal airway for most children, but the data for adults suggest that this cosmetic surgical procedure may, in fact, hinder further growth in the critical area of the nasal valve, especially if muscle disinsertion or denervation occurs. We are currently assessing this disturbing finding.

Table 11–2 also lists the percentage of individuals with impaired nasal airways by type of cleft. Studies of normal and nasally impaired adults,[115] modeling studies,[98,116] and extrapolation of data from nasal resistance studies[117–119] suggest that airway impairment in adults occurs when the smallest cross-sectional area anywhere in the nose is less than 0.40 cm². Areas greater than 0.40 cm² during rest breathing usually meet respiratory requirements without physical constraints imposed by the relationship of area to airflow rate.[115] Other studies indicate that adults with cross-sectional areas less than 0.40 cm² mouthbreathe to some extent.[116,117,120,121]

Effects of Secondary Procedures on the Nasal Airway

Secondary procedures for velopharyngeal inadequacy such as the pharyngeal flap alter the nasopharyngeal airspace, increase nasal airway resistance,[122] decrease airway size,[103] and increase the prevalence of mouthbreathing.[104] Because most individuals with palatal clefts are oral-nasal breathers from birth, the placement of a flap does not mean that an individual will notice or complain of increased airway resistance, because the addition of a flap really does not often change breathing behaviors in most individuals. However, the effect might be significantly different in an individual whose airway and breathing mode were fairly normal prior to the flap but were impaired after the flap. Under such circumstances, the individual would have to switch to some oral breathing and probably notice that breathing was more difficult. In some instances, pharyngeal flaps may even result in sleep apnea, especially in children.[122–124] Similarly, when adenoid tissue hypertrophies around the flap or when enlarged tonsils are present, the ports may become obstructed. The removal of both tonsils and adenoid tissue prior to pharyngeal flap surgery should be considered in light of possible life-threatening consequences.[125]

Effects of Maxillary Expansion on the Nasal Airway

Individuals with cleft palate often have maxillary arch constriction that requires further treatment. In some cases, expansion by orthodontic means is sufficient but in others surgical expansion may be necessary. Both procedures appear to have a beneficial effect on nasal respiration.[112,126,127] An increase in the range of 45% to 55% can be expected, although in many instances this increase is still not great enough to ensure a change to nasal breathing.

Both procedures apparently alter the nasal valve area, which in the normal nose presents the smallest nasal cross-sectional area and provides the most significant airflow resistance during breathing.[110] Aerodynamic studies of the nasal airway support this assumption. Turvey and colleagues[112] and Guenthner and associates[113] suggested that maxillary repositioning opens the nasal valve, thus reducing nasal resistance. They observed that the external nares change in shape from narrow slits to more ovoid forms postoperatively. Rapid maxillary expansion probably has a similar effect because suture opening is greatest in the anterior palate.[128] A reasonable assumption is that maxillary constriction produces a narrow nasal valve. Although nasal airway resistance may be increased by turbinate hypertrophy, nasal polyps, extremely large adenoids, and a deviated septum, maxillary expansion should have little effect on such factors. Expansion does appear to improve airway patency by increasing alar width and nasal valve size.[112, 113, 127, 129]

An interesting additional finding was that nasal breathing also improves after expansion. Walker and coworkers[130] noted a considerable change toward nasal breathing in most subjects after performing a maxillary osteotomy. They noted that although individuals who were oral-nasal breathers for a long period of time, such as in the cleft population, tend to remain oral breathers even with improvement in nasal airway patency, this was not the case in their study. They suggested that maxillomandibular fixation for a period of 6 to 8 weeks may have encouraged a change to nasal breathing. Faced with high oral airway impedance due to fixation, many may have changed to lower resistance nasal breathing, thereby modifying a long-term habit.

Craniosynostosis

Reports dealing with airway problems associated with craniosynostosis indicate that in almost every instance, the airway is impaired. Unfortunately, the literature is replete with anecdotal reports but little hard data. Our own unpublished database suggests that the upper airway in these patients is about 70% smaller than in normals. There are several reasons why the airway is reduced, and most relate to morphological differences. For example, midfacial hypoplasia reduces the nasopharyngeal airspace.[131] Bilateral choanal atresia may be present, and this condition totally obstructs the nose.[132] Oropharyngeal airway obstruction may result from glossoptosis associated with retrognathia or micrognathia.[132] The almost universal presence of airway impairment in this population produces predominant oral breathing in almost every instance, and an open-mouth posture is common. Episodes of apnea often affect children with craniofacial anomalies, and adenoidectomy has been reported to be useful in some instances. Tonsillectomy is also effective when the oropharyngeal airway is small, especially in the presence of glossoptosis.

Although it is evident from physical examination, including radiologic assessments, that the airway is diminished in individuals with craniosynostosis, quantitative studies linking specific morphologic features with airway impairment and breathing behaviors have not been performed despite the fact that the necessary technology is available. Without this information, this population will continue to be treated symptomatically and intuitively.

Effects of the Nasal Airway on Speech

Speech is a modified breathing behavior that uses the respiratory system to provide an energy source and involves structures within the respiratory tract to modulate this energy into meaningful sounds. The oral, nasal, and pharyngeal structures that are affected by cleft lip and palate during breathing are often compromised for speech as well.

Cleft palate speech is usually characterized by two major distortions, one of resonance and the other of articulation.[133-137] Both relate to an inability to attain adequate velopharyngeal closure.[138-141] The articulation errors associated with velopharyngeal inadequacy are of particular interest to clinicians and researchers because the problems they pose usually remain after surgical repair, and the reasons they appear may have important implications for speech-motor control. It is paradoxical that although velopharyngeal inadequacy stimulates compensatory speech behaviors, such responses tend to undermine rather than enhance speech performance.

There are several compensatory strategies used by cleft palate speakers.[97, 142, 143] Individuals with velopharyngeal inadequacy use greater respiratory effort or air volumes during speech. Their volumes are approximately twice those of normal speakers.

The two factors responsible, that is, airflow rate and duration of production, are both increased in cleft palate speakers. The implications of this are of interest because of the relationship between respiratory effort and speech performance. For example, in the presence of velopharyngeal inadequacy, the use of larger volumes of air increases nasal emission. However, the relationship between nasal emission, voice quality, and sound intelligibility is complex and determined to an extent by the magnitude of nasal airway resistance. As discussed earlier, nasal resistance is considerably higher in the cleft population.[97] This suggests that certain cleft palate speakers can compensate somewhat for velopharyngeal inadequacy by increasing respiratory effort because high nasal resistance should raise intraoral pressure. On the other hand, nasal turbulence also occurs when airway resistance is high. Thus an individual with nasal obstructions could conceivably produce undesirable turbulent noises and thereby decrease intelligibility with greater respiratory effort.

Compensatory changes in speech timing and alterations in tongue carriage also occur among cleft palate speakers.[117, 144] Apparently the level of intelligibility attained by cleft speakers is determined by the manner in which the various articulatory structures of the vocal tract respond to inadequacy rather than the specific degree of velopharyngeal impairment.

An important question among clinicians who treat speech problems associated with cleft palate is why compensatory speech behaviors that undermine performance develop. Recent studies suggest that these behaviors may be attempts to satisfy the requirements of a regulating system.[116, 145–148] The production of speech requires a relatively constant subglottal pressure, which serves as the energy source.[149–152] Intraoral pressures for consonants also appear to be fairly constant within subjects, although they do vary according to speaker age[153, 154] and sex.[153, 155, 156] In addition, they have been found to vary by word position,[157–160] voicing characteristics,[152, 161–167] vowel context,[168–170] utterance length,[160, 171, 172] and syllabic stress.[172, 173] Among cleft palate speakers, although peak intraoral pressure falls as the extent of velopharyngeal impairment increases, it usually remains above 3 cm H_2O.[98, 174]

Comparison of these findings with model simulations[121, 174] suggests that speakers make adjustments to velar impairment that tend to maintain pressure at levels thought to be necessary for obstruent consonant productions. One study[175] indicated that the ability to achieve adequate speech pressures depends upon total upper airway resistance; that is, successful maintenance of consonant pressures depends upon velar and nasal resistance. Specifically, individuals with velopharyngeal impairment use different respiratory volumes that are adjusted somewhat to the magnitude of upper airway resistance.

On the basis of these studies, Warren suggested that speech aerodynamics follows the rules of a regulating system.[148] Specifically, for speech aerodynamics subglottal pressure is kept relatively constant by checking or enhancing elastic forces and by compensating for sudden changes in respiratory load that occur with opening and closing of the upper airway. Precise control over the movement of upper airway structures and airflow tends to keep subglottal pressures regulated.[147] There is evidence that movements of the speech structures follow patterns that result in generally controlled vocal tract resistance and stable intraoral pressures.[148]

The significance of a regulating system in terms of cleft palate relates to the loss of velar resistance with inadequate palate function. If nasal resistance is low, upper airway resistance could be supplemented by articulatory adjustments that increase airway resistance at other levels of the vocal tract. This implies that articulatory gestures may be modified by aerodynamic needs, and speech performance may be compromised. Indeed, a recent study by Peterson-Falzone[176] tends to support this assumption. Peterson-Falzone found that the type of cleft affects the prevalence of compensatory articulation errors associated with velopharyngeal impairment. Errors were more frequent for those with bilateral cleft lip/palate, followed by cleft palate only, and least frequent in those individuals with unilateral cleft lip/palate. Interestingly, children with unilateral cleft lip/palate have the most compromised airways, and those with bilateral clefts of the lip and palate have the least compromised airways. This supports the thesis that articulatory patterns may be modified by aerodynamic needs. The pharyngeal fricative, glottal stop, nasal grimace, and high tongue carriage may be examples of such responses. Speakers increase airway resistance but undermine intelligibility. Whether these behaviors are prompted by low nasal resistance is a question of significant clinical relevance.

References

1. Clifford E: Psychological aspects of cleft lip and palate. *In* Bzoch KR (ed): Communicative Disorders Related to Cleft Lip and Palate, 2nd ed, pp 37–51. Boston: Little, Brown, 1979.
2. Richman LC, Eliason M: Psychological characteristics of children with cleft lip and palate: Intellectual, achievement, behavioral and personality variables. Cleft Palate J 1982; 19:249–257.
3. Tobiasen JM: Psychosocial correlates of congenital facial clefts: A conceptualization and model. Cleft Palate J 1984; 21:131–139.
4. Cohn ER, Hesky EMO, Bradley WF, et al: Life response to Crouzon's Disease. Cleft Palate J 1985; 22:123–131.
5. Oller DK, Wieman LA, Doyle W, et al: Infant babbling and speech. J Child Lang 1976; 3:1–11.
6. Oller DK: The emergence of sound of speech in early infancy. *In* Yeni-Komshian GH, Kavanagh JF, Ferguson CA (eds): Child Phonology, vol I, pp 93–112. New York: Academic Press, 1980.
7. Locke J: Phonological Acquisition and Change. New York: Academic Press, 1983.
8. Vihman M, Macken M, Miller R, et al: From babbling to speech: A reassessment of the continuity issue. Language 1985; 61:397–445.
9. Smith B: The emergent lexicon from a phonetic perspective. *In* Smith MD, Locke JL (eds): The Emergent Lexicon: The Child's Development of a Linguistic Vocabulary, pp 75–106. San Diego, CA: Academic Press, 1988.
10. Vihman MM: Individual differences in babbling and early speech: Predicting to age three. *In* Lindblom B, Jetterstrom R (eds): Precursors of Early Speech, pp 135–143. Basingstoke, Hampshire, England: MacMillan, 1986.
11. Landahl KL, Rasco RA, Mishra V, et al: Speech Development in Children with Craniofacial Malformation. Paper presented at the 43rd anniversary meeting of the American Cleft Palate Association in New York, 1986.
12. Smith BL, Oller DK: A comparative study of pre-meaningful vocalizations produced by normally developing and Down's syndrome infants. J Speech Hear Disord 1981; 46:46–51.
13. Smith BL: Some observations concerning pre-meaningful vocalizations of hearing-impaired infants. J Speech Hear Disord 1982; 47:439–441.
14. Smith BL: Implications of infant vocalizations for assessing phonological disorders. *In* Lass NJ (ed): Speech and Language: Advances in Basic Research and Practice, vol 11, pp 169–195. New York: Academic Press, 1984.
15. O'Gara MM, Logemann JA: Phonetic analyses of the speech development of babies with cleft palate. Cleft Palate J 1988; 25:122–134.
16. O'Gara MM, Logemann JA: Early speech development in cleft palate babies. *In* Bardach J, Morris HL (eds): Multidisciplinary Management of Cleft Lip and Palate, pp 717–721. Philadelphia: WB Saunders, 1990.
17. Salas-Provance M, Kuehn DP, Marsh J: Acoustic-Phonetic Analysis of the Prespeech Vocalizations of 13 Month Old Children with Cleft Palate. Paper presented at the American Cleft Palate-Craniofacial Association convention, St. Louis, Missouri, 1990.
18. Chapman KL: Vocalizations of toddlers with cleft lip and palate. Cleft Palate Craniofacial J 1991; 28:172–178.
19. Dalston, RM: Communications skills of children with cleft lip and palate: A status report. *In* Bardach J, Morris HL (eds): Multidisciplinary Management of Cleft Lip and Palate, pp 746–749. Philadelphia: WB Saunders, 1990.
20. Fein DJ: Population data from the U.S. Census Bureau. Speech Hearing Assoc 1983; 25:47.
21. Trost JE: Articulatory additions to the clinical description of the speech of persons with cleft palate. Cleft Palate J 1981; 18:193–203.
22. Peterson-Falzone SJ: Personal communication, 1991.
23. Pannbacker M: Oral language skills of adult cleft palate speakers. Cleft Palate J 1975; 12:95–106.
24. Whitcomb L, Ochsner G, Wayte R: A comparison of expressive language skills of cleft palate and non-cleft palate children: A preliminary investigation. J Oklahoma Speech Hear Assoc 1976; 3:25.
25. Kommers MS, Sullivan MD: Written language skills of children with cleft palate. Cleft Palate J 1979; 16:81–85.
26. Shames G, Rubin H: Psycholinguistic measures of language and speech. *In* Bzoch KR (ed): Communicative Disorders Related to Cleft Lip and Palate, 2nd ed., pp 202–223. Boston: Little, Brown, 1979.
27. Leeper HA Jr, Pannbacker M, Roginski J: Oral language characteristics of adult cleft palate speakers compared on the basis of cleft type and sex. J Commun Disord 1980; 13:133–146.
28. Richman LC: Cognitive patterns and learning disabilities in cleft palate children with verbal deficits. J Speech Hear Res 1980; 23:447–456.
29. Wasserman GA, Allen R, Linares LO: Maternal interaction and language development in children with and without speech-related anomalies. J Commun Disord 1988; 21:319–328.
30. Nation JE, Wetherbee MA: Cognitive-communicative development of identical triplets, one with unilateral cleft lip and palate. Cleft Palate J 1985; 22:38–50.
31. Scherer NJ, D'Antonio LL, Snyder LS: Language Disorders in Children with Cleft Palate: Do They Exist and How Early Can They Be Identified? Paper presented at the 48th annual meeting of the American Cleft Palate-Craniofacial Association, Hilton Head, South Carolina, 1991.
32. Fox W, Lynch J, Brookshire B: Selected development factors of cleft palate children between two and thirty-three months of age. Cleft Palate J 1978; 15:239–245.
33. Long NV, Dalston RM: Paired gestural and vocal behavior in one-year-old cleft lip and palate children. J Speech Hear Disord 1982; 47:403–406.
34. Long NV, Dalston RM: Gestural communication in twelve-month-old cleft lip and palate children. Cleft Palate J 1982; 19:57–61.
35. Long NV, Dalston RM: Comprehension abilities of one-year-old infants with cleft lip and palate. Cleft Palate J 1983; 20:303–306.

36. Bates E, Benigni L, Bretherton I, et al.: Cognition and communication from 9-12 months: A correlational study. Boulder, CO: Institute for the Study of Intellectual Behavior, University of Colorado, 1977.
37. Richman LG, Eliason M: Development in children with cleft lip and/or palate: Intellectual, cognitive, personality and parental factors. Semin Speech Lang 1986; 7:225–240.
38. McWilliams BJ, Morris HL, Shelton RL: Cleft Palate Speech. Philadelphia: BC Decker, 1990.
39. Elfenbein J, Waziri M, Morris HL: Verbal communication skills of six children with craniofacial anomalies. Cleft Palate J 1981; 18:59–64.
40. Musallam S, Poley J, Riley H: Apert's syndrome (acrocephalosyndactyly): A description and a report on seven cases. Clin Pediatr 1975; 14:1054–1062.
41. Noetzel MJ, Marsh JL, Palkes H, et al: Hydrocephalus and mental retardation in craniosynostosis. J Pediatr 1985; 107:885–892.
42. Stovin JJ, Lyon JA, Clemmens RL: Mandibulofacial dysostosis. Radiology 1960; 74:225–231.
43. McGill T: Otolaryngologic aspects of Apert syndrome. Clin Plast Surg 1991; 18:309–313.
44. Selder A: Hearing disorders in children with otocraniofacial syndrome. In Wertz RT (ed): Orofacial Anomalies: Clinical and Research Implications (ASHA Report #8), pp 95–110. Washington DC: American Speech and Hearing Association, 1973.
45. Baldwin J: Dysostosis craniofacialis of Crouzon: A summary of recent literature and case reports with emphasis on involvement of the ear. Laryngoscope 1968; 78:1660–1667.
46. Holborow C: Deafness and the Treacher Collins syndrome. J Laryngol Otol 1961; 75:978–984.
47. Jahrsdoerfer RJ: Congenital malformations of the ear: Analysis of 94 operations. Ann Otol Rhinol Laryngol 1980; 89:348–352.
48. Caldarelli DD, Hutchinson JC, Pruzansky S, et al: A comparison of microtia and temporal bone anomalies in hemifacial microsomia and mandibulofacial dysostosis. Cleft Palate J 1980; 17:111–115.
49. Pron G, Galloway C, Armstrong D, et al: Ear malformation and hearing loss in patients with Treacher Collins syndrome. Cleft Palate Craniofac J 1993; 30:97–103.
50. Phillips SG, Miyamoto RT: Congenital conductive hearing loss in Apert syndrome. J Otolaryngol 1986; 95:429–433.
51. Gould HJ, Caldarelli DD: Hearing and otopathology in Apert syndrome. Arch Otolaryngol Head Neck Surg 1982; 108:347–349.
52. Too-Chung MA: The assessment of middle ear function and hearing by tympanometry in children before and after early cleft palate repair. Br J Plast Surg 1983; 36:295–299.
53. Soudijn ER, Huffstadt AJC: Cleft palates and middle ear effusions in babies. Cleft Palate J 1975; 12:229–233.
54. Yules RB: Current concepts of treatment of ear disease in cleft palate children and adults. Cleft Palate J 1975; 12:315–322.
55. Paradise JL: Management of middle ear effusions in infants with cleft palate. Ann Otol Rhinol Laryngol Suppl 1976; 85(Suppl 25):285–288.
56. Musgrave RR, McWilliams BJ, Matthews HP: A review of the results of two different surgical procedures for the repair of clefts of the soft palate only. Cleft Palate J 1975; 12:281–290.
57. Bess FH, Schwartz DM, Redfield N: Audiometric, impedance and otoscopic findings in children with cleft palates. Arch Otolaryngol Head Neck Surg 1976; 102:465–469.
58. Bergstrom L: Congenital and acquired deafness in clefting and craniofacial syndromes. Cleft Palate J 1978; 15:254–261.
59. Caldarelli DD: Incidence and type of otopathology associated with congenital palatopharyngeal incompetence. Laryngoscope 1978; 88:1970–1984.
60. Heller J, Gens GW, Croft CB, et al: Conductive hearing loss in patients with velopharyngeal insufficiency. Cleft Palate J 1978; 15:246–253.
61. Forner LL, Hixon TJ: Respiratory kinematics in profoundly hearing-impaired speakers. J Speech Hear Res 1977; 20:373–408.
62. Monsen RB: Acoustic qualities of phonation in young hearing-impaired children. J Speech Hearing Res 1979; 22:270–288.
63. Zimmermann G, Rettaliata P: Articulatory patterns of an adventitiously deaf speaker: Implications for the role of auditory information in speech production. J Speech Hear Res 1981; 24:169–178.
64. Horii Y: Some voice fundamental frequency characteristics of oral reading and spontaneous speech by hard-of-hearing young women. J Speech Hear Res 1982; 25:608–610.
65. Binnie CA, Daniloff RG, Buckingham HW: Phonetic disintegration in a five-year-old following sudden hearing loss. J Speech Hear Disord 1982; 47:181–189.
66. Mahshie JJ, Conture EG: Deaf speakers' laryngeal behavior. J Speech Hear Res 1983; 26:550–559.
67. Whitehead RL, Barefoot SM: Airflow characteristics of fricative consonants produced by normally hearing and hearing-impaired speakers. J Speech Hear Res 1983; 26:185–194.
68. Metz DE, Whitehead RL, Whitehead BH: Mechanics of vocal fold vibration and laryngeal articulatory gestures produced by hearing-impaired speakers. J Speech Hear Res 1984; 27:62–69.
69. Goehl H, Kaufman DK: Do the effects of adventitious deafness include disordered speech? J Speech Hearing Disord 1984; 49:58–64.
70. Shriberg LD, Smith AJ: Phonological correlates of middle-ear involvement in speech-delayed children: A methodological note. J Speech Hear Res 1983; 26:293–297.
71. Potsic WP, Cohen M, Winchester R: The types of hearing loss and ear pathology noted in screening craniofacial patients. Cleft Palate J 1979; 16:164–166.
72. Moller P: Hearing, Middle ear pressure and otopathology in a cleft palate population. Acta Otolaryngol 1981; 92:521–527.
73. Crysdale WS: Rational management of middle ear effusions in the cleft palate patient. J Otolaryngol 1976; 5:463–467.
74. Freeland AP, Evans DM: Middle ear disease in the cleft palate infant: Its effect on speech and language development. Br J Plast Surg 1981; 34:142–143.

75. Webster JC, Eldis F: Ear disease in relation to age in the cleft palate child and adolescent. Clin Otolaryngol 1978; 3:455–461.
76. Caldarelli DD: Incidence and type of otologic disease in the older cleft palate patient. Cleft Palate J 1975; 12:311–314.
77. Swigart E: Hearing sensitivity of adults with cleft lip and/or palate. Cleft Palate J 1979; 16:72–80.
78. Doyle WJ, Cantekin EI, Bluestone CD: Eustachian tube function in cleft palate children. Ann Otol Rhinol Laryngol 1980; 89(Suppl 68):34–40.
79. Lawrence CW, Philips BJ: A telefluoroscopic study of lingual contacts made by persons with palatal defects. Cleft Palate J 1975; 12:85–94.
80. Lynch JI, Fox DR, Brookshire BL: Phonological proficiency of two cleft palate toddlers with school-age follow-up. J Speech Hear Disord 1983; 48:274–285.
81. Terashima T: Acoustic studies of nasal snort in cleft palate patients. J Jpn Cleft Palate Assoc 1982; 4:46–62.
82. Dahl E, Hanusardottir B, Bergland O: A comparison of occlusions in two groups of children whose clefts were repaired by three different surgical procedures. Cleft Palate J 1981; 18:122–127.
83. Ranta R, Rintala AE: Correlations between microforms of the Van der Woude syndrome and cleft palate. Cleft Palate J 1983; 20:158–162.
84. Schwartz BH, Long RE, Smith RJ, et al: Early prediction of posterior crossbite in the complete unilateral cleft lip and palate. Cleft Palate J 1984; 21:76–81.
85. Bishara SE, Van Demark DR, Henderson WG: Relation between speech production and oro-facial structures in individuals with isolated clefts of the palate. Cleft Palate 1975; 12:452–460.
86. Turvey T, Journot V, Epker B: Correction of anterior open bite deformity: A study of tongue function, speech changes and stability. J Maxillofac Surg 1976; 4:93–101.
87. Vallino LD: Speech, velopharyngeal function, and hearing before and after orthognathic surgery. J Oral Maxillofac Surg 1990; 48:1274–1281.
88. Schwarz C, Gruner E: Logopedic findings following advancement of the maxilla. J Maxillofac Surg 1976; 4:40–55.
89. Bralley RC, Schoeny ZG: Effects of maxillary advancement on the speech of a submucosal cleft palate patient. Cleft Palate J 1977; 14:98–101.
90. McCarthy JG, Coccaro PJ, Schwartz MD: Velopharyngeal function following maxillary advancement. Plast Reconstr Surg 1979; 64:180–189.
91. Garber SR, Speidel TM, Marse G: The effects on speech of surgical premaxillary osteotomy. Am J Orthod 1981; 79:54–62.
92. Dalston RM, Vig PS: Effects of orthognathic surgery on speech: A prospective study. Am J Orthod 1984; 86:291–298.
93. Zimmermann G, Kelso JAS, Lander L: Articulatory behavior pre and post full-mouth tooth extraction and alveoloplasty: A cinefluorographic study. J Speech Hear Res 1980; 23:630–645.
94. Arvystas M, Shprintzen RJ: Craniofacial morphology in Treacher Collins syndrome. Cleft Palate Craniofac J 1991; 28:226–230.
95. Grayson BH, Weintraub N, Bookstein FL, et al: A comparative cephalometric study of the cranial base in craniofacial anomalies: Part 1. Tensor analysis. Cleft Palate J 1985; 22:75–87.
96. Drettner B: The nasal airway and hearing in patients with cleft palate. Acta Otolaryngol 1960; 57:131–142.
97. Warren DW, Duany LF, Fischer ND: Nasal airway resistance in normal and cleft palate subjects. Cleft Palate J 1969; 6:134–140.
98. Warren DW: A quantitative technique for assessing nasal airway impairment. Am J Orthod 1984; 86:306–314.
99. Siegel MI, Monney MP, Kimes KR: Analysis of the size variability of the human normal and cleft palate fetus nasal capsule by means of three-dimensional computer reconstruction of histologic preparations. Cleft Palate J 1987; 24:190–199.
100. Schendel SA, Pearl RM, DeArmond SJ: Pathophysiology of cleft lip muscle. Plast Reconstr Surg 1989; 83:777.
101. Schendel SA, Pearl RM, DeArmond SJ: Pathophysiology of cleft lip muscles following the initial surgical repair. Plast Reconstr Surg 1991; 88:197–200.
102. Hairfield WM, Warren DW, Hinton VA: Inspiratory and expiratory effects of nasal breathing. Cleft Palate J 1987; 24:183–189.
103. Warren DW, Hairfield WM, Dalston ET: The relationship between nasal airway size and nasal-oral breathing in cleft lip and palate. Cleft Palate J 1990; 27:46–51.
104. Hairfield WM, Warren DW, Seaton DL: Prevalence of mouthbreathing in cleft lip and palate. Cleft Palate J 1988; 25:135–138.
105. Uddstromer M: Nasal respiration. Acta Otolaryngol 1940; 42:3–146.
106. Saibene F, Mognoni P, Lafortuna CL: Oronasal breathing during exercise. Pflugers Arch 1978; 378:65–69.
107. Niinimaa V, Cole P, Mintz S: Oronasal distribution of respiratory airflow. Respir Physiol 1981; 43:69–75.
108. Warren DW, Hairfield WM, Dalston ET, et al: Effects of cleft lip and palate on the nasal airway in children. Arch Otolaryngol 1988; 114:987–992.
109. De Wit CA, Kapteyn TS, van Bochove W: Some remarks on the physiology, the anatomy and the radiology of the vestibulum and the isthmus nasi. Int Rhinol 1965; 3:37–42.
110. Bridger GP: Physiology of the nasal valve. Arch Otolaryngol Head Neck Surg 1970; 92:543–553.
111. Hinderer KH: Surgery of the valve. Int Rhinol 1970; 8:60–67.
112. Turvey TA, Hall DJ, Warren DW: Alterations in nasal airway resistance from superior repositioning of the maxilla. Am J Orthod 1984; 85:109–114.
113. Guenthner TA, Sather AH, Kern EB: The effect of LeFort I maxillary impaction on nasal airway resistance. Am J Orthod 1984; 85:308–315.

114. Kern EB: Surgery of the nasal valve. *In* Sisson GA, Tardy ME (eds): Plastic and Reconstructive Surgery of the Face and Neck: Rehabilitative Surgery, Vol 2, pp 43–59. New York: Grune & Stratton, 1977.
115. Warren DW, Hinton VA, Pillsbury HC, et al: Effects of size of the nasal airway on nasal airflow rate. Arch Otolaryngol Head Neck Surg 1987; 113:405–406.
116. Warren DW, Allen G, King HA: Physiologic and perceptual effects of induced anterior open bite. Folia Phoniatr 1984; 36:164–173.
117. Watson RM, Warren DW, Fischer ND: Nasal resistance, skeletal classification and mouthbreathing in orthodontic patients. Am J Orthod 1968; 54:367–379.
118. McCaffrey TV, Kern EB: Clinical evaluation of nasal obstruction. Arch Otolaryngol Head Neck Surg 1979; 105:542–545.
119. Warren DW, Hairfield WM, Seaton DL, et al: The relationship between nasal airway cross-sectional area and nasal resistance. Am J Orthod 1987; 92:390–395.
120. Hinton VA, Warren DW, Hairfield WM, et al: The relationship between nasal cross-sectional area and nasal air volume in normal and nasally impaired adults. Am J Orthod 1987; 92:294–298.
121. Warren DW, Hairfield WM, Seaton DL, et al: The relationship between nasal airway size and nasal-oral breathing. Am J Orthod 1988; 93:289–293.
122. Warren DW, Trier WC, Bevin AG: Effect of restorative procedures on the nasopharyngeal airway in cleft palate. Cleft Palate J 1974; 11:367–373.
123. Guilleminault C, Eldridge FL, Tilkian A, et al: Sleep apnea syndrome due to upper airway obstruction: A review of 25 cases. Arch Intern Med 1976; 137:296–300.
124. Kravath RE, Pollack CP, Borowiecki B, et al: Obstructive sleep apnea and death associated with surgical correction of velopharyngeal incompetence. Pediatrics 1980; 96:645–648.
125. Gray S: Airway obstruction and apnea in cleft palate patients. *In* Bardach J, Morris HL (eds): Multidisciplinary Management of Cleft Lip and Palate, pp 418–425. Philadelphia: WB Saunders, 1990.
126. Hershey HG, Stewart BL, Warren DW: Changes in nasal airway resistance associated with rapid maxillary expansion. Am J Orthod 1976; 69:274–284.
127. Warren DW, Hershey HG, Turvey TA, et al: The nasal airway following rapid maxillary expansion. Am J Orthod 1987; 91:111–116.
128. Wertz RA: Changes in nasal airflow incident to rapid maxillary expansion. Angle Orthodont 1968; 38:1–11.
129. Turvey TA, Warren DW: Impact of maxillary osteotomies on nasal breathing. Oral Maxillofac Surg Clin North Am 1990; 2:831–841.
130. Walker DA, Turvey TA, Warren DW: Alterations in nasal respiration and nasal airway size following superior repositioning of the maxilla. J Oral Maxillofac Surg 1988; 46:276–281.
131. Goldberg JS, Enlow DH, Whitaker LA, et al: Some anatomical characteristics in several craniofacial syndromes. J Oral Surg 1981; 39:489–498.
132. Crysdale WS: Otorhinolaryngologic problems in patients with craniofacial anomalies. Otolaryngol Clin North Am 1981; 14:145–155.
133. McWilliams BJ: Some factors in the intelligibility of cleft palate speech. J Speech Hear Dis 1954; 19:524.
134. Spriestersbach DC: Assessing nasal quality in cleft palate speech of children. J Speech Hear Dis 1955; 20:266.
135. Spriestersbach DC, Moll KL, Morris HL: Subject classification and articulation of speakers with cleft palate. J Speech Hear Dis 1961; 4:362.
136. Riski JE: Articulation skills and oro-nasal resonance in children with pharyngeal flaps. Cleft Palate J 1979; 16:421.
137. VanDemark DR: Predictability of velopharyngeal competency. Cleft Palate J 1979; 16:429.
138. Shelton RL, Brooks AR, Youngstrom KA: Articulation and patterns of palatopharyngeal closure. J Speech Hear Dis 1964; 29:390.
139. Brooks AR, Shelton RL, Youngstrom KA: Compensatory tongue palate-posterior pharyngeal wall relationships in cleft palate. J Speech Hear Dis 1965; 30:166.
140. Pitzner JC, Morris HL: Articulation skills and adequacy of breath pressure ratios of children with cleft palate. J Speech Hear Dis 1966; 31:26.
141. Shelton RL, Morris HL, McWilliams BJ: Anatomical and physiological requirements for speech. *In* McWilliams BJ, Wertz RT (eds): Speech, Language and Psychosocial Aspects of Cleft Lip and Palate: The State of the Art (ASHA report #9), pp 2–18. Washington, DC: American Speech and Hearing Association, 1973.
142. Warren DW: Nasal emission of air and velopharyngeal function. Cleft Palate J 1967; 4:148–156.
143. Warren DW, Mackler SB: Duration of oral port constriction in normal and cleft palate speech. J Speech Hear Res 1968; 11:391–401.
144. Claypoole WH, Warren DW, Bradley DP: The effect of cleft palate on oral port constriction during fricative productions. Cleft Palate J 1974; 11:95–104.
145. Warren DW, Nelson G, Allen GD: Effects of increased vertical dimension on oral port size and fricative intelligibility. J Acoust Soc Am 1980; 67:1828–1831.
146. Warren DW, Hall DJ, Davis J: Oral port constriction and pressure airflow relationships during sibilant productions. Folia Phoniatr 1973; 33:380–394.
147. Warren DW: Aerodynamics of speech. *In* Lass NJ (ed): Speech, Language, and Hearing. Philadelphia: WB Saunders, 1982.
148. Warren DW: Compensatory speech behaviors in individuals with cleft palate: A regulation/control phenomenon? Cleft Palate J 1986; 23:251–260.
149. Ladefoged P: Subglottal activity during speech. *In* Proceedings of the Fourth International Congress on Phonetic Sciences, pp 73–91. The Hague: Mouton, 1962.
150. Ladefoged P: Linguistic aspects of respiratory phenomena. *In* Bouhuys A (ed): Sound Production in Man, pp 141–151. New York: Ann N Y Acad Sci, 1968.

151. Mead J, Bouhuys A, Proctor DF: Mechanisms generating subglottic pressure. *In* Bouhuys A (ed): Sound Production in Man, pp 177–181. New York: Ann N Y Acad Sci, 1968.

152. Netsell R: Subglottal and intraoral air pressure during intervocalic contrast of /t/ and /d/. Phonetica 1969; 20:68–73.

153. Bernthal JE, Beukelman DR: Intraoral air pressure during the production of /p/ and /b/ by children, youths, and adults. J Speech Hear Res 1978; 21:361–371.

154. Stathopoulos ET, Weismer G: Oral airflow and intraoral air pressure: A comparative study of children, youths and adults. Folia Phoniatr 1985; 37:152–159.

155. Subtelny J, Worth J, Sakuda M: Intraoral pressure and rate of flow during speech. J Speech Hear Res 1966; 9:498–518.

156. Lotz WK, Netsell R: Developmental patterns of laryngeal aerodynamics for speech. Paper presented at the Midwinter Meeting of the Association for Research in Otolaryngology, Clearwater Beach, FL, 1986.

157. Malecot A: An experimental study of force of articulation. Studia Linguistica 1955; 9:35–44.

158. Malecot A: The force of articulation of American stops and fricatives as a function of position. Phonetica 1968; 19:95–102.

159. Arkebauer H, Hixon TJ, Hardy J: Peak intraoral pressure during speech. J Speech Hear Res 1967; 10:196–208.

160. Brown W, McGlone R: Constancy of intraoral air pressure. Folia Phoniatr 1969; 21:332–339.

161. Black J: The pressure component in the production of consonants. J Speech Hear Res 1950; 15:207–210.

162. Malecot A: The effectiveness of intraoral air pressure pulse parameters in distinguishing between stop cognates. Phonetica 1966; 14:65–81.

163. Lubker J, Parris P: Simultaneous measurements of intraoral air pressure, force of labial contact, and labial electromyographic activity during production of the stop cognates /p/ and /b/. J Acoust Soc Am 1970; 47:625–633.

164. Lisker L: Supraglottal air pressure in the production of English stops. Language Speech 1971; 13:215–230.

165. Warren DW, Hall DJ: Glottal activity and intraoral pressure during stop consonant productions. Folia Phoniatr 1973; 25:121–129.

166. Weismer G, Longstreth D: Segmental gestures at the laryngeal level in whispered speech: Evidence from an aerodynamic study. J Speech Hear Res 1980; 23:383–392.

167. Stathopoulos ET: Relationship between intraoral air pressure and vocal intensity in children and adults. J Speech Hear Res 1986; 29:71–74.

168. Brown W, McGlone R, Proffit W: Relationship of lingual and intraoral air pressure during syllable production. J Speech Hear Res 1973; 16:141–151.

169. Karnell M, Willis C: The effect of vowel context on consonantal intraoral air pressure. Folia Phoniatr 1982; 34:1–8.

170. Klich RJ: Effects of speech level and vowel context on intraoral air pressure in vocal and whispered speech. Folia Phoniatr 1982; 34:33–40.

171. Prosek RA, House A: Intraoral air pressure as a feedback cue in consonant production. J Speech Hear Res 1975; 18:133–147.

172. Flege JE: The influence of stress, position, and utterance length on the pressure characteristics of English /p/ and /b/. J Speech Hear Res 1983; 26:111–118.

173. Malecot A: The lenis-fortis opposition: Its physiologic parameters. J Acoust Soc Am 1970; 47:1588–1592.

174. Dalston RM, Warren DW, Morr KE, et al: Intraoral pressure and its relationship to velopharyngeal inadequacy. Cleft Palate J 1988; 25:210–219.

175. Warren DW, Dalston RM, Dalston ET: Maintaining speech pressures in the presence of velopharyngeal impairment. Cleft Palate J 1990; 27:53–58.

176. Peterson-Falzone SJ: A cross-sectional analysis of speech results following palatal closure. *In* Bardach J, Morris HL (eds): Multidisciplinary Management of Cleft Lip and Palate, pp 750–757. Philadelphia: WB Saunders, 1990.

12 | Management of Middle Ear Disease and Malformations

Vincent N. Carrasco

INTRODUCTION

Children with craniofacial abnormalities frequently have associated abnormalities of adjacent sensory organs. This has significant impact on their ability to learn and acquire language. Development of the central auditory system occurs through a process of central integration of external stimuli that are presented to the neonate through these sensory organs. The processing of this information is not well understood, but disruption of this system, either peripherally, through the input organs, or within the central nervous system, causes delays.[1] Many of these associated abnormalities, including ear disease, are defined and should be aggressively pursued. Children with craniofacial abnormalities have a high incidence of otitis media and hearing loss early in life.[2] Early intervention is of paramount importance, and all patients with craniofacial abnormalities should have an otologic evaluation as an early part of their management.[3]

This chapter discusses middle ear disease, specifically the anatomy and pathophysiology of the eustachian tube, its dysfunction and relationship to craniofacial disorders, otitis media, and hearing loss. Cleft palate, because of its frequency, will be used as the prototypical midface abnormality throughout this discussion. Included are middle ear malformations and treatment strategies.

ANATOMY OF THE EUSTACHIAN TUBE

The eustachian tube (ET) serves three functions. It ventilates the middle ear space, serves as a barrier to reflux of nasopharyngeal secretions, and drains secretions from the middle ear space. The ET is a channel that extends from the middle ear cavity to the nasopharynx. It has a cartilaginous and an osseous portion, and in the adult it is approximately 36 mm in length. The first 12 mm are osseous, beginning in the tympanic cavity and sharing a common wall with the internal carotid artery (within the anterior or the carotid wall of the tympanic cavity; Fig. 12–1). On the superior portion of this wall is the semicanal for the tensor tympani muscle with the tympanic orifice of the eustachian tube immediately below it. A triangular plate of fibrocartilage invests the next portion of the eustachian tube and attaches to the jagged edge of the osseous canal. The cartilage lies in a groove in the petrous portion of the temporal bone and greater wing of the sphenoid. It extends for approximately 24 mm medially, with the cartilage forming a submucous elevation in the nasopharynx called the torus tubarius. The torus is the posterior portion of the pharyngeal orifice of the eustachian tube. The superior portion of the cartilaginous tube hooks over the top of the ET but does not close around it. The cartilage remains open inferolaterally, forming a groove with the edge closed by a fibrous membrane. The ET lies within this groove. The angle of descent of the ET, from the ear to the nasopharynx, is approximately 35° from the horizontal plane and 45° medially from the sagittal plane.

The ET is narrowest in a region called the isthmus (see Fig. 12–1). This is located at the junction of the cartilaginous and osseous eustachian tube. The pharyngeal portion is the widest. The tube is lined with ciliated epithelium that is contiguous with the nasal part of the pharynx. The epithelium is thick here with many mucus-producing glands. In the osseous portion it is much thinner and tightly invested to the bone.

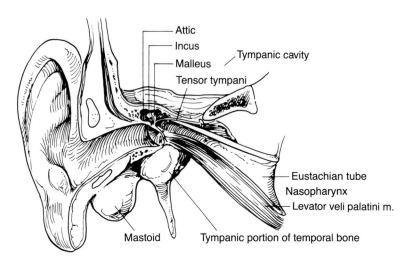

Figure 12–1. The relationship of the middle ear and the eustachian tube, as well as general anatomic points of the ear and its surrounding structures.

The pharyngeal orifice also has much adenoid tissue surrounding it known as the tubal tonsil.

The muscles that have the most influence on the ET are the levator veli palatini (LVP) and the tensor veli palatini (TVP). The tensor tympani and salpingo pharyngeus muscles also play a role in middle ear ventilation and pressure regulation. This anatomy is important because it is directly affected in cleft palate as part of the anomaly as well as after repair of the defect. The function of these muscles is also significantly affected in maxillary and mandibular orthognathic surgery for other mid-face abnormalities.[4]

The LVP arises from the inferior surface of the temporal bone as well as the medial portion of the cartilaginous ET. It is lateral to the choanae and deep to the torus tubarius. It inserts into the palatine velum, with both sides blending in the midline.

The TVP is the muscle that dilates the eustachian tube.[5] The TVP muscle is lateral and anterior to the LVP, arising from the base of the medial pterygoid plate, the spine of the sphenoid, and the lateral wall of the cartilaginous ET. The tendon of the TVP muscle inserts into the perichondrium of the lateral lamina of the tubal cartilage in normal individuals (Fig. 12–2). It then descends vertically between the medial pterygoid muscle and the medial pterygoid plate, ending in a tendon that winds around the pterygoid hamulus and inserting into the palatine aponeurosis on the horizontal part of the palatine bone.[6]

In the cleft palate patients, the TVP muscle has a reduced number of fibers inserting into the aponeurosis of the soft palate, and the bulk of the muscle deviates to the posterior nasal spine and posterior portion of the palatine bone.[7] Also, the major portion of the TVP tendon blends with the anterior portion of the LVP muscle at the cleft edge of the velum. This anatomic derangement of the TVP muscle is hypothesized to eliminate its firm anchor, reducing its ability to adequately open the ET (Fig. 12–3).

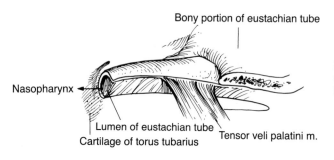

Figure 12–2. The muscle attachment of the tensor veli palatini and the cartilaginous portion of the torus tubaris and the nasopharynx.

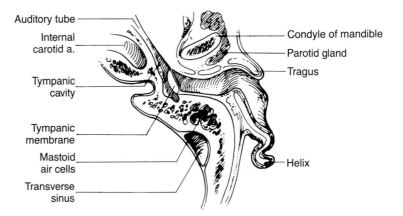

Figure 12–3. Axial view demonstrating the anterior portion of the auditory tube, the close relationship of the internal carotid artery and the transverse sinus to the middle ear, and the relationship of the condyle of the mandible to the anterior canal wall of the exterior auditory canal.

EFFECT OF PRIMARY CLOSURE OF CLEFT PALATE AND SURGICAL CORRECTION OF MAXILLARY HYPOPLASIA

In a longitudinal study of children with cleft palate (CP) before and after palatoplasty, Doyle and coworkers[8] observed that preoperative passive ET function was abnormal and improved postoperatively. This was attributed to malpositioning of the LVP muscle in CP, which results in constriction of the inferior tubal floor and increased extraluminal pressure. Passive opening of the ET is less likely because of increased opening pressure. During palatoplasty the LVP muscle is freed and rotated to the midline. This removes the inferior constriction of the ET and eliminates the added extraluminal pressure. In addition, Doyle and coworkers observed that eustachian tube function controlled by the TVP was minimally altered and remained poor following palatoplasty. The anatomy of the TVP muscle, after palatoplasty, does not change unless it is divided during surgery, at which point its function is reduced.[4]

Surgical correction of midfacial deformities may involve manipulation of the pterygoid plates. Potentially this can have profound effects on the structures within the nasopharynx. In a short-term study (6 to 8 weeks postoperatively) Butow and associates[7] indicated that the addition of a TVP muscle sling at the time of cleft palate surgery improves ET function. They emphasized the importance of maintaining the integrity of the hamulus as well as the tendons of the TVP muscle during corrective CP surgery. These maneuvers, in addition to the TVP muscle sling, may improve ET patency. Controlled trials are necessary to determine the efficacy of this procedure.

Audiologic testing indicated that nearly 50% of noncleft patients have persistent poor ET function after orthognathic maxillary surgery.[4] This was manifested by poor middle ear ventilation and fluid retention. Maxillary mobilization and pterygoid plate disruption result in altered function of the TVP, tensor tympani, and salpingo pharyngeus muscles. Reduced eustachian tube function occurred after mandibular setback surgery as well. The etiology of this is attributed to displaced tissues gathering around and below the ET. It has been observed that 10% of cleft palate patients undergoing cleft repair surgery had improved ET function postoperatively on the noncleft side. No long-term studies of the effects of these procedures on ET function have been performed to date.

OTITIS MEDIA

Children with midface hypoplasia and craniofacial anomalies have otitis media with effusion at such a high rate of frequency that many practitioners consider this a universal phenomenon.[2] Included in this group are the Pierre Robin sequence, trisomy 21, Treacher Collins syndrome, and Crouzon syndrome (Table 12–1).

Patients with diminished ET function are susceptible to recurrent acute otitis media (AOM). The most common organisms in acute otitis media are pneumococcus, *Haemophilus influenzae,* and B-hemolytic streptococci. These organisms generally respond

Table 12-1. SYNDROMES WITH CRANIOFACIAL ANOMALIES WITH HIGH RISK FOR
OTITIS MEDIA

Albers-Schonberg disease (osteopetrosis)
Apert syndrome (acrocephalosyndactyly)
Crouzon disease (craniofacial dysostosis)
Down syndrome (trisomy 21)
Goldenhar syndrome (oculoauriculovertebral dysplasia)
Hunter syndrome (mucopolysaccharidosis)
Hurler syndrome (mucopolysaccharidosis)
Mohr syndrome (orofacial-digital)
Parrot disease (achondroplasia)
Patau syndrome (trisomy 13–15)
Pierre Robin anomaly (cleft palate, micrognathia, glossoptosis)
Pyle disease (craniometaphyseal dysplasia)
Treacher Collins syndrome (mandibulofacial dysostosis)
Turner syndrome (gonadal dysgenesis)

to first line antibiotic treatment with more resistant strains of *H. influenzae,* for example, responding well to B-lactamase resistant antibiotics.

Recurrent bouts of AOM, chronic middle ear effusion, and chronic otitis media with development of cholesteatoma are characteristic of untreated disease (see glossary). Anything that interferes with the function of the eustachian tube causes otitis media. This includes adenoid hypertrophy, allergic swelling, obstruction secondary to nasal packing, and cleft palate. The first three conditions cause AOM because of eustachian tube obstruction, but in cleft palate the eustachian tube fails to open. Temporal bone studies[5] on specimens from individuals with cleft palate demonstrated no insertion of the TVP muscle in 40% of specimens and diminished insertion in the remaining 60%. Consideration of this is critical when the current theories of tubal dilation are examined. Proctor[9] stated that the eustachian tube is rotated and opened by coordinated contraction of the TVP and LVP muscles. Another theory postulates that the eustachian tube is fixed to the skull base and is opened by contraction of the TVP muscle.[5] Nonetheless, derangement of function of the TVP muscle is a significant factor in eustachian tube dysfunction.

Histologic sections of eustachian tube cartilage in infants, individuals with cleft palate, and microtia indicate immature development. This immaturity results in cartilaginous hypercompliance (''floppy cartilage''), providing poor support for the ET and resulting in poor function. Yamaguchi and colleagues offered this as an explanation for the ventilatory dysfunction observed in these groups.[10] They found that in normals, ET cartilage matured to adult densities by 8 to 12 years of age correlating to the age, at which the incidence of otitis media is found to decrease.[10] This intrinsic cartilaginous abnormality, coupled with the anomalous muscular attachment observed in cleft palate, sets the stage for poor auditory tube function and subsequent otitis media.

Middle ear effusion after AOM can take from 3 to 6 weeks to resolve in individuals with normal ET function. Conductive hearing loss is associated with middle ear effusion (type B tympanogram). If the effusion does not resolve, as in the case in eustachian tube dysfunction, it develops into chronic serous otitis media. The effusion in this setting is typically thick and gelatinous (so-called glue ear).

If the middle ear is not re-aerated periodically, as it is in individuals with normal ET function, the air present is eventually absorbed by the lining of the middle ear, creating a vacuum. This can be measured by impedance audiometry as a type C tympanogram. The air is generally replaced by fluid (hence recurrent or chronic serous otitis media) from the epithelial lining and microvasculature. If the cavity maintains a persistent negative pressure compared to ambient atmospheric pressure and does not develop effusion, the middle ear becomes atelectatic. This is characterized by progressive retraction of the tympanic membrane (TM) over the lateral surface of the ossicles and promontory. The result is one of two scenarios. The first is that the TM (particularly the pars flaccida portion) erodes the ossicles, resulting in a large conductive hearing loss. Typically the long process of the incus is gradually destroyed, eventually fracturing, with the TM resting on the capitulum of the stapes.

The other scenario is continued growth of the TM into the epitympanum or additus of the middle ear. As it becomes more atelectatic, a retraction pocket forms. The deepening retraction pocket develops into a narrow-necked squamous epithelial lined sac. Initially it cleans itself, shedding the squamous debris, but as the size increases and the neck narrows, it loses this ability. The desquamated epithelium becomes trapped and infected, developing into a cholesteatoma. This progresses to chronic otitis media, characterized by tympanic membrane perforation, constant purulent drainage, and bone destruction. It should also be noted that a TM perforation, typically a marginal one in an otherwise normal eardrum, can lead to development of a cholesteatoma by migration of squamous epithelium around the edge of the perforation into the middle ear space, where it continues to grow.

Ear drainage that is recurrent or long-standing is a sign of chronic otitis media. Patients who develop TM perforation with middle ear granulation tissue or cholesteatoma frequently have associated mastoid disease. The process responds to local care in the form of antibiotic drops and systemic antibiotics, but it is an operative problem requiring surgical intervention to restore the normal physiology of the ear. Chronic ear disease is associated with a mastoid that harbors nonaerated air cells that are poorly vascularized and are sequestered from the middle ear. This allows them to retain a mixed bacterial population that includes *Pseudomonas aeruginosa* discharging into the middle ear and is seen as drainage.

A study by Ovesen and associates[11] summed up the extent of ear disease in children with clefts. The incidence of hearing impairment, abnormal middle ear pressure, tympanic membrane retraction (pars flaccida), and abnormal TM appearance was 24%, 44%, 23%, and 12%, respectively, in 11-year-old children with CP. This was compared with 0%, 12.5%, 6%, and 12%, respectively, in age-matched healthy controls.

HEARING LOSS

Children with congenital anomalies frequently have hearing loss. The type of loss —conductive, sensorineural, or mixed—depends upon the anomalies. Conductive hearing losses can be from congenital ossicular disorders, ossicular discontinuity, tympanic membrane perforation, or tympanosclerosis. There also is an incidence of sensorineural hearing loss in syndromic children. Table 12-2 is a relatively complete list, compiled from the literature by Bergstrom,[12] of craniofacial syndromes that have an association with hearing loss. Detection requires a high index of suspicion and careful monitoring. Typically, children with mild (25 to 40 db) to moderate (40 to 65 db) hearing loss and normal intelligence can acquire some speech. This occurs at a slower pace than normal and is characterized by word and sound substitutions. These children compensate well and go undetected for long periods of time. Discovery occurs when the demands of learning make the handicap more obvious. This usually is identified when they start school.

A child with serous otitis media has a hearing loss that can be as great as 25 to 30 db.[12] Hearing loss from chronic otitis media or middle ear anomalies falls into the moderate or 40 to 65 db range. Children with sensorineural hearing loss (SNHL) can fall anywhere along the spectrum. Those in the severe (65 to 95 db) or profound (>95 db) range generally have SNHL but may also have a mixed hearing loss.

Individuals treated with myringotomy and tubes for serous otitis media who nonetheless retain significant CHL postoperatively require further evaluation for underlying middle ear anomalies. These take the form of ossicular malformations characterized by poorly formed ossicular masses, congenital stapes footplate fixation, or aberrant facial nerves.

Atresia and microtia are obvious causes of conductive hearing loss. But superimposed SNHL occurs with some level of frequency in the affected as well as a normal appearing contralateral ear. Any child with hearing loss, whether conductive or sensorineural, benefits from hearing aids. Placement as early as possible optimizes environmental stimulation, which promotes language development. This should be done unless immediate intervention relieving the hearing loss is planned.

TREATMENT

Effusion secondary to ET dysfunction in children with CP generally does not resolve with antimicrobial therapy alone. It tends to recur or persist, making myringotomy and PE tube placement necessary to relieve the conductive hearing loss and to permit proper aeration of the middle ear space. This procedure is performed as soon as

Table 12–2. SYNDROMES AND ASSOCIATED HEARING LOSS

Sensorineural

Marshall syndrome
Sticker
Lop ears, imperforate anus, triphalangeal thumbs
General cortical hyperostosis
Cleidocranial dysostosis
Stippled epiphyses and goiter
Agenesis of carotid artery
Craniodiaphyseal dysplasia

Conductive

Pierre Robin
Treacher Collins
Cleft palate
"Cleft palate plus"
Apert
Oral facial digital II
Pfeiffer
Hallermann-Streiff
Otofaciocervical
Malformed, low-set ears
Otopalatodigital
Hemifacial microsomia
First and second branchial syndrome
Frontonasal dysplasia
Oculodentodigital
Ocular hypertelorism
Chondrodystrophia calcificans
Congenital facial palsy
Lop ears, micrognathia
Kniest syndrome

Conductive, Sensorineural, or Mixed

Goldenhar
Crouzon
Möbius
Microtia
Wildervanck
Acrodysostosis
Partial deletion of chromosome 18
Osteopetrosis
Thalidomide
Cup ears, lacrimo-auriculo-dento-digital
Pre-auricular pits, cervical fistula syndromes
Facial hemihypertrophy
Fibrous dysplasia
Mucopolysaccharidosis
Craniometaphyseal dysplasia
Dominant and recessive "ear-kidney syndromes"
Diastrophic dwarfism
Frontometaphyseal dysplasia
Klippel-Feil
Rubella syndrome
Sclerosteosis

From Bergstrom L: Congenital and acquired deafness in clefting and craniofacial syndromes. Cleft Palate J 1978; 15:354–361.

feasible in a child who shows signs of disease. In an individual with CP whose disease is not too severe, the procedure is coordinated with repair of the cleft defect, sparing the child an additional general anesthetic.

Adenoidectomy in addition to myringotomy with PE tube placement is used to improve ET function and to reduce episodes of OM in normal children.[13] This is generally reserved for children who require multiple PE tube placement for chronic or recurrent disease. In cleft palate patients with recurrent or chronic otitis media, adenoidectomy does not relieve the problem.[14] The etiology of recurrent otitis media in CP is secondary to failure of ET opening. This is different from noncleft patients, where there is some component of decreased ET tube opening but there exist additional components of ET obstruction and reflux of infected material from the adenoids.

Adenoidectomy in children with cleft palate and submucous cleft palate is contraindicated because of the importance the adenoid pad plays in reducing velopharyngeal incompetence.[15] Another consideration in cleft patients is peritubal adenoidectomy, which removes peritubal tonsillar tissue only and leaves the adenoid pad undisturbed.[16] The procedure does little for ET function unless the tissue mass is large and obstructive. Peritubal adenoidectomy may reduce ET tube contamination from a chronically infected tubal tonsil without the consequences of adenoidectomy in the child with cleft or velopharyngeal inadequacy (VPI). The goal is to reduce the reflux of infected material from the tonsil up the ET and avoid contamination of the middle ear. However, the main etiology of ET dysfunction in CP is its failure to open. The efficacy of the procedure is not well documented.

Chronic otitis media implies tympanic membrane perforation, and this exists with or without cholesteatoma. The typical scenario is a patient with a history of eustachian type dysfunction who has a chronic draining ear and is subsequently found to have a tympanic membrane perforation. This is a surgical problem necessitating at least tympanoplasty if not tympanomastoidectomy. The patient is evaluated by physical examination of the ear looking for tympanic membrane perforation and squamous debris indicative of cholesteatoma. An audiogram is performed to assess the hearing and computed tomography (CT) of the temporal bone is performed to assess the anatomy and extent of the disease. The CT should be done with fine cuts (1 mm) in the axial and coronal planes. The CT provides information on the condition of the middle ear and surrounding structures, such as bone erosion, ossicular destruction, lateral semicircular canal dehiscence, facial nerve involvement, and spread of disease to the middle or posterior cranial fossae.

At this point the surgical treatment plan is designed, with the options, risks, and benefits discussed with the patient or family. The goals of treatment are eradication of disease, production of a safe ear, followed by conservation of hearing. Destruction of the ossicles occurs in multiple settings. Cholesteatoma formation and atelectasis were mentioned earlier, but, additionally, trauma can cause disruption of the ossicular chain. During cholesteatoma surgery, part of the incus, malleus, or stapes superstructure is frequently involved with disease, and eradication of disease necessitates removal of these bones.

Reconstruction of the middle ear can be performed immediately or delayed for 6 months, depending upon the extent of disease and the surgeon's ability to eradicate it. Reconstruction can take many forms. The patient's own ossicles can be reshaped and used as a strut to obtain continuity between the tympanic membrane, the stapes superstructure, or the stapes footplate. Reconstruction is highly dependent upon the condition of the ear as well as the remaining portions of the ossicular chain. In the case of massive cholesteatoma, the ossicles in totality may be completely eroded, leaving only the stapes footplate. In this setting, the operation is performed in two stages, with the first stage being designed for eradication of disease and the second stage performed 6 months later for reconstruction. The reconstruction can be performed from ossicular remnants that are autoclaved and banked in the mastoid cavity or from biocompatible materials.

Prostheses that contact the neotympanic membrane are generally made from hydroxyapatite. If there is only a stapes footplate remaining, a total ossicular reconstruction prosthesis (TORP) is placed. If the stapes superstructure is intact, a partial ossicular reconstruction prosthesis (PORP) is placed. Hearing results from these prostheses are frequently quite good and can return the patient's hearing to within 10 db of its maximum potential.

Congenital anomalies of the ear associated with craniofacial anomalies may be treated by auricular reconstruction or a prosthesis secured with endosseous implants. When auricular reconstruction is undertaken, the process begins at age 5. The external ear is reconstructed first and often multiple stages are required. The external auditory canal and middle ear structures are subsequently reconstructed. The external auditory canal is formed by drilling the mastoid bone and grafting it with a split-thickness skin graft. The tympanic membrane is constructed from temporalis fascia with preservation of the ossicular mass. Ossicular reconstruction may be necessary to provide continuity of the sound-conducting mechanism of the middle ear. In unilateral atresia, the option of middle ear reconstruction is usually delayed until the patient reaches an age at which he or she can decide whether the risk of inner ear and facial nerve injury as well as maintenance of a cavity is worthwhile. To potentially create a problem in a unilateral atresia in the form of facial paralysis, deafness, or a draining ear in a situation where no problem exists is best done in the setting where the patient can directly participate in the decision-making process.

CONCLUSIONS

The anatomy and pathophysiology of the eustachian tube, its relationship to craniofacial disorders, otitis media, middle ear disease, and hearing loss were presented. Early detection and intervention are the keys to the treatment of affected patients. Reconstitution of anatomy helps to restore the normal physiology of the region. This, coupled with intervention for recurrent otitis media and preservation of hearing, aids in appropriate speech and language development for children with these anomalies.

GLOSSARY

Atelectasis: Retraction and draping of the tympanic membrane over the ossicles. This is believed to occur as a result of chronic eustachian tube dysfunction resulting in long-standing negative pressure within the middle ear space. Cholesteatoma can form from pars flaccida retraction pocket formation or the ossicles can become eroded by the TM. Both can result in conductive hearing loss.

Cholesteatoma: A cystic mass lined with keratinizing squamous epithelium. It becomes filled with desquamated debris and enlarges within the mastoid and middle ear. It can be congenital (rare) or acquired. In the acquired form it arises either from squamous epithelium at the edge of a TM perforation in chronic otitis media that migrates into the middle ear space, or from a retraction pocket, which has a gradually narrowing orifice as it enlarges. This typically develops in the pars flaccida region of the tympanic membrane in an atelectatic or poorly ventilated ear.

Conductive Hearing Loss: Hearing loss secondary to disruption of the conductive mechanism of the middle ear, which includes the tympanic membrane and ossicles. The inner ear is normal. This can be acquired through a destructive process or can be congenital with fixation or absence of certain portions of the ossicular chain (i.e., congenital stapes footplate fixation).

Mixed loss: A combination of sensorineural and conductive hearing loss. This can be congenital, acquired, or both.

Myringoplasty: Tympanic membrane repair.

Scutum: Medial edge of the posterior canal wall of the external auditory canal at the level of the fibrous annulus of the tympanic membrane.

Sensorineural Hearing Loss: "Neural" hearing loss in which there is loss of function of the inner ear either congenitally or from destruction.

Tympanomastoidectomy: Tympanoplasty plus drilling of the mastoid bone.

Tympanoplasty: Surgical procedure that involves restoration of the conductive mechanism of the middle ear. This can include tympanic membrane repair as well as ossicular reconstruction.

Tympanosclerosis: A descriptive term identifying hard, dense connective tissue around the ossicles. This causes significant conductive hearing loss. This also describes white, firm plaques seen on the TM in patients with recurrent or chronic otitis media. There is typically no hearing loss as a result of the TM variety. These can be unrelated disorders.

References

1. Pillsbury HC, Grose JH, Hall JW: Otitis media with effusion in children: binaural hearing before and after corrective surgery. Arch Otolaryngol Head Neck Surg 1991; 117:718–723.

2. Paradise JL, Bluestone CD, Felder H: The universality of otitis media in fifty infants with cleft palate. Pediatrics 1969; 44:35.

3. Anonymous: Parameters for the evaluation and treatment of patients with cleft lip-palate or other craniofacial anomalies. Cleft Palate Craniofacial J 1993; 30(Suppl 1):S2–S12.

4. Barker G: Auditory tube function and changes following corrective orthognathic maxillary and mandibular surgery in cleft and non-cleft patients. Scand J Plast Reconstr Surg 1987; 21:113–138.

5. Matsune S, Sando I, Takahashi H: Insertion of the tensor veli palatini muscle into the eustachian tube cartilage in cleft palate cases. Ann Otol Rhinol Laryngol 1991; 100:439–446.

6. Gray H: Anatomy of the Human Body, 29th American ed (Goss CM, ed), p 1194. Philadelphia: Lea and Febiger, 1973.

7. Butow K-W, Louw B, Hugo SAR, Grimbeck RJ: Tensor veli palatini muscle tension sling for eustachian tube function in cleft palate. J Cranio-Max Fac Surg 1991; 19:71–76.

8. Doyle W, Reilly J, Jardini L, Rovnak S: Effect of palatoplasty on the function of the eustachian tube in children with cleft palate. Cleft Palate J 1986; 23:63–68.

9. Proctor B: Anatomy of the eustachian tube. Arch Otolaryngol 1973; 97:2–8.

10. Yamaguchi N, Sandu I, Takahashi H, et al: Histologic study of eustachian tube cartilage with and without congenital anomalies: A preliminary study. Ann Otol Rhinol Laryngol 1990; 99:984–987.

11. Ovesen T, Blegvad-Andesen O: Alteration in tympanic membrane appearance and middle ear function in 11 year old children with complete unilateral cleft lip and palate with healthy age matched subjects. Clin Otolaryngol 1992; 17:203–207.

12. Bergstrom L: Congenital and acquired deafness in clefting and craniofacial syndromes. Cleft Palate J 1978; 15:354–361.

13. Bluestone CD, Wittell RA, Paradise JL, Felder H: Eustachian tube function as related to adenoidectomy for otitis media. Trans Am Acad Ophthalmol Otolaryngol 1972; 76:1325–1339.

14. Severeid LR: A longitudinal study of the efficacy of adenoidectomy in children with cleft palate and secondary otitis media. Trans Am Acad Ophthalmol Otolaryngol 1972; 76:1319.

15. Gereau S, Shprintzen RJ: The role of adenoids in the development of normal speech following palate repair. Laryngoscope 1988; 98:299–303.

16. Drake AF, Fischer ND: Peritubal adenoidectomy. Laryngoscope 1993; 103:1291–1292.

Prosthodontic Management | 13

Michael R. Arcuri and William E. LaVelle

The patient with congenital facial clefting requires a multiple disciplinary team approach to care throughout life. A maxillofacial prosthesis may be used to restore deglutition, mastication, speech, and cosmesis. The prosthetic treatment will depend upon the coordinating efforts of numerous specialties including, but not limited to, surgeons, speech pathologists, orthodontists, psychologists, and prosthodontists. Prosthetic needs will vary with each patient from presurgical orthopedic appliances, speech aids, single tooth replacements, multiple tooth replacements, complete dentures with a speech aid and prosthetic replacement of missing facial units.

The ultimate goal of treatment for the patient with facial clefting is rehabilitation, with a modality of treatment that results in normal function and excellent cosmesis without the use of a removable prosthesis. This ideal is not always obtainable, regardless of the quality of care. Prosthetic treatment for cleft patients may be classified into three phases: (1) early treatment (birth to teens), (2) interim treatment (teens to adulthood), and (3) adult treatment (20s throughout life).

Presurgical orthopedic appliances designed to move maxillary segments into near normal positions are fabricated within the first 2 weeks postpartum. An impression is made with a nonridged material, such as irreversible hydrocolloid or rubber bases, to produce a cast on which a variety of appliances may be made.[1] The bottle appliance is constructed to be used while the patient suckles. The appliance is fabricated by applying relief on the cast, to create a space where the desired movement of the segment is to occur. The acrylic appliance thus produces movement through pressure being applied to the opposite side of the arch during feeding. The appliance will require readaption at 2 week intervals as the desired alignment takes place. Surgery is scheduled as normal arch alignment is achieved. The surgery can usually be scheduled at 3 months of age. The goal of the appliance is to enhance primary lip closure with less lip tension and to improve hard and soft tissue alignment. Since the bony structure is in a more normal position, a more definitive preliminary lip repair is possible; thus the need for secondary surgical procedures can be minimized (Fig. 13–1).[2, 3]

Appliances to assist in feeding may be constructed in a similar fashion. Fabricated in clear acrylic resin, the appliance covers the cleft of the alveolus and palate with a small extension posteriorly. This type of prosthesis, if used, may only be needed temporarily until normal feeding is stimulated. In general, feeding appliances are unnecessary with proper feeding instructions from the pediatric nurse or staff.[4] The necessity of a speech aid appliance is indicated as speech develops and surgery cannot be performed due to systemic problems, or if surgical dehiscence has occurred. A speech aid or speech bulb can only be constructed successfully if deciduous teeth have erupted and if the child is cooperative with placement of orthodontic bands and impressions. The earliest treatment can usually be accomplished is at 2½ to 3 years of age. Orthodontic bands with a single edgewise buccal tube are placed on the second deciduous molars, and an irreversible hydrocolloid impression is made. This appliance has three segments: the palatal section (clear acrylic resin) with .030 wrought wire clasp, the velar section, and the pharyngeal or bulb section. When the palatal section is finished, a wire loop is added for the velar section to act as a carrier for impression compound. The level of the speech bulb will be at the level of the palatal shelf or atlas, or approximately at the point of greatest muscle activity of the superior constrictor muscle, resulting in Passavant's pad or ridge. The impression for the speech bulb is formed by muscle movement during speech and head movements, and during deglutition. Once acceptable closure is achieved, mouth temperature impression wax (Iowa wax) is added for final adaptation. The impression is then processed in clear acrylic resin (Fig. 13–2). Speech therapy is then undertaken to achieve normal speech. The

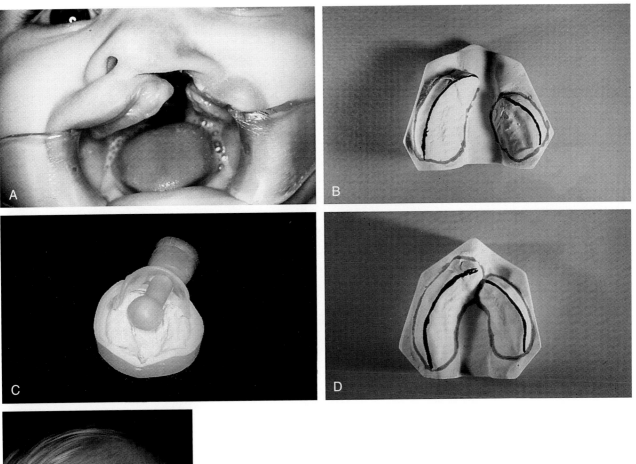

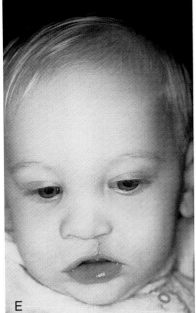

Figure 13–1. Orthopedic feeding appliance. *A,* Infant with cleft lip and palate. *B,* Initial cast of palate. Gray outlines alveolar ridges, black indicates ridge crest. *C,* Presurgical orthopedic feeding appliance on cast. *D,* Final cast showing position of alveolar ridges before lip closure. *E,* Infant after lip closure.

speech aid appliance, when properly fabricated and used in conjunction with a speech therapist, can enable the patient to produce normal speech. The speech aid will require revision periodically to compensate for growth or loss and eruption of teeth during the mixed dentition stage.

The interim stage of prosthetic treatment, during the teen years, may involve a speech aid if surgery cannot be performed, replacement of teeth, correcting the vertical dimension of occlusion, and preserving the arch position. Adolescence changes the needs of treatment from functional to cosmetic, as self-image becomes more important. The patient during this phase of treatment may be undergoing orthodontic treatment

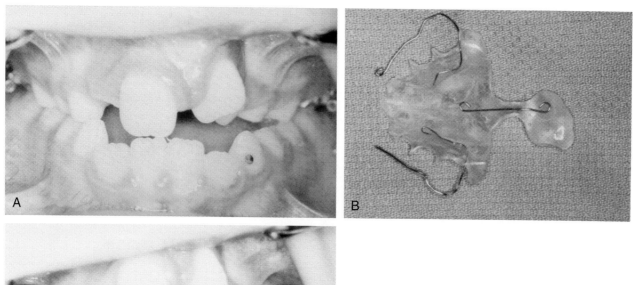

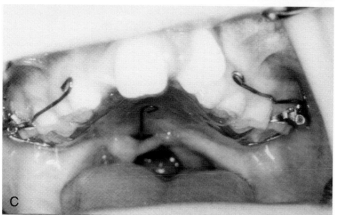

Figure 13–2. Pediatric speech aid. *A,* Cleft palate in a child with orthodontic bands containing edgewise buccal tubes on permanent first molars. *B,* Speech air prosthesis. *C,* Speech aid prosthesis in place.

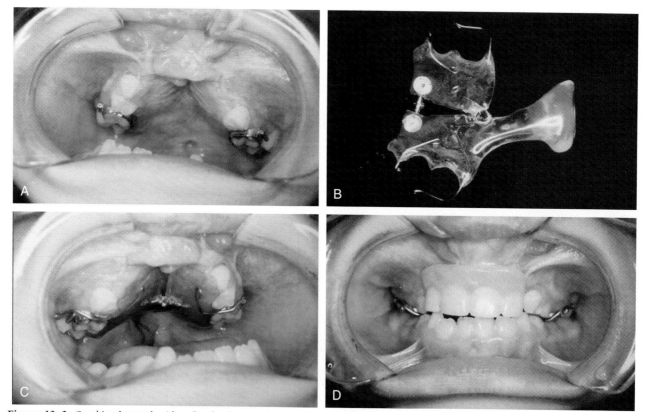

Figure 13–3. Combined speech aid and palatal expansion appliance. *A,* Repaired cleft palate. *B,* Speech aid with anterior jack screw and posterior hinge for expansion. *C,* Appliance in place. *D,* Appliance in place with acrylic resin teeth added to cosmetically enhance appearance.

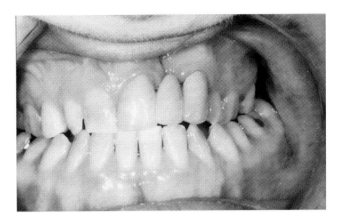

Figure 13–4. Fixed partial denture replacing tooth 10 over a cleft alveolus.

and possible secondary surgical revisions, and prosthodontics. Orthodontic needs, which include maxillary expansion with a speech aid appliance, will require close cooperation between the orthodontist and prosthodontist. The facial cleft patient desiring and needing orthodontic care to improve esthetics and function cannot go without the speech appliance. The combination of maxillary expansion and the speech aid can be fabricated to perform maxillary expansion and to incorporate the speech bulb (Fig. 13–3).[5] Interim partial dentures to replace missing teeth are constructed during this period to enhance cosmesis until a definitive fixed or removable partial, dentures, or implant prosthesis can be fabricated.

The adult phase of treatment, from the late teens throughout life, may consist of fixed or removable partial dentures, overdentures, complete dentures, and a speech aid. The ideal rehabilitation should result in decreasing the necessity of these prosthodontic replacements. The facial cleft patient completing orthodontic treatment may only need prosthodontic replacement of missing dentition, whether it be a single tooth or multiple teeth. The treatment of choice would be an implant-supported single tooth or a fixed

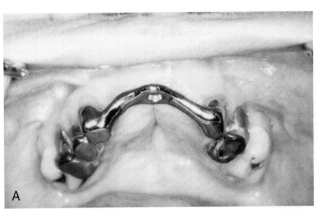

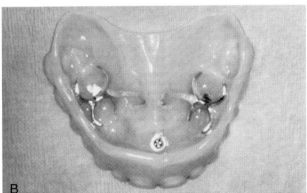

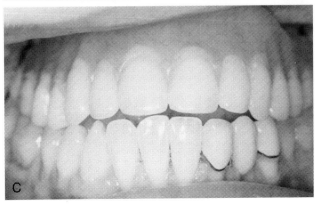

Figure 13–5. Repaired cleft palate and maxillary overdenture. *A,* Repaired cleft palate, with cast restorations on teeth connected by a tissue bar.[6] *B,* Overdenture with internal cast gold clasps and Ceka attachment. *C,* Overdenture in place.

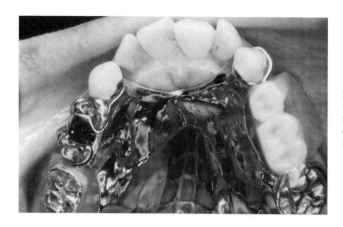

Figure 13–6. Partial denture soft palate obturator. Anterior retentive clasp placed into mesial buccal undercuts resist upward movement of the pharyngeal bulb. Posterior retentive clasps into distal buccal undercuts resist downward movements of the pharyngeal bulb.

partial denture. The prosthodontic rehabilitation is based on conventional prosthodontic principles of replacing missing teeth, arch stabilization and preservation of the remaining dentition. Fixed partial denture prosthesis may also be used to restore and enhance dental alveolar deficiencies that have not been successfully repaired surgically (Fig. 13–4). Maxillary overdentures with or without a speech bulb may be necessary in the adult cleft patient to restore vertical dimension of occlusion, functional mastication, and midface deficiency. The design of the overdenture prosthesis will vary with the severity of maxillary constriction and with quality and quantity of the supporting structures. The preservation of the natural dentition is of primary importance for this type of prosthetic rehabilitation (Fig. 13–5).[6]

Obturators that obtain their support, retention, and stability from the existing dental-alveolar structures may be used by the patient in excess of 15 hours per day. This frequency of use may cause significant damage to the supporting tissues. It is also not uncommon to encounter a patient who reports continuous use of their prosthesis, only removing it for daily cleaning. While in use, an obturator has a variety of forces placed upon it that are transmitted to associated hard and soft tissues. During deglutition the posterior tongue is elevated and may contact the velar portion of the prosthesis. This action places an upward force on the posterior extension of the prosthesis, causing it to rotate in a ''teeter-totter''-like fashion, about the most posterior tooth with which it is in contact. Anterior to this point of rotation, the prosthesis will move inferiorly. This downward movement is resisted by the placement of a retentive cast metal retention clasp anterior to the point of rotation. In a similar fashion, any downward force placed upon the velar extension, as from residual soft palate structure, would require a retention mechanism posterior to the point of rotation to resist this movement (Fig. 13–6). This persistent anterior-posterior movement of the prosthesis can develop into a traumatic cycle that results in chronic inflammation of the periodontal structures, leading to loss of associated alveolar bone and teeth.

To resist these potentially destructive forces, teeth used to retain and support an obturator are often treated with cast restorations. These restorations may involve two adjacent teeth that are splinted together, thus enhancing their ability to resist horizontal or vertical movements. The palatal aspects of these restorations may have parallel

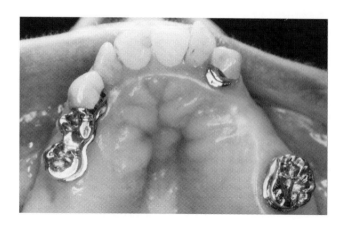

Figure 13–7. Ledge rest on cast restorations. Ledge rest provides support and indirect retention for the prosthesis shown in Figure 13–6.

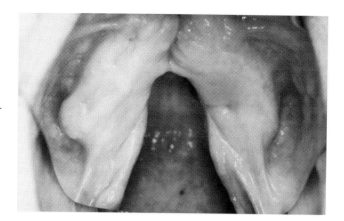

Figure 13–8. Unrepaired cleft palate in an edentulous 76-year-old.

guide planes and a ledge rest that enhance stability and retention (Fig. 13–7).[7] Cast restorations also enable the development of contours within the tooth for incorporation of the partial denture clasps, which are inconspicuous and placed into precisely developed undercuts for retention.

The framework for a removable partial denture (RPD) obturator is fabricated in acrylic resin, chrome, or gold alloy. The use of metal instead of acrylic resin allows the framework to remain thin (0.3 to 0.5 mm) with excellent physical properties and provide a more accurate fit to the tissues. This increase in accuracy provides increased stability and enhanced stress distributed to the teeth.

In the edentulous patient, forces applied to the velar and pharyngeal extensions are the same as with the dentate population. However, all support, retention, and stabilization must come from the residual alveolar mucosa and palatal structures (Fig. 13–8). Individuals who have undergone various surgical procedures for closure of pharyngeal, velar, palatal, and alveolar defects often present with significant amounts of scar tissue in these areas (Fig. 13–9). The presence of this less resilient tissue can make the fabrication of a retentive denture prosthesis difficult. Procedures used to close palatal and floor-of-nose defects may result in oral antral fistulas. These fistulas vary in size and number, and are often surrounded by dense fibrous scar tissue. Fistulae that remains after attempted repair of the floor of the nose may enter the oral cavity in the mucobuccal fold, be extremely small, and thus difficult to identify. The location and size of these defects in an area responsible for providing the peripheral denture seal may inhibit the fabrication of a retentive prosthesis and allow nasal leakage of air and fluids. The fistula must be sealed with the peripheral border of the prosthesis if the prosthesis is to remain in place without the use of adhesives.

The fabrication of a complete denture obturator is divided into two separate stages. First, the palatal portion of the prosthesis is fabricated similar to a conventional denture. The prosthesis is delivered to the patient and used for 2 to 3 weeks. During this time adjustments concerning fit, retention, and occlusion are made. Posterior tooth forms usually involve rational teeth (flat) to enhance prostheses stability and to aid in reducing undesirable lateral forces being applied to the prosthesis and underlying

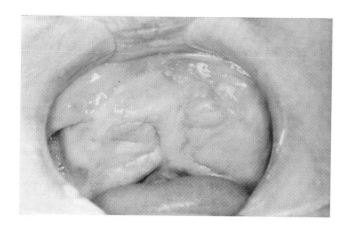

Figure 13–9. Edentulous repaired cleft palate.

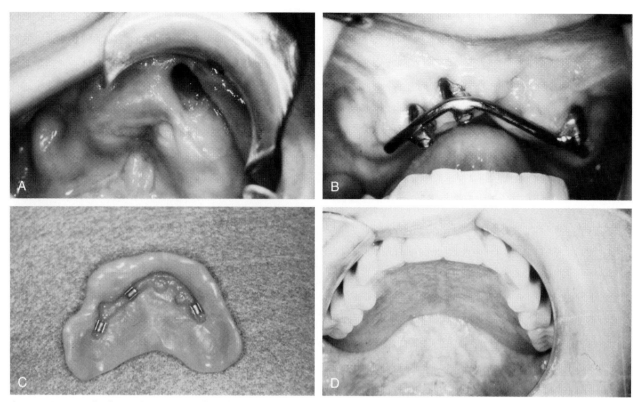

Figure 13–10. Palatal prosthesis retained with implant. *A,* Edentulous maxilla with anterior oral antral fistula. *B,* Retention bar connected to three titanium implants. *C,* Maxillary prosthesis with retention clips. *D,* Prosthesis intraorally retained by implant system.

alveolus. Once the patient is functioning adequately, the velar-pharyngeal portion is added with the aid of a speech pathologist. The impression for the speech bulb is the same as for the interim speech aid prosthesis.

The persistence and magnitude of the dislodging forces produced by soft tissues may make the successful use of a complete denture difficult if not impossible. The successful use of titanium interosseous screw–type implants for dental rehabilitation has led to their use in restoring cleft palate defects. Arcuri and associates reported the use of Nobelpharma self-tapping implants into residual maxillae and pterygoid plates of cleft palate patients, with 87% of the implants placed used to retain a palatal prosthesis.[8] The use of dental implants enables the development of retention systems that can provide adequate retentive forces to counter the dislodging forces of soft tissue (Fig. 13–10).

Hypoplastic horizontal and vertical growth of the maxilla is common with clefts of the palate. The horizontal component of this deficiency may result in a flattened midface, accompanied by unilateral or bilateral crossbites. Correction of these features may be accomplished through a combination of orthodontic and orthognathic surgical procedures. Vertical deficiencies are less apparent and may appear clinically insignificant. However, if severe they may result in deficient midface height, producing a pseudo "Andy Gump" appearance. This situation may be corrected with surgical management. With less significant vertical deficiencies, clinical signs may not be apparent; however, symptoms may exist. A decrease in vertical growth of the alveolar segments may result in an individual functioning at a decreased vertical dimension of occlusion (VDO). These patients may complain of facial fatigue during and/or following mastication, and/or headaches. Patients may also complain that their mouth appears collapsed or that their lips turn down at the commissures.

Correction of a discrepancy in vertical height inevitably leads to increasing the patient's vertical dimension of occlusion (VDO). Through speech assessment an approximation can be made of the amount of increase in the VDO the patient may tolerate. To verify the acceptance of any change in the VDO, occlusal splint therapy should be used.[9] If the patient uses the splints routinely for an 8 to 12 week period without complaints, then the probability that the individual could function at the new vertical provided by the splints is good (Fig. 13–11).

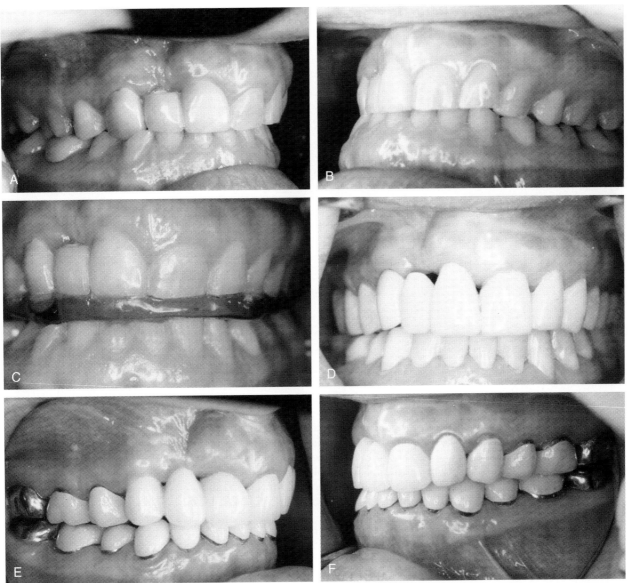

Figure 13–11. Repaired unilateral cleft lip and palate with insufficient vertical dimension of occlusion (VDO). *A* and *B*, Pre-treatment dentition. *C*, Interocclusal splint used to evaluate the patient response to an increase in the VDO. *D*, Provisional restorations made to the new VDO. *E* and *F*, Definitive restorations at the new VDO.

When a patient is partially edentulous in the anterior maxilla and an increase in the VDO is desired, then the use of an overdenture may suffice. The use of this type of restoration is easily fabricated, may produce excellent esthetic results, and is relatively inexpensive. In a more fully dentate patient, an overdenture may not be feasible. In these situations the placement of cast restorations on all teeth in the maxilla and mandible may be necessary (see Fig. 13–5).

With the advancement of surgical techniques, the enhancement or correction of facial malformations has greatly improved. Even large tissue defects can be reconstructed with the use of vascularized free tissue grafts. These vascularized grafts can produce impressive functional and esthetic results in restoring structures in the midface and intraoral regions. Unfortunately, even with these grafting techniques, not all tissue defects lend themselves to surgical reconstruction. Several craniofacial syndromes involve the development of the external ear.[10] Because of its complex anatomy, this structure is often difficult to reconstruct and position so that it corresponds to the contralateral ear. Even after several surgical revisions, the resulting structure may not resemble the desired anatomy and position. It is common for a patient to undergo numerous staged surgical procedures, extending over several years, and find that the

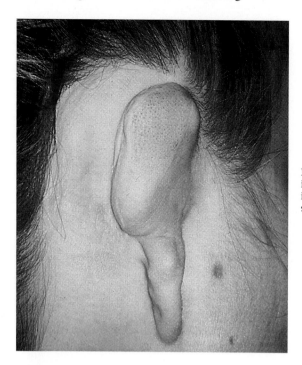

Figure 13–12. After multiple surgeries to reconstruct a congenitally missing ear, this is the disappointing result.

auricular structure is unacceptable (Fig. 13–12). An alternative to surgical auricular reconstruction is prosthetic replacement.

Advantages of prosthetics include little to no surgical intervention, little or no hospitalization, and less financial burden. The disadvantage of this therapy is the daily requirement to place, remove, and clean the prosthesis. In addition, the life span of a prosthesis may be as short as 24 to 36 months, and replacement may be required. Current fabrication techniques involve the use of acrylic resins and silicones that are colored by the incorporation of various pigments. Ultraviolet radiation from sunlight has a detrimental effect on acrylic resin, silicones, and pigments, reducing the life span of the prosthesis. A life style that involves excessive exposure to the sun may necessitate more frequent prosthesis replacement.

Historically, auricular prostheses have been retained by mechanical devices (headgear, eye glasses) or adhesives. The use of mechanical devices may detract from the

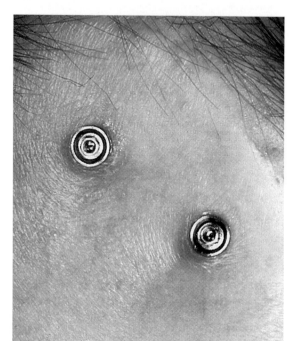

Figure 13–13. Titanium screw implant abutments penetrating skingrafted surface over the temporal bone.

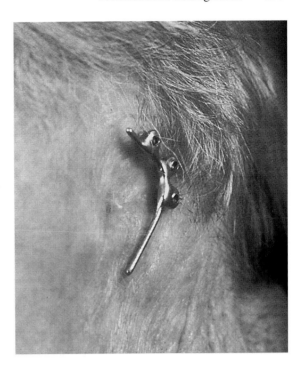

Figure 13–14. Retention bar connected to implant abutments for an auricular prosthesis. (Credit for bar, Dr. Robert Jons, University of Iowa.)

esthetic quality of the prosthesis. In addition, they are cumbersome and often difficult to position and maintain in the correct alignment. Adhesives are messy and may make positioning of the prosthesis difficult. They collect dust and oil, which may become difficult to remove from the prosthesis and cause skin irritations. Chronic rubbing of the prosthesis to remove adhesive during cleaning procedures increases the risk of damaging thin margins that aid in camouflaging the prosthetic junction with the skin.

One technique, developed from the intraoral use of titanium screw interosseous implants, has alleviated many of the problems previously encountered with mechanical or adhesive retention systems. This technique in auricular prosthetics involves the placement of an implant screw (fixture) into the temporal bone. The placement of the fixture is aided by a surgical guide developed from a diagnostic wax-up of the proposed prosthesis. After a 4- to 6-month healing period, the fixture is surgically

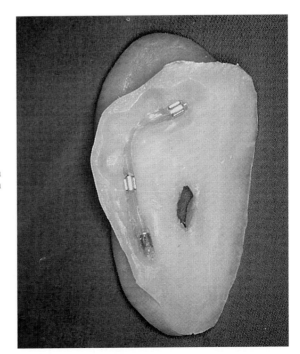

Figure 13–15. Clip retention system in auricular prosthesis that will attach to bar in Figure 13–14.

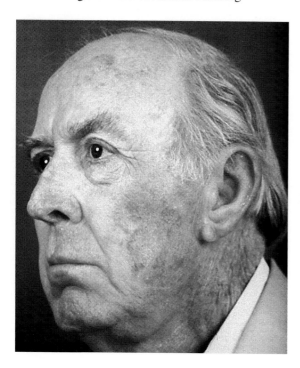

Figure 13–16. Implant retained auricular prosthesis in place. (Credit for prosthesis, Dr. Ann Fyler, University of Iowa.)

exposed and an abutment is attached. During the abutment placement procedure, the soft tissue surrounding the abutment is reduced in thickness or removed and replaced with a split-thickness skin graft. The purpose of this tissue reduction is to limit the amount of soft tissue movement (Fig. 13–13). Excessive soft tissue movement around transcutaneous implants has been associated with chronic soft tissue inflammation.

After the placement of the abutments, a retention mechanism that incorporates magnets or clips is developed (Fig. 13–14). The corresponding component to the retention system is placed within the prosthesis (Fig. 13–15). This type of retention system allows for greater retention while reducing the amount of tissue contact with the prosthesis (Fig. 13–16). Implant retention has reduced the need for adhesives, has simplified hygiene procedures, and has enhanced the retention and stability of the prostheses. Many patients who have undergone this treatment express increased confidence that their prostheses will remain in place even during athletic activities. In addition to their use in auricular prostheses, transcutaneous implants have also been used effectively in the prosthetic treatment of oculofacial and midface defects.

Regardless of age or stage of treatment, a patient suffering from facial clefting has a better prognosis for obtaining optimal esthetics and function if the treatment is directed by a team approach. Unilateral treatment, without evaluation and input by associated specialties, may no doubt result in an individual receiving acceptable treatment. However, the goal of treatment should not be to reach the realm of acceptability but to obtain the highest quality of care possible for our patients.

References

1. Rahn AO, Boucher LJ: Maxillofacial Prosthetics: Principles and Concepts, p 190. Philadelphia: WB Saunders, 1970.
2. McNeil CK: Orthodontic procedure in the treatment of congenital cleft palate. Dent Rec 1950; 70:126–132.
3. Salyer KE: Presurgical orthopedic treatment. *In* Surgical Techniques in Cleft Lip and Palate, pp 4–7. St. Louis, MO: Mosby Year Book, 1991.
4. Rogers BO: Facial Dysfigurement; A Rehabilitation Problem, p 83. Washington, DC: U.S. Department of Health Education and Welfare, Vocational Rehabilitation Administration, 1963.
5. LaVelle WE, Vandemark D: Construction of a maxillary orthopedic appliance to obtain simultaneous maxillary expansion and obturation. J Prosthet Dent 1976; 36:665–670.
6. LaVelle WE, Zach G: The tissue bar as an aid in cleft palate rehabilitation. J Prosthet Dent 1973; 30:321–325.

7. Henderson D, McGivney GP, Castleberry DJ: Ledges on abutment crowns. *In* McCracken's Removable Partial Prosthodontics, 7th ed, pp 265–269. St. Louis, MO: CV Mosby, 1985.
8. Arcuri MR, LaVelle WE, Higuchi KW, Svec BR: Implant-supported prosthesis for treatment of adults with cleft palate. J Prosthet Dent 1994; 71:375–378.
9. Tumer KA, Missirlian DM: Restoration of the extremely worn dentition. J Prosthet Dent 1990; 52:467–474.
10. McCarthy JG: Plastic Surgery: Volume 4. Cleft Lip and Palate and Craniofacial Anomalies, pp 2437–3174. Philadelphia: WB Saunders, 1990.

14

Early Considerations in the Orthodontic Management of Skeletodental Discrepancies

Per Rygh and Rolf S. Tindlund

CENTER: TEAMWORK

There has been consensus since the early 1950s that a multidisciplinary team within a center takes care of craniofacial anomalies. The success of the interaction between different specialties depends on the active coordination of the sequence and timing of the various aspects of treatment. It is vital that the team members have detailed insight into the different aspects of their collective treatment concept. The team must function as an organization with authority, under a general policy for the treatment of patients with a combination of certain disorders, to delegate the many tasks in a realistic and efficient manner. An optimal treatment result is dependent on the approach, the capacity, and the experience of the team. The following discussion is limited to the monitoring of patients with cleft lip and palate (CLP).

Overall Treatment Goals

The optimal goal of rehabilitation of a child with CLP is to enable the patient to grow up with potentials and possibilities equal to those of the child without clefts. Treatment ambitions and policies have changed since the 1950s. According to Bergland and associates,[1] three eras in the history of rehabilitation of CLP patients can be distinguished: (1) the prosthodontic, (2) the orthodontic/prosthodontic, and (3) the non-prosthodontic biologic. In general, the current goal is to eliminate the need for prosthetic intervention: tooth replacement and segmental stabilization. Any alveolar defect of magnitude sufficient to restrict orthodontic closure of the cleft space should be treated with bone graft.

Optimal function and *attractiveness* are key words. Breathing, sucking, swallowing, chewing, hearing, and speech are vital. Dentofacial appearance is a major component of the self-concept.[2-5] Children who are bullied, harassed, or rejected by family and peers may develop a negative and self-deprecating attitude. Early adolescence is a time of change and uncertainty and a period of special importance, because negative self-esteem in these years is likely to persist.[6,7] Therefore, early rehabilitation of the CLP child, preferably before start of school, should be a major goal.

Jaw Orthopedics and Orthodontics

Orthopedics/orthodontics has a place in the interdisciplinary management of skeletal discrepancies. In CLP patients, the treatment tasks are coordinated with those of several other participants: clinical specialists in plastic and craniofacial surgery, hearing, speech, pediatrics, and psychology.

The role of the orthodontist in the craniofacial team in treatment of patients with CLP mainly concerns deviations in the individual's long-term growth and development

---

Dedicated to Dr. Gunnar E. Johnson, Department of Plastic and Reconstructive Surgery, Haukeland sykehus, University Hospital of Bergen, Norway, the plastic surgeon who performed the primary surgery in all patients with cleft lip and palate by the same procedure from 1972 to 1986, including the patients shown in this chapter (except the patient in Fig. 14–23, who was born in 1968).

and is based on the ability to register, recognize, prevent, and treat dentofacial and, to some extent, craniofacial deformities. The orthodontist is usually responsible for

1. Supervision of growth and development of the jaws.
2. Collection of standardized records.
3. Dentofacial orthopedics.
4. A decision on the need for bone grafting.
5. Conventional orthodontics (straightening of the teeth).
6. Follow-up studies concerning growth and development.
7. Administration of nonorthodontic dental care.

(In Bergen, the orthodontist directs the coordination of the team efforts in patients over the age of 6 years.)

Documentation at regular intervals during the growth period by plaster models, photographs, standardized radiography, and cephalometry enables longitudinal studies of dentofacial growth and dysmorphology and comparison with standardized cephalometric normative growth studies. Such studies have contributed to a better understanding of postnatal growth and development of CLP patients. Limitations include the lack of consistent age-related documentation, the great variety of diagnostic and treatment methods, different ethnicity, the small size of samples, and limited access to intercenter comparison. There is a need for a standardized prospective investigation on homogeneous materials.[8,9] Randomized clinical trials are considered the optimal design for clinical research on multidimensional long-term outcomes of the primary surgery on CLP patients.[8,10,11] However, if current knowledge on different responses to orthodontic treatment in different facial types and growth patterns in CLP patients is disregarded, the results may be inaccurate and inconclusive.

Orthopedic/orthodontic management consists of restoring the morphologic forms of the jaws that are affected in abnormal development and thereby restoring function. Prevention or intervention, passive or active guidance, and modification of growth may involve the application of external force systems. Thus dentofacial appearance and good occlusion should be considered parallel goals of orthodontic treatment. Orthopedic/orthodontic intervention should occur at an appropriate time, not only to avoid psychological consequences, but also to influence growth processes in an optimal way.

Orthodontic/orthopedic treatment of dentofacial problems in the child without clefts depends on the nature of the normal biologic variation and the craniofacial type on which the developing malocclusion is superimposed. The ability to establish a diagnosis and time-optimal treatment intervention depends on the rationale for growth modification. Orthodontic stimulation, in contrast to restraint of growth of the craniofacial complex, necessitates differentiated timing; for example, the temporomandibular joint and the sutural system do not simultaneously react optimally to applied stress and strain. In the CLP child in whom pathogenesis with clefting is superimposed on the normal biologic variation, the ability to treat depends on (1) the nature of the craniofacial anomaly, (2) the postnatal deformities that have been imposed by the surgical closure of the cleft(s) and continue to be expressed as long as craniofacial growth continues, and (3) the original craniofacial type, as in non-CLP children.

Collaboration with the orthognathic surgeon has solved many problems for patients for whom, as experience has shown, heroic orthodontic treatment alone was not the optimal solution.

Dental care by preventive measures and caries control is often undertaken by the pediatric dentist collaborating with the orthodontist. The deciduous as well as the permanent teeth are important for normal function and as anchorage for orthopedic/orthodontic appliances. Emphasis should therefore be given to caries-preventive and conservative treatment measures.

GENERAL PRINCIPLES OF ORTHOPEDIC/ ORTHODONTIC TREATMENT

No universal orthodontic intervention or appliance can treat all forms of malocclusion. Even in non-CLP patients with malocclusions that appear very similar, the treatment responses to a particular appliance may vary. Orthodontic treatment planning is therefore based on an accurate diagnosis for the individual patient and on an understanding of biomechanics directly influenced by empiric knowledge and research. The potential of an appliance system depends on several factors, including the variable response of the patient.

These principles are also valid for CLP patients. Even if one plastic surgeon performs all the surgery by identical procedures and treatment protocol, the individual outcome may vary from excellent to rather poor. In Bergen, one plastic surgeon performed all primary surgery on all CLP patients from 1972 to 1986 (see the section on surgical procedures). On this basis it was assumed that the great variation in long-term treatment outcome resulted from different growth patterns related to (1) different clefting pathogeneses that caused different degrees of prenatal maxillary hypoplasia and (2) the individual hereditary craniofacial growth pattern.

Clinical considerations on whether, when, and how to treat CLP patients require an understanding of the variations of facial types, growth patterns, and associated malocclusions in the normal population as well as of facial growth trends, local dentoalveolar disturbances, and functional considerations in CLP patients. The interaction between craniofacial morphology and clefting warrants further consideration.

Normal Population: Craniofacial Types

There is evidence that different facial types are inherited and that the growth pattern is also influenced by factors outside the dentoalveolar system. In non-CLP patients, the different facial types and individual growth patterns are not readily changed by current orthopedic or surgical treatment procedures. Reports indicate that the original growth pattern continues after treatment intervention, which may contribute to relapse in the growing patient. This intrinsic growth pattern may be explained partly by craniofacial morphology and its associated postural position with the cervical column.[12, 13] Persons with a wide angle between the cranium and the cervical column were characterized on average by a large anterior facial height, maxillary and mandibular retrognathism, and an increased angle between the mandibular plane and the palatal and anterior cranial base planes.

Relationship Between the Cranial Base and the Facial Skeleton

The interdependence of the facial skeleton and the cranial base is reflected in the angle NSBa between the nasion–sella turcica (NSL) line and the basion (mean value, 130°). If the cranial base angle is acute, the entire face is positioned anteriorly (Fig. 14–1A). If the cranial angle is obtuse, the face is positioned more posteriorly (Fig. 14–1C). By using metallic implants as stable landmarks in conjunction with lateral and anteroposterior cephalometry, Björk[14, 15] and Björk and Skieller[16] demonstrated with longitudinal studies that changes occurred in the individual during growth, but the pattern of growth was maintained. Solow[17] also studied the pattern of craniofacial associations by using cephalometry, based on defined reference points and lines (Fig. 14–2A,B,C), which is important for orthodontic considerations concerning individual diagnosis and treatment planning as well as follow-up studies.

The individual craniofacial complex in profile (see Figs. 14–1A,B,C; 14–2A,B,C) can be classified by

1. Facial type (angles sella–nasion–A point [SNA], sella–nasion–B point [SNB]).
2. Sagittal-basal maxillomandibular jaw relationship (angle ANB).
3. Vertical-basal inclination of the maxillary palatal plane and mandibular plane to the cranial base (angles NSL-NL, NSL-ML).

Facial type represents the relationship between the cranial base and the sagittal position of the maxilla and mandible (the degree of prognathism), which indicates how far forward the facial complex is situated under the cranium, as expressed by angles SNA and SNB. It may be classified as prognathic, orthognathic, or retrognathic:[18]

Facial Type	Maxilla	Mandible
Prognathic	SNA > 85°	SNB > 83°
Orthognathic	79° ≤ SNA ≤ 85° (mean, 82°)	77° ≤ SNB ≤ 83° (mean, 80°)
Retrognathic	SNA < 79°	SNB < 77°

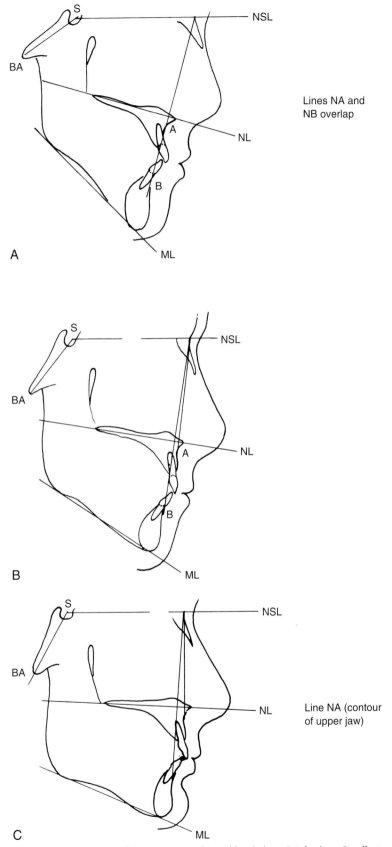

Figure 14–1. Craniofacial types in profile. *A*, Prognathic; *B*, orthognathic; *C*, retrognathic. *Abbreviations: BA*, basion; *S*, sella turcica; *A*, subspinale (point A); *B*, supramentale (point B); *NSL*, line through sella and nasion; *NL*, nasal line; *ML*, mandibular line.

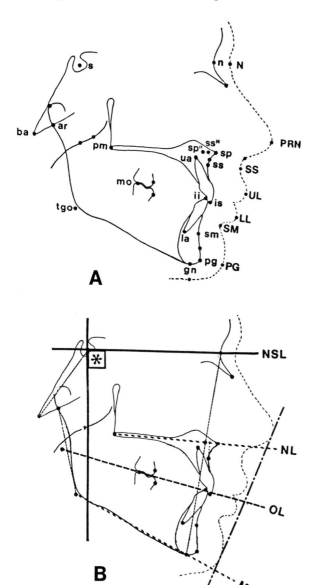

Cephalometry:	Description of Variables	Variables in Case Reports
Sagittal basal jaw relations:	s-n-ss° s-n-sm° ss-n-sm° s-n-pg° n-s-ba°	SNA° SNB° ANB° SNPg° NSBa°
Vertical basal jaw inclinations:	n.s-pm.sp° n.s-mo.(is.ii)° n.s-tgo.gn° pm.sp-tgo.gn°	NSL-NL° NSL-OL° NSL-ML° NL-ML°
Mandibular angle:	gn-tgo-ar°	Gonial°
Maximal length:	pm-ss projected to NL-line	pm-ss″(mm)
Facial heights:	Upper face height Lower face height	n-sp″ (mm) sp″-gn (mm)
Incisors* Inclinations:	ua.is-ii.la° ua.is-n.ss°* la.ii-n.sm°*	Inter: 1-1° Max: 1-NA°* Mand: 1-NB°*
Soft tissue relations:	Soft."ANB"° UL.PG-n.sm° UL-PRN.PG LL-PRN.PG	SS-N-SM° H-angle° UL-EL (mm) LL-EL (mm)

*Permanent incisors, including the unerupted incisors, are registered in measurements and cephalometric tracings. The incision points (is and ii) indicate the degree of eruption.

C

Figure 14–2. Cephalometric evaluation. *A,* Reference points; *B,* reference lines; *C,* variables used in case reports. For explanation of abbreviations, see text.

The anteroposterior jaw length is often shorter in the retrognathic face than in the prognathic face. The prognathism may be harmonious for both jaws or, if of different degrees in the upper and lower portions of the face, may represent a sagittal-basal jaw discrepancy.

Sagittal-basal maxillomandibular jaw relationship is the difference in prognathism of the jaws (angle ANB) (see Fig. 14–1). The sagittal-basal jaw relationship expressed by angle ANB (mean, 2°) may be classified according to Hasund's categories:[18]

Neutral basal jaw relationship: $0° \leq ANB \leq 4°$
Distal basal jaw relationship: $ANB > 4°$
Mesial basal jaw relationship: $ANB < 0°$

A neutral (normal) relationship indicates that the jaws protrude equally under the cranium (Fig.14–3A); a distal (postnormal) relationship means that the lower jaw is smaller than or situated posteriorly in relation to the base of the upper jaw (see Fig. 14–3B); a mesial (prenormal) relationship means that the lower jaw is larger than or situated anteriorly to the base of the upper jaw (see Fig. 14–3C). The mandible is defined as the variable.

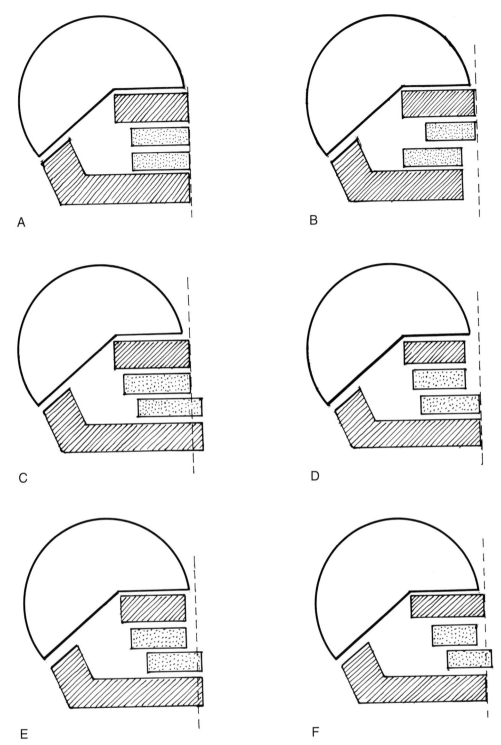

Figure 14–3. Jaw relationships. *A,* Neutral basal; *B,* distal basal; *C,* mesial basal; *C, D, E, F,* combinations resulting in anterior crossbite.

In these combinations of basal jaw relationship, the dentition and the supporting alveolus (dentoalveolar system) may be situated neutrally, anteriorly (protrusion or proclined incisors), or posteriorly (retrusion or retroclined incisors), accentuating or compensating for a basal discrepancy between the jaws. The value of the ANB angle in determining sagittal relationships is influenced by vertical facial height and the position of the incisors.

Vertical-basal inclination of maxillary palatal plane and mandibular plane to the cranial base (see Fig. 14–1) is the vertical relationship between the anterior cranial base and (1) the upper jaw, represented by the palatal plane or nasal line (NL) and assessed by angle NSL-NL (mean, 8.5°), and (2) the lower jaw, represented by the mandibular plane or line (ML) and assessed by angle NSL-ML (mean, 32°). These angles of maxillomandibular inclination are included in evaluating facial growth rotation.[15] Low values indicate a counterclockwise (anterior) rotation of the jaws, whereas high values indicate a clockwise (posterior) rotation of the mandibular base. The vertical-basal jaw relationship is represented by angle NL-ML (mean, 23.5°). High values may indicate a skeletal open configuration, and low values, in which the planes may be almost parallel, indicate a skeletal deep-bite configuration. The vertical jaw relationship should also be interpreted by linear measures with the facial index (n-sp″/sp″-gn × 100) of the anterior upper and lower facial heights. Prognathic faces reveal low to moderate anterior and high posterior facial heights (see Fig. 14–1A), whereas retrognathic faces reveal high anterior and low posterior facial heights (see Fig. 14–1C).

It is essential that standardized mean cephalometric values indicating an orthognathic face should not necessarily be used as the norm for the individual patient, because of biologic variation. Each facial pattern is typified by selected normative values.[18, 19] Thus, a retrognathic face may be associated with higher angular values of jaw inclination, whereas the prognathic face may be associated with lower values.

Facial Types and Growth Patterns

Prognathic faces (see Fig. 14–1A) are often associated with an anteriorly directed growth pattern and retrognathic faces (see Fig. 14–1C) with a posteriorly directed growth pattern.[15] Analysis of growth of the maxillomandibular complex may be complicated by remodeling occurring particularly at the nasal floor and at the lower margin of the mandible. Counterclockwise (anterior) growth rotation may be characterized by an apparent lowering of the posterior parts of maxilla and the mandible. Björk reported that anterior growth rotation of the mandible (Fig. 14–4A) is characterized by (1) upward and forward development of the condyles; (2) a curved canalis mandibularis; (3) an acute gonial angle; (4) convexity of lower border of the mandible, like a rocking chair; (5) an increased interincisal angle; (6) thicker cortical symphysial bone; (7) distally directed axes of the molars directed; and (8) reduced anterior lower face height (distance from nasal spine to gnathion). Posterior growth rotation of the mandible is characterized by the opposite features (see Fig. 14–4B).

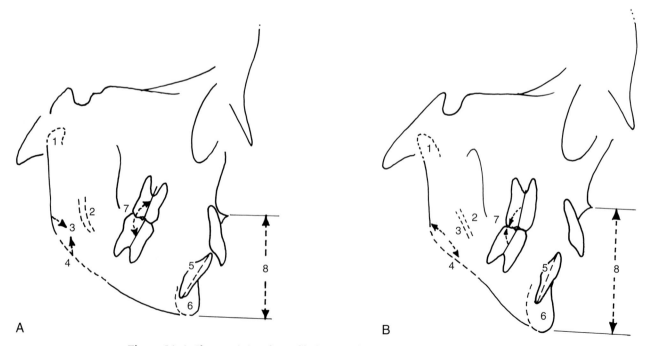

A   B

Figure 14–4. Characteristics of mandibular growth patterns. A, Anterior; B, posterior.

Dental Occlusion

The occlusion represents the relationship between the upper and lower dental arches and is commonly described in relation to the sagittal, vertical, and transverse dimensions:

Sagittal (Classification after Angle[20]):
Molar relationship: Angle class I occlusion (normal or neutral)
Angle class II occlusion (postnormal or distal)
Angle class III occlusion (prenormal or mesial)
Incisor relationship: Normal overjet (2 to 3 mm), increased overjet, or anterior crossbite
Vertical: Posterior and incisor segments: normal overbite (2 to 3 mm), deep bite, open bite
Transverse: Posterior relationship: normal or posterior crossbite(s): lingual or buccal
Incisal segment: midline deviation, dental axis inclination
Dental arch form, dental space or crowding conditions, symmetry

Growth Timing

The velocity of growth is characterized by developmental and individual variation. This may be considered during the infantile, juvenile, pubertal, and postpubertal periods on the basis of mean annual increments.[21] During the infantile period, the differential growth rates in boys and girls are similar but decline until the third year. During the juvenile period, the growth declines until during the prepubertal minimum until the pubertal growth spurt occurs at ages 11 to 13 years in girls and 13 to 14 years in boys. Somatic growth and craniofacial growth are related, and mandibular growth stabilizes at approximately 15 to 16 years in girls and 18 to 19 years in boys. Condylar growth occurs during the pubertal growth spurt, which is considered an optimal time for functional appliance therapy to modify and redirect growth.

Therapeutic alterations of the circummaxillary sutural systems should be considered earlier, preferably at ages 6 to 8 years. The rationale for earlier intervention in the maxillary complex is the responsive nature of the sutures during this period. By the time of the pubertal growth spurt, the development of the interdigitated maxillary sutural systems is resistant to orthopedic changes.[22,23]

Functional aspects, including nasal airflow resistance, are thought to be associated with facial growth. In non-CLP children with large adenoids and impeded nasal airflow, a narrow maxillary arch and high incidence of crossbite may be associated with an increased anterior facial height, reduced size of the nasopharynx, and a narrow alar base to the nose, with lowered tongue position and retroclination of upper and lower incisors. Linder-Aronson[24] reported that after adenoidectomy there was an increase in nasal airflow with continued growth of the mandible, which on average, revealed greater anterior rotation than in the control group and a reduction of the lower facial height. The characteristic non-CLP mouth-breather's face shows many similarities to the typical CLP appearance.[25] Early interceptive treatment enabling growth and development to take place under more normal functional impulses may reduce the severity of growth disorders.

Malocclusion

Overjet, overbite, and postnormal occlusion (Angle class II) are found in about 12% to 15% of Scandinavian non-CLP children,[26, 27] whereas negative overjet (anterior crossbite) is found in about 3% to 7%, often combined with lack of space in the maxillary arch. Anterior open bite is seen in about 2% to 4% of the children, and posterior crossbite in 6% to 9%.[28, 29]

Anterior and lateral crossbites in the family anamnesis are of particular interest with regard to CLP because maxillary deficiency in the sagittal, transverse, and vertical dimensions is common in CLP patients. This deficiency results in a growth pattern that contributes to the dental malocclusion, leading to anterior and often posterior crossbites. Figure 14–3C,D,E,F shows various dentoskeletal combinations that result in anterior crossbite: Figure 14–3C shows mandibular excess and anterior positioning in relation to the cranial base, resulting in dentoalveolar malocclusion. In Figure 14–3D, the mandible is of normal size and position in relation to the cranial base, but the maxillary skeletal pattern and dentition are situated posteriorly (retruded) in relation to the cranial base. In Figure 14–3*E*, skeletal maxillary deficiency is combined with mandibular skeletal excess. Figure 14–3*F* demonstrates upper dentoalveolar retrusion combined with lower dentoalveolar protrusion on normal jaw bases.

Anterior crossbite malocclusion may be found in all skeletal patterns and facial types (prognathic, orthognathic, and retrognathic); in different sagittal skeletal jaw configurations, mainly prenormal and normal; in deep or open vertical skeletal configurations; and in association with varying degrees of hypoplasia and hyperplasia of the jaws.[30,31] Furthermore, inherently different growth potentials may affect treatment responses related to age and function. Guyer and colleagues[31] showed that non-CLP class III patients at age 10 years represented a variety of combinations; maxillary skeletal retrusion was present in almost two thirds of the children. This is of clinical interest because orthopedic treatment seems more effective on the maxillary suture system than in restraining mandibular growth.[25,32–37] However, it is difficult to accurately predict the amount of mandibular excess, maxillary retrusion, and dentoalveolar discrepancies before puberty.[31,38–42]

GENERAL PRINCIPLES OF ORTHODONTIC TREATMENT FOR CLP PATIENTS

Orthodontic monitoring of CLP patients lasts from birth to adulthood, when growth is completed. The treatment program, however should consist of defined periods of active treatment rather than continuous ongoing treatment. The patient's cooperation should be conserved for active treatment; cost-benefit assessments support this policy. Early intervention should have a clear interceptive goal: to take advantage of the ages optimal for restoring and correcting morphology and function. Consistent treatment of patients with moderate skeletal discrepancies can yield stable results (Fig. 14–5).

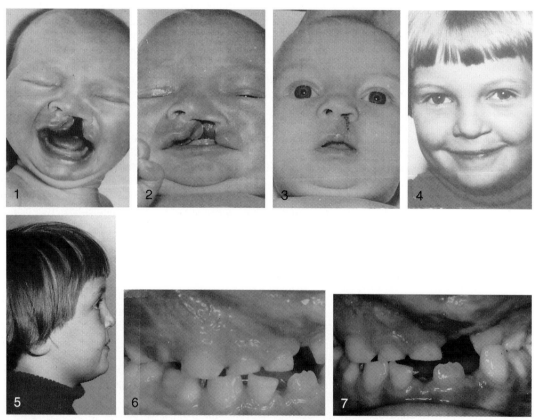

Figure 14–5. Complete UCLP, category 2A. *1, 2,* At birth, April 1971. *3,* Lip closure at age 3 months. *4 to 7,* At 6 years, moderate anterior and unilateral posterior crossbites with a tendency for concave profile. *8 to 16,* Interceptive orthopedics from age 6, for 8 years, including transverse expansion (3 months) followed by protraction (6 months) to alleviate spontaneous eruption of upper permanent incisors into normal position; retention by fixed palatal arch wire. *17 to 22,* Conventional orthodontics from age 12.5 years of 18 months' duration; adjustments for 3 months at age 18 retained by bonded retainers. *23 to 25,* X-rays at age 15 years.

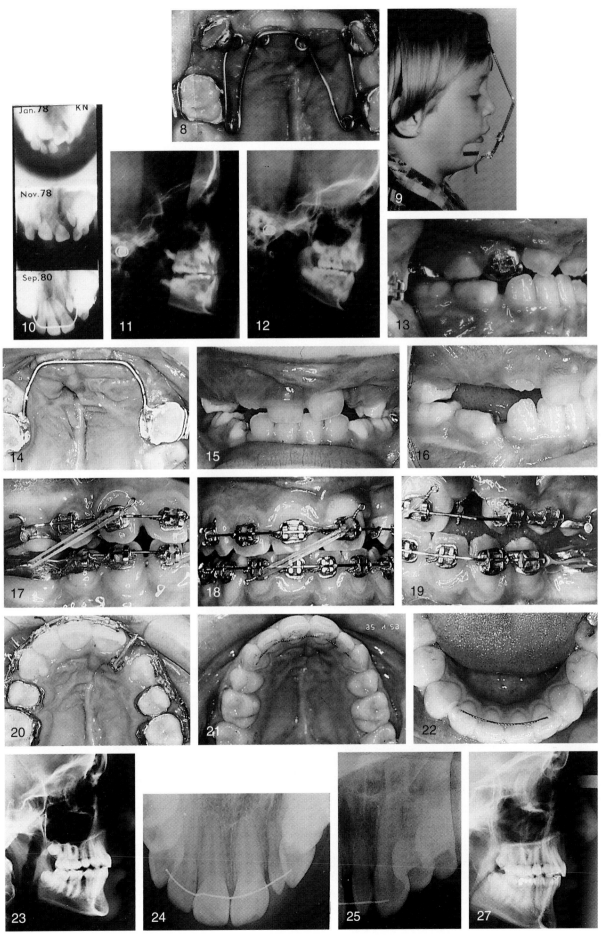

Figure 14–5 *Continued. See legend on opposite page.*

Illustration continued on following page

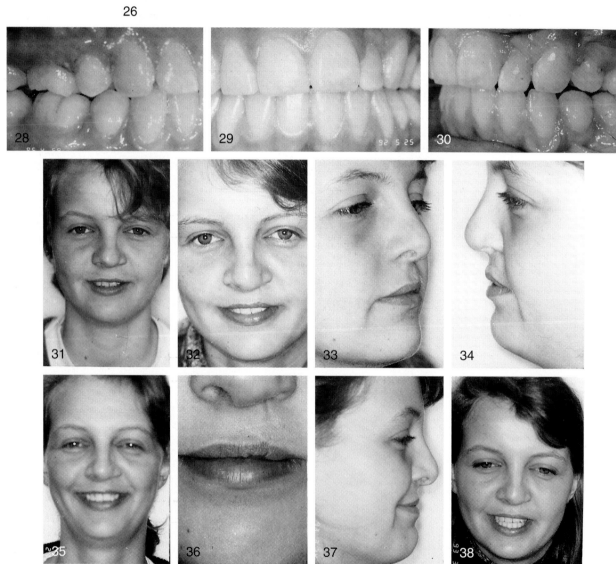

N.K.	6 years	15 years
SNA°	71.5	70.5
SNB°	72.0	71.0
ANB°	−0.5	−0.5
SNPg°	72.0	73.0
NSBa°	130.0	130.0
NSL-NL°	5.0	7.5
NSL-OL°	19.5	16.5
NSL-ML°	31.0	32.0
NL-ML°	26.0	30.0
Gonial°	112.0	115.5
pm-ss″ (mm)	39.0	43.5
n-sp″ (mm)	38.5	43.5
sp″-gn (mm)	54.0	63.0
1-1°	175.5	135.0
1-NA°	−4.5	29.0
1-NB°	9.5	16.5
SS-N-SM°	2.5	3.0
H-angle°	7.0	4.0
UL-EL (mm)	2.2	4.0
LL-EL (mm)	−0.5	2.5

770426 ———
860426 – – –

26

Figure 14–5 *Continued. 26,* Cephalometric analysis at ages 6 and 15 years. *27* to *30,* Dental occlusion at age 21 years. *31* to *38,* Facial development from ages 15 to 22 years.

The aim of orthopedic treatment is to improve the relationship of the jaw bases by relieving the upper jaw of restraining forces resulting from occlusal dysfunction by using active orthopedic/orthodontic forces to influence the amount and direction of growth and development of the facial components. A normal occlusal relationship with intercuspidation is a primary goal of treatment.

Orthopedic/orthodontic treatment of skeletal discrepancies is possible only during active growth. However, the treatment outcome depends on individual craniofacial characteristics and on the severity of primary and secondary problems related to clefting. The individual growth pattern influences the treatment objectives for each patient. Patients with maxillary clefts and retrognathic faces with an increased vertical lower facial height (high-angle cases) have sagittal discrepancies that may be more difficult to treat than those in patients with predominantly sagittal prognathic or orthognathic faces. In patients with sagittal mandibular prognathism, rotation of the mandible to a more downward, posteriorly directed posture may yield acceptable results in prognathic and orthognathic faces, but it is contraindicated in a retrognathic convex facial profile with an increased anterior facial height.

Within the policy of a scheduled CLP treatment program, the status of the individual patient at any time depends on the previous nonactive or active intervention. This is the basis for planning treatment objectives in the interactive team management, and a checklist is generated at different ages and stages in development. In general, this checklist may call for a set of different orthodontic treatment phases, each with a distinct beginning and end, in order to meet defined objectives and not to overburden the patient's cooperation (Fig. 14–6).

Bergen Treatment Protocols

Two CLP teams have been established in Norway since the 1950s: one in Oslo and one in Bergen, serving a population of 4.2 million. The treatment costs and travel expenditures are covered by the government social security program.

The Bergen Cleft Palate–Craniofacial Team treats patients from the western and northern parts of Norway; travel distances are up to 2000 km. Practical procedures are coordinated by the Department of Plastic and Reconstructive Surgery and the Department of Ear-Nose-Throat, University Hospital of Bergen (Haukeland); the Department of Orthodontics and Facial Orthopedics, Dental Faculty, University of Bergen; and the Eikelund Center for Speech Pathology.

To illustrate considerations of orthodontic management, several case reports from infancy to adulthood are presented. Final treatment evaluations are delayed until the end of growth: for girls, at age 15 years, and for boys, at age 18 years. The interaction between surgery and orthopedics/orthodontics is shown in Figure 14–6; however, this is only part of the multidisciplinary team context in which patients are treatment planned.

Neonatal Period

All Norwegian children born with facial clefts are registered with the National Birth Register. Infants born with complete clefts of the lip and palate are seen at the University hospital shortly after birth, preferably within 1 week. The need for presurgical maxillary orthopedics is decided at the first visit. These infants, as well as those with only cleft lip (CL) or isolated cleft palate (CP) are invited to a monthly full-day counseling session at Haukeland Hospital. All CLP team members participate.

Counseling for Parents

It is vital that professional counseling and care of parents and family be implemented soon after the birth. The parents should be informed that the rehabilitation program will ensure that their baby's esthetics, functional concerns, and expectations may nearly equal those of a child without a cleft. Many parents need time to accept the new situation and have instruction and information on immediate needs such as feeding. They should not be overwhelmed with excessively detailed information during the first few days, and well-illustrated informational material on short- and long-term treatment results from CLP patients is available.

Checklist Concerning Administration of Cleft Lip and Palate Patients,
Bergen Cleft Palate—Craniofacial Center, University of Bergen, Norway

Age	Duration	Orthodontics	Plastic Surgery
After birth		? Presurgical orthopedics for a few patients with wide clefts or asymmetry of jaw segments	
3 months			Closure of lip and anterior palate BCLP at 5-week interval (Millard technique)
12 months			Closure of soft palate (von Langenbeck technique)
4 years		Control	BCLP: Sulcus-plasty, columella-plasty
6 years		Clinical CLP Conference days: 1. The complete team diagnoses all patients of this age group 2. Team assembly discusses all individual treatment plans 3. Individual letters of treatment plan to all patients	
6–7 years	1 year	? Dentofacial orthopedics? 1. Transverse expansion 2. Anterior protraction 3. Fixed retention	
7–9 years	½ year	? Alignment of upper incisors	
10 years		Control	Secondary bone grafting?
11–13 years	1½ years	Conventional orthodontic treatment	
13 years		Fixed retention of upper jaw?	
15 years		Clinical CLP Conference days: same procedures as at 6 years	
15–16 years			Adjustment: lip and nose?
18–19 years		? Dental adjustments? Preprosthetic orthodontics (bridgework, implants) Presurgical orthodontics	Adjustment: lip and nose? Orthognathic surgery?

Figure 14–6. Overview of interaction between orthodontics and plastic surgery.

Team Evaluation Documentation

The Children's Department of Haukeland Hospital administers the registration of anamnestic and clinical data, as well as evaluation by a pediatric geneticist, to rule out any possible association with other syndromic conditions. A pediatrician also checks the patient's fitness for primary surgical intervention and other risky procedures.

A thorough clinical evaluation of the topographic anatomy of the cleft, plaster models of the cleft area (including the nose), and photographic registration should provide the basis of the documentation of the patient. Additional information may be supplemented during all future team evaluations and treatment by the different team members.

OPTIONAL ORTHOPEDIC/ORTHODONTIC INTERVENTION PERIODS

The timing and sequencing of orthodontic treatment is an essential component of team management. The orthopedic/orthodontic treatment program of the Bergen CLP team (see Fig. 14–6) has been based on periods of active focused treatment followed by intervals of observation and fixed retention, as recommended by the American Cleft Palate–Craniofacial Association (ACPA).[43] Because of the wide range of severity of malocclusions in CLP patients, it is very important to determine the treatment objectives for each individual case. The following treatment options may be regarded as an individual checklist:

1. Presurgical neonatal maxillary orthopedics.
2. Orthodontic considerations in growth developments.
3. Interceptive orthopedics in the late primary/early mixed dentition: transverse expansion and protraction.
4. Alignment of maxillary incisors.
5. Secondary bone grafting of the cleft alveolar process.
6. Conventional orthodontics in the permanent dentition.
7. Adjunctive orthodontics related to prosthodontics or orthognathic surgery (17 to 19 years).

Presurgical Neonatal Maxillary Orthopedics

Presurgical orthopedic treatment is undertaken to assist the surgeon in repairing the lip and the anterior part of the alveolar process, by providing better anatomic orientation of maxillary segments in order to allow closure with less strain to the tissue. Burston[2] pioneered and introduced neonatal maxillary orthopedics in the 1950s, and many teams adopted the method.

In patients with complete bilateral cleft lip and palate (BCLP), the forward-displaced anterior premaxillary segment was brought back into the arch after the medially placed posterior segments had been expanded to provide space into which the premaxillary segment could be repositioned. Similarly, severe asymmetries in patients with complete unilateral cleft lip and palate (UCLP) were treated by aligning the laterally placed greater segment on the noncleft side while expanding the palatally placed lesser segment on the side of the cleft. This aligning of the segments provided the surgeon with a simpler primary surgical repair of the cleft lip while supporting the alar base on the affected side.

In Bergen the use of presurgical orthopedics is recommended in selected cases, and strapping for retrusion of the protruded premaxilla in BCLP is not done. The need for presurgical orthopedics is determined by the plastic surgeon and orthodontist, and this treatment starts as soon as possible after birth until the primary lip closure. Figure 14–7 shows a UCLP patient who benefited from such treatment because of the wide cleft. The rationale for recommending maxillary orthopedics includes the following aims:

• Reposition the severely displaced maxillary segments.
• Reduction in width of wide clefts.
• Improved symmetry of nose and cleft maxilla.

Primary Surgical Repair

Surgery is performed at the Department of Plastic and Reconstructive Surgery, University Hospital of Bergen. Since 1986, the following protocols have been established: The cleft lip and the cleft area of the hard palate are closed when the child is approximately 3 months old, if the child is in good general health and has a body weight of 4 to 5 kg (see Fig. 14–6). A Millard procedure is used for the lip closure, combined with a single-layer vomerplasty for the closure of the anterior part of the palate. In patients with BCLP, the clefts are closed in two stages with an interval of approximately 5 weeks. The bony clefts of the dentoalveolar process are left open until 8 to 11 years of age, when alveolar bone grafts are recommended. The soft palate and isolated palatal clefts are closed at 12 months of age by the von Langenbeck technique.

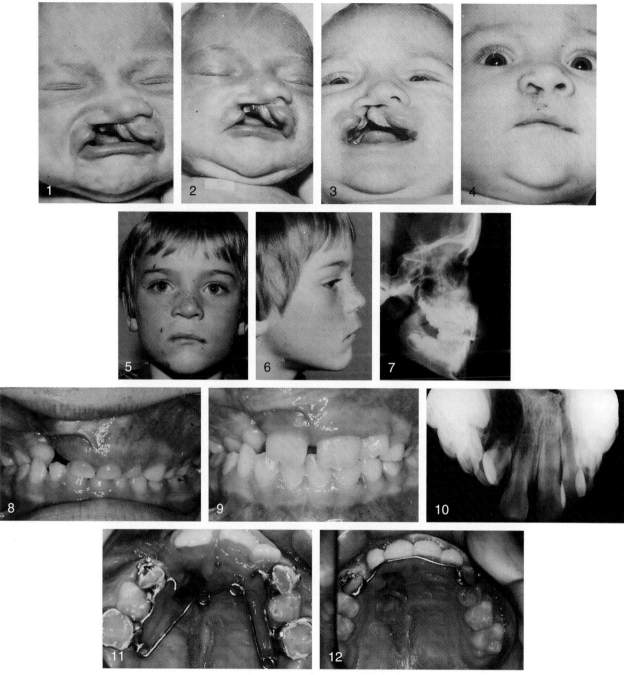

Figure 14–7. Complete UCLP, category 1. *1*, At birth, August 1973. *2, 3,* After presurgical orthopedics. *4,* Lip closure at age 3 months. *5* to *8*, At age 6 years, favorable sagittal development, unilateral crossbite. *9* to *12*, Transverse expansion at age 8 years, followed by fixed retention.

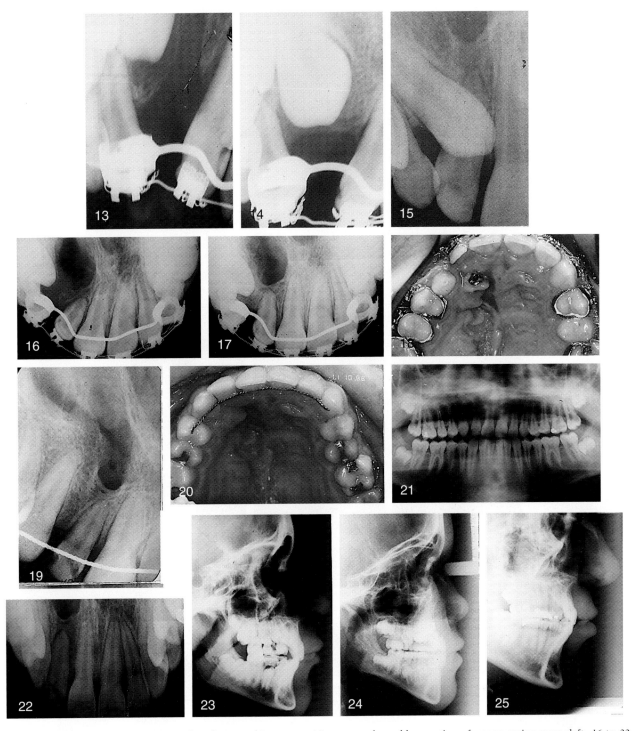

Figure 14–7 *Continued. 13* to *15,* Secondary bone grafting at age 10 years; unfavorable eruption of upper canine near cleft. *16* to *22,* Conventional orthodontics at age 12 years lasting for 18 months, followed by bonded retainer. *23* to *25,* Lateral cephalograms from ages 11 to 20 years.

Illustration continued on following page

K.E.	6 years	15 years	19.5 years
SNA°	81.5	79.0	79.5
SNB°	75.5	77.5	78.5
ANB°	6.0	1.5	1.0
SNPg°	75.5	79.5	80.5
NSBa°	128.0	133.0	133.5
NSL-NL°	7.5	7.0	5.0
NSL-OL°	22.0	15.0	13.5
NSL-ML°	33.5	30.5	27.5
NL-ML°	26.0	23.5	22.5
Gonial°	126.5	117.5	118.0
pm-ss″ (mm)	39.5	47.5	48.0
n-sp″ (mm)	37.5	47.5	48.5
sp″-gn (mm)	52.0	69.5	72.5
1-1°	160.5	133.0	128.5
1-NA°	8.0	23.0	27.0
1-NB°	5.5	23.0	23.5
SS-N-SM°	10.0	5.5	4.5
H-angle°	16.5	9.5	4.5
UL-EL (mm)	-1.5	2.5	5.0
LL-EL (mm)	0.0	1.0	2.0

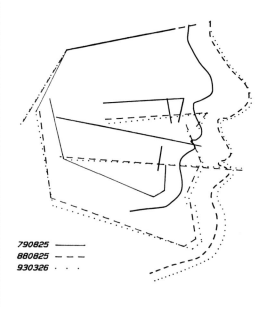

790825 ———
880825 – – –
930326 · · ·

26

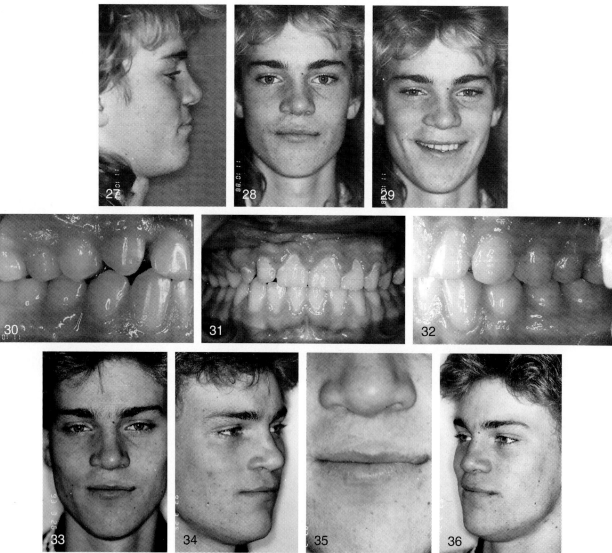

Figure 14–7 *Continued. 26,* Cephalometric analysis at ages 6, 15, and 19.5 years. *27 to 32,* Facial appearance and dental occlusion at age 15 years. *33 to 36,* Facial appearance at age 20 years.

Peripolasty and Alveolar Bone Grafting

Between 1971 and 1986, primary periosteoplasty on the cleft alveolar process was performed before primary lip closure. All primary surgery (lip and palate closure) in this period was performed by one plastic surgeon. By mobilizing mucoperiosteal flaps, "bony bridges" were induced in the cleft alveolar process in more than 50% of the cases.[44] All patients described in this chapter underwent the surgery program with primary periosteoplasty. Figure 14–8 shows the potential for total bony healing of clefts by this method, and the result may be thought-provoking in future considerations of methods of surgical intervention in alveolar bone grafting. Figure 14–9 with a wide cleft before presurgical orthopedics illustrates the healing potential of a mucoperiostal flap on the cleft side in comparison with the noncleft side.

Text continued on page 257

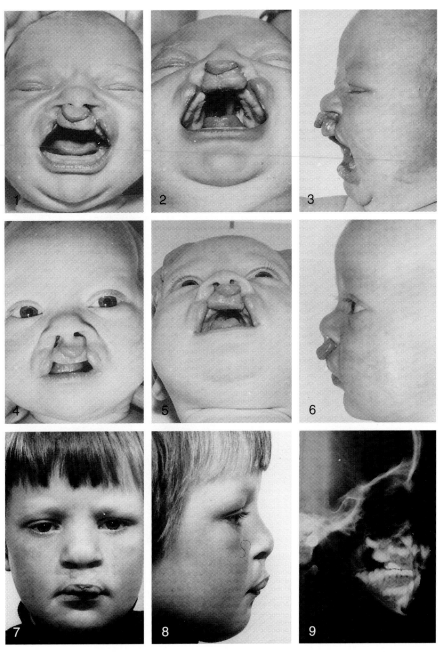

Figure 14–8. Complete BCLP, category 1. *1* to *3*, At birth, December 1971. *4* to *6*, After presurgical orthopedics. *7* to *9*, At age 6 years, favorable sagittal development, bilateral crossbite.

Illustration continued on following page

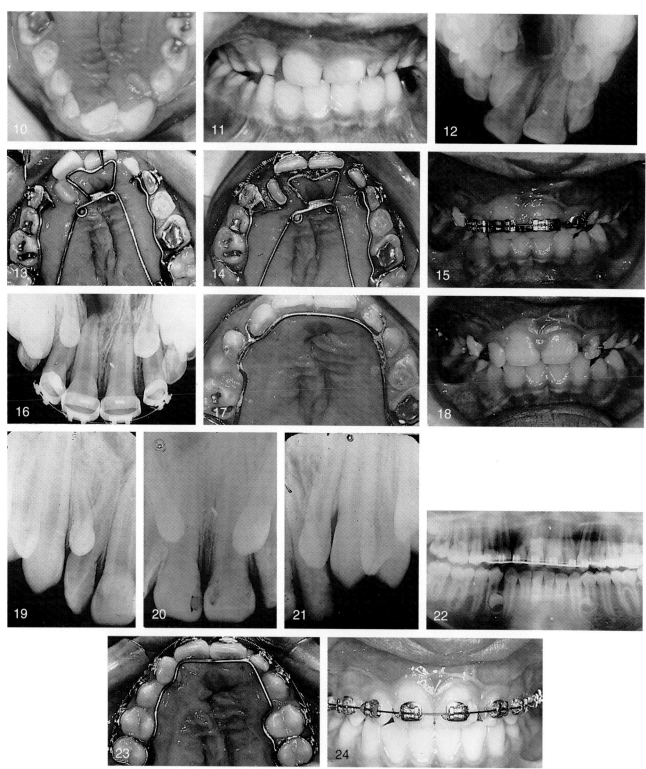

Figure 14–8 *Continued. 10* to *13*, Transverse expansion at age 9 years, followed by fixed retention. *14* to *18*, Alignment of upper incisors over 7 months, followed by a fixed palatal retention arch wire. *19* to *22*, Note two supernumerary upper lateral incisors of good size and two supernumerary premolar buds in the lower jaw; supernumeraries were removed. *23, 24*, Conventional orthodontics from age 12.5 years lasting 8 months, followed by Hawley retainer; no retention after age 15.

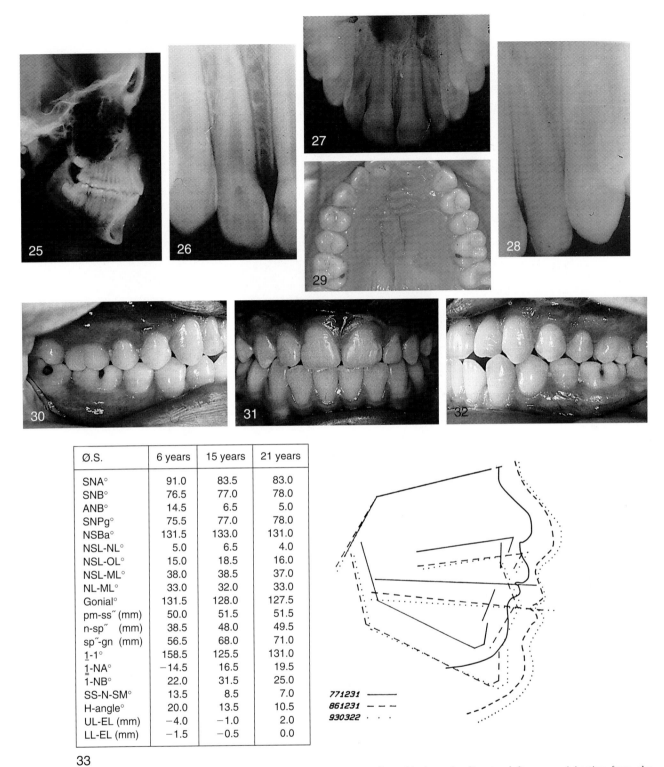

Ø.S.	6 years	15 years	21 years
SNA°	91.0	83.5	83.0
SNB°	76.5	77.0	78.0
ANB°	14.5	6.5	5.0
SNPg°	75.5	77.0	78.0
NSBa°	131.5	133.0	131.0
NSL-NL°	5.0	6.5	4.0
NSL-OL°	15.0	18.5	16.0
NSL-ML°	38.0	38.5	37.0
NL-ML°	33.0	32.0	33.0
Gonial°	131.5	128.0	127.5
pm-ss″ (mm)	50.0	51.5	51.5
n-sp″ (mm)	38.5	48.0	49.5
sp″-gn (mm)	56.5	68.0	71.0
1-1°	158.5	125.5	131.0
1-NA°	−14.5	16.5	19.5
1-NB°	22.0	31.5	25.0
SS-N-SM°	13.5	8.5	7.0
H-angle°	20.0	13.5	10.5
UL-EL (mm)	−4.0	−1.0	2.0
LL-EL (mm)	−1.5	−0.5	0.0

771231 ———
861231 — — —
930322 · · ·

33

Figure 14–8 *Continued. 25* to *32,* Dental occlusion at age 21 years; note favorable bone healing in cleft areas originating from the primary periosteoplasty at age 3 months (no secondary bone grafting was performed). *33,* Cephalometric analysis at ages 6, 15, and 21 years.

Illustration continues on following page

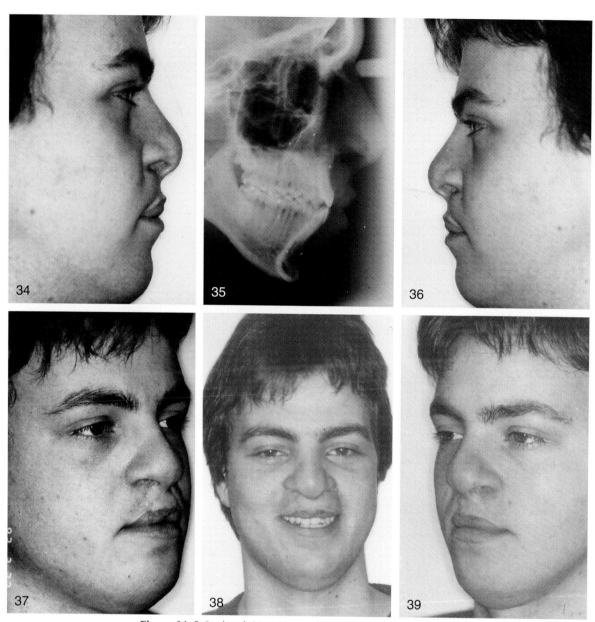

Figure 14–8 *Continued. 34* to *39,* Facial appearance at age 21 years.

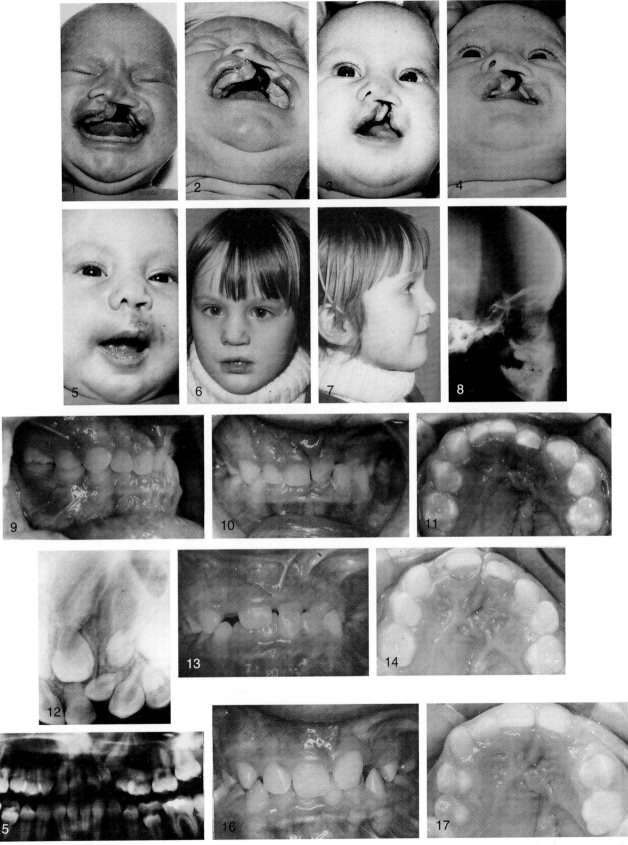

Figure 14–9. Complete UCLP, category 0. *1, 2,* At birth, September 1976. *3, 4,* After presurgical orthopedics. *5,* Lip closure at age 3 months. *6* to *12,* At age 6 years, favorable sagittal and transverse development except dentoalveolar crossbite of the deciduous canine. *13* to *17,* Lingually positioned permanent upper central incisor was protruded by a plate; no retention.

Illustration continued on following page

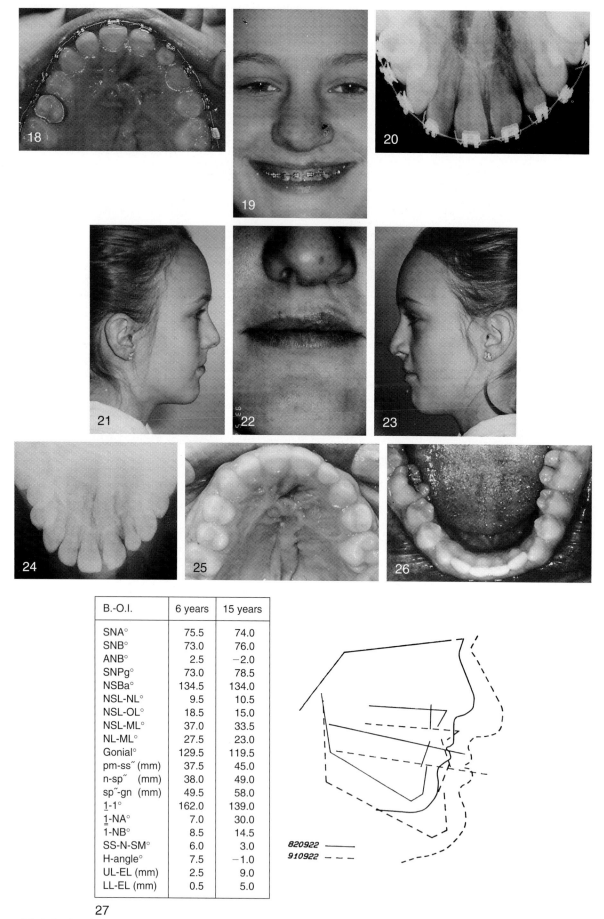

B.-O.I.	6 years	15 years
SNA°	75.5	74.0
SNB°	73.0	76.0
ANB°	2.5	−2.0
SNPg°	73.0	78.5
NSBa°	134.5	134.0
NSL-NL°	9.5	10.5
NSL-OL°	18.5	15.0
NSL-ML°	37.0	33.5
NL-ML°	27.5	23.0
Gonial°	129.5	119.5
pm-ss″ (mm)	37.5	45.0
n-sp″ (mm)	38.0	49.0
sp″-gn (mm)	49.5	58.0
1-1°	162.0	139.0
1-NA°	7.0	30.0
1-NB°	8.5	14.5
SS-N-SM°	6.0	3.0
H-angle°	7.5	−1.0
UL-EL (mm)	2.5	9.0
LL-EL (mm)	0.5	5.0

820922 ——
910922 - - -

27

Figure 14–9 *Continued. 18* to *20,* Conventional orthodontics from age 12.5 years for 20 months; no secondary bone grafting. *21* to *26,* Facial appearance and dental occlusion at age 15 years (left upper second premolar was missing). *27,* Cephalometric analysis at ages 6 and 15 years.

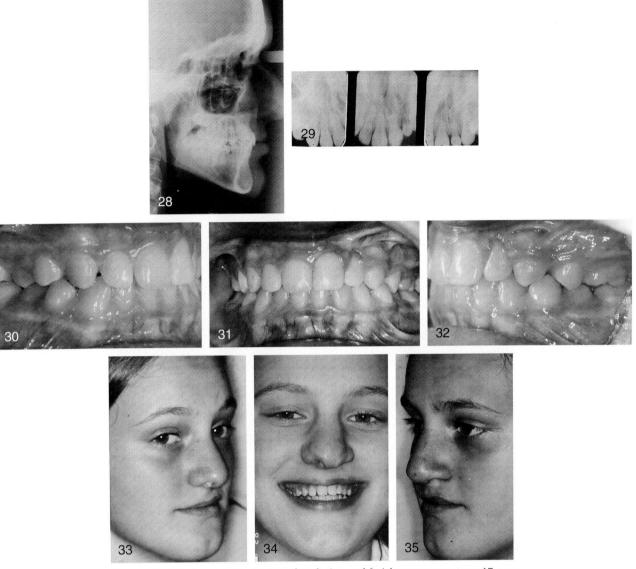

Figure 14–9 *Continued.* 28 to 35, Dental occlusion and facial appearance at age 17 years.

Since 1980, additional bone grafting into the cleft area has been undertaken at the age of 8 to 11 years if the amount of bone was insufficient for adequate tooth eruption or orthodontic movement of teeth. Figure 14–10 illustrates how bone developed in a patient with bilateral cleft lip and alveolus (BCLA) after the mucoperiosteal flap over the right cleft area and the result after secondary bone grafting in the left cleft area. The upper incisors were moved orthodontically into the correct positions.

Secondary Revision

Secondary corrective surgery may be needed. BCLP patients would require an elongation of the columella to lift the nasal tip and a sulcusplasty of the maxillary vestibulum. This procedure is performed at approximately 4 years of age, and the lip is mobilized from the alveolar crest. In cases in which the speech therapist makes a diagnosis of velopharyngeal incompetence, a pharyngeal flap–plasty is recommended at 5 years of age or later. When the patient is 8 to 11 years of age, the orthodontist takes a major role in the decision to perform alveolar bone grafting (see Fig. 14–6). Nasal deformities are revised according to individual needs, most often after 15 years of age.

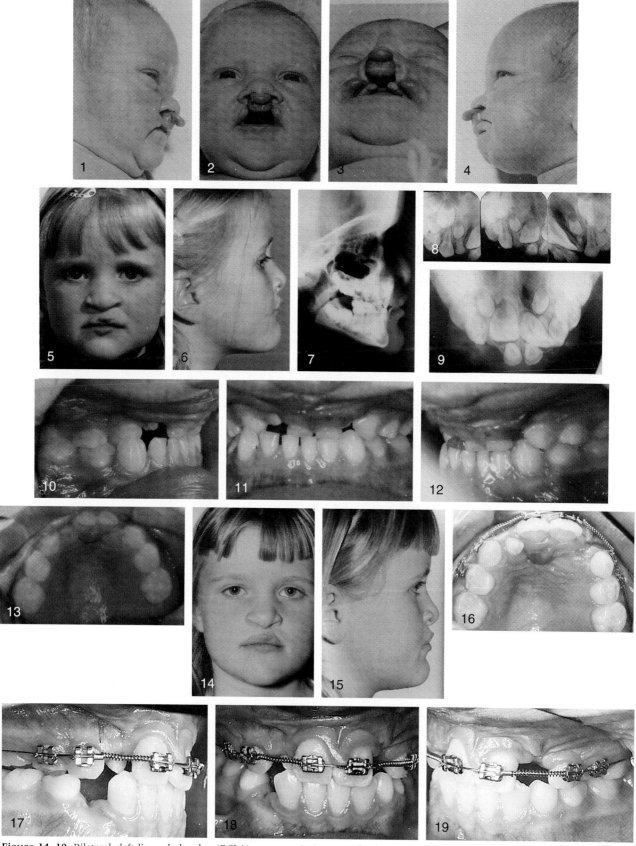

Figure 14–10. Bilateral cleft lip and alveolus (BCLA), category 0. *1* to *4*, At birth, July 1975. *5* to *13*, At age 6 years, favorable sagittal and transverse development except dentoalveolar crossbite of the deciduous canine. *14* to *19*, At age 8 years, secondary bone grafting (left side only), followed by alignment of upper incisors at age 9.5 years.

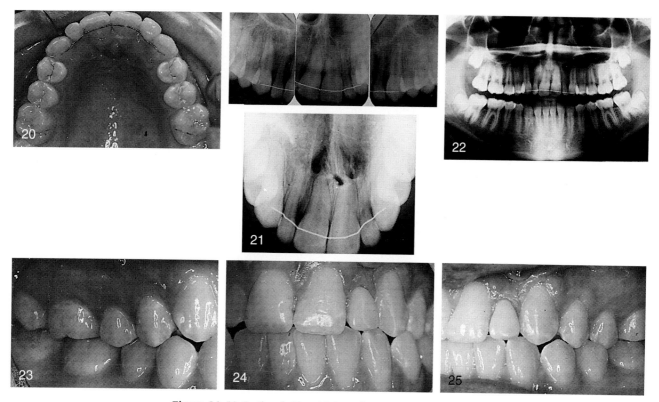

Figure 14–10 *Continued. 20* to *25,* Dental occlusion at age 15 years.

Illustration continued on following page

Orthodontic Considerations in Growth Development

Clefts of the lip and/or palate can be superimposed on any facial type. For this reason, it is essential to distinguish between (1) the different craniofacial types and related growth patterns that are normally distributed in the noncleft population and on which CLP is superimposed (see Figs. 14–1A,B,C) and (2) the secondary growth deviations and compensations that develop in patients with CLP (Fig. 14–11). Clefting that occurs in certain facial types may result in combinations of growth patterns in which discrepancies between the jaws are more difficult to repair.

Facial Growth in Patients with Cleft Lip and Palate

Regardless of treatment rationale, a certain number of patients with complete clefts reveal an unfavorable growth pattern of the craniofacial complex. In UCLP, the general tendency is for underdevelopment and/or posterior positioning of the maxilla and mandible in relation to the anterior cranial base, increased steepness of the mandibular plane, a more obtuse gonial angle, and other differences.[25, 36, 45–48] There is also a reduction in maxillary length in relation to the cranial base and in maxillary height in relation to the anterior facial height.[25, 36, 46–52] A sagittal discrepancy between the upper and lower jaws, with the maxilla in a more retruded position, often characterizes these patients.

Ross,[47] in a survey of 528 white males with complete UCLP from 15 centers around the world, reported decreased midface depth as a result of a shorter maxilla, more upright maxillary incisors, a less prominent and smaller mandible, and an increased mandibular plane angle. These characteristics resulted in unfavorable sagittal basal jaw relations even in patients whose deformities were considered mild in comparison with normal control material. In patients with poor facial growth, the shorter basal maxilla was, in addition, positioned posteriorly, often in association with a narrow pharynx. This resulted in a more severe difference in sagittal jaw relations, with reduced maxillary height, increased lower facial height, and an unfavorable effect on facial vertical proportion and balance.

Facial form in BCLP patients also differed from that of non-CLP subjects. Semb[53] found that although initially prominent, the maxilla receded over time, reaching a

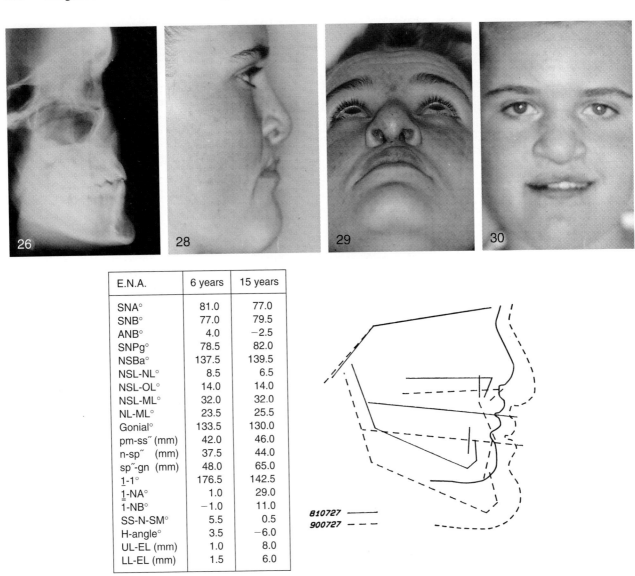

E.N.A.	6 years	15 years
SNA°	81.0	77.0
SNB°	77.0	79.5
ANB°	4.0	−2.5
SNPg°	78.5	82.0
NSBa°	137.5	139.5
NSL-NL°	8.5	6.5
NSL-OL°	14.0	14.0
NSL-ML°	32.0	32.0
NL-ML°	23.5	25.5
Gonial°	133.5	130.0
pm-ss″ (mm)	42.0	46.0
n-sp″ (mm)	37.5	44.0
sp″-gn (mm)	48.0	65.0
1-1°	176.5	142.5
1-NA°	1.0	29.0
1-NB°	−1.0	11.0
SS-N-SM°	5.5	0.5
H-angle°	3.5	−6.0
UL-EL (mm)	1.0	8.0
LL-EL (mm)	1.5	6.0

810727 ———
900727 - - - -

27

Figure 14-10 *Continued. 26,* Radiographic appearance at 15 years. *27,* Cephalometric analysis at ages 6 and 15 years. *28 to 30,* Facial appearance at age 17 years.

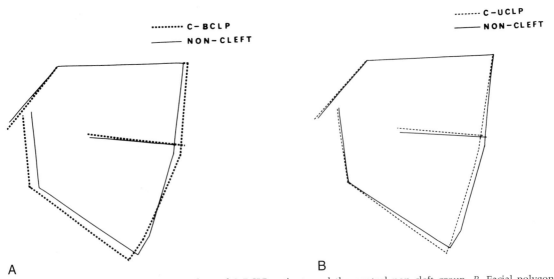

A

B

Figure 14-11. *A,* Facial polygons of the mean values of 9 BCLP patients and the control non-cleft group. *B,* Facial polygons of the mean values of 20 UCLP patients and the control group.

sagittal jaw relation somewhat similar to that of patients with UCLP by the late teen years. The mandible was retrusive and exhibited a steep mandibular plane and increased gonial angle. Anterior lower face height was often increased and posterior face height reduced.[52,53]

The frequency and degree of such growth disturbances were greatly reduced after introduction of modern surgical procedures.[54] Nevertheless, maxillary growth deficiencies in sagittal, vertical, and/or transverse dimensions develop in some patients. This in turn may cause skeletal as well as dentoalveolar discrepancies between the upper and lower jaws, characterized by anterior and posterior crossbite.[52,55–59]

Dental Considerations: Hypodontia in Patients with Cleft Lip and Palate

Hypodontia (congenitally missing teeth) occurs in 5% to 10% of the general population (the lower second premolar in 2.5%, the upper lateral incisor in 1.2%, the upper second premolar in 1.3%). This does not include third molars.[60] Hypodontia has been shown to occur more commonly in CLP children.[61,62] The incidence of hypodontia in the permanent dentition is increased with greater severity of the cleft.[63] In a study of 96 complete clefts, Fleiner and coworkers[64] found that the upper lateral incisor was missing before lip repair in 6% of patients. A single upper lateral incisor, dysplastic or normal, was present in 48% of the subjects (far more often distal to the cleft), and two upper lateral incisors (one tooth on each side of the cleft) were found in 46%.

Combinations of hypodontia and malformed teeth are also common. Figure 14–12 illustrates cleft lip and alveolus in which the upper central incisors, which were of

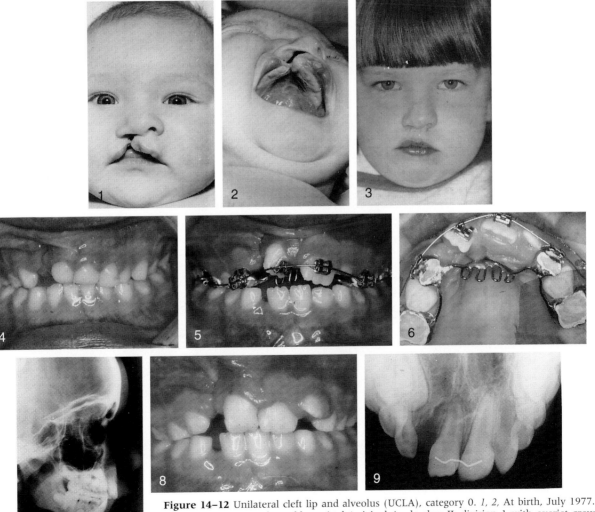

Figure 14–12 Unilateral cleft lip and alveolus (UCLA), category 0. *1, 2,* At birth, July 1977. *3, 4,* At age 6 years, favorable sagittal (original Angle class II, division 1 with overjet grew into class I occlusion) and transverse development. *5 to 9,* Alignment of upper incisors from age 8 years for 6 months after a fixed palatal arch wire with tongue-crib alleviated spontaneous eruption of the central incisors.

Illustration continued on following page

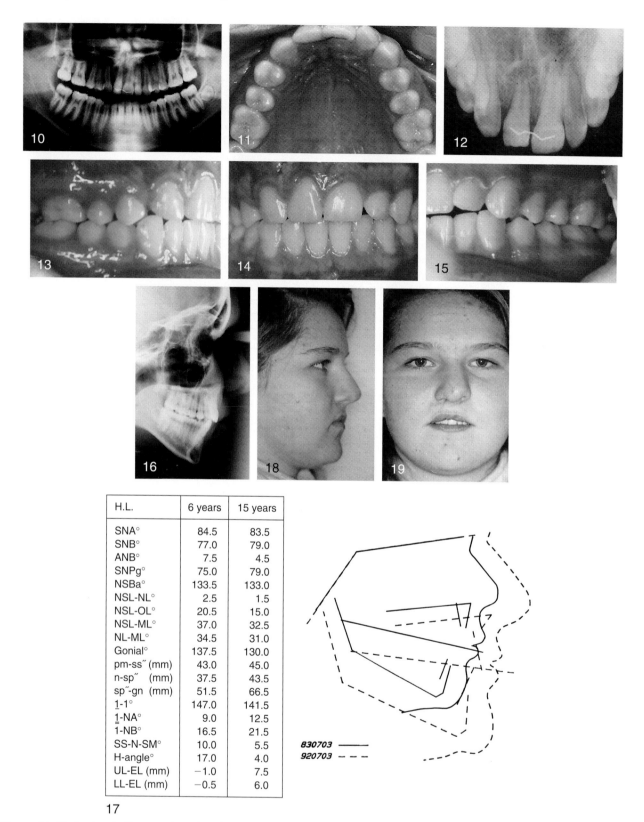

H.L.	6 years	15 years
SNA°	84.5	83.5
SNB°	77.0	79.0
ANB°	7.5	4.5
SNPg°	75.0	79.0
NSBa°	133.5	133.0
NSL-NL°	2.5	1.5
NSL-OL°	20.5	15.0
NSL-ML°	37.0	32.5
NL-ML°	34.5	31.0
Gonial°	137.5	130.0
pm-ss″ (mm)	43.0	45.0
n-sp″ (mm)	37.5	43.5
sp″-gn (mm)	51.5	66.5
1̲-1̲°	147.0	141.5
1̲-NA°	9.0	12.5
1-NB°	16.5	21.5
SS-N-SM°	10.0	5.5
H-angle°	17.0	4.0
UL-EL (mm)	−1.0	7.5
LL-EL (mm)	−0.5	6.0

830703 ———
920703 - - - -

17

Figure 14–12 *Continued.* *10* to *16,* Dental occlusion at age 15 years (secondary bone grafting at 10 years); the upper right canine erupted spontaneously into position of missing lateral incisor. *17,* Cephalometric analysis at ages 6 and 15 years. *18, 19,* Facial appearance at age 15 years.

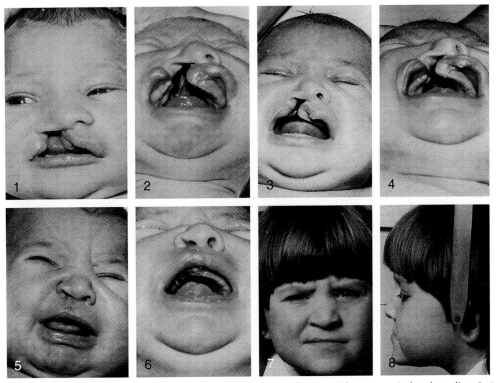

Figure 14–13. Complete UCLP, category 2A. *1, 2,* At birth, September 1975. *3, 4,* After presurgical orthopedics. *5, 6,* Lip closure at age 3 months. *7 to 12,* At age 6 years, concave profile and marked anterior and unilateral posterior crossbite.

Illustration continued on following page

different sizes, were accommodated into a dental arch and one lateral incisor was missing. Figure 14–13 shows how a malformed central incisor was orthodontically brought into position and reshaped after endodontic treatment.

Form/Function Considerations: Orofacial Dysfunction and Growth Pattern

The tendency for attenuated growth and retropositioning of the midface and for an increased anterior lower face height may contribute to (1) disturbance of nasal respiration, (2) low and forward posture of the tongue complex, and (3) lack of correct stimuli from proper mastication. Nasal airway resistance to breathing is often increased among CLP patients. This has been attributed to nasal deformities and maxillary growth deficits, both of which tend to reduce the size of the nasal airspace.[65] In CLP patients, reduced nasal respiratory function has been found to contribute to the increased anterior facial height.[24, 66]

Orthopedic expansion of the median palatine suture in noncleft mouth-breathers lowers the nasal resistance to normal values and is thought to enhance nasal respiration.[67–70] There is clinical evidence that lateral expansion of the maxilla may also enhance increased nasal respiration in CLP patients; this finding is supported by studies reported by Harvold and associates[71, 72] on monkeys. With complete occlusion of the nasal airway to provide an oral airway, the tongue adopted a lower position with lowering of the mandible and an increase of the lower anterior facial height.

The situation in CLP patients with some collapse of the maxillary dental arch may be similar. The repaired palatal vault is lower than in non-CLP children, and crossbite of the maxillary segments reduces the lateral space available for the tongue. The vertical, transverse, and sagittal underdevelopment of the maxillary alveolar processes may partly explain the lower tongue position in CP children.[52] Low posture of the

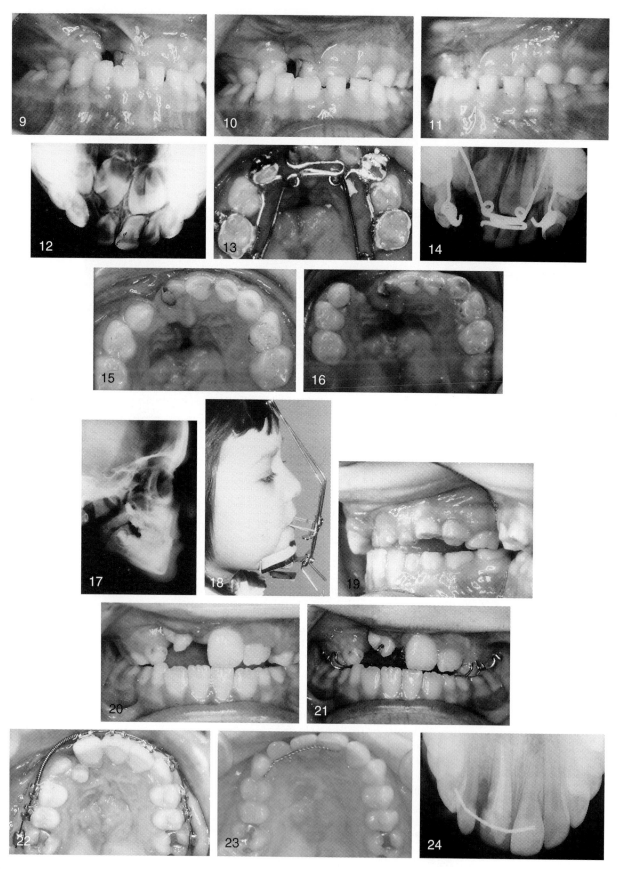

Figure 14–13 *Continued. 13* to *19,* Interceptive orthopedics from age 6.1 years: transverse expansion (3 months) followed by protraction (8 months) to alleviate spontaneous eruption of upper permanent incisors into normal position; retention by a fixed palatal arch wire. *20* to *22,* Alignment of upper incisors at age 8 years; right upper central incisor was malformed and had to be moved orthodontically down into position and reshaped; the incisor was treated endodontically because of an extreme invagination and fixed by a bonded retainer; secondary bone grafting at age 10.5 years. *23, 24,* Upper dentition with bonded retainer at age 15.

U.L.	6 years	15 years
SNA°	79.0	78.5
SNB°	81.0	80.5
ANB°	−2.0	−2.0
SNPg°	80.0	82.0
NSBa°	134.5	134.5
NSL-NL°	3.5	0.0
NSL-OL°	16.5	15.0
NSL-ML°	26.5	24.0
NL-ML°	23.0	24.0
Gonial°	111.5	108.5
pm-ss″ (mm)	37.0	42.5
n-sp″ (mm)	35.5	42.0
sp″-gn (mm)	48.5	61.5
$\underline{1}$-$\underline{1}$°	176.5	137.0
$\underline{1}$-NA°	−2.5	25.5
$\overline{\underline{1}}$-NB°	7.5	19.5
SS-N-SM°	2.0	2.0
H-angle°	3.5	1.0
UL-EL (mm)	5.0	6.5
LL-EL (mm)	1.0	4.5

25

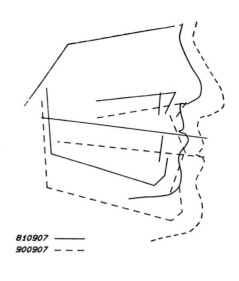

810907 ———
900907 – – –

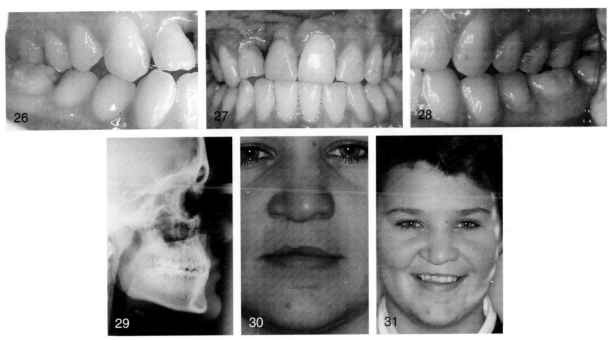

Figure 14–13 *Continued. 25,* Cephalometric analysis at ages 6 and 15 years. *26 to 31,* Dental occlusion and facial appearance at age 17 years.

tongue, resulting from lack of nasal respiration and from restrained sagittal and vertical growth of the midface, is a further indication for both posterior mandibular rotation and maxillary retrognathism.[49]

Subtelny and Brodie[73] found that early establishment of normal intermaxillary relationships in CLP patients by simple expansion techniques affords better conditions for future rehabilitation. The maxilla is enabled to grow in a more normal manner and allows the tongue to assume a more normal position.[74] Thus early orthopedic treatment, including transverse expansion and protraction, may increase the dimensions of the nasal and the intermaxillary space, allowing a higher position of the tongue. This may contribute to breaking the form-function interaction.

In view of the generally accepted association between form and function, the correct relationship of the primary dentition may be considered important for growth and development of the anterior part of the maxilla. CLP patients with midface deficiency often lack normal occlusal relationships and occlusal forces.[52, 75] Furthermore, anterior and posterior dental crossbites may cause dental interferences with associated mandibular shifts into habitual occlusion. The eruption, the direction of eruption, and the position of teeth are closely associated with the development of the dentoalveolar process in conjunction with the number, size, and position of the teeth.[76–78]

Reduced Response if Treatment Is Postponed

Collapse of segments of the maxillary dental arch prevents surface apposition and thereby prevents segment growth and arch length increase. Because sutural growth of the upper jaw is very active at 6 to 7 years of age and then declines to the prepubertal minimum,[16] the potential for maxillary growth is best promoted under the influence of occlusal forces from mastication. The observation that basal maxillary changes are seen mainly with protraction therapy instituted before the age of 8 years in non-CLP patients[66] and in CLP patients[37, 79–81] has been explained by complexity of maxillary sutural systems before the onset of puberty.[22, 23]

Treatment Considerations: Ages 1 to 6 Years

Lack of regular dental care, caries prophylaxis, and conservative treatment of the deciduous dentition may jeopardize ensuing orthopedic/orthodontic treatment. In general, tooth extractions may be linked to alveolar atrophy and loss of the dentoalveolar process. Implementation of dental care programs by the craniofacial team requires evaluation in the early primary dentition.

Interceptive Orthopedic Intervention: How Early?

Early rehabilitation of appearance and function of CLP children has been considered a major goal.[48, 82, 83] At age 4, all CLP patients are evaluated by the orthodontist for skeletodental components of the developing malocclusion. Although intervention may result in an excellent response at age 5 years or earlier, the better cooperation that can be expected of children at age 6 years is a factor in establishing that age as an appropriate time to start treatment. Tindlund[37, 81] found significantly better skeletal response when maxillary protraction was started at a mean age 6.3 years than later. The goal was to allow the permanent maxillary incisors to erupt spontaneously into a normal overjet and overbite relationship. The treatment intervention was therefore dependent on the severity of the discrepancy in individual cases. Protraction during the late deciduous dentition period reduces the unwanted dentoalveolar protrusive effect on the permanent incisors.[25, 84] In general, the youngest patients were more enthusiastic and cooperative than those who started treatment at about 10 years of age.

Team Evaluation of All Patients with Cleft Lip and Palate at 6 Years

The Bergen CLP team evaluates all patients at the ages of 6 and 15 years (see Fig. 14–6). The different specialists undertake individual examinations, the problems are prioritized and discussed by the team, and recommendations are conveyed to the parents. At this time, standardized records are obtained for all patients with clefts: collection of lateral and frontal cephalograms, an orthopantomogram, occlusal films and periapical views of the maxillary frontal and cleft area(s), x-ray videograms to register the function of the soft palate and lips, intraoral and extraoral color slides, two black-and-white portraits, and plaster study models with occlusal registration. These diagnostic records are used for evaluation of dental and facial growth and development and form the basis for longitudinal studies. After assessment of the records, the whole team reconvenes to discuss the information obtained and develop individual treatment plans and recommendations for the patients and parents, who are informed by letters.

Orthodontic Evaluation at 6 Years

The results of the orthodontic inspection and the various analyses may be outlined in the following form:

1. Soft tissue facial appearance: full face and profile.
2. Type of face: prognathic, orthognathic, or retrognatic.

3. Basal jaw configuration: sagittal, vertical, or transverse.
4. Dental occlusion: frontal (overjet, overbite) or lateral (Angle classification).
5. Dental space conditions.
6. Disturbances of dental development and occlusion.
7. Orofacial dysfunction.
8. Vestibular, periodontal, and mucosal abnormalities.

Treatment Considerations at and After Age 6 Years

When a patient is 6 years of age, the craniofacial growth and occlusal development give some indications of what can be expected later. For each patient, the orthopedic/orthodontic treatment needs, treatment options, implementation, and timing must be considered in relation to the patient's other needs, and overall team management with the risks, costs, and benefits of alternative treatment options is discussed.

The development of Angle class III occlusion in non-CLP members of the family may indicate that clefting has been superimposed on a growth pattern that may contribute negatively to orthodontic/orthopedic treatment. Figure 14–14 shows a patient with a malformed left upper central incisor, a missing lateral incisor, and anterior and posterior crossbite (the mother, grandfather, and uncle had class III malocclusion). This case demonstrates how the right central incisor was moved into the position of the extracted malformed left central incisor and how the right lateral incisor was moved into the position of the right central incisor. Orthognathic surgery was performed when the patient was 16. Figure 14–15 depicts a patient whose father had received orthognathic surgery for class III occlusion. This case illustrates an acceptable response and a stable result after orthopedic/orthodontic treatment without orthognathic surgery.

Cephalometric Analysis

The mandible may be considered a main reference in relation to the cranial base (or Frankfort horizontal) because the primary clefting defect affects the maxillary complex and is only moderately influenced sagittally and vertically. However, a few CLP patients may reveal genuine mandibular prognathism (see Fig. 14–14). Therefore, the position of the lower jaw, its relationship to the cranial base, and its size, form, and height in relation to total face height contribute to the diagnosis and treatment plan. The size and relationship of the maxilla (sagittal, vertical, and transverse) to the cranial base indicate the degree of underdevelopment and the treatment possibilities. The skeletal and dental components of the resulting malocclusion are important factors in determining treatment needs and recommendations.

Dental Occlusion, Space Conditions, and Extractions

In non-CLP patients, the space considerations in the lower jaw often dictate extraction or nonextraction therapy. The relationships between size of the dental arch and the sum of the widths of the teeth, the position of the lower incisor teeth, the curve of Spee, and the possibility for distal movement of the molars are considered. These considerations also apply to CLP patients. The space conditions in the affected upper jaw with clefting and the possibilities for expansion of the upper dental arch are other decisive factors. Hypodontia in such cases may be resolved by orthodontic space closure or space maintenance, depending on the degree of maxillary deficiency and the number and distribution of missing teeth. Most important are that (1) the protrusion of the upper incisors not exceed the normal sagittal-axial inclination on the maxillary base and (2) the lower incisors not be retruded more than to normal position to compensate for the underdeveloped upper jaw. Therefore, extractions in the lower jaw to compensate for a small upper jaw should be considered in the context of a continuing discrepancy until mandibular growth has stabilized. At that time, it is important for the clinician to distinguish between (1) cases in which the patient can be treated by dentoalveolar compensation to camouflage the skeletal discrepancy, such as uprighting of the lower incisors after extractions, and (2) cases in which the patient would benefit from a combined orthodontic/orthognathic surgery approach. Presurgical orthodontic treatment is often necessary to procline the lower incisors when decompensation precedes surgery, if early

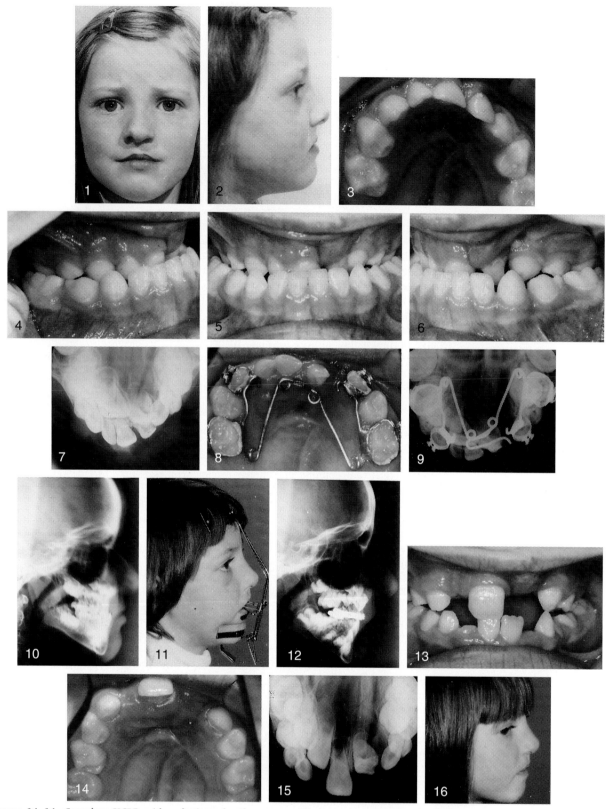

Figure 14–14. Complete UCLP with soft tissue band, category 2B: born August 1976, familial mandibular prognathism (mother, maternal grandfather, and maternal uncle), left upper lateral incisor missing, left upper central incisor malformed. *1* to *7*, At age 5.5 years: marked anterior and bilateral crossbites. *8* to *16*, Interceptive orthopedics from age 5.5 years: transverse expansion (3 months) followed by protraction (9 months) to alleviate spontaneous eruption of upper right permanent incisor into normal position.

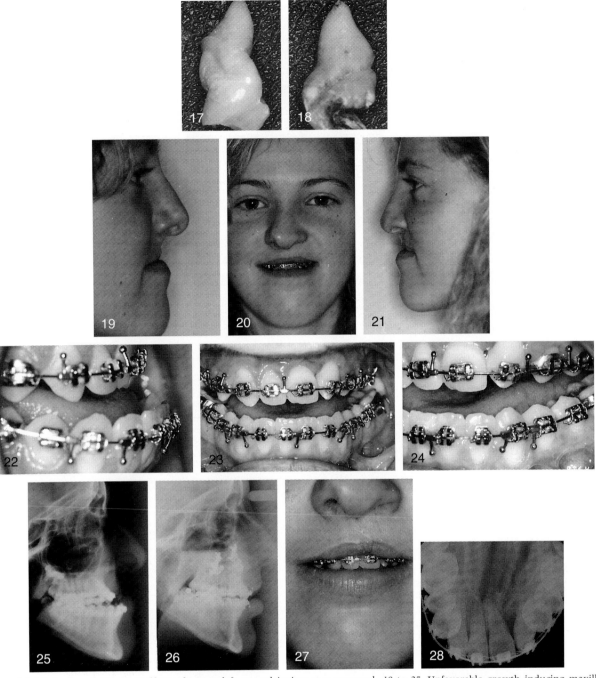

Figure 14–14 *Continued. 17, 18,* Malformed upper left central incisor was removed. *19* to *25,* Unfavorable growth inducing maxillary retrognathism and mandibular severe overdevelopment with an anterior crossbite; the right upper central incisor was moved into the position of the removed left central incisor, whereas the upper right lateral incisor serves as right central incisor.

Illustration continued on following page

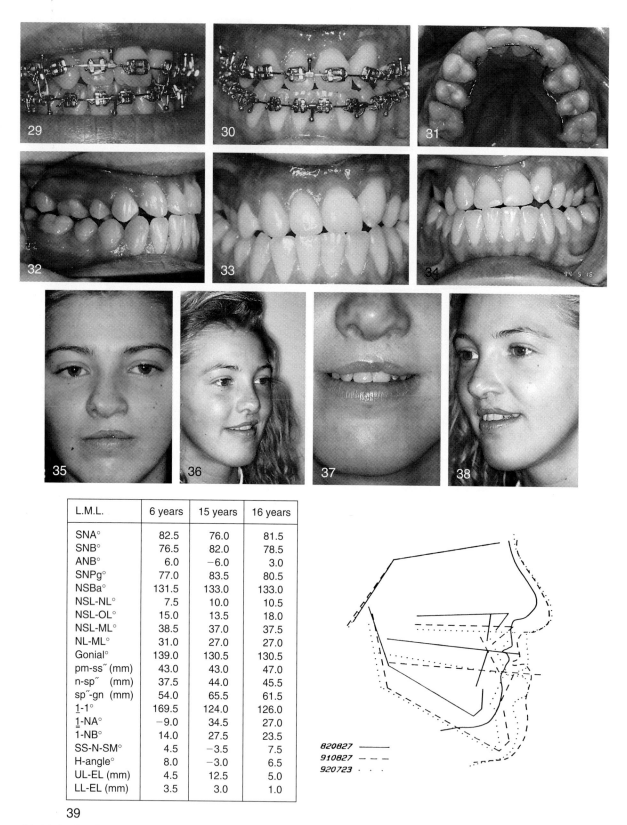

L.M.L.	6 years	15 years	16 years
SNA°	82.5	76.0	81.5
SNB°	76.5	82.0	78.5
ANB°	6.0	−6.0	3.0
SNPg°	77.0	83.5	80.5
NSBa°	131.5	133.0	133.0
NSL-NL°	7.5	10.0	10.5
NSL-OL°	15.0	13.5	18.0
NSL-ML°	38.5	37.0	37.5
NL-ML°	31.0	27.0	27.0
Gonial°	139.0	130.5	130.5
pm-ss″ (mm)	43.0	43.0	47.0
n-sp″ (mm)	37.5	44.0	45.5
sp″-gn (mm)	54.0	65.5	61.5
1-1°	169.5	124.0	126.0
1-NA°	−9.0	34.5	27.0
1-NB°	14.0	27.5	23.5
SS-N-SM°	4.5	−3.5	7.5
H-angle°	8.0	−3.0	6.5
UL-EL (mm)	4.5	12.5	5.0
LL-EL (mm)	3.5	3.0	1.0

820827 ———
910827 – – –
920723 · · ·

39

Figure 14–14 *Continued. 26 to 33,* Dental occlusion after bimaxillary orthognathic surgery at age 16 years (LeFort I osteotomy and mandibular vertical ramus osteotomy); *34 to 38,* Dental occlusion and facial appearance after space opening and reshaping of upper right lateral incisor into upper right central form. *39,* Cephalometric analysis at ages 6, 15, and 16 years (after orthognathic surgery).

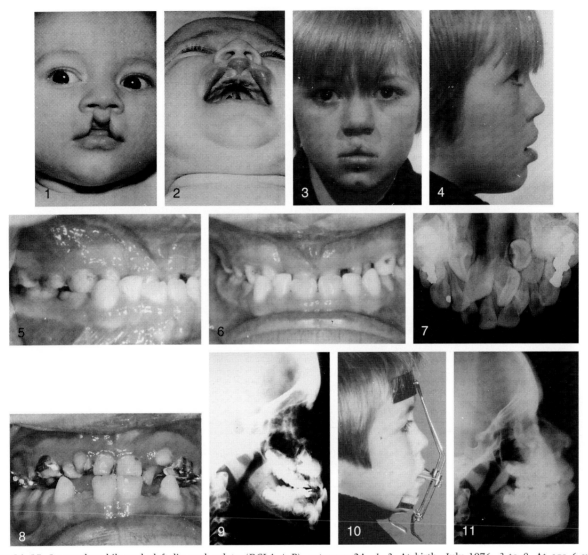

Figure 14–15. Incomplete bilateral cleft lip and palate (BCLA + P), category 2A. *1, 2,* At birth, July 1976. *3* to *9,* At age 6 years, marked anterior crossbite. *10, 11,* Protraction for 14 months from age 6.1 years.

Illustration continued on following page

compensation for the skeletal pattern has been attempted before the extent of future growth could be predicted.

Treatment Aims in Early Mixed Dentition

Orthopedic/orthodontic treatment may contribute to early rehabilitation of dentofacial appearance by reducing discrepancies between upper and lower jaw and by establishing correct occlusion before the patient starts school. If the clefting and surgical repair have affected maxillary growth, posterior and/or anterior dental crossbites and vertical maxillary deficiency may result in overclosure, which enhances the class III skeletal pattern. Even if this is localized to a few teeth, deviation of the mandible to the crossbite side and/or anteriorly into an incisal crossbite may have an effect similar to that created by a functional appliance and result in the stereotypical concave profile of patients with clefts.

The aim of treatment is that all CLP patients have a long period of normal facial growth stimuli by establishing, from the age of 6–7 years,

- Symmetry within the upper dentition and related to the facial midline (Fig. 14–16*A*).
- Normally functioning occlusion with (1) correct position of upper incisor teeth and (2) favorable transverse and sagittal posterior occlusion (see Fig. 14–16*B*).

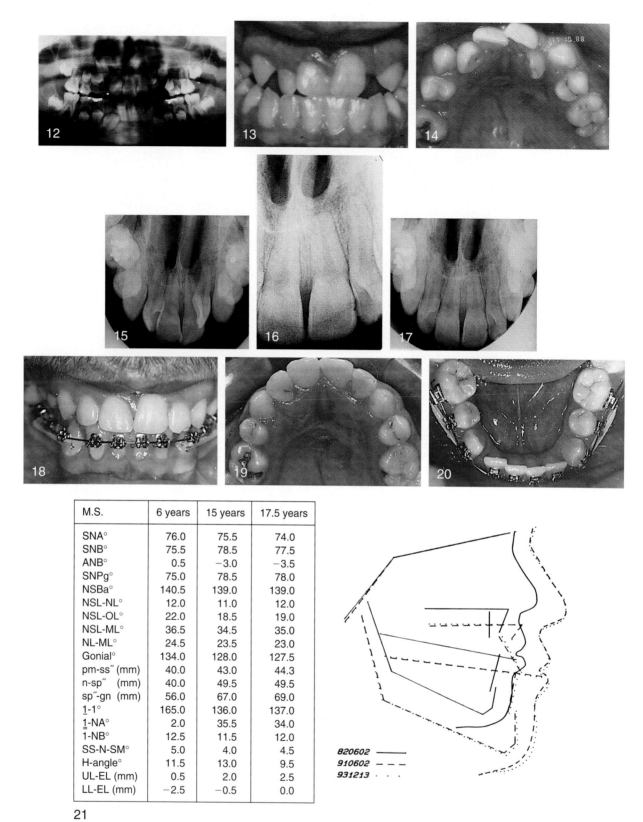

M.S.	6 years	15 years	17.5 years
SNA°	76.0	75.5	74.0
SNB°	75.5	78.5	77.5
ANB°	0.5	−3.0	−3.5
SNPg°	75.0	78.5	78.0
NSBa°	140.5	139.0	139.0
NSL-NL°	12.0	11.0	12.0
NSL-OL°	22.0	18.5	19.0
NSL-ML°	36.5	34.5	35.0
NL-ML°	24.5	23.5	23.0
Gonial°	134.0	128.0	127.5
pm-ss″ (mm)	40.0	43.0	44.3
n-sp″ (mm)	40.0	49.5	49.5
sp″-gn (mm)	56.0	67.0	69.0
1-1°	165.0	136.0	137.0
1-NA°	2.0	35.5	34.0
1-NB°	12.5	11.5	12.0
SS-N-SM°	5.0	4.0	4.5
H-angle°	11.5	13.0	9.5
UL-EL (mm)	0.5	2.0	2.5
LL-EL (mm)	−2.5	−0.5	0.0

820602 ———
910602 − − −
931213 · · ·

21

Figure 14–15 *Continued. 12* to *20,* Conventional orthodontics from age 12.5 years for 24 months, followed by a Hawley retainer until age 17.5 years; upper left second premolar missing; supernumerary upper left lateral incisor and three first premolars were removed. *21,* Cephalometric analysis at ages 6, 15 and 17.5 years.

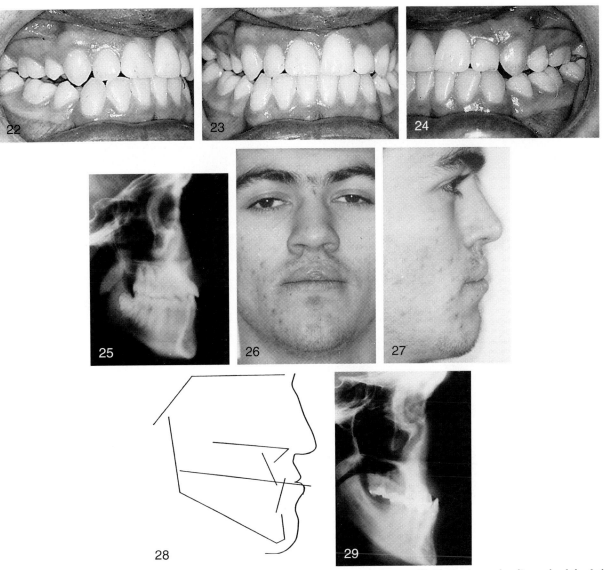

Figure 14-15 *Continued. 22* to *27*, Dental occlusion and facial appearance at age 17.5 years; *28, 29*, Tracing and radiograph of the father, who underwent orthognathic surgery to correct mandibular prognathism.

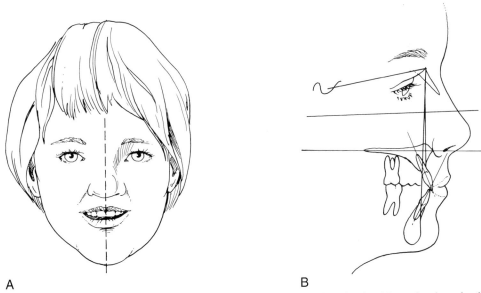

A   B

Figure 14-16. Treatment aims in early mixed dentition. *A*, Correct symmetry within the dentition related to the facial midline; *B*, correct inclination of the incisors and stable intercuspidation in the lateral segments.

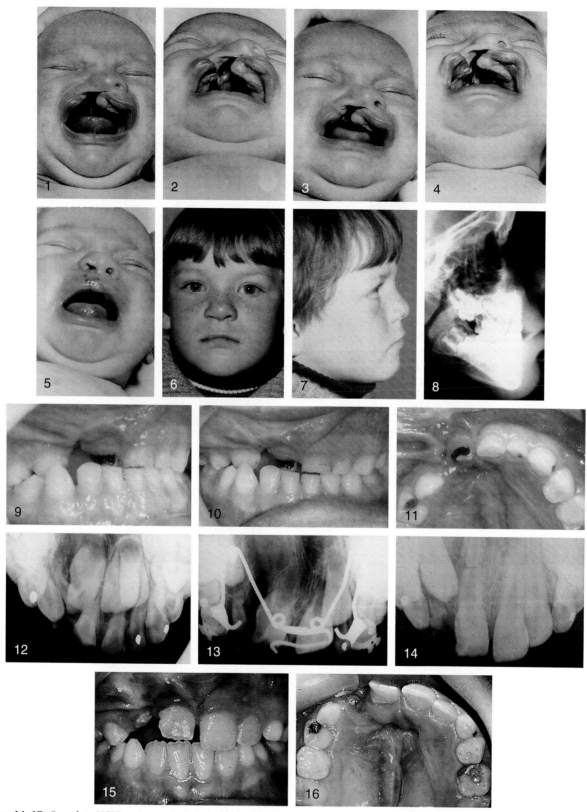

Figure 14–17. Complete UCLP, category 1. *1, 2,* At birth, July 1975. *3, 4,* After presurgical orthopedics. *5,* Lip closure at age 3 months. *6* to *12,* At age 6 years, favorable sagittal development; unilateral posterior crossbite with lack of space for eruption of incisors; upper right permanent lateral incisor missing. *13* to *16,* Transverse expansion (4 months) at age 7 years.

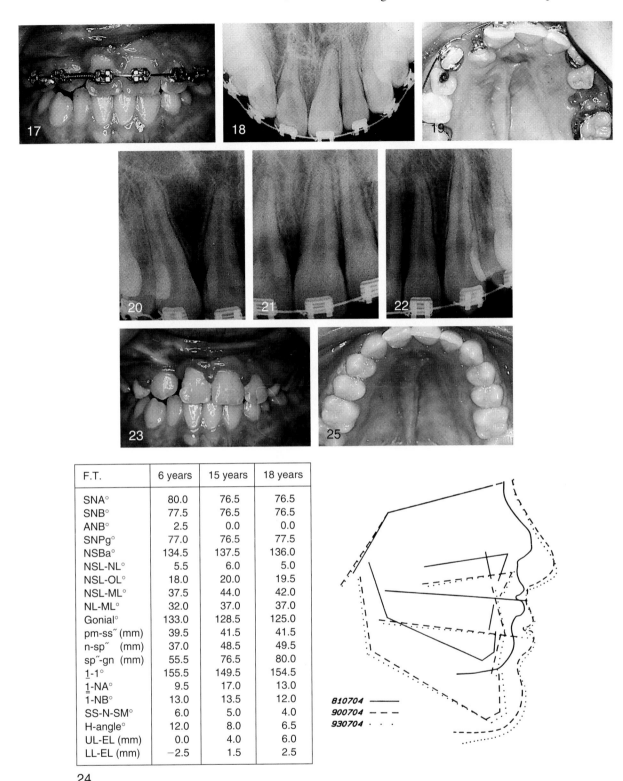

F.T.	6 years	15 years	18 years
SNA°	80.0	76.5	76.5
SNB°	77.5	76.5	76.5
ANB°	2.5	0.0	0.0
SNPg°	77.0	76.5	77.5
NSBa°	134.5	137.5	136.0
NSL-NL°	5.5	6.0	5.0
NSL-OL°	18.0	20.0	19.5
NSL-ML°	37.5	44.0	42.0
NL-ML°	32.0	37.0	37.0
Gonial°	133.0	128.5	125.0
pm-ss″ (mm)	39.5	41.5	41.5
n-sp″ (mm)	37.0	48.5	49.5
sp″-gn (mm)	55.5	76.5	80.0
1-1°	155.5	149.5	154.5
1-NA°	9.5	17.0	13.0
1-NB°	13.0	13.5	12.0
SS-N-SM°	6.0	5.0	4.0
H-angle°	12.0	8.0	6.5
UL-EL (mm)	0.0	4.0	6.0
LL-EL (mm)	−2.5	1.5	2.5

810704 ———
900704 – – –
930704 · · ·

24

Figure 14–17 *Continued.* *17* to *23,* Secondary bone grafting at age 10 years, followed by movement of the right upper canine into the position of the lateral incisor. *24,* Cephalometric analysis at ages 6, 15, and 18 years.

Illustration continued on following page

Treatment Indications

At age 6 years, patients with cleft lip and/or palate may be classified according to four categories, regardless of the type of clefting.

Category 0

This category includes minor clefts, CL, CP, and complete UCLP and BCLP but minimal skeletal discrepancy.

Normal skeletal facial morphology:

Class I sagittal jaw relationship with normal molar and incisal relationship (Angle class I) or distal sagittal occlusion (Angle class II) with moderate overjet; minor dental irregularities in the cleft site are inevitable but with harmonious basal transverse jaw relationship and normal width of upper and lower jaws (see Fig. 14–9).

Need for treatment:

No need for early orthopedic treatment.

Alignment of permanent incisors in the cleft area(s) at 7 to 8 years of age.

Bone grafting at 8–11 years of age.

Conventional orthodontic treatment at 11 to 13 years of age.

Category 1

This category includes UCLP, BCLP, and CP.

Normal skeletal/facial morphology with posterior dental crossbite(s):

Normal overbite or overjet, class I sagittal jaw relationship combined with dentoalveolar transverse discrepancy with partial or complete posterior crossbite, which may be unilateral or bilateral (see Figs. 14–7, 14–8, 14–17, 14–18).

Need for treatment:

Skeletal and/or dentoalveolar transverse expansion of the upper jaw.

Alignment of permanent incisors in the cleft area(s) at 7 to 8 years of age. Bone grafting at 8–11 years of age.

Conventional orthodontic treatment at 11 to 13 years of age.

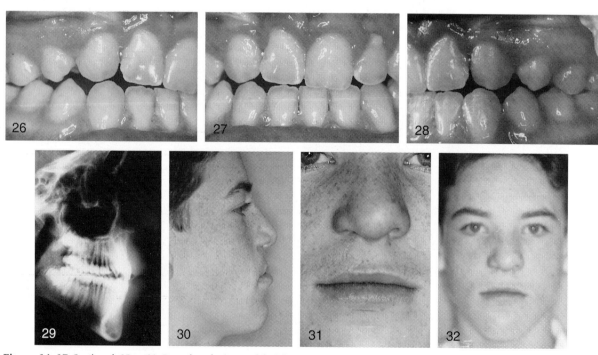

Figure 14–17 *Continued. 25 to 32,* Dental occlusion and facial appearance at age 18 years; no retention since age 16 years.

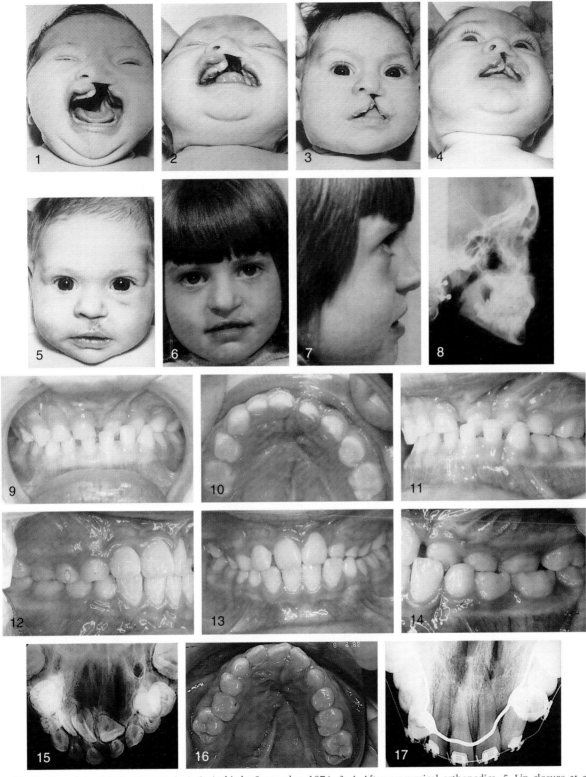

Figure 14–18. Complete UCLP, category 1. *1, 2,* At birth, September 1976. *3, 4,* After presurgical orthopedics. *5,* Lip closure at age 3 months. *6* to *11,* At age 6 years, favorable sagittal development, unilateral posterior crossbite; no early transverse expansion because of acceptable space conditions; upper left permanent lateral incisor was missing. *12* to *16,* Spontaneous eruption of upper permanent incisors into normal position; no secondary bone grafting. *17,* Transverse expansion at age 13 when the left canine was to be moved orthodontically into the arch; conventional orthodontics for 16 months.

Illustration continued on following page

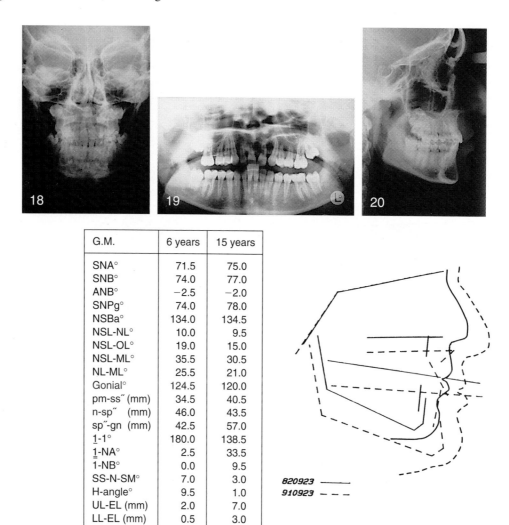

G.M.	6 years	15 years
SNA°	71.5	75.0
SNB°	74.0	77.0
ANB°	−2.5	−2.0
SNPg°	74.0	78.0
NSBa°	134.0	134.5
NSL-NL°	10.0	9.5
NSL-OL°	19.0	15.0
NSL-ML°	35.5	30.5
NL-ML°	25.5	21.0
Gonial°	124.5	120.0
pm-ss″ (mm)	34.5	40.5
n-sp″ (mm)	46.0	43.5
sp″-gn (mm)	42.5	57.0
1-1°	180.0	138.5
1-NA°	2.5	33.5
1-NB°	0.0	9.5
SS-N-SM°	7.0	3.0
H-angle°	9.5	1.0
UL-EL (mm)	2.0	7.0
LL-EL (mm)	0.5	3.0

820923 ———
910923 – – –

21

Figure 14–18 *Continued.* *17* to *20,* X-ray status at age 17 years. *21,* Cephalometric analysis at ages 6 and 15 years.

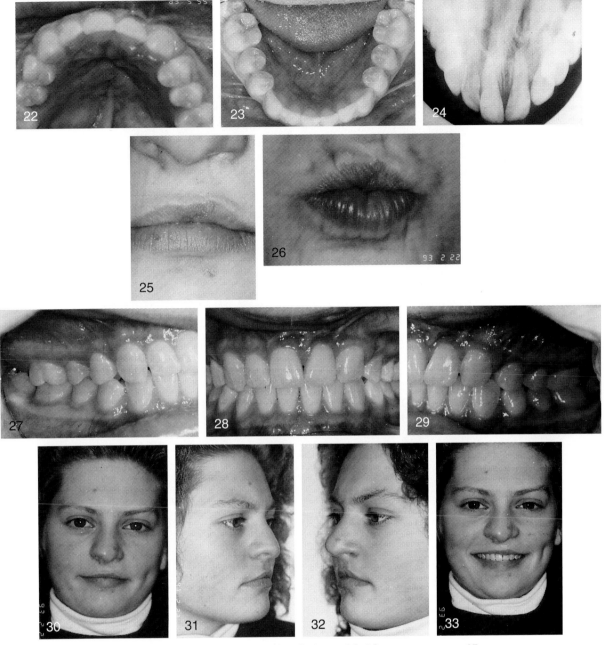

Figure 14-18 *Continued. 22* to *33,* Dental occlusion and facial appearance at age 17 years.

Category 2A

This category includes total UCLP and BCLP, and occasionally CP.

Moderate skeletal facial discrepancies:

Moderate underdevelopment of upper jaw (sagittal, vertical, transverse); normal or increased height of lower jaw; moderate discrepancy of the basal sagittal, vertical, transverse jaw relationship; Angle class III occlusion with moderate anterior crossbite and normal to deep overbite; partial or total posterior crossbite.

The patient illustrated in Figure 14–19 underwent presurgical orthopedics, transverse expansion for 3 months, protraction for 1 year, and orthodontic tooth alignment with a stable end result. The patients illustrated in Figures 14–5, 14–13, and 14–15

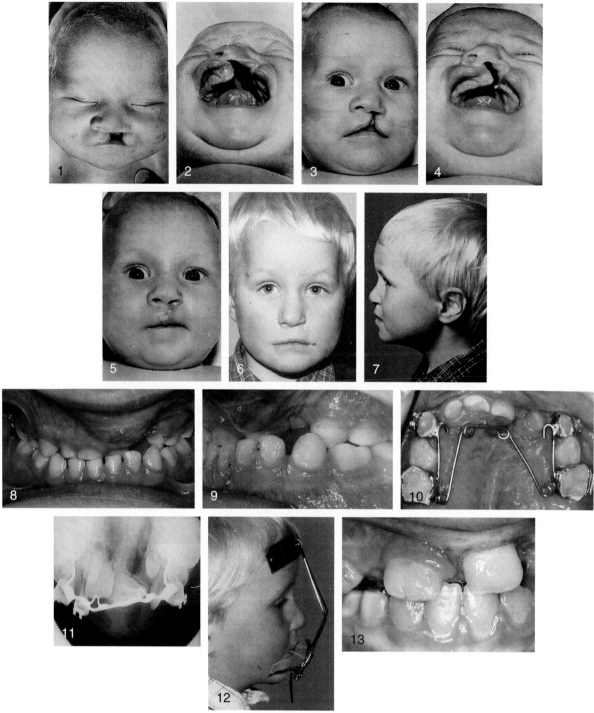

Figure 14–19. Complete UCLP, category 2A. *1, 2,* At birth, January 1974. *3, 4,* After presurgical orthopedics. *5,* Lip closure at age 3 months. *6 to 9,* At age 6 years, moderate anterior and unilateral posterior crossbites. *10 to 13,* Interceptive orthopedics from age 5 years: transverse expansion (3 months) followed by protraction (12 months) to alleviate spontaneous eruption of upper permanent incisors into normal position; retention by a fixed palatal arch wire.

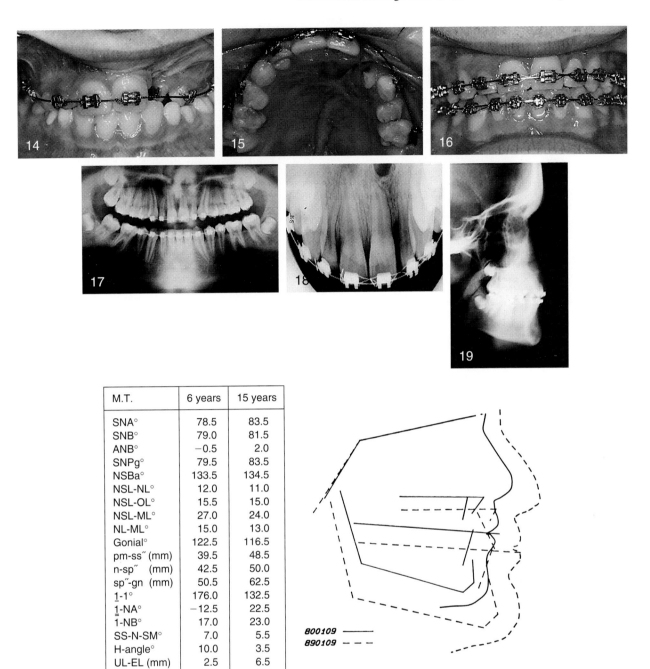

M.T.	6 years	15 years
SNA°	78.5	83.5
SNB°	79.0	81.5
ANB°	−0.5	2.0
SNPg°	79.5	83.5
NSBa°	133.5	134.5
NSL-NL°	12.0	11.0
NSL-OL°	15.5	15.0
NSL-ML°	27.0	24.0
NL-ML°	15.0	13.0
Gonial°	122.5	116.5
pm-ss″ (mm)	39.5	48.5
n-sp″ (mm)	42.5	50.0
sp″-gn (mm)	50.5	62.5
1-1°	176.0	132.5
1-NA°	−12.5	22.5
1-NB°	17.0	23.0
SS-N-SM°	7.0	5.5
H-angle°	10.0	3.5
UL-EL (mm)	2.5	6.5
LL-EL (mm)	2.0	4.0

800109 ———
890109 – – –

20

Figure 14–19 *Continued. 14, 15,* Alignment of upper central incisors at age 8 years; secondary bone grafting at age 10 years. *16* to *19,* Conventional orthodontics for 24 months until 15 years. *20,* Cephalometric analysis at ages 6 and 15 years.

Illustration continued on following page

underwent similar treatment strategies in this category. Figure 14–20 illustrates a patient with UCLP who underwent transverse expansion, protraction, and secondary bone grafting. Space had to be provided for upper incisors, and the left cuspid was moved into the space of the left lateral incisor.

Need for treatment:

Interceptive orthopedics: transverse expansion and anterior protraction of the upper jaw at 6 to 7 years of age.

Alignment of permanent incisors in the cleft area(s) at 7 to 8 years of age.

Bone grafting at 8–11 years of age.

Conventional orthodontic treatment at 11 to 13 years of age.

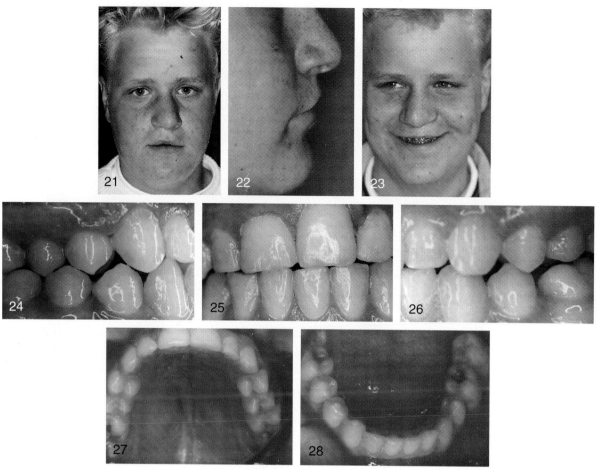

Figure 14–19 *Continued.* *21* to *28,* Dental occlusion and facial appearance at age 16 years (patient moved abroad; no later registration).

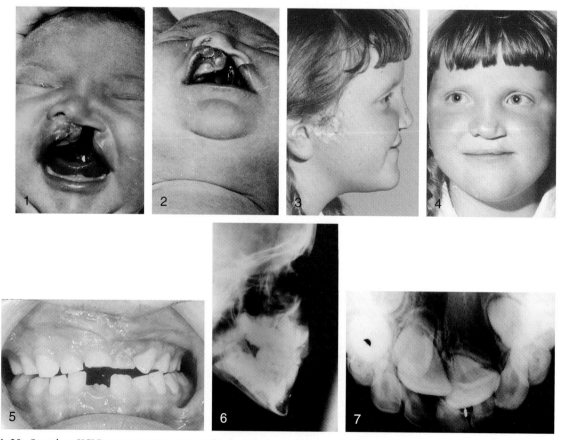

Figure 14–20. Complete UCLP, category 2A. *1, 2,* At birth, February 1971. *3* to *7,* At age 6 years, moderate anterior and unilateral posterior crossbites and lack of space for optimal eruption of upper incisors.

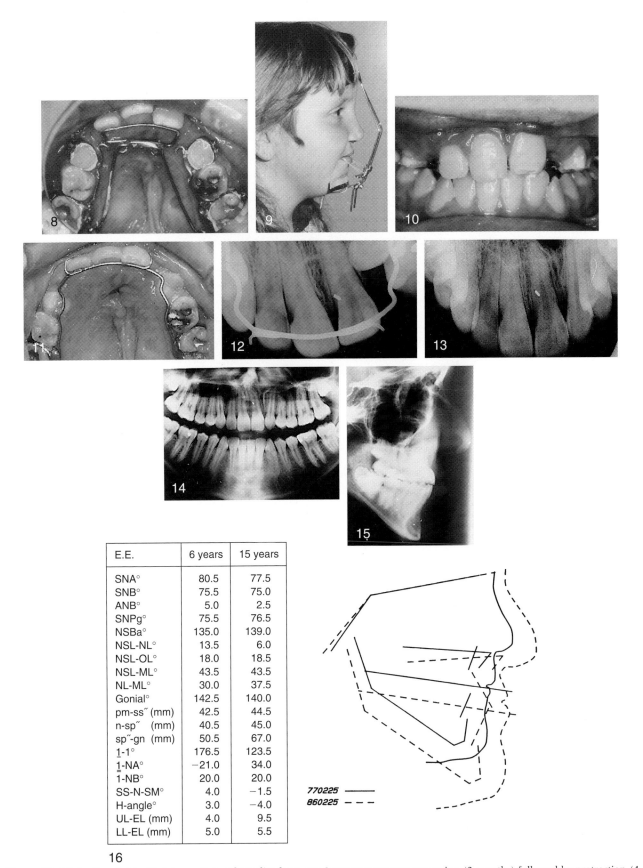

E.E.	6 years	15 years
SNA°	80.5	77.5
SNB°	75.5	75.0
ANB°	5.0	2.5
SNPg°	75.5	76.5
NSBa°	135.0	139.0
NSL-NL°	13.5	6.0
NSL-OL°	18.0	18.5
NSL-ML°	43.5	43.5
NL-ML°	30.0	37.5
Gonial°	142.5	140.0
pm-ss″ (mm)	42.5	44.5
n-sp″ (mm)	40.5	45.0
sp″-gn (mm)	50.5	67.0
1-1°	176.5	123.5
1-NA°	−21.0	34.0
1-NB°	20.0	20.0
SS-N-SM°	4.0	−1.5
H-angle°	3.0	−4.0
UL-EL (mm)	4.0	9.5
LL-EL (mm)	5.0	5.5

770225 ⎯⎯⎯
860225 ⎯ ⎯ ⎯

16

Figure 14–20 *Continued. 8 to 12,* Interceptive orthopedics from age 8 years: transverse expansion (2 months) followed by protraction (4 months) to alleviate spontaneous eruption of upper permanent incisors into normal position; retention by a fixed palatal arch wire; secondary bone grafting at age 8 years; left upper lateral incisor missing; improvement of the occlusion through opening of a space for bridgework between left upper cuspid and first premolar was rejected. *13 to 15,* X-ray status at age 15 years. *16,* Cephalometric analysis at ages 6 and 15 years.

Illustration continued on following page

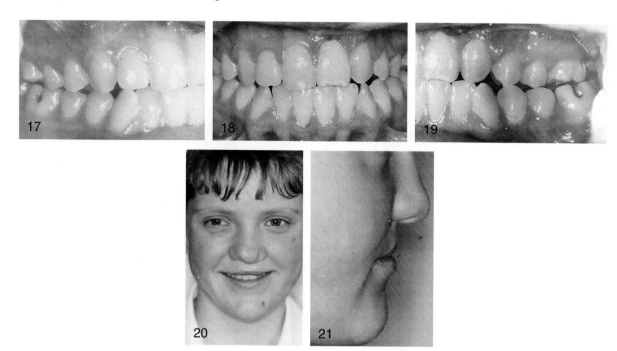

Figure 14–20 *Continued. 17* to *21,* Dental occlusion and facial appearance at age 15.

Category 2B

This category, which cannot be diagnostically differentiated from category 2A until patients are 13 to 15 years of age, includes total UCLP, BCLP, and occasionally CP.

Severe skeletal facial discrepancies:

Severe underdevelopment of upper jaw (sagittal, vertical, transverse), mandibular excess that results in Angle class III occlusion with anterior and posterior cross-bites and vertical skeletal open bite.

The patient illustrated in Figure 14–21 has complete UCLP with an anterior cross-bite and deep overbite that were treated by transverse expansion for 3 months, protraction headgear for 9 months, and then orthodontic tooth alignment. Further growth will determine whether orthognathic surgery is needed to improve the facial appearance and dental occlusion. The patient with BCLP shown in Figure 14–22 had the lower left second premolar transplanted to the space for the upper right second premolar. Orthognathic surgery was performed at 20 years. The patient shown in Figure 14–23 had BCLP with a severe anterior crossbite in the permanent dentition, which was corrected with a protraction headgear for 2 years starting at the age of 12 years with a good response in spite of his age. The patient illustrated in Figure 14–14 underwent transverse expansion and wore protraction headgear to correct the maxillary sagittal deficiency in preparation for the orthognathic surgery.

Need for treatment:

Interceptive orthopedics: transverse expansion and anterior protraction of the upper jaw at 6 to 7 years of age.

Alignment of permanent incisors in the cleft area(s) at 7 to 8 years of age.

Bone graft at 8–11 years of age.

Conventional orthodontic treatment at 11 to 13 years of age.

Combined orthognathic and surgical correction in adulthood after completion of growth.

Text continued on page 295

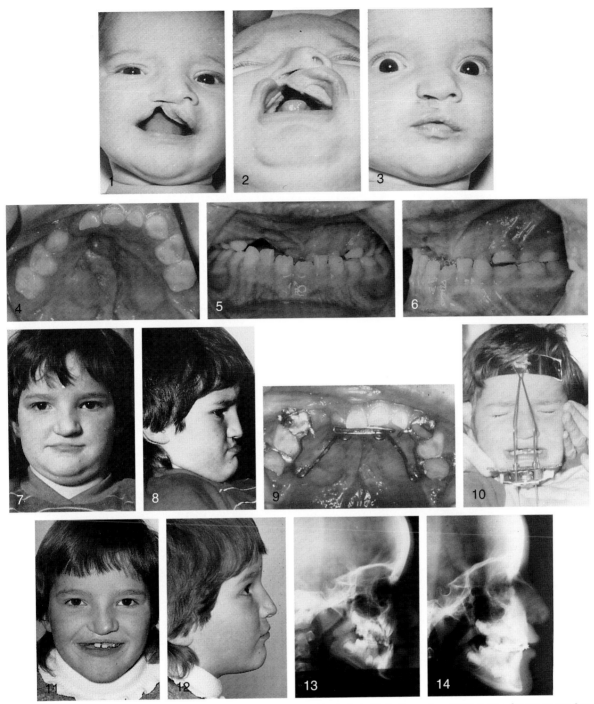

Figure 14–21. Complete UCLP except for a soft tissue band, category 2B. *1, 2,* At birth, December 1978; *3,* Lip closure at age 3 months; *4 to 8, 13,* At age 5.5 years, marked anterior and bilateral crossbites; no familiar mandibular prognathism known.

Illustration continued on following page

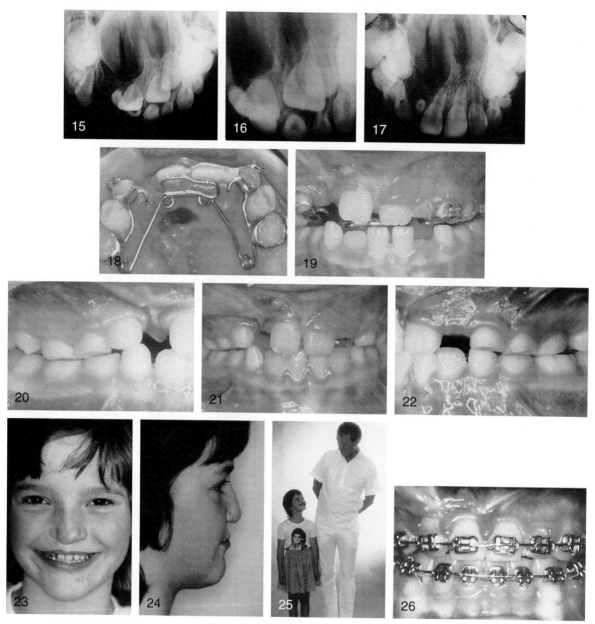

Figure 14–21 *Continued. 9* to *24,* Interceptive orthopedics from age 5.5 years: transverse expansion (3 months) followed by protraction (9 months) to alleviate spontaneous eruption of upper right permanent incisor into normal position; secondary bone grafting at age 8 years; right upper lateral incisor was missing. *25, 26,* Conventional orthodontics at age 11 years lasting for 25 months; bonded retainer.

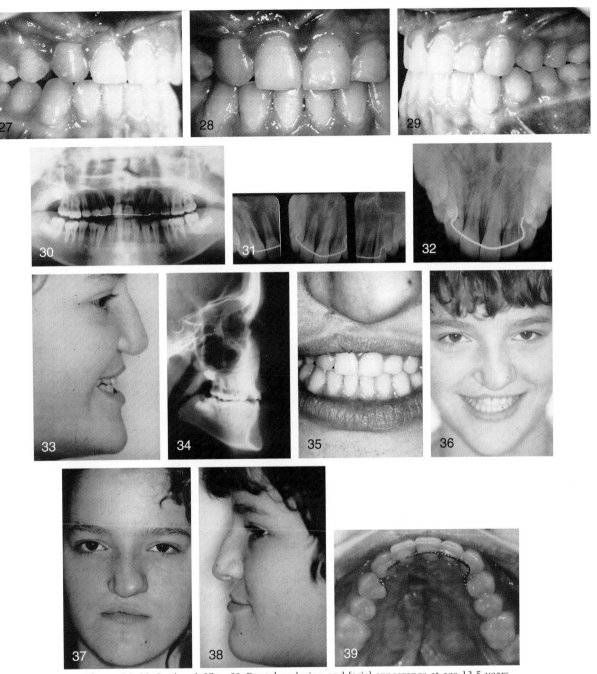

Figure 14–21 *Continued. 27 to 39,* Dental occlusion and facial appearance at age 13.5 years.

Illustration continued on following page

S.A.	6 years	15 years
SNA°	82.0	74.5
SNB°	76.0	79.0
ANB°	6.0	−4.5
SNPg°	77.5	81.0
NSBa°	129.0	135.5
NSL-NL°	6.5	5.0
NSL-OL°	15.0	15.5
NSL-ML°	34.5	32.5
NL-ML°	35.0	27.5
Gonial°	124.5	124.5
pm-ss″ (mm)	37.5	38.5
n-sp″ (mm)	36.5	43.5
sp″-gn (mm)	55.5	67.5
1-1°	139.0	141.5
1-NA°	15.5	28.5
1-NB°	19.5	14.5
SS-N-SM°	5.5	−1.0
H-angle°	11.0	−5.0
UL-EL (mm)	3.0	10.5
LL-EL (mm)	2.5	7.5

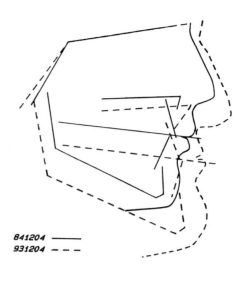

841204 ———
931204 — — —

40

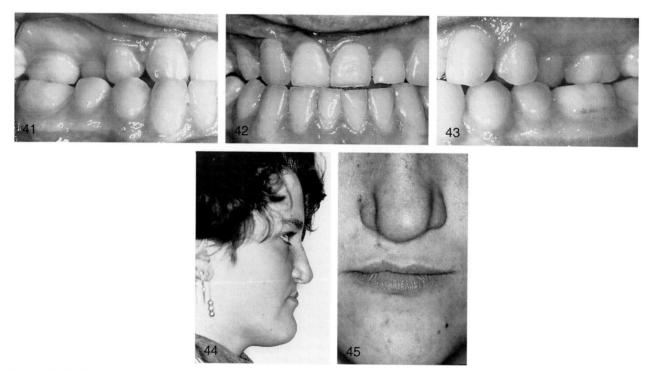

Figure 14–21 *Continued. 40,* Cephalometric analysis at ages 6 and 15 years. *41 to 45,* At age 15 years, unfavorable growth has generated maxillary retrognathism with an edge-to-edge bite and a concave profile, which probably indicate orthognathic advancement of the maxilla at age 16 years.

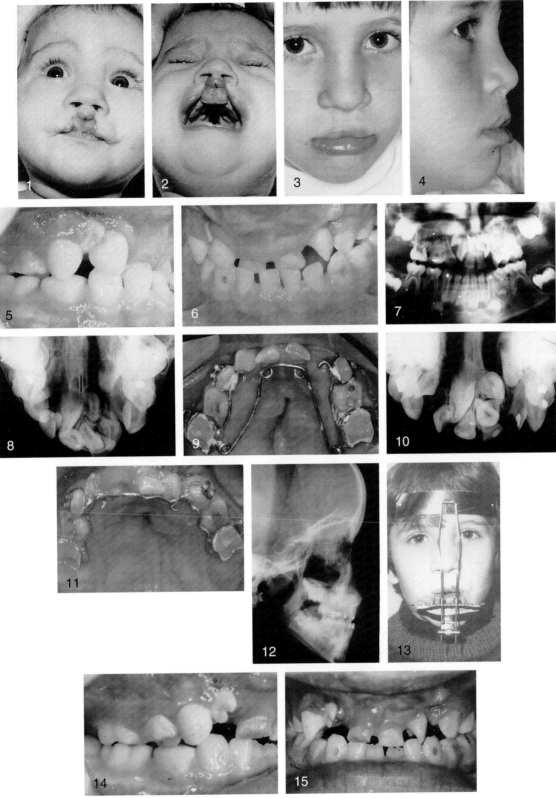

Figure 14–22. Complete BCLP except for soft tissue bands, category 2B. *1, 2,* At birth, November 1973. *3 to 8,* At age 6 years, marked anterior and unilateral crossbite; crowded incisor buds; the two upper and the right lower second premolars were missing. *9 to 15,* Interceptive orthopedics from age 6 years: transverse expansion (3 months) followed by protraction (12 months); malformed upper right lateral incisor was removed.

Illustration continued on following page

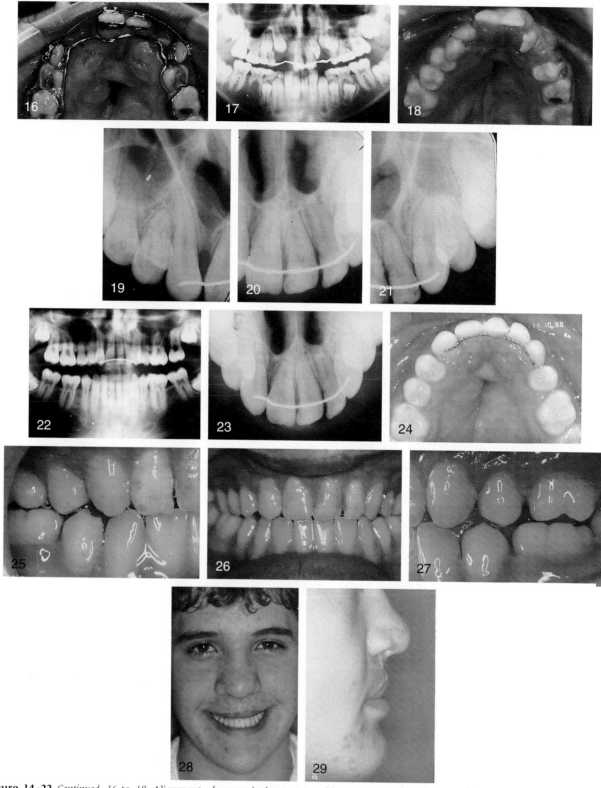

Figure 14–22 *Continued. 16* to *18,* Alignment of upper incisors at age 10 years; secondary bone grafting at age 10 years; left lower bicuspid transplanted to upper right region at age 12 years; conventional orthodontics from age 11 years (28 months); bonded retainer. *19* to *29,* Dental occlusion and facial appearance at age 15 years.

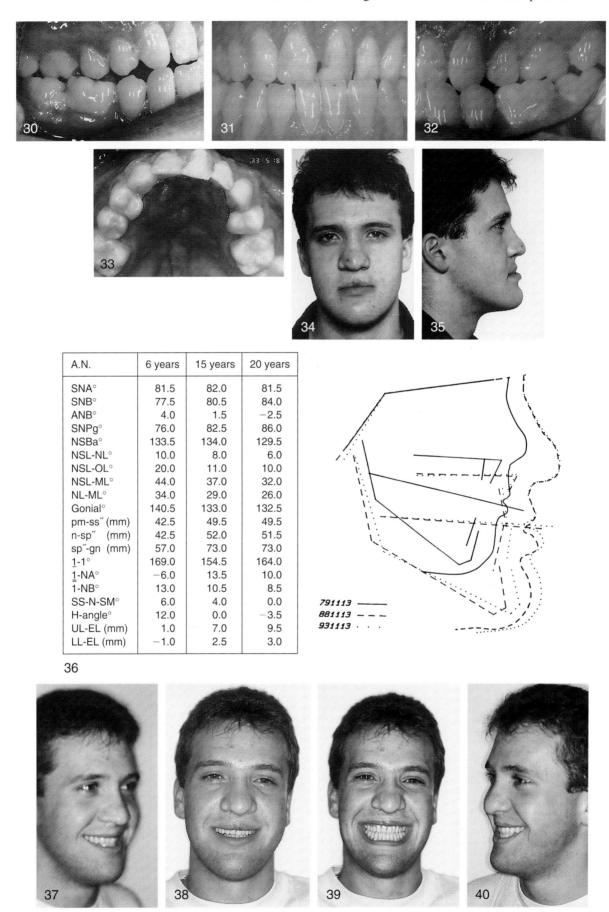

A.N.	6 years	15 years	20 years
SNA°	81.5	82.0	81.5
SNB°	77.5	80.5	84.0
ANB°	4.0	1.5	−2.5
SNPg°	76.0	82.5	86.0
NSBa°	133.5	134.0	129.5
NSL-NL°	10.0	8.0	6.0
NSL-OL°	20.0	11.0	10.0
NSL-ML°	44.0	37.0	32.0
NL-ML°	34.0	29.0	26.0
Gonial°	140.5	133.0	132.5
pm-ss″ (mm)	42.5	49.5	49.5
n-sp″ (mm)	42.5	52.0	51.5
sp″-gn (mm)	57.0	73.0	73.0
1-1°	169.0	154.5	164.0
1-NA°	−6.0	13.5	10.0
1-NB°	13.0	10.5	8.5
SS-N-SM°	6.0	4.0	0.0
H-angle°	12.0	0.0	−3.5
UL-EL (mm)	1.0	7.0	9.5
LL-EL (mm)	−1.0	2.5	3.0

791113 ———
881113 — — —
931113 · · · ·

36

Figure 14–22 *Continued. 30* to *35,* At age 20 years, unfavorable growth had generated maxillary retrognathism and mandibular overdevelopment with a moderate anterior crossbite. *36,* Cephalometric analysis at ages 6, 15, and 20 years. *37* to *43,* After orthognathic surgery at age 20.2 years (mandibular vertical ramus osteotomy, January 1994).

Illustration continued on following page

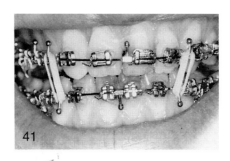

A.N.	20.2 years
SNA°	81.5
SNB°	80.5
ANB°	1.0
SNPg°	82.0
NSBa°	130.0
NSL-NL°	6.0
NSL-OL°	13.0
NSL-ML°	37.0
NL-ML°	30.5
Gonial°	136.5
pm-ss″ (mm)	49.5
n-sp″ (mm)	52.0
sp″-gn (mm)	74.5
1-1°	155.0
1-NA°	10.0
1-NB°	11.0
SS-N-SM°	5.5
H-angle°	1.0
UL-EL (mm)	8.0
LL-EL (mm)	4.0

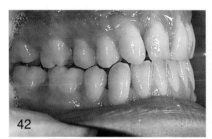
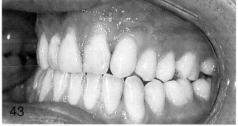

Figure 14–22 *Continued.*

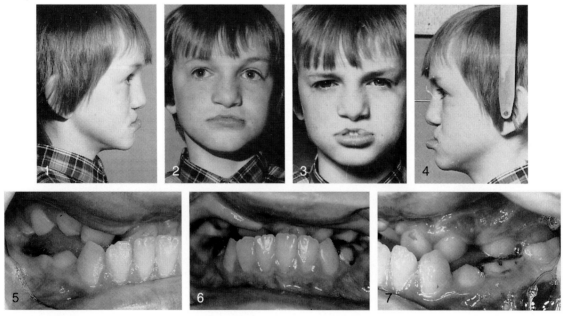

Figure 14–23. BCLP (complete right side and incomplete left side), category 2B: born November 1968; patient was not seen until age 10.5 years. *1* to *7*, Extreme anterior-bilateral crossbites in the late mixed dentition without adequate dental support for fixed interceptive orthopedics.

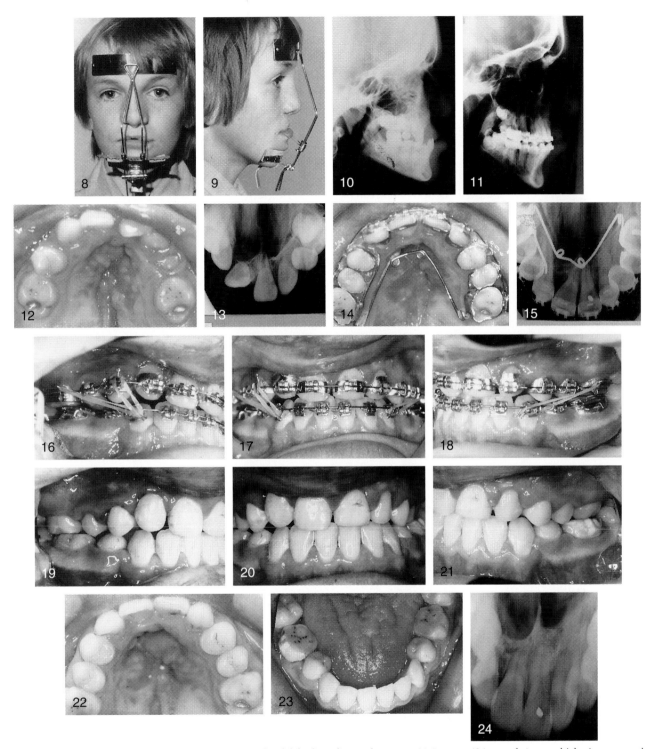

Figure 14–23 *Continued.* *8* to *13*, Protraction from fixed labial appliance from age 11.5 years (26 months), at which time normal proclination limited further protrusion. *14* to *18*, Conventional orthodontics, including transverse expansion; both maxillary lateral incisors were missing; both lower first premolars were removed; remaining anterior crossbite was corrected by retroclination of the lower incisors. *19* to *24*, Dentition at age 15.5 years.

Illustration continued on following page

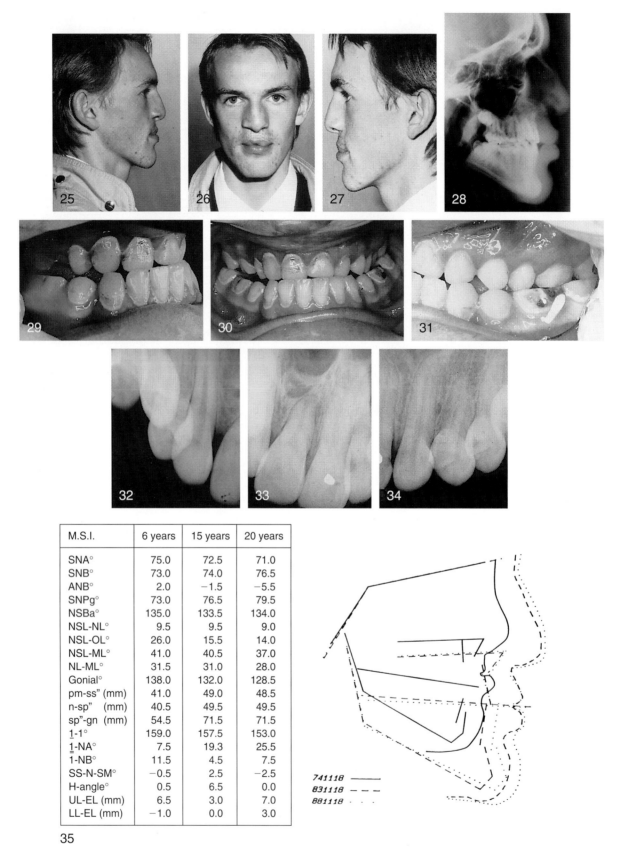

M.S.I.	6 years	15 years	20 years
SNA°	75.0	72.5	71.0
SNB°	73.0	74.0	76.5
ANB°	2.0	−1.5	−5.5
SNPg°	73.0	76.5	79.5
NSBa°	135.0	133.5	134.0
NSL-NL°	9.5	9.5	9.0
NSL-OL°	26.0	15.5	14.0
NSL-ML°	41.0	40.5	37.0
NL-ML°	31.5	31.0	28.0
Gonial°	138.0	132.0	128.5
pm-ss" (mm)	41.0	49.0	48.5
n-sp" (mm)	40.5	49.5	49.5
sp"-gn (mm)	54.5	71.5	71.5
1-1°	159.0	157.5	153.0
1-NA°	7.5	19.3	25.5
1-NB°	11.5	4.5	7.5
SS-N-SM°	−0.5	2.5	−2.5
H-angle°	0.5	6.5	0.0
UL-EL (mm)	6.5	3.0	7.0
LL-EL (mm)	−1.0	0.0	3.0

741118 ———
831118 — — —
881118 · · · ·

35

Figure 14–23 *Continued. 25 to 31,* Facial appearance and dental occlusion at age 19 years; unfavorable growth had produced a moderate anterior crossbite; the patient found this result acceptable and rejected orthognatic surgery. *32–34,* Radiographs. *35,* Cephalometric analysis at ages 6, 15, and 20 years.

Interceptive Orthopedic Treatment in the Late Primary/Early Mixed Dentition: Indications for the Protraction Face Mask

The aims of interceptive orthopedic treatment at this stage are to

• Correct midface skeletal deficiency.
• Eliminate anterior and/or posterior crossbite.
• Provide optimal space for spontaneous incisor eruption.
• Improve the soft tissue profile.

The introduction of the facial mask for early protraction by heavy forces to the maxillary complex in CLP patients was reported by Delaire and colleagues.[66,79] The facial mask provided a mechanism for influencing and promoting skeletal and dentoalveolar correction by influencing the circummaxillary sutures (Fig. 14–24A). Before 1970, the chin cup provided mainly dentoalveolar retroclination of the mandibular incisors to correct the class III incisal relationship with limited effect (see Fig. 14–24B). Extraoral forces from the facial mask can be directed forward and downward from the maxillary cuspid area of the alveolar process (Fig. 14–25). Use of a facial mask also allows the establishment of good vertical closure of the incisors after correction of an anterior crossbite and thereby increases posttreatment stability.

Since 1977, all CLP patients with anterior and/or posterior crossbites have received an interceptive orthodontic treatment phase during the deciduous and early mixed-dentition periods.[25,36,37,81,84,85]

The Bergen rationale has been predicated on early transverse, sagittal, and vertical modification and redirection of circummaxillary growth in all three dimensions:

1. Transverse expansion of the upper jaw.
2. Anterior protraction of the upper jaw.
3. Fixed retention by a palatal arch wire.

In order to obtain more favorable conditions for midfacial growth and development, transverse expansion followed by maxillary protraction allows the permanent incisors to erupt spontaneously into a positive overjet and overbite position. Thus the aim of the orthopedic forces to the maxilla is to improve the midface skeletal deficiency. This interceptive orthopedic treatment phase starts at age 6 years and lasts about 15 months (two visits for a transverse expansion of about 10 mm during 3 months, and additional four visits for protraction during 12 months) with an average of six visits.

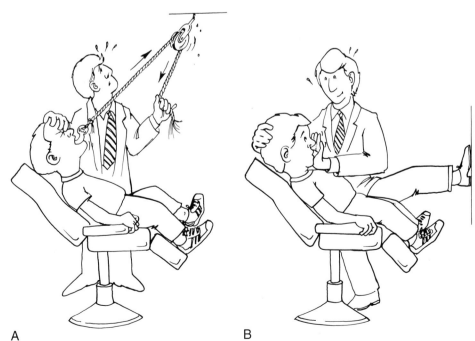

A   B

Figure 14–24. Results are obtained more readily by pulling forward *A*, and pushing backward *B*, at the same time.

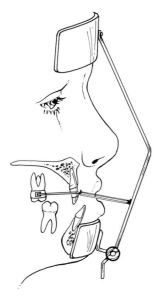

Figure 14–25. Facial mask supported by forehead and chin. Elastic bands from the maxillary cuspid area to the bar provides the force system (forward and downward).

The orthopedic/orthodontic treatment of a patient with CLP must be based on short, optimal periods of active, controlled, efficient orthodontic treatment.[43] Fixed appliances both during treatment and, to a large extent, during retention yield the most effective cost-benefit ratio.

Appliances

A fixed appliance system for both transverse expansion and protraction of the maxilla should provide controlled expansion, attachment for anterior traction by facial mask, and compatibility with edgewise appliance therapy and should allow good hygiene. The production of such an appliance is illustrated in Figure 14–26. A modified quad-helix* appliance is soldered to four bands (with tubes or brackets) on the second deciduous molars and cuspids (Fig. 14–27A,B). The first deciduous molar is thus locked and serves as additional anchorage was well. The permanent molars are used only when the second deciduous molars are missing or decayed. Bands on the deciduous cuspids allow the important downward-directed pull from the mask (Fig. 14–28). The fixed appliance is able to resist any counterclockwise rotational effect on the nasal (NL) and occlusion (OL) planes that typically results from using class III mechanics on upper molars.

Transverse Expansion

The typical expansion period lasts 3 months, with two activations at 6-week intervals. As a rule, transverse expansion is completed before protraction begins. Transverse expansion is achieved at a rate of approximately 3 mm per month, regardless of cleft type.[84,85] The appliances are individually activated extraorally before being recemented. A force of about 200 g on each side is considered optimal (see Figs. 14–7, 14–8, 14–17). Often the canine area needs more expansion than the molar areas. As there is a great tendency for relapse, some overexpansion is necessary. Hooks attached mesiolingually to the cuspid bands provide attachment for elastic bands connected to a facial mask if protraction is needed. The quad-helix appliance also allows the combined use of conventional labial orthodontic archwires for alignment of the incisors. Because there is no midpalatine suture to be split, the quad-helix appliance is well suited to gently applying forces to the scar tissue after surgical palatal repair. Rapid palatal expansion is a rational approach to splitting the midpalatal bony suture but is inappropriate for stretching the scar tissue and may result in creating an oronasal fistula.

No significant sagittal forward movement of maxilla was revealed after treatment was limited to transverse expansion. A downward clockwise rotation of the mandible had occurred.[84] By comparing the use of fixed quad-helix appliances with removable

---

* Rocky Mountain: Maxillary quad-helix appliance, 0.38 (0.965 mm) Blue Elgiloy (Ricketts).

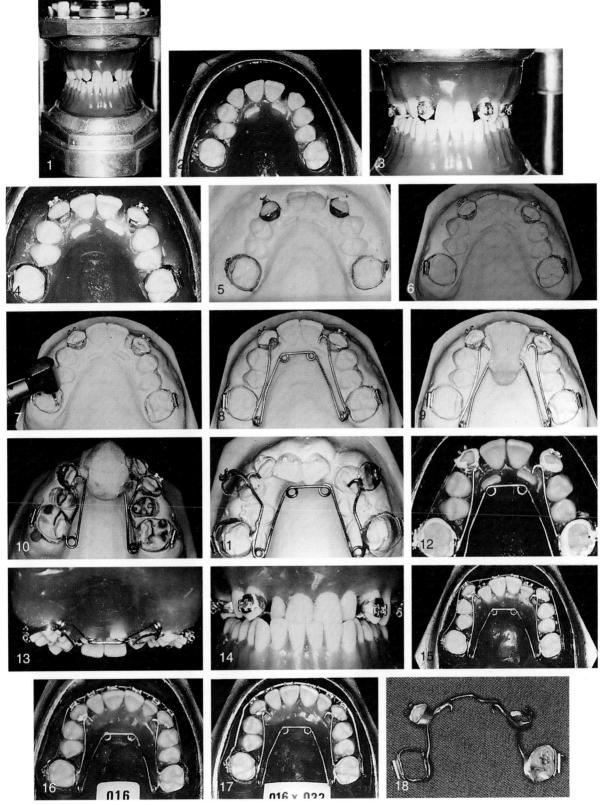

Figure 14–26. *1* to *10*, Production of a modified quad-helix appliance. *11* to *14*, Transverse expansion. *15, 16,* Combined with round labial arches for alignment of incisors. *17,* Labial root-torque of incisors by rectangular arch wire. *18,* Fixed palatal retention until shedding of the deciduous anchor teeth.

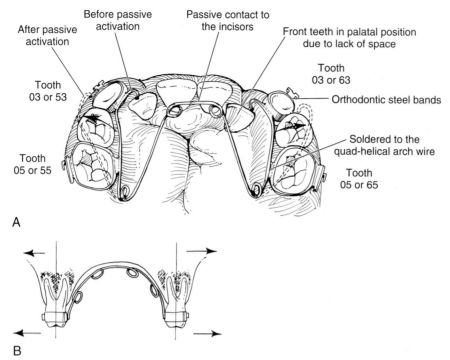

Figure 14–27. Modified quad-helix appliance. *A,* Occlusal view of quad-helix spring soldered to bands on deciduous cuspids and molars. Note hooks mesial to the cuspids. Drawn line is passive; stippled line was activated before cementation. *B,* Frontal view indicating position of the helices in relation to palate. The rigid appliance makes parallel expansion possible.

expansion plates on non-CLP patients, Hermanson and coworkers[86] found that the quad-helix appliance had better effects and entailed fewer visits, lower costs, and shorter treatment time. An acrylic plate would occupy more space, would tend to further lower the tongue position, and would not readily resist the forward-downward traction of the cuspid region from a facial mask.

Protraction

The quad-helix appliance is formed to contact the incisors passively (Fig. 14–27A), directly by bends or by a soldered-on extension (see Figs. 14–8, part 13; 14–13, part 13). In cases in which no transverse expansion is needed or when the quad-helix appliance is uncomfortable after the expansion period, a simple lingual arch is soldered to four bands on second deciduous molars and cuspids (see Figs. 14–26, part 18; 14–28, part 13).

The protraction starts when the maxillary expansion is complete. The quad-helix appliance is used as anchorage for the facial mask (Delaire)* (see Fig. 14–25). No other fixation of the mask is needed than the two intraoral elastic bands† from hooks in the canine regions to a bar on the mask. The force used for facial protraction is about 350 g on each side (thus a total of 700 g). The face mask is used mainly at night for 10 to 12 hours.

If the maxillary protraction is delayed until the permanent incisors are fully erupted and if a downward force component to the maxillary incisor teeth is indicated, the incisors are bonded. In cases in which the incisors should be protruded bodily to obtain labial bone deposition, the use of edgewise arch wires may be indicated, if necessary, with labial root torque.[80]

---

* Nichrominox: Masque orthodontique des Drs. Delaire et Verdon.
† Unitek: Latex ex-oral 1/4''LGT; Unitek/3M: ''Fran'' 8oz. 1/4'' (404-736)

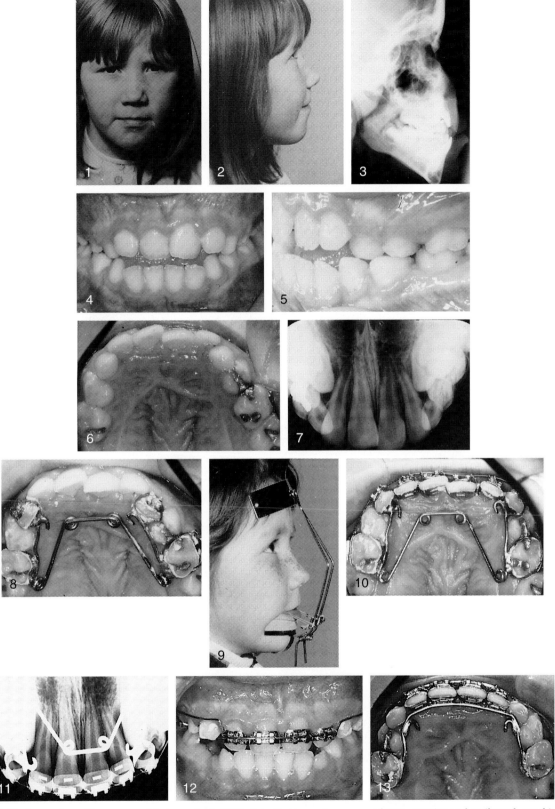

Figure 14-28. Incomplete CP, category 2A: born April 1971. *1* to *7,* At age 6 years, moderate anterior and unilateral crossbites and basal open bite configuration. *8* to *9,* Interceptive orthopedics from age 7.5 years: transverse expansion (3 months), followed by protraction (7 months); *10* to *13,* Alignment of upper incisors (6 months), retained by fixed palatal arch wire.

Illustration continued on following page

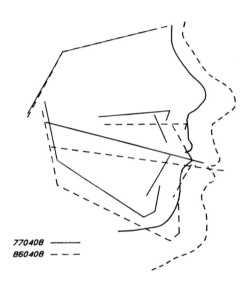

S.H.I.	6 years	15 years
SNA°	82.5	86.0
SNB°	78.0	80.5
ANB°	4.5	5.5
SNPg°	76.0	80.0
NSBa°	133.0	131.5
NSL-NL°	8.0	12.5
NSL-OL°	27.5	21.0
NSL-ML°	46.0	39.0
NL-ML°	38.0	26.5
Gonial°	135.0	127.5
pm-ss″ (mm)	36.0	43.1
n-sp″ (mm)	44.0	51.5
sp″-gn (mm)	55.5	62.0
1-1°	124.5	119.5
1-NA°	19.0	21.5
1-NB°	32.0	33.5
SS-N-SM°	4.5	9.5
H-angle°	15.0	14.0
UL-EL (mm)	1.0	2.0
LL-EL (mm)	-1.5	2.0

770408 ⎯⎯⎯
860408 ⎯ ⎯ ⎯

16

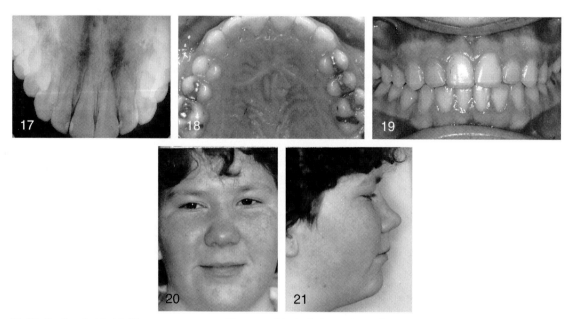

Figure 14–28 *Continued. 14, 15,* X-ray status at age 15 years. *16,* Cephalometric analysis at ages 6 and 15 years. *17 to 21,* Dental occlusion and facial appearance at age 15 years; no retention.

Clinical Results

The orthopedic/orthodontic forward traction of the upper jaw acting on the circummaxillary sutures and the resulting effect on the dentition is more effective[25, 36] than previous attempts to retrain mandibular growth with a chin cup.[32, 33] This means that insofar as the sagittal jaw discrepancy results from underdevelopment of the upper jaw, the prognosis is good.[37, 81] A fair response of the sagittal basal jaw relationship was found in 63% of the cases (mean increase of angle ANB, 3.3°), whereas a response of forward movement of maxilla was found in 44% of the cases (mean distance, 2.4 mm). A fair response of both skeletal combined maxillomandibular change and skeletal forward movement of maxilla was found in 35% of the cases.[37] Insofar as the discrepancy results from overgrowth of the mandible, the result is limited mainly to a concomitant downward and backward rotation of the mandible.

Predictor variables were associated mainly with maxillary underdevelopment, characterized by retrusion of the upper jaw, short sagittal length of maxilla that resulted in skeletal sagittal discrepancy, and counterclockwise inclination of the occlusal plane with retrusion of the upper lip, the nose tip, and the maxillary dentition.[83] Mandibular retrognathism was prevalent among patients with skeletal maxillomandibular discrepancy, whereas a normal mandibular position was associated with favorable skeletal forward movement of maxilla during protraction. Clinically, the most striking features indicating favorable skeletal response were maxillary retrusion and a concave facial profile.

Limitations

Of importance with regard to categories 2A and 2B is that patients in these groups may not be differentially categorized until the age of 13 years for girls and often later for boys. The diagnostic differences between mandibular excess, maxillary retrusion, and dentoalveolar discrepancies are not accurately predicted before puberty (see Fig. 14–3C,D,E,F).[31, 38–42] After an early orthopedic protraction period, the individual growth pattern tends to revert to the original tendency of reduced maxillary growth, and an anterior crossbite may become reestablished as a result of further growth.[35]

It is important that the permanent upper incisors are not proclined beyond normal axial inclination during a second period of orthopedics and/or during the conventional orthodontic treatment. Thus the inclination of the maxillary permanent incisors limits the protraction treatment,[25] indicating that cases showing a sagittal basal discrepancy beyond a certain degree call for a combined orthodontic and surgical procedure.[87] For a successful orthopedic/orthodontic result, it is essential that the incisor inclination in both jaws is normal. For the same reason, a treatment plan that includes extraction of mandibular premolars for retrusion of the mandibular incisors should not be recommended until the growth pattern can be determined.

Stability and Relapse

As a consequence of surgical repair, maxillary growth and development in CLP patients may be affected apart from any intrinsic growth deficiencies. The mandible is not directly affected, but compensatory growth may be influenced by the clefting. Depending on the scarring after the surgical repair, the growth of the upper jaw may be influenced. Although there appears to be minimal relapse of the upper jaw,[35] its relative position after protraction may be influenced by the normally growing lower jaw. The amount of occlusal discrepancy established at the age of 6 years (before treatment) is a useful predictor for treating CLP patients by protraction (see description of category 2A), but exceptions are seen (see description of category 2B).

Soft Tissue Profile

Protraction treatment improves the lower face soft tissue profile, often within a few months (Fig. 14–21, parts 8, 11 to 14).[25, 35, 36, 84] The soft tissue profile changes include increased protrusion of the upper lip as well as improved sagittal lip relationships in both the BCLP and UCLP groups. This is noteworthy because the non-CLP control group showed a slight reduction in these variables during the same period.[84] In spite of significantly different effects on the subjacent bony parts, namely, significant increase of the bony maxillary prognathism in the UCLP group only and mainly dentoalveolar treatment effects in the BCLP group,[36] the soft tissue responses were rather similar. The magnitude of the total hard tissue changes, skeletal or dentoalveolar, seems to be the prime factor for the soft tissue changes with a close relationship between the soft tissue profile and the supporting hard tissue structures. A further improvement of the lip position in CLP patients during protraction would require more effect on the subjacent bone[88] because the angle ss-n-sm (ANB) was found to be the only cephalometric variable displaying a significant linear correlation with the attractiveness scores in adult CLP patients.[89]

UCLP and BCLP Patients

Although these two groups at the age of 6 years show differences in skeletodental morphology, the treatment considerations and the treatment objectives of the individual patients are in principle the same. The individual need for interceptive orthopedics may differ as much within the groups as between the groups. As previously described, significant increase of maxillary prognathism by protraction was found only in the UCLP group, whereas the treatment effects in the BCLP group were mainly dentoalveolar.[25] These observations of significant differences between the UCLP and BCLP groups in Bergen are most likely associated with the formerly used primary surgical procedures, including a periosteoplasty, that induced a bony fusion of the arch segments on one or both sides that may have impaired further growth. However, after protraction there was no longer a significant difference of the maxillary prognathism between the two CLP groups, and the sagittal position of the upper molars was normalized in both groups. The upper incisors were still retroclined in both groups, significantly more in the BCLP groups. Increase of the upper facial height (n-sp″) and clockwise rotation of the occlusal line were significantly greater in the BCLP group. On average, the period of protraction lasted 12 months in the UCLP group and 15 months in the BCLP group.[25]

Fixed Retention

It is essential that the results obtained after the early orthopedic treatment are stabilized by a fixed palatal arch, which is discontinued at the time the anchoring deciduous teeth are shed (see Fig. 14-26, part 18). Supervision by the local dentist at the patient's regular check-up visits is the rule. However, in cases with an unfavorable growth pattern, a Function Corrector III (FR-3)[90] may be considered as an active retainer option.

Long-Term Treatment Outcome

Patients in category 0   Very good (Figs. 14-9, 14-10, 14-12, 14-18, 14-29, 14-31, and 14-33)
Patients in category 1   Very good (Figs. 14-7, 14-8, and 14-17)
Patients in category 2A Good/fair for a permanent result (Figs. 14-5, 14-13, 14-15, 14-19, 14-20, 14-28, 14-30, and 14-32)
Patients in category 2B Good regarding the upper dentition, arch form, and position of incisors
Good regarding the soft tissue profile
Poor regarding a permanent result until adult age
(Figs. 14-14, 14-21, 14-22, and 14-23)

Patients assigned to category 2B may be candidates for orthognathic surgery at an adult age. This is no contraindication to an early interceptive treatment period of maxillary protraction provided it does not lead to dentoalveolar compensations that complicate possibility of later optimal surgical intervention. Long-term clinical experi-

Text continued on page 312

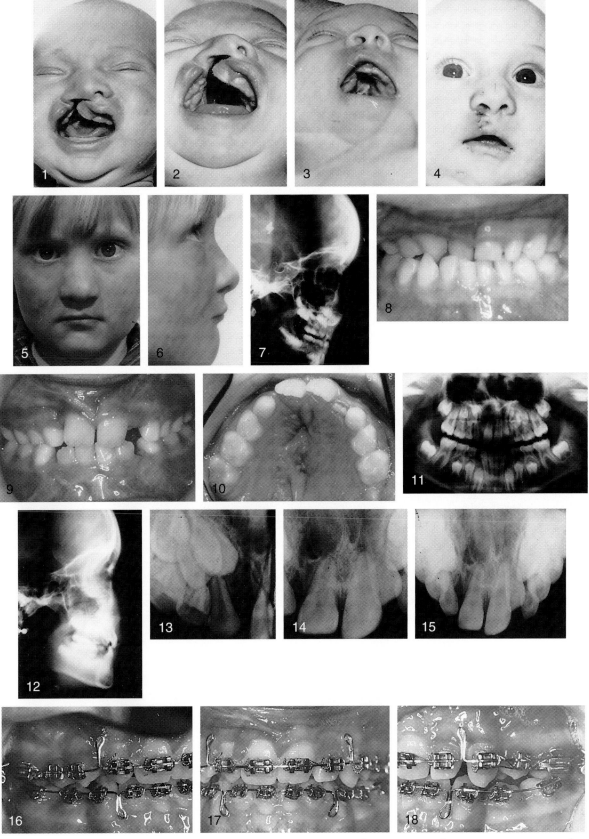

Figure 14–29. Complete UCLP, category 0. *1, 2,* At birth, June 1976. *3, 4,* Lip closure at 3 months. *5* to *8,* At age 6 years, favorable sagittal and transverse development except dentoalveolar crossbite of the right deciduous canine and central incisor (no early orthopedics); right upper lateral incisor missing. *9* to *15,* Inverted upper incisor protruded by a removable plate, no retention; secondary bone grafting at age 11 years to improve a tiny bony bridge.

Illustration continued on following page

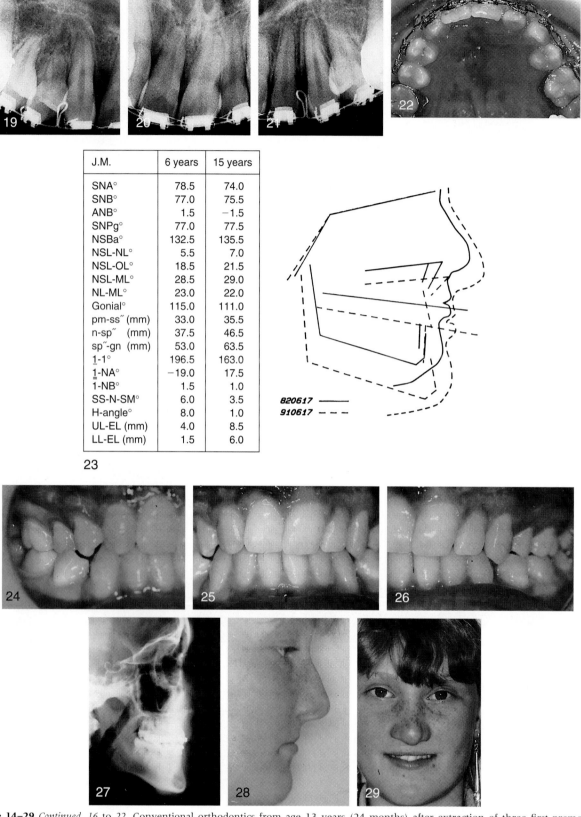

J.M.	6 years	15 years
SNA°	78.5	74.0
SNB°	77.0	75.5
ANB°	1.5	−1.5
SNPg°	77.0	77.5
NSBa°	132.5	135.5
NSL-NL°	5.5	7.0
NSL-OL°	18.5	21.5
NSL-ML°	28.5	29.0
NL-ML°	23.0	22.0
Gonial°	115.0	111.0
pm-ss″ (mm)	33.0	35.5
n-sp″ (mm)	37.5	46.5
sp″-gn (mm)	53.0	63.5
1-1°	196.5	163.0
1-NA°	−19.0	17.5
1-NB°	1.5	1.0
SS-N-SM°	6.0	3.5
H-angle°	8.0	1.0
UL-EL (mm)	4.0	8.5
LL-EL (mm)	1.5	6.0

820617 ———
910617 – – –

Figure 14–29 *Continued. 16* to *22,* Conventional orthodontics from age 13 years (24 months) after extraction of three first premolars. *23,* Cephalometric analysis at ages 6 and 15 years. *24* to *29,* Dental occlusion and facial appearance at age 17 years.

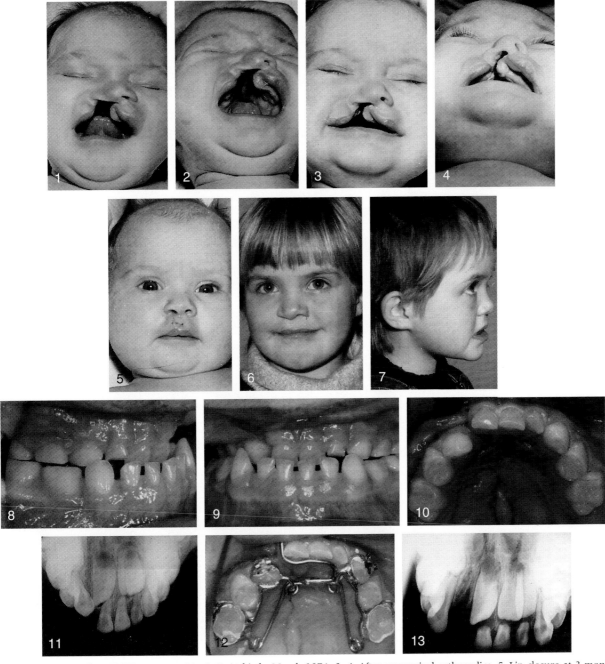

Figure 14–30. Complete UCLP, category 2A. *1, 2,* At birth, March 1976. *3, 4,* After presurgical orthopedics. *5,* Lip closure at 3 months. *6* to *11,* At age 6 years, moderate anterior and bilateral posterior crossbites with a tendency for dished-in profile; crowding as a result of lack of space; missing right upper lateral incision.

Illustration continued on following page

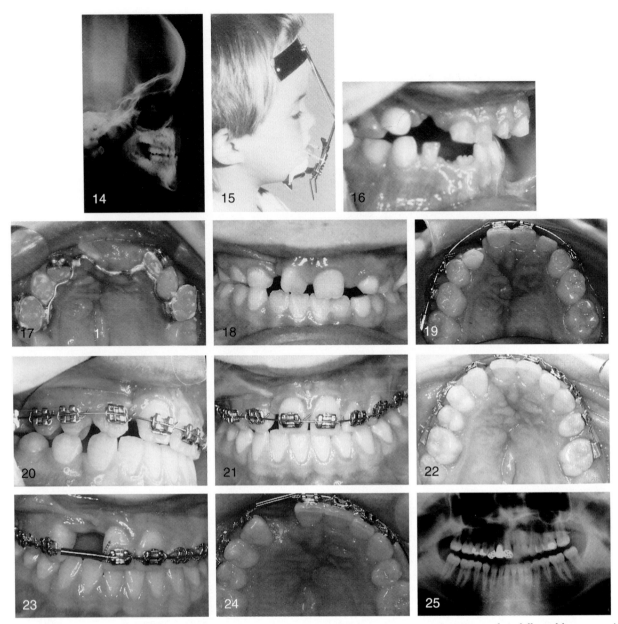

Figure 14-30 *Continued. 12* to *17,* Interceptive orthopedics from age 6 years: transverse expansion (3 months), followed by protraction (6 months); retention by fixed palatal arch wire. *18, 19,* Alignment of upper incisors (6 months); secondary bone grafting at age 11 years. *20* to *25,* Conventional orthodontics from age 13 years; left upper first premolar was extracted because of unilateral class II occlusion; space for right lateral incisor region was opened in order to establish correct position of maxillary incisors in accordance to facial midline, followed by a temporary bonded bridge.

M.C.	6 years	15 years
SNA°	75.5	73.0
SNB°	75.0	75.5
ANB°	0.5	−2.5
SNPg°	75.5	78.5
NSBa°	133.5	135.0
NSL-NL°	5.0	6.5
NSL-OL°	15.5	17.5
NSL-ML°	36.0	32.0
NL-ML°	31.0	25.5
Gonial°	128.5	119.5
pm-ss˝ (mm)	35.0	36.0
n-sp˝ (mm)	34.0	41.0
sp˝-gn (mm)	54.0	65.0
1-1°	162.0	144.5
1̲-NA°	10.0	25.5
1̄-NB°	7.5	13.0
SS-N-SM°	3.0	1.0
H-angle°	4.5	−2.5
UL-EL (mm)	2.0	6.5
LL-EL (mm)	1.5	4.5

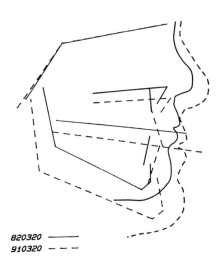

820320 ———
910320 − − −

26

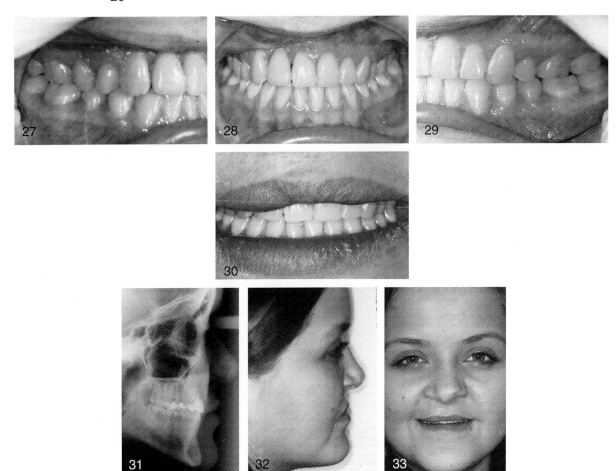

Figure 14–30 *Continued. 26*, Cephalometric analysis at ages 6 and 15 years. *27* to *33*, Dental occlusion and facial appearance at age 17 years.

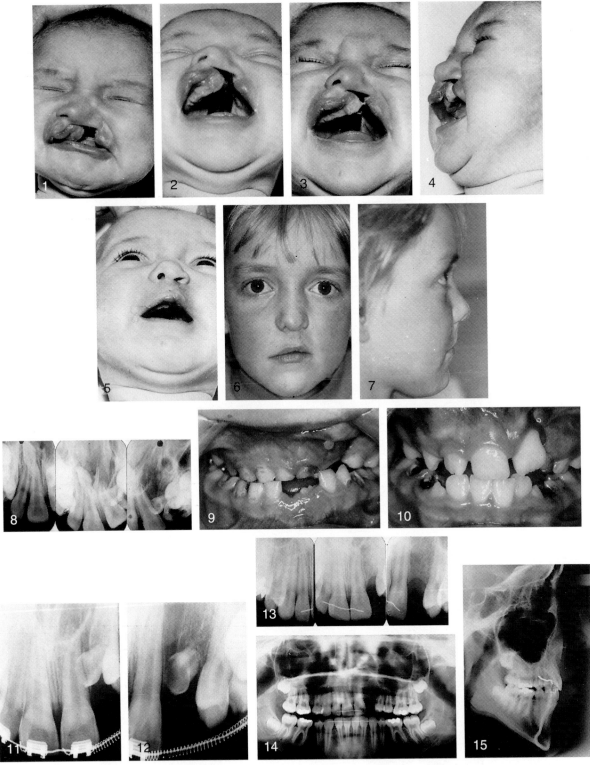

Figure 14–31. Complete UCLP, category 0. *1, 2,* At birth, April 1977. *3, 4,* After presurgical orthopedics. *5,* Lip closure at 3 months. *6 to 9,* At age 6 years, favorable growth; missing left upper lateral permanent incisor and canine; supernumerary mesiodens. *10 to 13,* Alignment of upper incisors at age 10; secondary bone grafting at age 11; conventional orthodontics at age 12 (12 months); three second premolars in the noncleft segments were removed; bonded retainers; in order to achieve correct midline, the space of upper left lateral incisor was left open for a future dental implant. *14, 15,* X-ray status at age 15.

S. E.	6 years	15 years
SNA°	76.5	73.0
SNB°	69.0	72.0
ANB°	7.5	1.0
SNPg°	68.5	72.0
NSBa°	132.0	131.5
NSL-NL°	7.5	8.5
NSL-OL°	22.5	21.5
NSL-ML°	47.0	46.0
NL-ML°	40.0	37.5
Gonial°	128.5	123.5
pm-ss″ (mm)	40.0	40.5
n-sp″ (mm)	43.0	51.5
sp″-gn (mm)	57.5	73.0
1-1°	−13.0	24.0
1̲-NA°	175.5	139.5
1̲-NB°	10.0	15.5
SS-N-SM°	8.5	3.5
H-angle°	7.0	1.0
UL-EL (mm)	2.5	7.5
LL-EL (mm)	2.5	4.0

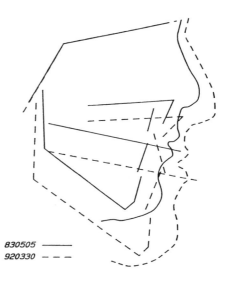

830505 ———
920330 - - -

16

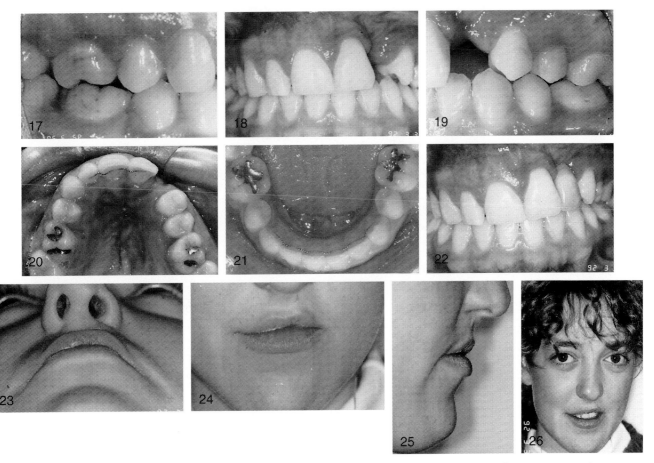

Figure 14–31 *Continued. 16*, Cephalometric analysis at ages 6 and 15 years. *17* to *26*, Dental occlusion (with a temporary replacement of left lateral incisor) and facial appearance at age 15 years.

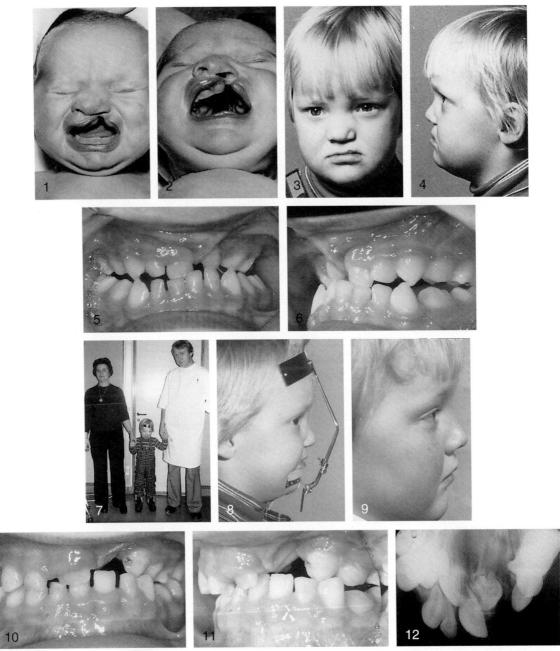

Figure 14–32. Complete UCLP with a tiny soft tissue band, category 2A. *1, 2,* At birth, July 1974. *4* to *6,* At age 4 years, moderate anterior-unilateral posterior crossbites; all four second permanent premolars were missing; *7* to *12,* Interceptive orthopedics from ages 4 and 5 years: transverse expansion (3 months) followed by protraction (5 months) to alleviate spontaneous eruption of upper permanent incisors to normal position.

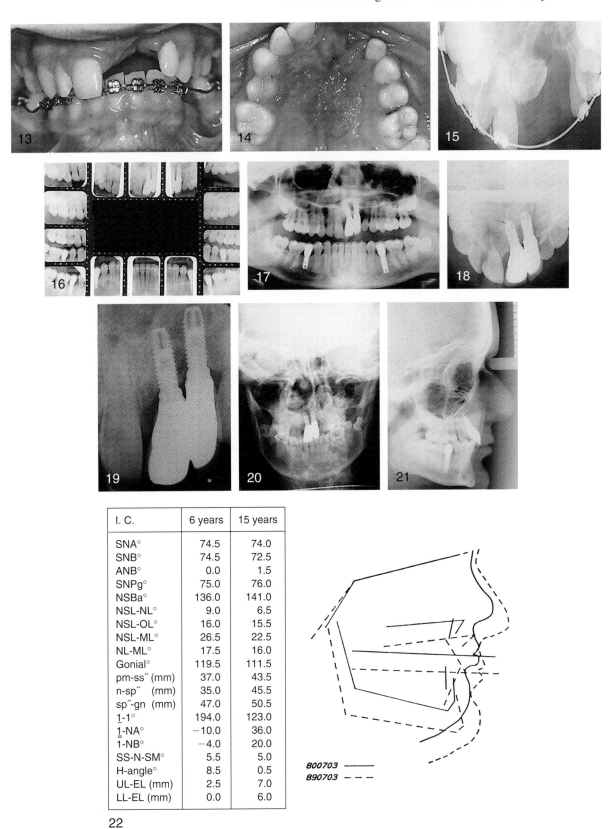

I. C.	6 years	15 years
SNA°	74.5	74.0
SNB°	74.5	72.5
ANB°	0.0	1.5
SNPg°	75.0	76.0
NSBa°	136.0	141.0
NSL-NL°	9.0	6.5
NSL-OL°	16.0	15.5
NSL-ML°	26.5	22.5
NL-ML°	17.5	16.0
Gonial°	119.5	111.5
pm-ss″ (mm)	37.0	43.5
n-sp″ (mm)	35.0	45.5
sp″-gn (mm)	47.0	50.5
1-1°	194.0	123.0
1-NA°	−10.0	36.0
1-NB°	−4.0	20.0
SS-N-SM°	5.5	5.0
H-angle°	8.5	0.5
UL-EL (mm)	2.5	7.0
LL-EL (mm)	0.0	6.0

800703 ———
890703 - - - -

22

Figure 14–32 *Continued. 13 to 15,* At age 15, during the period of conventional orthodontics, the severely malformed left central permanent incisor was removed at the time of secondary bone grafting. *16 to 21,* X-ray status at age 18.5 years; dental implants (fixtures) for replacement of left upper central and lateral incisors as well as both lower second premolars. *22,* Cephalometric analysis at ages 6 and 15.

Illustration continued on following page

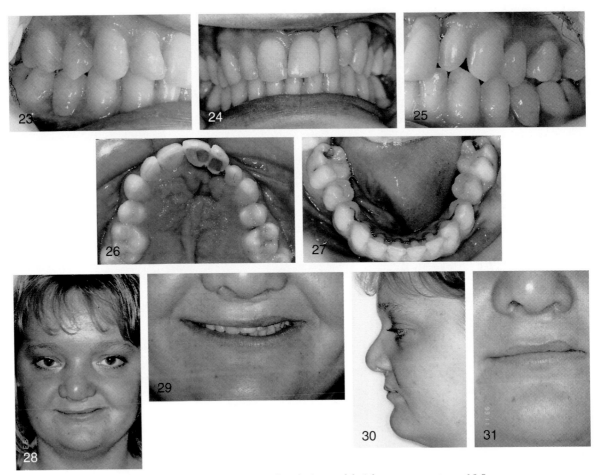

Figure 14–32 *Continued. 23* to *31,* Dental occlusion and facial appearance at age 18.5 years.

ence has shown the value of preparing an upper dental arch with correct number and inclination of the incisors (see Fig. 14–14). Care must be taken to prevent a forward, upward inclination of the occlusal plane, dental protrusion beyond normal values in the upper jaw, dental retrusion beyond normal values in the lower jaw, and lateral tipping of the posterior teeth. Establishing cost-benefit ratios in early treatment intervention is important in decision making when one-stage versus two-stage treatment interventions are considered.[25, 36, 37, 81, 84, 88]

Alignment of Maxillary Incisors

In spite of optimal space conditions after the transverse expansion treatment, the upper permanent incisors in CLP patients often erupt atypically, being tipped or rotated and palatally displaced. With optimal space conditions alignment of the incisors can be performed using a conventional technique with bonded brackets on the incisors. The palatal arch (or quad-helix) may remain during the aligning archwires (see Fig. 14–26, parts 15 to 17).

Aims of Treatment of Maxillary Incisors

- Alignment of malpositioned incisors, with caution taken not to move them into the cleft site, where supporting alveolar bone is required in order to prevent periodontal defects.
- Creation of optimal esthetic incisor positioning.

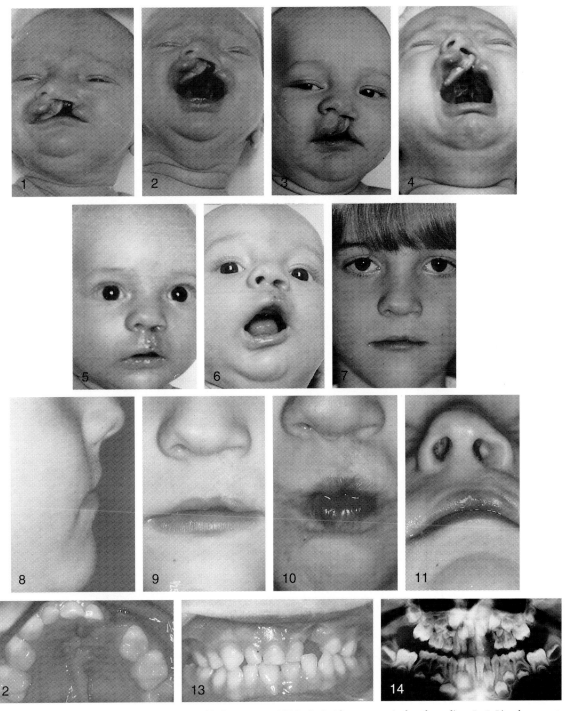

Figure 14–33. Complete UCLP, category 0. *1, 2,* At birth, January 1984. *3, 4,* After presurgical orthopedics. *5, 6,* Lip closure at age 3 months. *7* to *14,* At age 6 years, favorable growth and development.

Illustration continued on following page

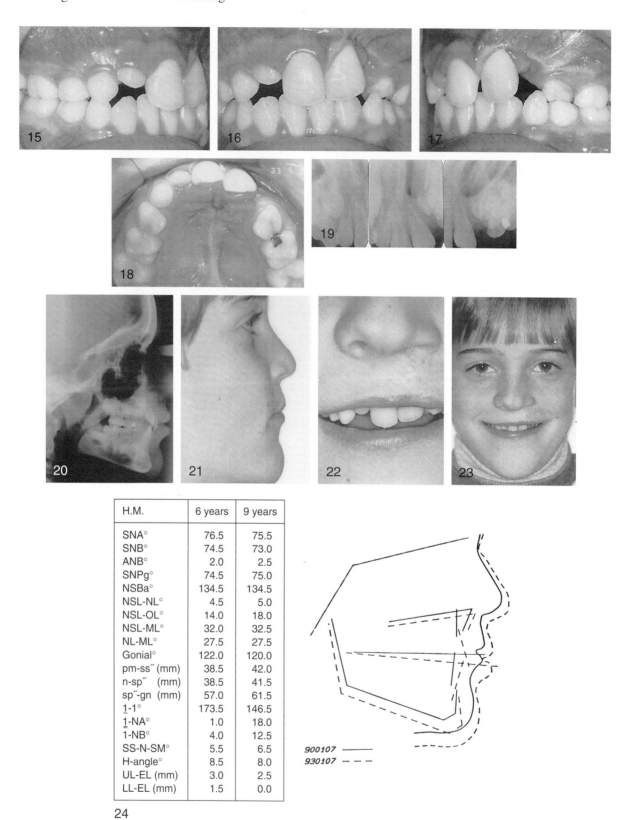

H.M.	6 years	9 years
SNA°	76.5	75.5
SNB°	74.5	73.0
ANB°	2.0	2.5
SNPg°	74.5	75.0
NSBa°	134.5	134.5
NSL-NL°	4.5	5.0
NSL-OL°	14.0	18.0
NSL-ML°	32.0	32.5
NL-ML°	27.5	27.5
Gonial°	122.0	120.0
pm-ss″ (mm)	38.5	42.0
n-sp″ (mm)	38.5	41.5
sp″-gn (mm)	57.0	61.5
1-1°	173.5	146.5
1̲-NA°	1.0	18.0
1̄-NB°	4.0	12.5
SS-N-SM°	5.5	6.5
H-angle°	8.5	8.0
UL-EL (mm)	3.0	2.5
LL-EL (mm)	1.5	0.0

900107 ———
930107 - - -

24

Figure 14–33 *Continued. 15* to *23,* At age 9 years, favorable facial growth and development of the dentition; no interceptive treatment or secondary bone grafting needed. *24,* Cephalometric analysis at ages 6 and 9 years.

Secondary Bone Grafting of the Cleft Alveolar Process

The introduction of secondary alveolar bone grafting procedures has resulted in excellent and reliable results.[1] Reevaluation of the primary periosteoplasty was necessary because an early bony fusion of the alveolar segments on one or both sides of the cleft may impair further growth and development.[91, 92] Therefore, primary periosteoplasty was terminated in 1986 in the Bergen CLP program. However, secondary bone grafting has been performed since 1980 in cases in which the primary periosteoplasty did not induce a bony bridge adequate for orthodontic space closure (see Fig. 14–29, parts 15, 19). Cancellous bony chips are harvested from the iliac crest and grafted to the alveolar cleft site at age 8 to 11 years, before eruption of the canine teeth.[1] When the lateral incisor is situated distal to the cleft, the bone grafting may be recommended early at age 8 years, to allow the eruption of the lateral incisor into the line of the arch. The role of the orthodontist on the team is to recommend the most appropriate time for alveolar bone grafting, depending on the dental requirements and developmental positions of the incisors and canines.

Aims of Alveolar Bone Grafts

- Elimination of remaining bony clefts.
- Orthodontic closure in cases of tooth agenesis in the cleft area.
- Stabilization of the segments.
- Closure of oronasal fistulas.
- Bony support to alar base in cases with nasal asymmetry.
- Elimination of mucosal recesses.

Conventional Orthodontics in the Permanent Dentition

The conventional orthodontic treatment objectives—normalizing the occlusion (see Fig. 14–29)—are generally the same in CLP patients as in non-CLP children, provided that (1) an undisturbed growth pattern (categories 0 and 1) or an acceptable basal jaw configuration has been obtained by an interceptive orthopedic treatment phase (category 2a) and (2) residual bony jaw clefts have been eliminated through primary periosteoplasty or secondary bone grafting. The orthodontic treatment plan should be coordinated with the team approach to overall management of the patient's needs. Cephalometric analyses, facial appearance, functional and dental occlusion, and space conditions should be considered in the three main time frames: primary, mixed, and permanent dentitions. Individual problems may prolong treatment time, but fixed appliances are indispensable for the orthodontic treatment of CLP patients both to obtain the detailed treatment objectives and for retention.

The patients described in this chapter were treated by the straight-wire edgewise-technique that is used in non-CLP children.[93] The implementation of a well-designed treatment plan with defined treatment goals at specified times may be delegated to the local orthodontists. This is important when patients travel distances of more than 3000 miles (2000 km) and requires good collaboration between the local care providers and the CLP team. Stability represents a special problem in CLP patients, and bonded palatal retainers are frequently used.

Aims of Treatment in the Permanent Dentition

- Improving the dentofacial relationship.
- Balancing the relationship between the dental and skeletal components.
- Establishing favorable maxillomandibular balance and proportion.
- Establishing normal incisal and buccal occlusion.
- Establishing harmonious dental arches in both jaws.
- Correcting axial inclinations of teeth.
- Correcting midlines.
- Avoiding prosthetic replacement of teeth when possible.
- Establishing functional occlusion in centric relations.
- Establishing optimal lip contour and contact.

Orthognathic Surgery (17 to 19 Years)

Ideally, space should be closed, to avoid prosthetic replacement. In a very few cases, however, there is a need for prosthetic bridgework. When lateral incisors are missing, the canine in most cases may be moved mesially to solve the problems (see Figs. 14–12, 14–17, 14–18, 14–20, 14–21, 14–22, 14–23, and 14–29). In patients with a tendency for a concave profile characteristic of midface deficiency, a full complement of maxillary teeth may be indicated. Space for the missing tooth or teeth is opened and retained with a temporary bonded bridge (see Fig. 14–30). However, if two or more teeth are absent in one segment (see Fig. 14–31), a small bridge is ordinarily needed, or implants may be considered. In the patient shown in Figure 14–32, who had UCLP with all second premolars and the left upper lateral incisor missing, the very malformed left upper central incisor was extracted. Implants to replace these incisors were inserted at age 18. Implants are likely to become an important aspect of future prosthetic replacements but should not be recommended until growth has stabilized. In cases of major basal maxillomandibular jaw discrepancies showing an unfavorable growth pattern, a combined orthodontic/orthognathic surgery treatment to achieve an esthetic and stable dental occlusion is indicated (see Fig. 14–14). The dental arches are orthodontically prepared so that after surgical repositioning, the general goals of normal occlusion are achieved.

Aims of Dental Adjustments

- Preprosthetic orthodontics related to small bridges or implants
- Combined treatment plan: orthodontics and orthognathic surgery if skeletal discrepancy has not been corrected by early intervention

CONCLUSIONS

Early orthodontic considerations concerning individual treatment plans for CLP patients imply evaluating the improvements of the patient against a checklist (see Fig. 14–6) of developmental objectives at each of the three main age intervals. The patient shown in Figure 14–33 needed no interceptive treatment or secondary bone grafting, because facial growth and development of the dentition were favorable at age 9 years. However, some patients do show inherent and/or acquired growth restraint with an unfavorable growth pattern of the craniofacial complex, most often expressed as anterior and/or posterior crossbite at an early age. The need for an interceptive orthopedic treatment period in these patients to correct the crossbite is based on the same orthodontic principles that are applicable for non-CLP children. In CLP children, the following treatment options may be considered:

1. Presurgical neonatal maxillary orthopedics (age 0 to 3 months).
2. Primary/early mixed dentition: interceptive orthopedics with protraction face mask (age 6 to 7 years).
3. Mixed dentition: bone grafting of the clefted alveolar process with presurgical alignment of maxillary incisors as necessary.
4. Permanent dentition: conventional orthodontics.
5. Adjunctive treatment: orthognathic surgery, prosthodontics, and so forth.

References

1. Bergland O, Semb G, Åbyholm FE: Elimination of the residual alveolar cleft by secondary bone grafting and subsequent orthodontic treatment. Cleft Palate J 1986; 23:175–205.
2. Burston WR: The pre-surgical orthopaedic correction of the maxillary deformity in clefts of both primary and secondary palate. In Wallace AB (ed): Transactions of the 2nd International Congress on Plastic Surgery. Baltimore: Williams & Wilkins, 1960.
3. Stricker G, Clifford E, Cohen LK, et al.: Psychosocial aspects of craniofacial disfigurement. A "state of the art" assessment conducted by the Craniofacial Anomalies Program Branch, the National Institute of Dental Research. Am J Orthod 1979; 76:410–422.
4. Shaw WC: The influence of children's dentofacial appearance on their social attractiveness as judged by peers and lay adults. Am J Orthod 1981; 79:399–415.
5. Shaw WC, Rees G, Dawe M, et al.: The influence of dentofacial appearance on the social attractiveness of young adults. Am J Orthod 1985; 87:21–26.
6. Alsaker FD, Olweus D: Assessment of global negative self-evaluations and perceived stability of self in Norwegian preadolescents and adolescents. J Early Adolesc 1986; 6:269–278.

7. Alsaker FD: Global negative self-evaluations in early adolescence [Thesis]. Bergen, Norway: Department of Psychosocial Science, University of Bergen, 1990.
8. Roberts CT, Semb G, Shaw WC: Strategies for the advancement of surgical methods in cleft lip and palate. Cleft Palate–Craniofac J 1991; 28:141–149.
9. Shprintzen RJ: Fallibility of clinical research. Cleft Palate–Craniofac J 1991; 28:136–140.
10. Vig KWL: Orthodontic considerations applied to craniofacial dysmorphology. Cleft Palate J 1990; 28:141–145.
11. Shaw WC, Dahl E, Asher-McDade C, et al.: A six-center international study of treatment outcome in patients with clefts of the lip and palate: Part 5. General discussion and conclusions. Cleft Palate–Craniofac J 1992; 29:413–418.
12. Solow B, Tallgren A: Head posture and craniofacial morphology. Am J Phys Anthrop 1976; 44:417–436.
13. Solow B: Upper airway obstruction and facial development. In Davidovitch E (ed): The Biological Mechanisms of Tooth Movement and Craniofacial Adaptation, pp 571–579. Columbus: Ohio State University Press, 1992.
14. Björk A: The face in profile [Thesis]. Sven Tandl Tidsk 1947; 40(Suppl 5b).
15. Björk A: Facial growth in man, studied with the aid of metallic implants. Acta Odontol Scand 1955; 13:9–34.
16. Björk A, Skieller V: Facial development and tooth eruption. An implant study at the age of puberty. Am J Orthod 1972; 62:339–383.
17. Solow B: The pattern of craniofacial associations. A morphological and methodological correlation and factor analysis study on young male adults. Acta Odont Scand 1966; 24(Suppl 46).
18. Hasund A: Clinical cephalometry for the Bergen technique. Bergen, Norway: Department of Orthodontics and Facial Orthopedics, School of Dentistry, University of Bergen, 1977.
19. Segner D: Floating norms as a mean to describe individual skeletal patterns. Eur J Orthod 1989; 11:214–220.
20. Angle EH: Treatment of malocclusion of the teeth: Angle's System, 7th ed. Philadelphia: SS White, 1907.
21. Björk A: The use of metallic implants in the study of facial growth in children. Method and application. Am J Orthod 1968; 29:243–260.
22. Melsen B: The cranial base. The postnatal development of the cranial base studied histologically on human autopsy material. Acta Odont Scand 1974; 32(Suppl 62).
23. Melsen B, Melsen F: The postnatal development of the palatomaxillary region studied on human autopsy material. Am J Orthod 1982; 82:329–342.
24. Linder-Aronson S: Effects of adenoidectomy on the dentition and facial skeleton over a period of five years. Trans Eur Orthod Soc 1972; pp 85–100.
25. Tindlund RS, Rygh P: Maxillary protraction: Different effects on facial morphology in unilateral and bilateral cleft lip and palate patients. Cleft Palate–Craniofac J 1993; 30:208–221.
26. Seipel CM: Variation in tooth position. Sven Tandläk Tidskr 1946; Suppl 39.
27. Rasmussen I, Helm S: Forekomsten af tannstillingsfeil i det primære tannsett. Tandlægebladet 1975; 79:383–388.
28. Telle ES: A study of the frequency of malocclusion in the county of Hedemark, Norway. Eur Orthod Soc Trans 1951; 27:192–198.
29. Helm S: Prevalence of malocclusion in relation to development of the dentition. Acta Odontol Scand 1970; 38(Suppl 58).
30. Wisth PJ: The sagittal head morphology of individuals with skeletal angle Class III malocclusions and changes subsequent to surgical treatment [Thesis]. Department of Orthodontics and Facial Orthopedics, University of Bergen, 1973.
31. Guyer EC, Ellis EE, McNamara JA, et al.: Components of Class III malocclusion in juveniles and adolescents. Angle Orthod 1986; 56:7–30.
32. Thilander B: Chin-cup treatment for Angle Class III malocclusion. Eur Orthod Soc Report 1965; 41:311–327.
33. Graber LW: Chin cup therapy for mandibular prognathism. Am J Orthod 1977; 72:23–41.
34. Ishii H, Morita S, Takeuch T, et al.: Treatment effect of combined maxillary protraction and chincap appliance in severe skeletal Class III cases. Am J Orthod Dentofac Orthop 1987; 92:304–312.
35. Tindlund RS: Orthopaedic protraction of the midface in the deciduous dentition—Results covering 3 years out of treatment. J Craniomaxillofac Surg 1989; 17(Suppl 1):17–19.
36. Tindlund RS, Rygh P, Bøe OE: Orthopedic protraction of the upper jaw in cleft lip and palate patients during the deciduous and mixed dentition periods in comparison with normal growth and development. Cleft Palate–Craniofac J 1993; 30:182–194.
37. Tindlund RS: Skeletal response to maxillary protraction in patients with cleft lip and palate before the age of 10 years. Cleft Palate–Craniofac J 1994; 31:295–308.
38. Tweed CH: Clinical Orthodontics, vol. 2. St. Louis: CV Mosby, 1966.
39. Vego L: Early orthopedic treatment for Class III skeletal patterns. Am J Orthod 1976; 70:59–69.
40. Ruhland A: The correlation between Angle Class III malocclusion and facial structures as diagnostic factors. Eur Orthod Soc Trans 1975; pp 229–240.
41. Schulhof RJ, Nakamura S, Williamson WV: Prediction of abnormal growth in Class III malocclusions. Am J Orthod 1977; 71:421–430.
42. Campbell PM: The dilemma of Class III treatment: Early or late? Angle Orthod 1983; 53:175–191.
43. American Cleft Palate–Craniofacial Association: Parameters for evaluation and treatment of patients with cleft lip/palate or other craniofacial anomalies. Cleft Palate–Craniofac J 1993; 30(Suppl 1).
44. Schjelderup H, Johnson GE: A six-year follow-up study of 155 children with cleft lip and palate. Br J Plast Surg 1983; 36:154–161.
45. Dahl E: Craniofacial morphology in congenital clefts of the lip and palate. An x-ray cephalometric study of young adult males. Acta Odontol Scand 1970; 28:(Suppl 57).

46. Chierici G, Harvold E, Vargervik K: Morphogenetic experiments in cleft palate: Mandibular responses. Cleft Palate J 1973; 10:51–61.

47. Ross RB: Treatment variables affecting facial growth in complete unilateral cleft lip and palate. Part I: Treatment affecting growth. Cleft Palate J 1987; 24:5–23.

48. Semb G: A study of facial growth in patients with unilateral cleft lip and palate treated by the Oslo CLP team. Cleft Palate–Craniofac J 1991; 28:1–21.

49. Ross RB: The clinical implications of facial growth in cleft lip and palate. Cleft Palate J 1970; 7:37–47.

50. Hotz M, Gnoinski W: Comprehensive care of cleft lip and palate children at Zürich University: A preliminary report. Am J Orthod 1976; 70:481–504.

51. Bishara S, Sierk DL, Huang K-S: Longitudinal changes in the dento-facial relationships of unilateral cleft lip and palate subjects. Cleft Palate J 1979; 16:391–401.

52. Sirinavin I: Cranio-facial and dental morphology of six-year-old Norwegian boys with complete cleft lip and palate [Thesis]. Bergen, Norway: Department of Orthodontics, University of Bergen, 1980.

53. Semb G: A study of facial growth in patients wth bilateral cleft lip and palate treated by the Oslo CLP team. Cleft Palate–Craniofac J 1991; 28:22–39.

54. Bergland O: Changes in cleft palate malocclusion after the introduction of improved surgery. Trans Eur Orthod Soc 1967; 43:383–398.

55. Pruzansky S, Aduss H: Prevalence of arch collapse and malocclusion in complete unilateral cleft lip and palate. Eur Orthod Soc Rep 1967; 43:365–382.

56. Bergland O, Sidhu SS: Occlusal changes from the deciduous to the early mixed dentition in unilateral complete clefts. Cleft Palate J 1974; 11:317–326.

57. Ranta R, Oikari T, Haataja J: Prevalence of crossbite in deciduous and mixed dentition in Finnish children with operated cleft palate. Proc Finn Dent Soc 1974; 70:20–24.

58. Dahl E, Hanusardottir B: Prevalence of malocclusion in the primary and mixed dentition in Danish children with incomplete cleft lip and palate. Eur J Orthod 1979; 1:81–88.

59. Chatkupt S: Craniofacial and dental morphology of six-year-old Norwegian children with isolated cleft palate [Thesis]. Bergen, Norway: Department of Orthodontics and Facial Orthopedics, University of Bergen, 1982.

60. Grahnen H: Hypodontia in the permanent dentition. Odontol Rev 1956; (Suppl 3).

61. Böhn A: Dental anomalies in harelip and cleft palate. Acta Odontol Scand 1963; 21(Suppl 38).

62. Ranta R: The development of the permanent teeth in children with complete cleft lip and palate. Proc Finn Dent Soc 1972; 68(Suppl 3).

63. Ranta R: A review of tooth formation in children with cleft lip/palate. Am J Orthod Dentofac Orthop 1986; 90:11–18.

64. Fleiner B, Hoffmeister B, Steckeler S: Frequency and localisation of the lateral incisors in UCLP and BCLP [Abstract]. Presented at the 50th meeting of the American Cleft Palate–Craniofacial Association, Pittsburgh, 1993.

65. Warren DW, Duany LF, Fischer ND: Nasal pathway resistance in normal and cleft lip and palate subjects. Cleft Palate J 1969; 6:449–469.

66. Delaire J, Verdon P, Flour J: Ziele und Ergebnisse extraoraler Züge in postero-anteriorer Richtung in Anwendung einer orthopädischen Maske bei der Behandlung von Fällen der Klasse III. Fortschr Kieferorthop 1976; 37:247–262.

67. Linder-Aronson S, Aschan G: Nasal resistance to breathing and palatal height before and after expansion of the median palatine suture. Odontol Rev 1963; 4:254–270.

68. Wertz RA: Changes in nasal airflow incident to rapid maxillary expansion. Angle Orthod 1968, 38:1–11.

69. Hershey G, Stewart B, Warren D: Changes in nasal airway resistance associated with rapid maxillary expansion. Am J Orthod 1976; 69:274–284.

70. Warren DW, Hershey HG, Turvey TA, et al.: The nasal airway following maxillary expansion. Am J Orthod Dentofac Orthop 1987; 91:111–116.

71. Harvold EP, Chierici G, Vargervik K: Experiments on the development of dental malocclusions. Am J Orthod 1972; 61:38–44.

72. Harvold EP, Vargervik K, Chierici G: Primate experiments on oral sensation and dental malocclusion. Am J Orthod 1973; 63:496–508.

73. Subtelny JD, Brodie AG: An analysis of orthodontic expansion in unilateral cleft lip and cleft palate patients. Am J Orthod 1954; 40:686–697.

74. Ohkiba T, Hanada K: Adaptive functional changes in the swallowing pattern of the tongue following expansion of the maxillary dental arch in subjects with and without cleft palate. Cleft Palate J 1989; 26:21–30.

75. Delaire J, Salagnac JM: Anatomie et physiologie du pilier antérieur maxillaire et architecture faciale. Rev Stomat (Paris) 1977; 78:447–464.

76. Harvold E: Cleft lip and palate: Morphologic studies on the facial skeleton. Am J Orthod 1954; 40:493–506.

77. Subtelny JD: The importance of early orthodontic treatment in cleft palate planning. Angle Orthod 1957; 27:148–158.

78. Ogidan O, Subtelny JD: Eruption of incisor teeth in cleft lip and palate. Cleft Palate J 1983; 20:331–341.

79. Delaire J, Verdon P, Lumineau J-P, et al.: Quelques résultats des tractions extra-orales à appui fronto-mentonnier dans le traitement orthopédique des malformations maxillo-mandibulaires de classe III et des séquelles osseuses des fentes labio-maxillaires. Rev Stomatol 1972; 73:633–642.

80. Subtelny JD: Oral respiration: Facial maldevelopment and corrective dentofacial orthopedics. Angle Orthod 1980; 50:147–164.

81. Tindlund RS: Prediction of sagittal skeletal response to maxillary protraction in patients with cleft lip and palate before the age 10 years. Cleft Palate–Craniofac J, in press.

82. Rygh P, Tindlund RS: Orthopaedic expansion and protraction of the maxilla in cleft palate patients—A new treatment rationale. Cleft Palate J 1982; 19:104–112.

83. Tindlund RS: Behandling av leppe/kjeve/ganespalte i Bergen—Teamwork. Nor Tannlegeforen Tid 1987; 97:360–369.

84. Tindlund RS, Rygh P: Soft-tissue profile changes during widening and protraction of the maxilla in patients with cleft lip and palate compared with normal growth and development. Cleft Palate–Craniofac J 1993; 30:454–468.

85. Tindlund RS, Rygh P, Bøe OE: Intercanine widening and sagittal effect of maxillary transverse expansion in patients with cleft lip and palate during the deciduous and mixed dentitions. Cleft Palate–Craniofac J 1993; 30:195–207.

86. Hermanson H, Kurol J, Rönnerman A: Treatment of unilateral posterior crossbite with quad-helix and removable plates. A retrospective study. Eur J Orthod 1985; 7:97–102.

87. Scheuer H: Indications for interrupting orthodontic treatment in UCLP-patients. Kieferorthop Mitteilung 1991; 3:5–13.

88. Segner D: Treatment goals for sagittal base relationship in CLP-patients. Kieferorthop Mitteilungen 1990; 2:5–14.

89. Segner D: Correlating cephalometric measurements and esthetic ratings of the profile in patients displaying clefts of the lip, alveolus and palate. Kieferorthop Mitteilungen 1992; 4:1–11.

90. Fränkel R: Maxillary retrusion in class III and treatment with the Function Corrector III. Trans Eur Orthod Soc 1970; 46:249–259.

91. Hellquist R, Linder-Aronson S, Norling M, et al: Dental abnormalities in patients with alveolar clefts, operated upon with or without primary periosteoplasty. Eur J Orthod 1979; 1:169–180.

92. Friede H, Lennartsson B: Forward traction of the maxilla in cleft lip and palate patients. Eur J Orthod 1981; 3:21–39.

93. Hasund A: The Bergen-Technique. Bergen, Norway: Department of Orthodontics, School of Dentistry, University of Bergen, 1972.

15

Diagnosis of and Treatment Planning for Facial Asymmetries

John Paul Stella and Bruce N. Epker

INTRODUCTION

Patients with facial clefts and/or craniosynostosis often have clinically significant facial asymmetry that must be addressed in the habilitation process. The intention of this chapter is to provide a quantitative and qualitative assessment protocol for determining soft and hard tissue components of facial asymmetry.

This chapter is intended to aid in (1) critically and objectively (quantitatively) evaluating patients with facial asymmetries; (2) identifying the specific location(s) of both the skeletal and soft tissue facial asymmetries; (3) according to the data accumulated in the evaluation of the patient, making a *quantitative diagnosis;* (4) formulating a rational treatment plan that considers both the skeletal and soft tissue components of the asymmetry; and (5) sequencing the skeletal and soft tissue surgery in a rational fashion.

All faces are inherently asymmetric when critically evaluated. However, for the purposes of this text, facial asymmetry is defined as the presence of clinically significant variations between the two halves of the face that the patient (or parents, in the instance of most congenital asymmetric facial disfigurements) is concerned about and that can be *quantified by the clinician.*

The more significant the facial asymmetry, the more easily it can be identified and measured (Fig. 15–1A,B,C).

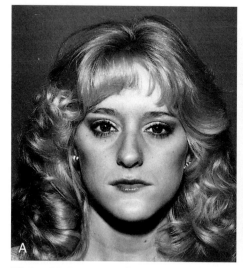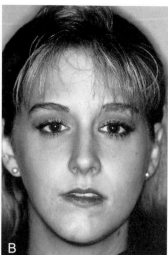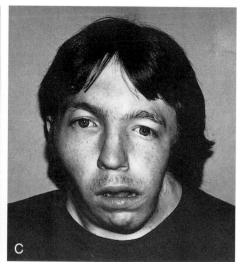

Figure 15–1. *A, B, C,* Illustrations of slight to moderate to severe facial asymmetries progressively involving the lower, middle, and upper thirds of the face.

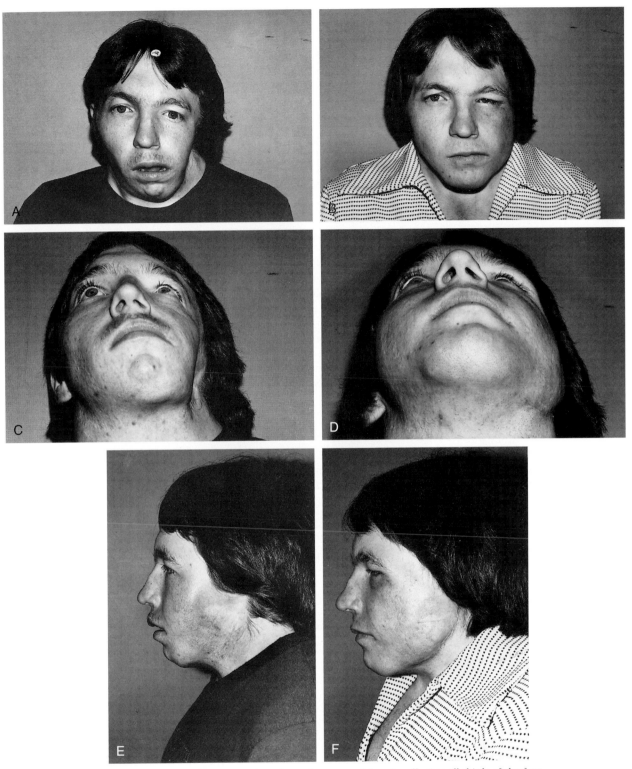

Figure 15–2. Pre- and postcorrection views of a severe deformity affecting all thirds of the face.

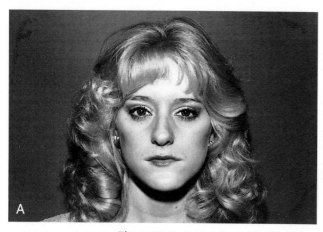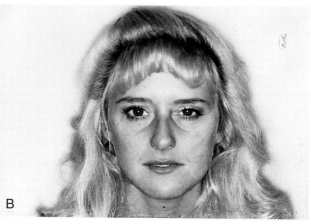

Figure 15–3. Pre- and postcorrection views of lower third face asymmetry deformity.

Improvements in individuals with severe facial asymmetries corrected via surgery are often judged by both the patient and surgeon to be satisfactory even when less-than-optimal results are obtained (Fig. 15–2*A,B,C,D,E,F*).

Conversely, the more minor the asymmetry is, the more precise the evaluation and treatment planning must be (Fig. 15–3*A,B*). Anything short of an optimal outcome will often result in dissatisfaction. In either case, knowing what to look for, how to plan, and how to execute surgery are critical elements in the production of satisfied patients and optimal esthetic outcomes.

This chapter is divided into three sections: (1) the initial examination and data collection, (2) qualitative and quantitative diagnosis, and (3) treatment planning for patients with facial asymmetries.

The algorithm depicted in Figure 15–4 summarizes the *initial evaluation* and *data collection* that patients with facial deformities undergo in order to comprehensively define the location and magnitude of the facial deformity. This results in the establishment of a definitive diagnosis.

Initial Examination and Data Collection

I.

Facial Symmetry

Standard Orthodontic/Surgical Evaluation

- Standard Facial Anthropometric Measurements
- Photos (occlusion in C.R.)
  - Frontal (repose and smiling)
  - Profile
  - Occlusals
- Lateral Cephalometric Radiograph
- Panorex
- Dental Models (C.R.)
- TMJ Examination

Evaluation

II.

Clinically Significant Facial Asymmetry

Detailed Evaluation of Asymmetry Patient

A. Correct Compensatory Head Posture

B. Identity Level(s) of Facial Asymmetry

Lower 1/3	Middle 1/3	Upper 1/3
1, 2, 3, 4, 5	2, 3, 4, 5	2, 5

1) Standard Orthodontic/Surgical
2) Detailed Anthropometric Measurements of Affected Level
3) Barium PA and Lateral Cephalometric Radiographs
4) Face Bow Mounted Models (C.R.)
5) Special Imaging

Figure 15–4.

Treatment Planning for Asymmetric Patients

I. Skeletal			II. Soft Tissue		
Lower 1/3	Middle 1/3	Upper 1/3	Lower 1/3	Middle 1/3	Upper 1/3
A, B	A, B	A, C	A, B	A, B	A, B

I. Skeletal

A) Esthetic Procedures
  ■ Augmentations
    • Autogenous Onlays
    • Alloplastic Onlays
  ■ Reductions
    • Skeletal Recontouring
    • Ostectomies
B) Orthognathic Surgery
C) Craniofacial Surgery

II. Soft Tissue

A) Repositioning
    • Primary (cleft lip-palate)
    • Secondary
B) Reductions:
  ■ Liposuction
    • Myectomies
C) Augmentation
  ■ Autogenous Grafts
    • Free Fat Transfers
    • Dermal Fat Grafts
    • Collagen—Gore-Tex

III.

Combination of Soft and Skeletal
Tissue Connection

Figure 15–5.

Figure 15–5 is an algorithm outlining a protocol for *treatment planning* for patients with facial asymmetries. Of importance, treatment planning for such patients involves identifying both skeletal and soft tissue components of the asymmetry, which will be discussed later.

INITIAL EXAMINATION AND DATA COLLECTION

This section will discuss and follow the algorithm depicted in Figure 15–4. In all patients being evaluated for correction of a facial deformity, the first assessment is for symmetry. If the face is symmetric, the standard orthodontic-surgical evaluation is performed (Fig. 15–4, left column). This evaluation includes a facial anthropometric evaluation, a lateral cephalometric radiograph, frontal and profile photographs (occlusion in centric relation), a panoramic evaluation, dental models (trimmed and articulated in centric relation), and a temporomandibular joint examination. Upon initial evaluation, if either the patient's chief complaint is facial asymmetry and/or visual examination by the clinician reveals the patient's face to be asymmetric, a different evaluation is performed (see Fig. 15–4, right column).

Correct Compensatory Head Posturing

When clinically significant facial asymmetry exists, the clinician must first carefully evaluate for "compensatory head posture" and, when it exists, position the patient's head so the habitual head posture is corrected (Fig. 15–6A,B).

Compensatory head posture likely exists to distract attention from the facial asymmetry. Compensatory head posture may take the form of the patient tipping the head slightly to either the right or the left (see Fig. 15–6A,B). A more subtle means of compensation can be manifest in hair style that distracts attention from the asymmetry. In either case, clinically assisted positioning of the patient's head to eliminate the compensation before any objective qualitative or quantitative evaluation is paramount. Effectively correcting for compensatory head posture is necessary to ensure accurate qualitative and quantitative identification of the asymmetry.

In those patients with asymmetric skull bases and symmetric external auditory canals and orbits, it is best to position the patient's head so that Frankfort horizontal

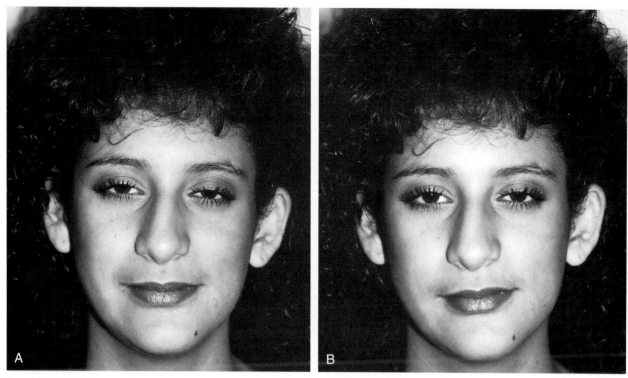

Figure 15–6. *A,* Patient with compensatory head posture. Note patient tipping her head to left (as evidenced by asymmetric eyes and ear levels) to straighten the chin. *B,* Patient with corrected head position. Note obvious chin asymmetry but level eye and ear postions.

and the patient's interpupillary lines are parallel to the floor. Patients who have asymmetric cranial bases with orbital dystopia and/or congenitally absent external auditory canals are provided a mirror and asked to look into the mirror so that they are peering directly into their own eyes (pupils). This establishes a *reproducible head position* (natural head position) with the interpupillary line as parallel to the floor as the patient's cranial base asymmetry will allow. After the patient's head is properly oriented, assessment of the qualitative and quantitative components of the patient's facial asymmetry can be made.

Identifying Level(s) of Facial Asymmetry

With compensatory head posture corrected, the clinician subjectively assesses the level(s) of the facial asymmetry: lower third, middle third, and upper third of the face (Fig. 15–4, right column). This is important because the indicated evaluations and data collection are predicated on the initial identification of the level(s) of the facial asymmetry. What follows is a brief discussion of the special evaluations for patients with facial asymmetries; select these evaluations as indicated, depending upon the level of asymmetry (Fig. 15–4, right column).

Standard Orthodontic-Surgical Evaluation

As noted previously, the clinical examinations, photographs, radiographs, models, and temporomandibular joint examinations are routinely performed for all individuals being evaluated for correction of facial deformities. Of importance, a detailed anthropometric assessment is helpful to more objectively assess facial esthetics. Tables 15–1, 15–2, 15–3, and 15–4 summarize suggested anthropometric measurements of the face that are useful.

Table 15–1.

Patient's expressed esthetic desires: _____

General facial characteristic	Frontal Facial Esthetics		
	Symmetry Asymmetry		
	Total Face Ratios	**Female**	**Male**
Vertical Ratios			
Head	V-Gn		
Neurocranium	V-N	50	
Facial height	N-Gn	50	
Total face	Tr-Gn		
Forehead	Tr-G	30	
Upper face	G-Sn	35	
Lower face	Sr-Gn	35	
Face	G-Gr		
Upper face	G-Sn	50	45
Lower face	Sr-Gn	50	55
Vertical/Horizontal Ratios			
Total face			
Forehead width/total face height	Ft-Ft/Tr-Gn	65	
Zygoma width/total face height	Zy-Zy/Tr-Gn	75	
Bigonial width/total face height	Go-Go/Tr-Gn	55	
Face			
Forehead width/face height	Ft-Ft/G-Gn	90	
Zygoma width/face height	Zy-Zy/G-Gn	105	
Bigonial width/face height	Go-Go/G-Gn	75	80
Total facial thirds			
Forehead width/forehead height	Ft-Ft/Tr-G	220	
Zygoma width/upper face height	Zy-Zy/G-Sn	220	230
Bigonial width/lower face height	Go-Go/Sn-Gn	140	

Table 15–2.

Upper Third Face			
Shape and symmetry of the	Calvaria _____		
	Temporal areas _____		
	Frontal areas _____		
	Eyebrows _____		
	Supraorbital rim _____		
Middle Third Face		**Females**	**Males**
Vertical Ratios			
Eyes			
Orbit height/upper face height	Os-Or/G-Sn	50	
Upper lid height/orbit height	Os-Ps/Os-Or	40	
Lid sulcus/lid margin	Sulcus/Ps	10 mm	
Eye fissure height/orbit height	Ps-Pi/Os-Or	35	
Upper lid/iris	Ps/Iris	2 mm	
Lower lid/iris	Pi/Iris	2 mm	
Lower lid height/orbit height	Pi-Or/Os-Or	25	
Nose			
Nose length/middle third height	N-Sn/G-Sn	90	
Dorsum length/middle third height	N-Prn/G-Sn	80	
Dorsum length/nose length	N-Prn/N-Sn	90	

Table continued on following page

Table 15–2. *Continued*

Middle Third Face *Continued*

Horizontal Ratios

Eyes
Biocular width/head width	Ex-Ex/Eu-Eu	60	
Intercanthal width/biocular width	En-En/Ex-Ex	34	
Intercanthal width/zygomatic width	En-En/Zy-Zy	25	
Fissure width/intercanthal width	En-Ex/En-En	95	
Fissure width/biocular width	En-Ex/Ex-Ex	33	
Interpupillary width/biocular width	Midpupil/Ex-Ex	70	
Eye fissure cant/horizon	En-Ex/Horizon	5	

Nose
Nasal root width/alar width	Mf-Mf/Al-Al	60	
Nasal root width/intercanthal width	Mf-Mf/En-En	60	
Alar width/intercanthal width	Al-Al/En-En	100	105
Columella width/alar width	Columella/Al-Al	25	

Vertical/Horizontal Ratios

Eyes
Orbit height/biocular width	Os-Or/Ex-Ex	35
Orbit height/fissure width	Os-Or/En-Ex	35
Fissure height/fissure width	Ps-Pi/En-Ex	35

Nose
Alar width/nose length	Al-Al/N-Sn	60

Nasal Base Ratios
Tip length/nasal protrusion	Prn-C (1)/Prn-Sn	45
Columella length/nasal protrusion	C (1)-Sn/Prn-Sn	55
Columella length/alar length	Sn-C (1)/Ac-Prn	35
Nasal tip width/alar width	Tip width/Al-Al	75
Nasal protrusion/alar width	Prn-Sn/Al-Al	60
Nasal protrusion/alar length	Prn-Sn/Ac-Prn	60
Alar thickness	Ala	5 mm
Columellar thickness	Columella	8 mm

Ear Ratios

Location
Vertical	V-Po	130 mm	135 mm
Horizontal	N-Obs	115 mm	120 mm

Proportions
Width to length	Pra-Pa/Sa-Sba	55	
Attachment length/vertical length	Obs-Obi/Sa-Sba	95	80

Angles
Medial long axis to horizontal	Sa-Sba/Horizontal	100
Lateral protrusion from malar bone		25

Lower Third Face		**Females**	**Males**
Vertical Ratios			
Lower face	Sn-Gn	100%	
Upper lip	Sn-Sto	30	
Lower lip	Sto-Sl	25	
Chin	Sl-Gn	45	
Lips			
Upper lip/lower lip	Sn-Sto/Sto-Sl	105	120
Skin upper/upper lip	Sn-Ls/Sn-Sto	70	65
Skin lower/lower lip	Li-Sl/Sto-Sl	60	
Vermilion upper/lower lip	Ls-Sto/Sto-Li	85	
Horizontal Ratios			
Mouth width/bigonial width	Ch-Ch/Go-Go	55	
Mouth width/zygoma width	Ch-Ch/Zy-Zy	40	
Mouth width/biocular width	Ch-Ch/Ex-Ex	60	
Alar base width/mouth width	Al-Al/Ch-Ch	60	65
Philtrum width/mouth width	Chp-Chp/Ch-Ch	20	
Columella width/philtrum width	Columella/Chp-Chp	75	
Vertical/Horizontal Ratios			
Upper lip height/mouth width	Sn-Sto/Ch-Ch	40	
Lower face height/mouth width	Sn-Gn/Ch-Ch	130	135

Table 15–3.

Balance

Subnasale-stomion: stomion-menton   (1:2) _____

Subnasale-vermilion: vermilion-menton   (1:1) _____

Lips

Symmetry (rest) _____   (smiling) _____
                    Intrinsic   Nerve   Dentoskeletal

Ratio of upper vermilion to lower vermilion (1:1/4) _____

Interlabial distance (up to 3 mm) _____

Commissure width _____   and symmetry _____

Teeth

Exposure upper teeth (mm) (rest) _____ _____   (smiling) _____ _____

   Symmetry _____

Exposure lower teeth (mm) (rest) _____ _____   (smiling) _____ _____

   Symmetry _____

Dental symmetry _____

Dental midlines _____

Chin

Symmetry: Left _____ mm   Right _____ mm

Shape _____

Mandibular Angles

Symmetry _____

Deficient _____   Hyperplastic _____

Table 15–4. PROFILE FACIAL ESTHETICS

		Females	Males
Lateral Total Face Angulations			
Forehead	Tr-G/Vertical	−5%	
General facial	G-Pg/Vertical	−5%	
Middle face	G-Sn/Vertical	0%	
Nasofrontal	N-Prn/N-G	135	
Nasomental	N-Prn/Prn-Pg	125	
Cervical mental	Gn-C/ant. neck		110
Upper Third of Face			
Forehead:	Frontal bossing	Supraorbital hypoplasia	
Supraorbital rim projection (5 to 10 mm) (relative to cornea)	_____		
Glabellar angle: Excessive		Absent	
Middle Third of Face			
Sagittal			
Nasal root/nasal protrusion	En/Dorsum/Sn-Prn	75%	
Vertical/sagittal			
Nasal protrusion/nasal length	Sn-Prn/N-Sn	40%	
Angulations			
Nasofrontal	N-Prn/N-Gt	135	130
Nasofacial	G-Pg/N-Prn	35	
Nasolabial	Sn-C'/Sn-Ls	100	
Nose			
Tip length/nasal protrusion	Prn-C (1)/Prn-Sn	45%	
Columella length/nasal protrusion	C (1)-Sn/Prn-Sn	55%	
Columella length/alar length	Sn-C (1)/Ac-Pr	35%	
Nasal protrusion/alar width	Prn-Sn/Al-A	60%	
Nasal protrusion/alar width	Prn-Sn/Ac-Prn	60%	

Table continued on following page

Table 15–4. PROFILE FACIAL ESTHETICS *Continued*

			Females	Males
Nose Continued				
Bridge projection (5 to 8 mm) ————				
(relative to cornea)				
Dorsum prominence: Convex Concave				
Supratip break: Present Absent				
Nasal tip: Upturned Downturned				
Nasolabial angle (90° to 110°) ————				
Columella: Angled upward Angled downward				
Cheeks (relative to cornea)				
Infraorbital rim projection (0 to 2 mm) ————				
Lateral orbital rim projection (8 to 12 mm) ————				
Convex Flat Concave				
Paranasal area				
Tip-subnasal: subnasale-alar base (2:1) ————				
Convex Flat Concave				
Lower Third of Face				
Upper lip/vertical	Sn-Ls/Vertical		0	
Lower half of face/vertical	Sn-Pg/Vertical		−15	
Lower third of face/vertical	Li-Pg/Vertical		−20	
Cervical mental	Gn-C/Ant. Neck		110	
Lips				
Upper (relative to subnasale perpendicular): Protrusive Retrusive				
Lower (relative to upper lip): Protrusive Retrusive				
Labiomental fold: Deficient Excessive				
Chin projection: Retrusive Protrusive				
Neck-chin area				
Angle: Deficient Excessive				
Length: Deficient Excessive				

Moreover, patients with cants to their maxillary occlusal plane are evaluated both in repose and smiling. The skeletal asymmetry may or may not be accompanied by commensurate soft tissue animation asymmetry. For example, a patient may exhibit 5-mm maxillary occlusal plane cant, but when smiling and/or animating, the cant is exaggerated (Fig. 15–7*A,B*).

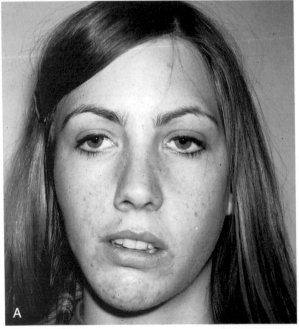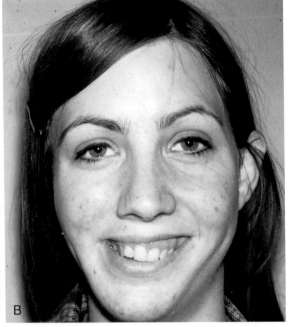

Figure 15–7. *A* and *B*, Patient with asymmetry that is accentuated by animation.

Detailed Anthropometric Measurements of Affected Level

A discussion of the utilization of the anthropometric data presented in Tables 15–1, 15–2, 15–3, and 15–4 follows. The illustrations in Figure 15–8A–I serve as a visual aid to identifying the necessary facial landmarks.

Emphasis is placed on the frontal anthropometric evaluations. The evaluation proposed in these tables is to quantitatively detect imbalance, disproportions, and angular facial abnormalities. In patients with facial asymmetry, the additional measurements must be made. In the asymmetric third or thirds of the face, a true facial midline is actually drawn on the patient's face (identical to that in the posteroanterior [PA] cephalometric radiograph) by bisecting the horizontal interpupillary level and establishing a perpendicular through the midpoint of the intercanthal area. From these lines, unilateral measurements are made in the asymmetric third or thirds of the face to each landmark, thereby quantifying the location and magnitude of the asymmetry. This information is integrated with that from the PA cephalometric data subsequently described to establish the quantitative diagnosis and enhance precision of surgical correction.

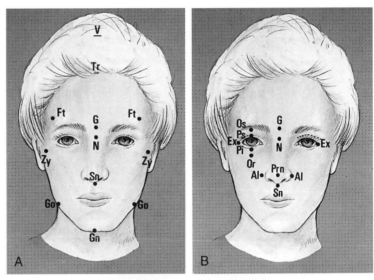

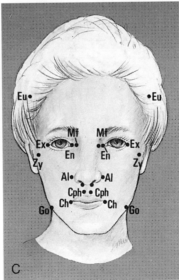

Figure 15–8.

Illustration continued on following page

Figure 15–8. *Continued*

PA and Lateral Barium Cephalometric Radiographs

To obtain these radiographs, the patient's head is properly oriented with the Frankfort horizontal and the interpupillary line parallel to the floor (natural head position). As previously noted, for those patients who have cranial base asymmetries, a mirror is provided and the patient is asked to look directly into his or her own pupils. With the head in this position, radiopaque barium cream is loaded into a monojet syringe, and a series of lines are scribed on the patient's face.

These lines are perpendicular to the Frankfort horizontal and are placed bilaterally. They include the following: (1) a line 1.5 cm anterior to the tragus of the ear, which extends over the angle of the mandible to the neck; (2) a line extending from the lateral canthus, down the cheek, under the submandibular area; and (3) a line from the commissure on one side and carried under the submental area to the opposing commissure. Midline points are placed at the midpoint of the glabella nasal tip, upper lip, and pogonion *independently of the rest of the face*. The midpoint of the chin is marked with the rest of the face blocked out with a white sheet of paper. Similarly, the midpoint of the upper lip, tip of the nose, and midglabella are marked. In this way, when the radiograph is obtained, the magnitude of, for example, chin asymmetry can be quantitatively determined.

With the patient's face marked as noted above, PA and lateral cephalometric radiographs are obtained. The PA barium tracing depicted in Figure 15–9C is used to quantitatively assess both the skeletal and soft tissue components of the asymmetry. The barium lateral cephalometric radiograph allows the examiner to critically determine the precise anterior-posterior location of each of the barium lines as they relate to the facial skeleton.

Face-Bow Mounted Models

The records of any asymmetry involving the lower third of the face include face-bow mounted models as a routine part of the work-up. These models are *anatomically trimmed* and articulated in centric relation position (Fig. 15–10A,B)

Feasibility model surgery is performed by releasing the models from the articulator and hand-articulating them to the desired occlusion. If by hand-articulating the models it is found that sectioning either one or both of the jaws in segments may be necessary to obtain class I cuspid occlusion and coordinated transverse relations, then duplicate models are made and the sectioning is performed. Once the teeth are in an acceptable position, the anatomically mounted and trimmed models can be used for definitive model surgery. This will be discussed later in this chapter.

Special Imaging

Special studies, including computed tomographic (CT) scans and/or magnetic resonance images (MRIs), are obtained at the surgeon's discretion. In general, CT scans with two- or three-dimensional reconstruction are best used to elucidate skeletal conditions that require greater radiographic definition and resolution. One example in which three-dimensional CT reconstruction is invaluable is in patients with congenital temporomandibular joint ankylosis. In such cases, the reconstructed scan can define those foramina in which the great vessels reside and the proximity of these vessels to the proposed surgical site. MRI is best used in those circumstances in which soft tissues (e.g., muscles, fat) are being evaluated.

QUANTITATIVE AND QUALITATIVE DIAGNOSIS

Anthropometric Data Utilization

All facial deformities, including asymmetries, are categorized into conditions of either excess or deficiency. By using the previously described anthropometric data, general ratios and then specific right-to-left measures of those asymmetric areas of the face are critically assessed. This permits definition and quantification of the excess of deficiency. Next, a millimetric determination of the magnitude of the asymmetry is obtained, by use of the right-to-left absolute measures. It should be appreciated that anthrometric measurements provide objective quantitative analysis of surface contours.

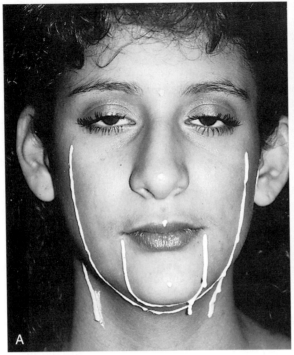
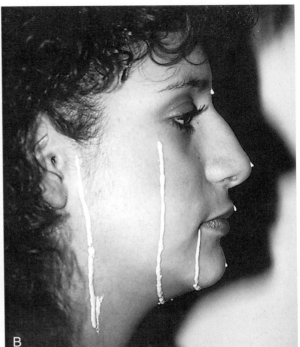

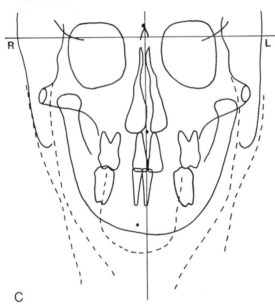

Figure 15–9.

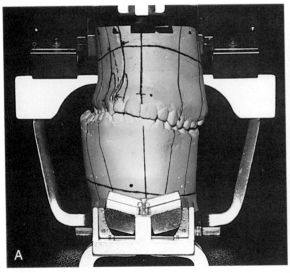
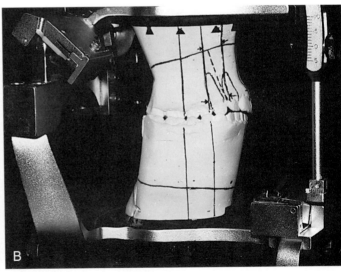

Figure 15–10.

They do not define the contributing components of the soft tissue and/or facial skeleton. Accordingly, these data are integrated with the PA cephalometric analysis to better elucidate the contribution of soft tissue and bone abnormalities to the asymmetry.

Special Cephalometric Data Utilization

PA and Lateral Barium Cephalometric Radiograph Utilization

Barium cephalometric radiographs include both the posterior-anterior and lateral cephalometric views. Figure 15–9C illustrates a tracing obtained from a PA barium cephalometric radiograph. This tracing was generated in the following manner: A horizontal referent line is drawn to intersect the most inferior aspect of the frontozygomatic suture bilaterally. A second referent line, drawn perpendicular to the horizontal referent line, is then made to approximate the facial midline. This midface reference is difficult to locate, but by integrating information obtained clinically, this line can be drawn in a clinically accurate position. The most useful clinical data to help establish this referent are the distance from the nasal tip to facial midline, and the upper and lower dental midlines and chin relative to the facial midline. The midfacial referent is drawn so that these clinical measurements are at their appropriate location in relation to the facial midline referent. A series of horizontal lines perpendicular to the midline facial referent may be drawn in the areas of the mandibular ramus, angle, body, and chin region. Distances from the midline to the bone and overlying soft tissue can be obtained by using barium markers to locate skin surfaces. By using the data from the specialized cephalometric diagnostic tracings, quantitative measurements of the skeleton, soft tissue thicknesses, and soft tissue contours can be made. These data can then be used to determine the size, shape, and dimensions of material(s) required for correction of facial asymmetry.

Utilization of Face-Bow Mounted Models

For facial asymmetries located in the lower third of the face, face-bow mounted models on an anatomic articulator must be analyzed. Qualitative and quantitative assessments are made by combining data obtained from these models, the PA cephalometric tracing, and clinical facial measurements. Before any referent lines or measurements are placed on the mounted models, these casts are evaluated and compared with the patient so that the accuracy of the face-bow mounting and occlusal bite in centric relation is assumed. This important step cannot be overemphasized because the asymmetry is related to the occlusion in all three planes of space. As with any mounted models, essential information such as the magnitude of transverse, anterior-posterior, and/or vertical discrepancy can be determined. The specifics of model marking and surgery are discussed in the later section *Definitive Model Surgery*.

TREATMENT PLANNING FOR PATIENTS WITH FACIAL ASYMMETRIES

Evolving and finalizing a treatment plan that will predictably produce symmetric and functional improvements depend on accurate quantitative and qualitative evaluation of the patient's facial deformity. The diagnosis is based on the accumulation of appropriate data. Appropriate data collection can be obtained only when the clinician accurately identifies those areas of the face that are either functionally compromised or esthetically unpleasing.

This section is divided into three parts: (1) facial skeletal surgery, (2) soft tissue surgery, and (3) planning the sequence of surgery for combined skeletal and soft tissue correction. It is understood that both the skeletal and soft tissue surgeries are intimately affected by one another; however, for the purpose of presentation, they will be discussed separately.

Facial Skeletal Surgery

Facial skeletal surgery can generally be considered to include (1) esthetic recontouring and (2) orthognathic surgery and craniofacial surgery.

Esthetic Recontouring Procedures

Esthetic recontouring maxillofacial skeletal surgery can be either augmentation or reduction. Augmentation may be accomplished by using either autogenous or alloplastic onlay materials.

Alloplastic Materials

Alloplastic onlay materials such as porous polyethylene,* hydroxyapatite, and custom-fabricated medical grade Silastic† have all been successfully employed in patients who have facial asymmetries (Fig. 15–11A,B).

The shape and dimensions of the alloplastic materials are determined from the detailed esthetic anthropometric data and barium cephalometric radiographic.

---

* Medpor Surgical Implant, Fairburn, GA.
† Dow Corning Wright, Arlington, TN.

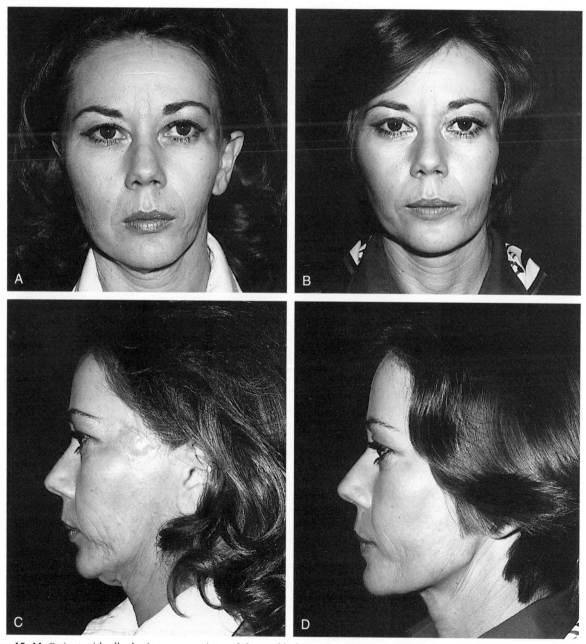

Figure 15–11. Patient with alloplastic augmentation to left mandibular angle. *A, B,* pre- and postoperative frontal views; *C, D,* pre- and postoperative left profile views.

Autogenous Materials

Autogenous onlay materials such as cranial or iliac crest bone have also been successfully employed as skeletal augmentation materials; however, the amount of resorption and final contour does not have the same predictability as that of alloplastic materials in most areas of the craniofacial skeleton. Two notable exceptions are reconstruction of the missing or hypoplastic zygoma-zygomatic arch and select secondary cleft lip–nose deformities, in which autogenous onlay materials appear to have greater long-term stability.

Skeletal Recontouring

In those cases in which the skeletal asymmetry is secondary to skeletal excess on the affected side, reduction osteoplasty is an excellent means of reestablishing symmetry (Fig. 15–12*A,B,C,D*).

Orthognathic Craniofacial Surgery

Lateral cephalometric prediction tracings are essential when planning treatment for facial deformities involving symmetric conditions. When planning treatment for patients with facial asymmetries, prediction tracings made from lateral cephalometric radiographs are less helpful. In these instances, the PA cephalometric radiographic prediction tracing is of primary importance. This, along with the definitive presurgical model surgery, provides the most helpful information required to accomplish an accurate reproduction of the treatment plan.

Prediction Tracings

PA Barium Cephalometric Radiographs

The PA barium cephalometric radiograph is diagnostically invaluable in determining both the skeletal asymmetric relationships and soft tissue thicknesses. It is this radiograph that aids in designing augmentation implants or reduction osteoplasties. The PA barium radiograph is most helpful when diagnosing and treatment planning asymmetries located in the middle and lower thirds of the face.

The quantitative data from the PA barium cephalometric radiograph must be combined with facial anthropometric measurements to be optimally useful in planning treatment for occlusal cants. Many patients who have skeletal or dental cants of the occlusal plane have asymmetry of the soft tissues around the perioral area. In some instances the patient's smile is asymmetric, or it may parallel the asymmetry. Therefore, to always correct the cant to the occlusal plane would visually intensify the patient's asymmetry in some instances. For example, a patient may have a 10-mm cant to the molar occlusal plane, but on animation, only 3 mm of excess tooth is demonstrated on one side. The amount of appropriate skeletal correction is 3 mm, not 10 mm.

A method to perform a PA prediction tracing of the changes in both hard and soft tissues follows. This section will discuss first the technique for isolated mandibular surgery and then the technique for combined maxillary and mandibular surgery.

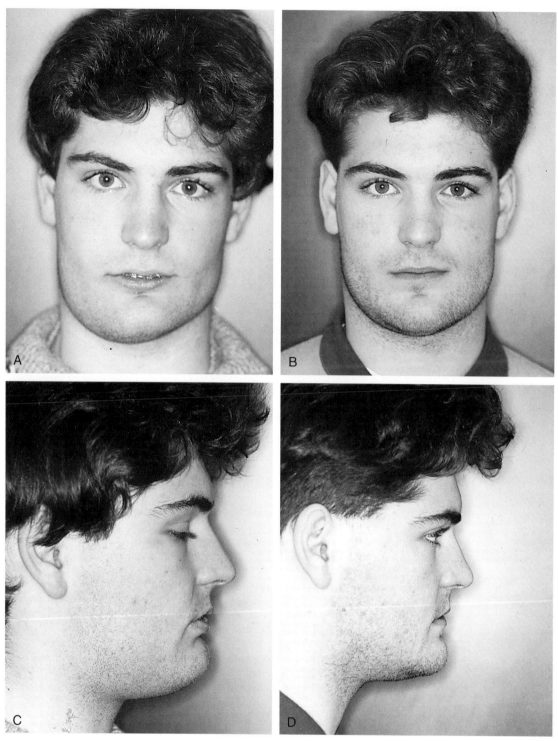

Figure 15–12. Patient with reduction osteoplasty of right mandibular inferior border. *A, B,* pre- and postoperative frontal views; *C, D,* pre- and postoperative right profile views.

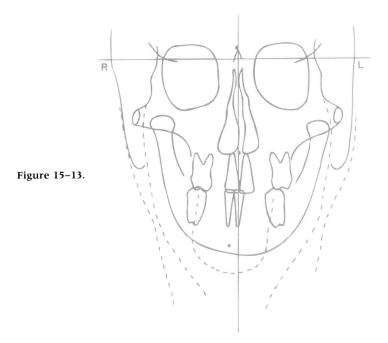

Figure 15–13.

Prediction Tracing: Mandibular Surgery

The presurgical PA cephalometric tracing of a patient who would benefit from an asymmetric mandibular advancement (setback) is seen in Figure 15–13.

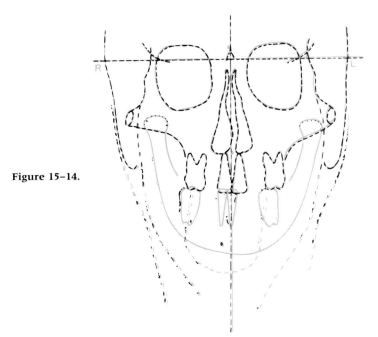

Figure 15–14.

1. Begin the prediction tracing (hereafter called the *prediction* and shown in black) by tracing on a clean piece of acetate tracing paper the facial midline, the upper horizontal referent line, the maxillary molars, the maxillary incisors, and the *soft tissue reference lines* above the molar crowns. Trace all other cephalometric features with the exception of the mandible and the soft tissue referent lines.

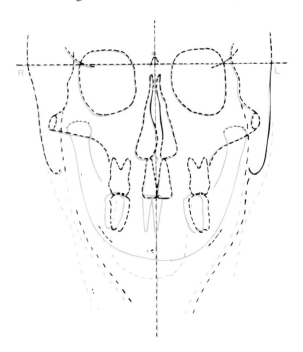

Figure 15–15.

2. Slide the *prediction* along the molar occlusal plane to achieve the best possible molar occlusion. Holding this superimposition, trace the mandibular molars, the lower border of the mandible at approximately the molar level, and the middle soft tissue reference line below the molar crown.

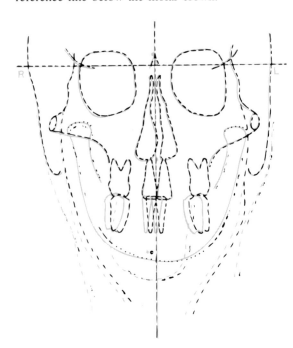

Figure 15–16.

3. Slide the *prediction* along the occlusal plane until the mandibular incisors achieve their optimal position in relation to the maxillary incisors. (Note: The occlusal plane cannot be tipped while this is done.) Holding this superimposition, trace the mandibular incisors and dot in the bony chin. This superimposition may be the same as the one above when the lower incisors and molars are equally asymmetric in relation to the upper teeth. Do not trace the soft tissue reference line at this time.

While holding the above superimposition, study the position of the bony chin and the soft tissue referent overlying it to determine whether the chin now lies in the midline. If the chin is now symmetric, trace the anterior soft tissue reference line and go to step 6. If the chin is not symmetric with the soft tissue referent lying on the facial midline, a genioplasty will be required to provide additional correction of the chin symmetry.

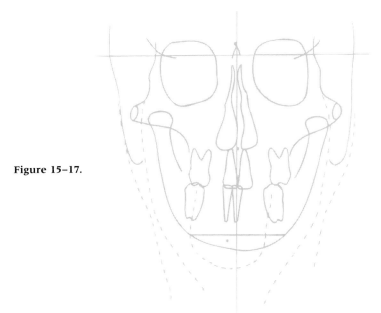

Figure 15–17.

4. Construct on the *tracing* a line to represent the position of the osteotomy for the proposed genioplasty (approximately 30 mm below the edge of the lower incisors and parallel to the occlusal plane).

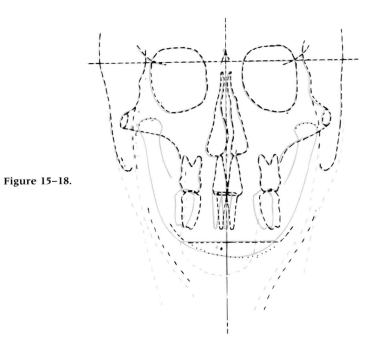

Figure 15–18.

5. Superimpose the *prediction* on the lower incisors and dotted chin, and trace the genioplasty line onto the *prediction*.

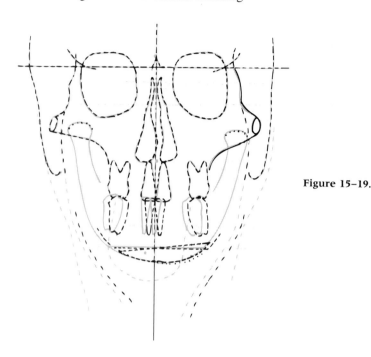

Figure 15–19.

6. Slide and/or rotate the *prediction* until the bony chin, soft tissue midline marker, and anterior soft tissue reference line of the *tracing* is in the desired position in relation to the *prediction*. Holding this superimposition, trace the bony chin, genio-plasty line, and anterior soft tissue reference line. (Note: The amount of overlapping of the genioplasty lines will indicate the amount of ostectomy necessary; divergence of these lines will indicate the amount of grafting necessary to produce the desired result.)

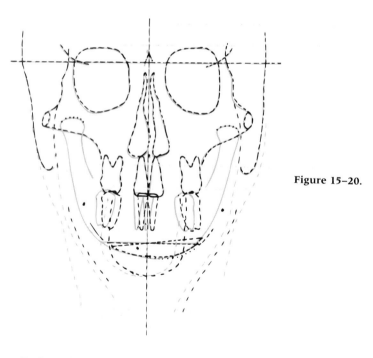

Figure 15–20.

7. Superimpose on the *fixed structures* (structures that are not surgically manipu-lated, such as the calvaria, cranial base, and orbits, and study the change in the molar and incisor positions. When lateral movement of the molars, the incisors, or both has been predicted, the rotation of the distal segment may produce some flaring or reduction in prominence of the proximal segments (i.e., mandibular angles) during surgery. Excessive flaring can be controlled by producing a medial displacing green-

stick fracture of the posterior aspect of the distal segment. Conversely, excessive reduction in mandibular angle prominence by a medial movement of the posterior aspect of the distal segment may necessitate interpositional grafting between the posterior aspect of the proximal segment. It is impossible to exactly predict these changes because the three-dimensional anatomy of the sagittal osteotomy cannot be determined before surgery. Nevertheless, the following guidelines will give the clinician some idea of what to expect at surgery so that adequate preparation can be made in advance, especially when there may be a need for grafting.

Tracing the proximal segments and the overlying soft tissues for prediction requires two assumptions and one piece of data. The first assumption is a 1:1 ratio of soft tissue change to bony movement in the area of the mandibular angles. The second assumption is that the condylar head remains within the confines of the glenoid fossa. The single piece of data is the change in the position of the mandibular proximal segments as measured on the definitive model surgery (which will be discussed later). These assumptions and information will allow a fairly accurate soft tissue prediction.

To complete the prediction as illustrated, the measurements required from the condylar grooves on the definitive model surgery indicate that these have moved 3 mm to the patient's left. While holding the superimposition on the fixed structures, place a dot on the *prediction* 3 mm to the left of the current mandibular angle.

Figure 15–21.

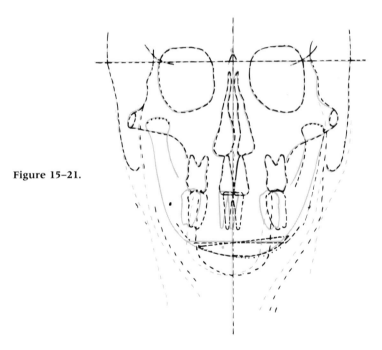

8. Slide and/or rotate the prediction, keeping the condyle in the fossa, until the mandibular angle of the *tracing* lies on the dot just made, and trace the proximal segment and the posterior soft tissue reference line to the angle of the mandible. Repeat on the opposite side (not illustrated).

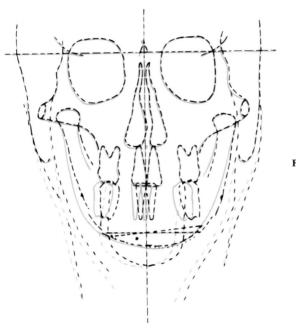

Figure 15–22.

9. Complete the *prediction* by (1) superimposing on the fixed structures, (2) tracing the lower portion of the posterior reference line, (3) connecting it to the upper portion by a smooth curve, and (4) smoothing out the middle reference line. The overall effect of the proposed surgery can now be studied.

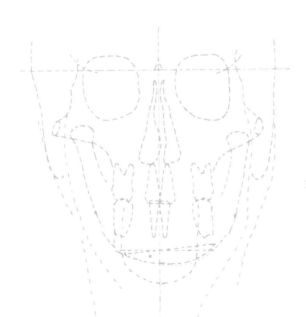

Figure 15–23.

The completed prediction seen above can now be studied to determine the need for adjunctive procedures or modification of the planned surgery needed to achieve the desired result.

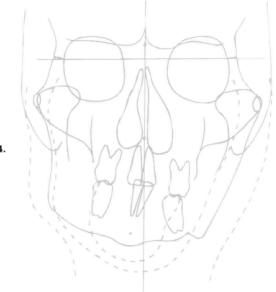

Figure 15–24.

PA Prediction Tracing: Combined Maxillary and Mandibular Surgery

Figure 15–24 shows the pretreatment PA cephalometric tracing of a patient who would benefit from a maxillary surgical procedure to level the occlusal plane and place the anterior teeth in the proper position to the midline and the lip *commissure* and an asymmetric mandibular setback.

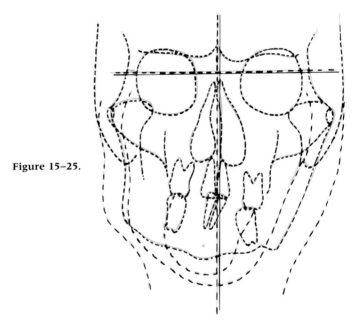

Figure 15–25.

1. Begin the *prediction* (black) by tracing a horizontal and a vertical reference line from the *tracing* (gray) on a new piece of tracing acetate.

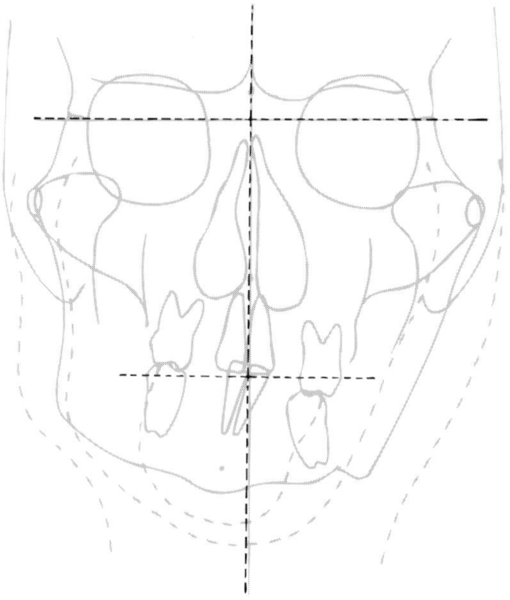

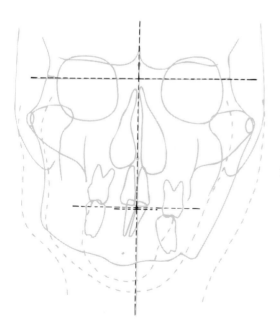

Figure 15–26.

2. Without moving the *prediction,* draw a horizontal line at the level of the desired molar occlusal plane. *The position of this line is determined on the basis of the esthetic considerations for the individual patient.* If the patient does not animate the corners of the mouth symmetrically, as may be the case in hemifacial microsomia, it may be best not to make this plane perfectly perpendicular to the facial midline. When animation is symmetric, this line is perpendicular to the facial midline. One side may move superiorly in a patient who has asymmetric vertical maxillary excess; one side may move inferiorly in a patient who has asymmetric vertical maxillary deficiency; or one side may move up and the other down, as in the example.

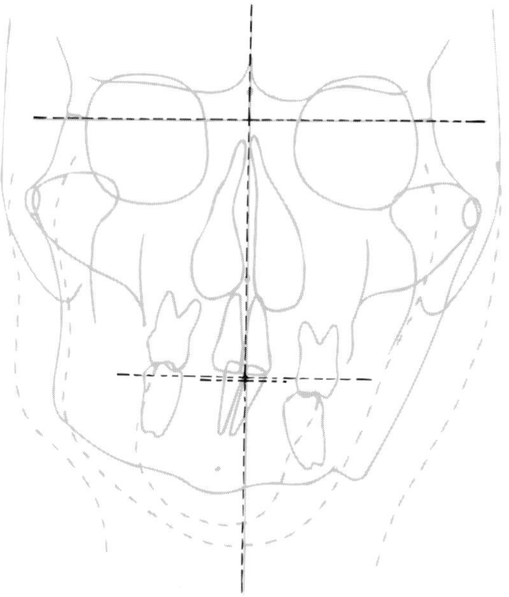

Figure 15–27.

3. Draw on the *prediction* a line to indicate the desired vertical position of the upper incisal edge. This line is parallel to the molar occlusal plane (drawn in step 2 above), and its vertical position is determined on the basis of the upper tooth-to-lip relation. For a patient who shows too much incisor, make it above the current level of the incisors. For a patient who shows too little incisor, make it below the current incisor level.

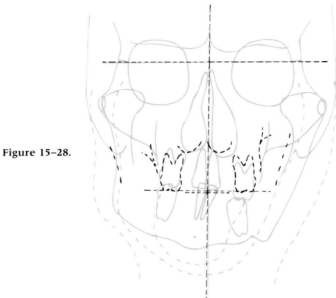

Figure 15–28.

4. Rotate the *prediction* until the predicted molar occlusal plane is coincident with the existing molar occlusal plane on the *tracing*. Then slide the *prediction* along the molar occlusal plane until the facial midline on the *prediction* is equidistant from the upper molars on the *tracing*. While holding this superimposition, trace the upper molars, the nasal floor, the lateral maxillary walls, and the portion of the middle soft tissue reference line that lies between the zygomatic arch and the molar occlusal plane.

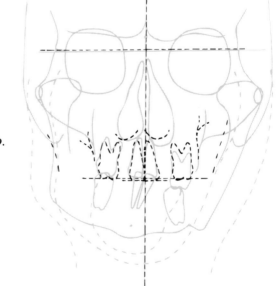

Figure 15–29.

5. Keeping the molar occlusal plane on the *prediction* parallel with that on the *tracing,* slide the *prediction* over the *tracing* until the upper incisors are in the midline and their incisal edges lie on the line drawn to indicate their optimal vertical level. While holding this superimposition, trace the upper incisors.

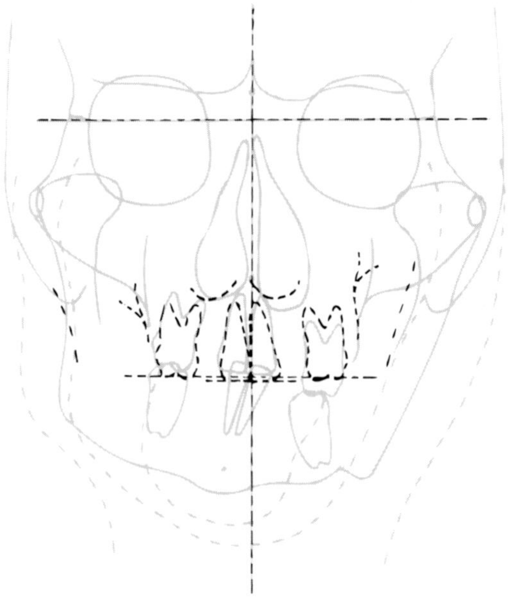

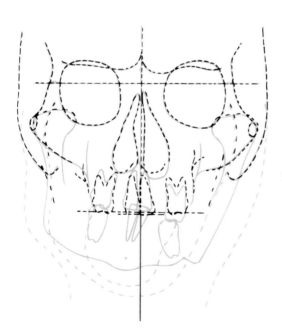

Figure 15–30.

6. Place the *prediction* on the *tracing* so that the horizontal and vertical referent lines traced at the beginning are coincident. Study the changes shown in the upper molars and incisors to ensure that the desired changes (as determined on facial esthetics) are coincident with the *prediction*.

Figure 15–31.

If this is so, trace the stable portions of the *tracing,* including the orbits, cranium, nasal cavity, and all other cephalometric features except the mandible and the remaining soft tissue reference. (Note: The soft tissue reference lines are traced in segments and likely will not be aligned. These will be smoothed out later in the prediction process.) Trace the heads of the condyles with dashed lines for reference in placing the distal segments of the mandible later in the process.

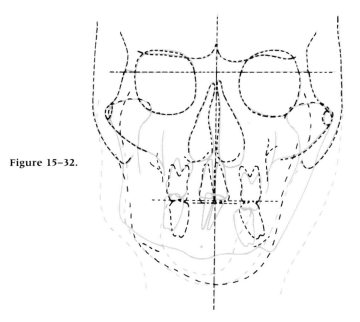

Figure 15–32.

7. Slide the *prediction* along the molar occlusal plane to achieve the best possible molar occlusion. Holding this superimposition, trace the mandibular molars and the lower border of the mandible at approximately the molar level and the middle soft tissue reference line below the molar crown.

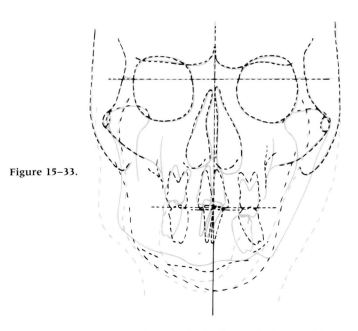

Figure 15–33.

8. Slide the *prediction* along the occlusal plane until the lower incisors achieve their optimal position in relation to the maxillary incisors. (Note: The occlusal plane cannot be tipped.) Holding this superimposition, trace the lower incisors and bony chin with a dashed line, because the position of the bony chin may be subsequently altered by the addition of a genioplasty. This superimposition may be the same as that in step 7 when the lower incisors and molars are equally symmetric. Do not trace the soft tissue reference line at this time.

While holding this superimposition, study the position of the bony chin and the soft tissue referent overlying it to determine whether the chin now lies in the midline. If the chin is now symmetric, trace the anterior soft tissue referent line and go to step 12. If the chin is *not* symmetric with the facial midline (as is usual), a genioplasty will be required in order to provide additional correction of the chin symmetry.

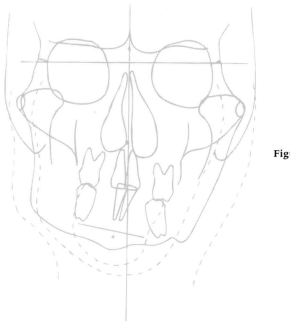

Figure 15–34.

9. Construct on the *tracing* a line to represent the position of the osteotomy for the proposed genioplasty (approximately 30 mm below the edge of the lower incisors and parallel to the molar occlusal plane).

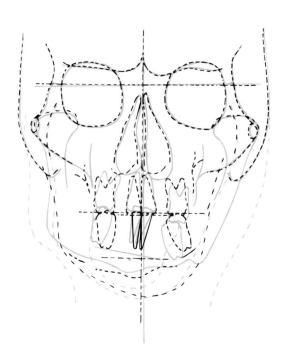

Figure 15–35.

10. Place the *prediction* on the *tracing* superimposing on the mandibular incisors and bony chin as traced in the preceding step, and trace the genioplasty line onto the *prediction*.

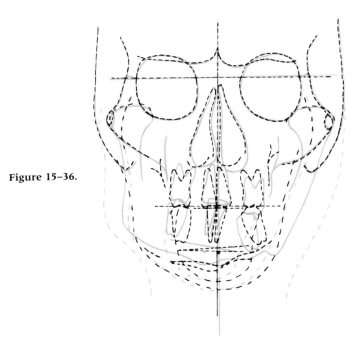

Figure 15–36.

11. Slide and/or rotate the *prediction* until the bony chin, soft tissue midline marker, and anterior soft tissue reference line of the *tracing* are in the desired position in relation to the *prediction*. Holding this superimposition, trace the bony chin, osteotomy line, and anterior soft tissue reference line. (Note: The amount of overlapping of the osteotomy lines will indicate the amount of ostectomy necessary; divergence of these lines will indicate the amount of grafting necessary to produce the desired result.)

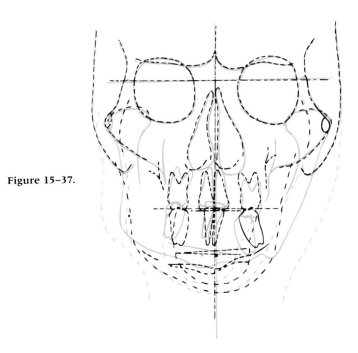

Figure 15–37.

12. Superimpose on the fixed structures and study the change in the molar and incisor positions. When lateral movement of the molars, the incisors, or both has been predicted, the rotation of the distal segment may produce flaring or reduction in prominence of the proximal segments (i.e., mandibular angles) during surgery. Excessive flaring can be controlled by producing a medial displacing greenstick fracture of the posterior aspect of the distal segment. Conversely, excessive reduction in mandib-

ular angle prominence by a medial movement of the posterior aspect of the distal segment may necessitate interpositional grafting between the posterior aspect of the distal segment and the anterior aspect of the proximal segment. It is impossible to exactly predict these changes because the three-dimensional anatomy of the sagittal osteotomy cannot be determined before surgery. Nevertheless, the following guidelines will give the clinician some idea of what to expect at surgery so that adequate preparation can be made in advance, especially when there may be a need for grafting.

To complete the *prediction* herein illustrated, the measurements required from the condylar grooves on the definitive model surgery indicate that these have moved 6 mm to the patient's left. While holding the superimposition on the fixed structures, place a dot on the *prediction* 6 mm to the left of the correct mandibular angle.

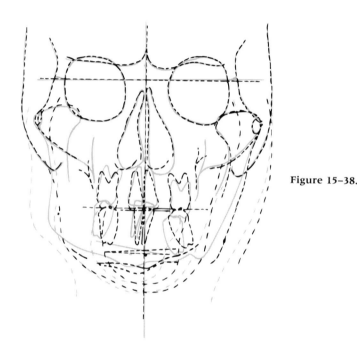

Figure 15–38.

13. Slide and/or rotate the *prediction,* keeping the condyle in the fossa, until the mandibular angle of the *tracing* lies on the dot just made, and trace the proximal segment and the posterior soft tissue reference line down to the angle of the mandible. Repeat on the opposite side (not illustrated).

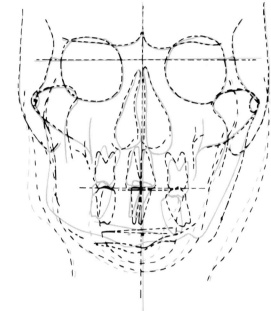

Figure 15–39.

14. Complete the *prediction* by (1) superimposing on the fixed structures, (2) tracing the lower portion of the posterior reference line, (3) connecting it to the upper portion by a smooth curve, and (4) smoothing out the middle reference line. The overall effect of the proposed surgery can now be studied.

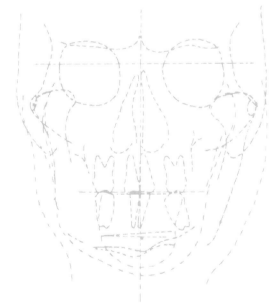

Figure 15–40.

The completed prediction tracing is shown above. It can now be studied to determine the need for modification of the proposed surgical procedure or the addition of adjunctive procedures.

Lateral Barium Cephalometric Radiograph

The lateral barium cephalometric radiograph for prediction tracing for the correction of facial asymmetries has limited value but is helpful from two standpoints. First, it confirms the specific anterior-posterior locations of the barium markers in relation to the underlying facial skeleton. This is helpful in examining the PA barium cephalometric radiograph in that the various barium marker lines can be related to specific skeletal anatomic locations.

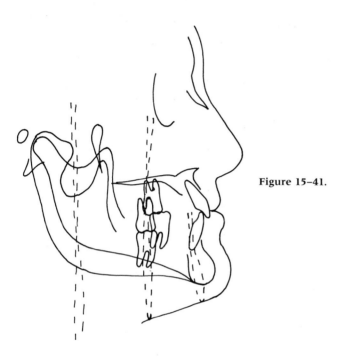

Figure 15–41.

Second, although using the lateral cephalometric radiograph to produce a prediction tracing is not entirely reliable in patients with facial asymmetry, it will give *average* skeletal anterior-posterior movements.

In summary, any definitive treatment plans involving the lower third of the face is best made by combining data from the anthropometric measurements, PA barium cephalometric radiograph, and the definitive immediate presurgical model surgery.

Definitive Model Surgery

As noted earlier, the model surgery is the most important means of identifying the movements required in order to correct asymmetry in the lower third of the face. After the models are checked for accuracy in relation to the actual patient, they are mounted and trimmed anatomically, and reference marks are made. It is noteworthy that reference marks on the definitive surgery models are helpful only if they are accurately transferred from the models to the patient intraoperatively. Arbitrarily determining horizontal or vertical references at the time of surgery can disorient the surgeon during the actual surgery. Therefore, any modality by which the model surgery references can be accurately transferred to the patient should be employed.

This text will not describe step by step the basics of model surgery; however, there are several noteworthy points in regard to asymmetric model surgery. It is suggested that the vertical reference marks on the lateral maxillary walls be made perpendicular to the occlusal plane, not to the Frankfort horizontal, both on the model surgery and on the patient. This allows for more accurate transfer of information from the models to the patient, since producing vertical reference marks in the mouth perpendicular to the occlusal plane is far easier than making reference marks perpendicular to the Frankfort horizontal. This transfer of lateral maxillary wall vertical reference marks can be easily accomplished with the use of a maxillary reference device such as that pictured in Figure 15–42.

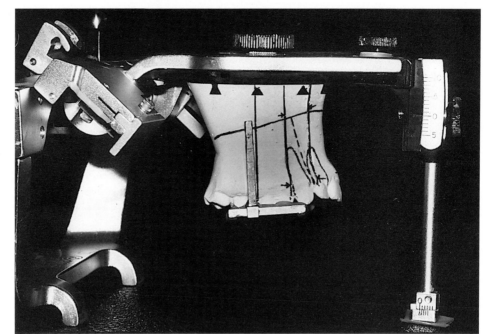

Figure 15–42. Epker-Stella Maxillary Reference Device. (Courtesy of Walter Lorenz Surgical Instruments, Jacksonville, FL.)

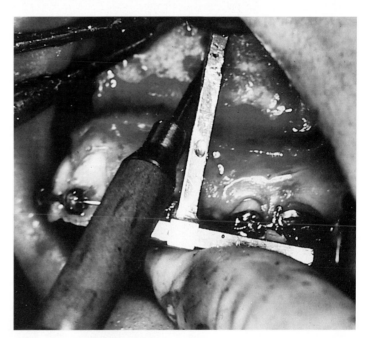

Figure 15–43.

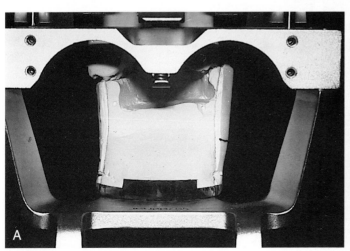

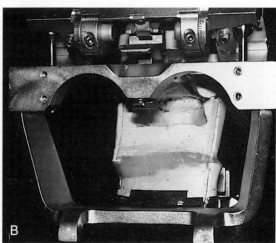

Figure 15–44.

The reference device is fabricated with two flat surfaces and a vertical component that is hinged on a bar. On one side of the flat surface, a wax occlusal registration of the patient's maxillary right side from cuspid to molar is made; on the opposing flat surface, the contralateral wax registration bite is made.

This device is used to transfer vertical references from the models to the patients (Fig. 15–43).

In patients who undergo asymmetric mandibular surgery, the model surgery provides essential information about the amount of mediolateral discrepancies that will exist between the condylar and dentoalveolar segments. This is best appreciated by placing a shallow condylar groove in the most posterolateral aspects of the mandibular models. This condylar groove extends from the most superior aspect of this area down to the mounting ring. In this way, when the mandibular model is sectioned and manipulated, the magnitude of the discrepancy that exists between the condylar segment and dentoalveolar segment can be appreciated.

This also enables the surgeon to strategically plan ramus surgery (Fig. 15-44A,B).

The model surgery is invaluable in determining the position of pogonion. Since orthognathic surgery on asymmetric patients is a three-dimensional event, the location of the chin after osteotomies of the maxilla and/or mandible is difficult to accurately predict. Appreciation of information obtained from the model surgery is the only means by which this can be predicted in cases of asymmetry. In order to accurately treatment plan and surgically position the chin, transference of information from the model surgery to the patient is critical.

The distance from the mandibular central incisal edge to pogonion as noted on the lateral cephalometric radiograph should be transferred to the models (Fig. 15–45A). From the frontal view of the patient, the mediolateral position of pogonion in relation to the facial midline is recorded on the models (Fig. 15–45B). The horizontal distance from pogonion to the incisal guide pin is also noted (Fig. 15–45C). In this way, the pogonion may be located on the models in all three dimensions.

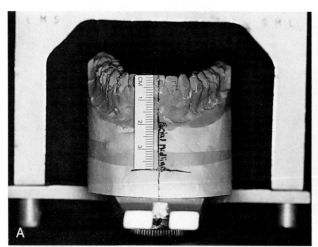

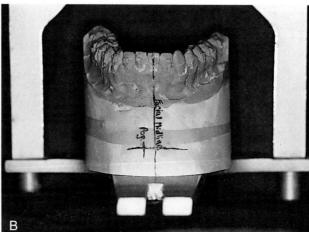

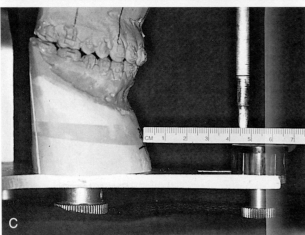

Figure 15–45.

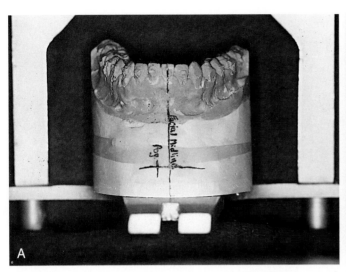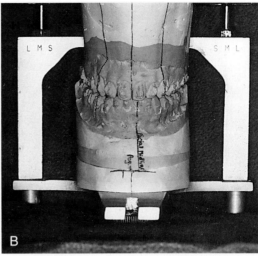

Figure 15–46. *A,* Preoperative position of pogonion (Pog) is 5 mm to the right of facial midline. *B,* Position of pogonion (Pog) after mandibular surgery. In this case, Pog has moved to the facial midline reference on the base of models. Note that the maxillary dental midline, mandibular dental midline, and Pog are all on the facial midline, which remains as a referent on the plaster of the mandibular mounting ring. At this point, symmetry is good, and only anterior-posterior chin position needs to be determined cephalometrically.

After the completion of the definitive model surgery, the measurements of the chin are reexamined. It is from this "new" chin position (Fig. 15–46*B*) that a genioplasty, if necessary, can be accurately planned and reproduced at surgery. In the case illustrated, the pogonion (Pog) has been brought to the facial midline by the ramus surgery alone. A straightening genioplasty would not be necessary.

Soft Tissue Surgery

As with skeletal surgery, soft tissue corrections of the face are accomplished by either primary or secondary repositioning, by reduction, or by augmentation.

Repositioning (Rearrangement)

Primary

A classic example of repositioning tissue to correct facial asymmetry is the primary correction of the cleft lip-nose deformity (Fig. 15–47*A,B*). The accepted anthropometric norm can assist in the repositioning of asymmetric tissues to produce the ideal result.

Secondary

Although many examples exist in this category (congenital, acquired, or developmental deformities), anthropometric assisted correction is helpful in producing an improved result (Fig. 15–48*A,B*).

Reduction

The primary methods of facial soft tissue reduction are liposuction and myectomy. Liposuction may be accomplished by two methods: open and closed techniques.

Liposuction

Closed liposuction techniques involve a small incision through which a small liposuction cannula is introduced and manipulated. The indications for closed liposuction are excessive deposits of fat and sufficient elasticity of the overlying soft tissues to properly redrape the underlying muscle after fat removal.

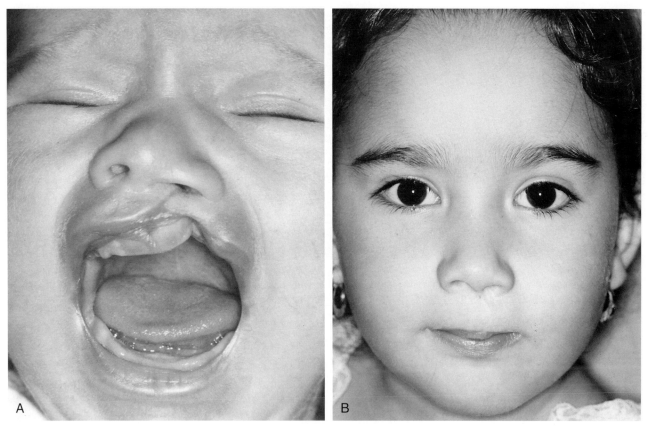

Figure 15–47.

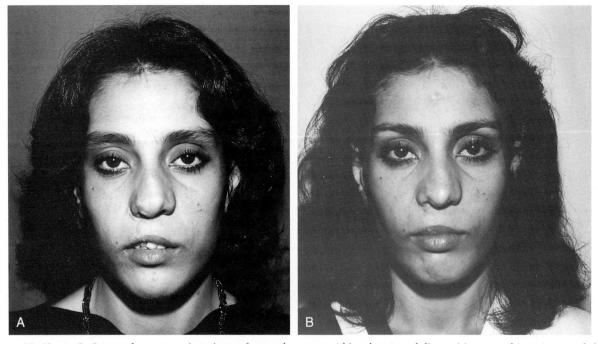

Figure 15–48. *A, B,* Pre- and postoperative views of secondary nose (rhinoplasty) and lip revision to achieve improved facial symmetry.

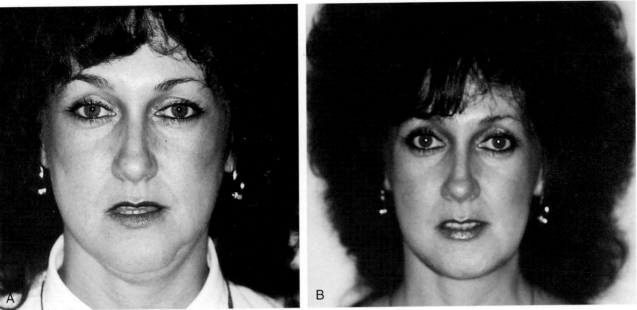

Figure 15–49. *A, B,* Pre- and postoperative appearances; combined osteotomies and soft tissue surgery, including lipectomy, were performed to correct facial asymmetry.

Closed liposuction can also be performed in those cases in which skin redundancy exists, if the planned facial skeletal surgery will stretch the soft tissue matrix to remove residual redundancy.

Open liposuction techniques involve larger incisions in which the fat and underlying muscle are directly visualized and surgically manipulated. Open approaches to fat removal are indicated when excessive adipose tissue exists in an environment of redundant skin and/or when underlying muscle surgery is anticipated. The open technique allows for fat removal with simultaneous muscle resection and/or repositioning, as well as resection of redundant skin (Fig. 15–49*A,B*).

Myectomy

This is used in cases of benign masseteric hypertrophy. The procedure is almost always conducted in concert with skeletal reduction surgery.

Augmentation

Soft tissue augmentation in patients with various soft tissue deficiencies in the maxillofacial region can be categorized into three basic types: free fat transfers, free dermal fat grafts, and alloplastic implants (e.g., collagen, Gore-Tex).

Free Fat Transfer

The primary indication for free fat transfer is to improve contour or asymmetric soft tissue defects. The technique for free fat transfer includes aspiration of fat into a sterile syringe by using small, rigid suction lipectomy cannulas. The donor site may be directly adjacent to the proposed contour defect or relatively distant, such as the abdomen or medial knee area. Excess fluid and/or local anesthesia is then expressed from the harvested fat. A large-bore 16- to 18-gauge needle is used to reinject the harvested fat to the small soft tissue defect (Fig. 15–50*A,B*).

Dermal Fat Grafts

Full dermal fat grafts are best used in larger soft tissue defects. Dermal fat may be harvested from either the abdomen or the buttocks. The shape and size of the harvested dermal fat graft are determined by the size and shape of the soft tissue contour defect. The recipient site is prepared by developing a soft tissue envelope in the area

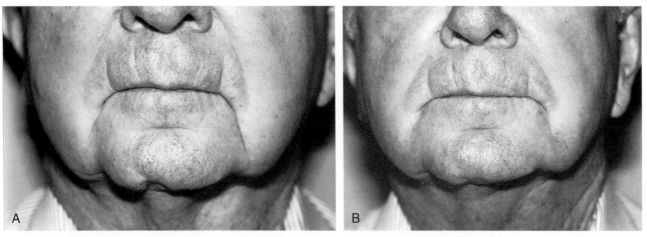

Figure 15–50. *A,* Preoperative view: Free fat transfer indicated to improve asymmetric deep orolabial folds and depressed chin scar. *B,* Postoperative view: Free fat injected into left orolabial fold and depressed chin scar to improve symmetry.

of the defect, as Figure 15–51 illustrates. The harvested dermal fat graft is placed and secured with strategically placed stent sutures. The graft is oriented at the recipient site so that the dermal aspect of the graft contacts the deeper underlying soft tissue vascular bed.

Planning the Sequence of Surgery for Combined Skeletal and Soft Tissue Correction

This topic is often overlooked, and its value is underestimated. Many symmetric patients require a variety of skeletal and soft tissue procedures to improve their facial deformities. By determining the sequence before surgery, operating time and blood loss can be minimized and the predictability of the final surgical result can be appreciated. In general, when combined skeletal and soft tissue surgeries are performed, it is usual to complete the skeletal surgery and close the access sites before addressing soft tissue augmentation or reduction. This sequence minimizes the potential for hematoma formation by allowing the immediate placement of pressure dressings.

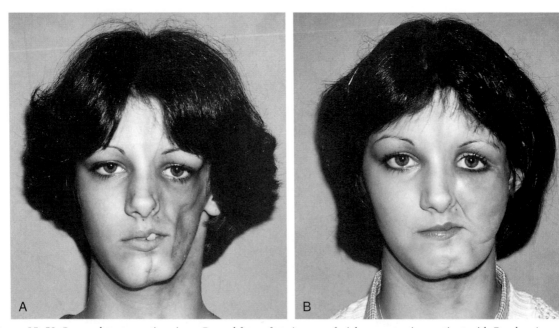

Figure 15–51. Pre- and postoperative views: Dermal fat graft to improve facial symmetry in a patient with Romberg's syndrome.

More specifically, when *profound* soft tissue deficiencies or excesses exist, performing combined skeletal and soft tissue surgeries in a single operation is advised. Six to twelve months later, refinements of the soft tissues may be done. Conversely, when more *subtle* soft tissue deficiencies or excesses exist, it is prudent to complete the skeletal and/or hard tissue procedures first. Six to twelve months later, residual soft tissue asymmetry may be evaluated.

CONCLUSIONS

This chapter presents an objective protocol for the evaluation, data collection, diagnosing, treatment planning, and surgical sequencing of patients with facial asymmetries.

Routine adherence to such a protocol will predictably and repeatedly produce quality results in a patient population with facial deformities.

References

1. Adams WM: Bilateral hypertrophy of masseter muscle. An operation for correction. Br J Plast Surg 1949; 2:78.
2. Adamson JE, Horton CE, Crawford HH: The surgical correction of the "turkey gobbler" deformity. Plast Reconstr Surg 1964; 34:598.
3. Adrien AE: Augmentation cheiloplasty. Plast Reconstr Surg 1991; 88:222.
4. Beckers HL: Masseteric muscle hypertrophy and its intraoral surgical correction. J Maxillofac Surg 1977; 5:28.
5. Bikhazi HB, Antwerp RV: The use of Medpor in cosmetic and reconstructive surgery: Experimental and clinical evidence. Plast Reconstr Surg 1990; 6:271.
6. Czarnecki ST, Nanda RS, Currier GF: Perceptions of a balanced facial profile. Am J Orthod Dentofac Orthop 1993; 104:180.
7. Davis WM: A simple method to gain symmetry of the intraoral genioplasty. J Oral Maxillofac Surg 1988; 48:710.
8. Elam MV, Berkowitz F: Submental and submandibular lipectomy by lipo-suction surgery. Am J Cosmet Surg 1988; 2:3.
9. Epker BN, Fish LC: Dentofacial Deformities: An Integrated Orthodontic-Surgical Approach. St. Louis: CV Mosby, 1986.
10. Epker BN, Stella JP: Transoral submental lipectomy: An adjunct to orthognathic surgery. J Oral Maxillofac Surg 1989; 47:795.
11. Epker BN, Stella JP: Systematic aesthetic evaluation of the neck for cosmetic surgery in cosmetic oral and maxillofacial surgery. Oral Maxillofac Surg Clin North Am 1990; 2:217–231.
12. Farkas LG: Anthropometrics of the Head and Face in Medicine, pp 8–59, 108–202. New York: Elsevier, 1981.
13. Farkas LG: Anthropometrics of the normal and defective ear. Clin Plast Surg 1990; 17:213.
14. Farkas LG, Hreczko TA, Kolar JC, et al: Vertical and horizontal proportions of the face in young adult North American Caucasians: Revision of neoclassical canons. Plast Reconstr Surg 1985; 75:328.
15. Farkas LG, Katie MJ, Hreczko TA, et al: Anthropometric proportions in the upper-lower lip-chin area of the lower face in young white adults. Am J Orthod 1984; 86:52.
16. Farkas LG, Kolar JC: Anthropometrics and art in the aesthetics of women's faces. Clin Plast Surg 1987; 14:599.
17. Farkas LG, Sohm P, Kolar JC, et al: Inclination of the facial profile: art versus reality. Plast Reconstr Surg 1985; 75:509.
18. Ginwalla MS: Bilateral benign hypertrophy of masseter muscle. J Oral Surg 1961; 19:482.
19. Kempf KK, Seyfer AE: Facial defect augmentation with a dermal-fat graft. Oral Surg Oral Med Oral Pathol 1985; 59(4):340–343.
20. Koury ME, Epker BN: Maxillofacial esthetics: Anthropometrics of the maxillofacial region. J Oral Maxillofac Surg 1992; 50:806–820.
21. Mackay DR, Manders EK, Saggers GC, et al: The fate of dermal and dermal-fat grafts. Ann Plast Surg 1993; 31(1):42–46.
22. Masters FN, Georiade KP: Surgical treatment of benign masseteric hypertrophy. Plast Reconstr Surg. 1955; 15:215.
23. Mordick TG 2d, Larossa D, Whitaker L: Soft tissue reconstruction of the face: A comparison of dermal-fat grafting and vascularized tissue transfer. Ann Plast Surg 1992; 29(5):390–396.
24. Nicolle FV, Matt BA, Scamp T: Dermaland facial autografts in facial aesthetic surgery. Aesthetic Plast Surg 1992; 16(3):219–225.
25. Rosenberg L, Mercer D: The preparation of small dermal grafts. Ann Plast Surg 1985; 15(3):270–271.
26. Rubin LR: Polyethylene as a bone and cartilage substitute: A 32 year retrospective. Biomater Plast Surg 1982; 30:472.
27. Singer R: Improvement of the "young" fatty neck. Plast Reconstr Surg 1984; 73:582.
28. Teimourian B: Face and neck suction–assisted lipectomy associated with rhytidectomy. Plast Reconstr Surg 1983; 72:627.
29. Turvey TA, Epker BN: Soft tissue procedures adjunctive to orthognathic surgery for improvement of facial balance. J Oral Surg 1974; 32:572.
30. Weisman PA: Simplified technique in submental lipectomy. Plast Reconstr Surg 1971; 48:443.

III

Surgical Management

16 | Principles and Management of the Soft Tissues in Facial Clefts

Jefferson U. Davis

The spectrum of the severity of oblique facial clefts is as wide as that allowed by the human phenotype; new variations in clefts are catalogued with each additional case report and series. Therefore, diagnostic evaluation, treatment planning, and medical or surgical intervention must be customized in all instances to fulfill the unique requirements of each case. In spite of the individualization of therapy mandated by such phenotypic variance in morphopathology, adherence to an underpinning core of management principles is essential for providing comprehensive patient care. The general principles described in this chapter are intended to be used as adjuncts in bringing clarity, order, and systematic thinking into the safe and effective management of such complex congenital abnormalities.

GENERALIZED APPROACH

As with all other types of craniofacial deformity, the potential for associated regional and remote pathology is great, and such pathology therefore must be suspected. Many anomalies may have a significantly adverse impact on the infant physiologically or functionally or may even be life-threatening. For this reason, it is efficacious to carry out first a primary survey, in which the infant is thoroughly examined, all abnormalities are listed, and immediate life-threatening problems are addressed. A secondary survey of all regions then uncovers additional problems of less immediate threat. Appropriate imaging techniques can then be safely employed in the stabilized infant in order to define more comprehensively and with greater resolution the anomalies thus identified.

The information derived from these systematic and comprehensive surveys is useful in the formulation of a guiding treatment plan. The relative severity of problems is characterized by the degree of threat to functional integrity. The sequence of treatment and the type of therapeutic interventional modality are then determined accordingly.

TIMING

The relative urgency for repair depends on the severity of any given anomaly as defined by the degree of threat to functional or anatomic integrity. For example, exposure of the globe in an infant with a severe coloboma of the lower eyelid and with a poor or nonexistent Bell phenomenon heralds corneal ulceration and opacification with scarring or possibly globe rupture and therefore mandates urgent intervention. Conversely, the same defect in a healthy infant with an effective Bell phenomenon may be temporized medically with the use of lubricating ointments, moisture chambers, bandage soft contact lenses, and surgical repair carried out semielectively when the child has adjusted to extrauterine life. In neonates who are physiologically unstable or have other more threatening anomalies, such steps may be delayed until repair can be done safely. Surgical reconstruction may then be technically less difficult, inasmuch as component tissues have grown larger and less friable.

SPECIFIC APPROACH; APPLICATION OF PRINCIPLES

List All Affected Tissues and Characterize the Cleft

Simply stated, this is the answer to the question "What's missing or damaged?" In the working list of structures and tissues that require reconstruction, make sure each component tissue and functional structure for a given anatomic unit is evaluated systematically as follows: skin of the lip, cheek, nose, and eyelids; orbicularis sphincter muscle of the lip, and eyelids; oral, nasal, and conjunctival mucosal lining tissue; supporting structural tissues such as bone of alveolus, maxilla, pyriform rim, orbital rim, orbital floor, and alar cartilage; and special tissues, including the vermilion border and white roll and wet line of the lip, the ciliary line, the ciliary margin, the tarsal plate, the medial canthus, and the lacrimal drainage tissues.

In a complete Tessier type 3 cleft, for example, there is a deficiency of skin and a decrease in vertical dimension along the cleft that extends from the lateral alar margin to the medial third of the lower lid, resulting in superior displacement of the ala and coloboma of the lid. In this example, all of the tissues mentioned earlier are involved. It should be recognized that all layers are involved to some degree in such defects, and therefore all layers should be repaired in order to prevent a depressed scar or a hypodynamic effect.

Combine All Essential First-Stage Soft Tissue Repairs as Much as Possible to Restore the Functional Effect of the Tissue Envelope

However, manage each component defect as if it were an isolated flaw while restoring anatomic continuity and functional integrity according to the requirements of the region affected. In general, as with cleft lip repair alone, early restoration of soft tissue continuity across the facial cleft by a layered anatomic repair results in earlier normalization of functional molding forces that dynamically influence the growth of proximate and underlying supportive tissues and, ultimately, facial morphology. Conversely, any advantage to be gained by early repair must be weighed against the deleterious effects of resultant scarring upon dento-orbitofacial growth.

Respect Anatomic Landmarks for Optimal Esthetic Outcome

In the upper lip cleft, this means careful alignment of the white roll and vermilion border, as well as myoplastic functional repair, whereas in the lower eyelid it means meticulous attention to alignment of the ciliary margin and line and repair of the orbicularis muscle, tarsal plate, and medial canthus. As is the case with repair of isolated cleft lips and coloboma, white roll–vermilion mismatch or notching of the ciliary margin is esthetically undesirable. Careful planning and early attention to landmarks not only restore anatomic and functional integrity but also minimize the necessity for secondary procedures.

Address the Lacrimal Drainage Vestiges

Obstruction of any aspect of the lacrimal drainage system results in inspissation of bacteria-rich tears and can lead to chronic infection or acute dacryocystitis. Nasolacrimal infections are frequent nidi for orbital cellulitis and as such can potentially jeopardize orbital bone grafts. Any existing nasolacrimal infection must be addressed before bone grafting if the procedure is to be done safely. Antibiotic eyedrops can be used to suppress bacteria, prevent acute flares to some degree, and prevent dacryocystitis and can act as prophylaxis against infection in preparation for orbital surgery. As with any chronic antimicrobial use, resistant strains can develop; therefore, rotation of antibiotics is suggested. The lacrimal drainage system may be extirpated if cannulation or reconstruction of existing elements is not possible and if chronic infection is a risk as a result of ductal disruption by the cleft. Secondary lacrimal drainage procedures, such as conjunctivorhinostomy, can be performed if epiphora is present.

Preserve Any and All Ocular Elements and Orbital Contents

The ocular vestige provides a better stimulus for growth than does an enucleation sphere. The coloboma that results from eyelid involvement with the cleft may seriously threaten the integrity and function of the eye because of corneal ulceration, scarring, or even globe rupture in severe instances. In such cases, early intervention to preserve ocular elements is warranted. If the physiologic condition of the infant prevents acute surgical management, moisture chambers, lubricating ointments, and moist-bandage soft contact lenses provide temporizing solutions until surgery can be performed.

Congenital clinical anophthalmia and microphthalmia are characterized by a shallow sloping orbital floor. The deformities are compounded by the bony cleft of the orbital floor, which allows what meager orbital contents there are to prolapse, resulting in dystopia. Similarly, the smallness of the globe and orbit results in a relatively contracted conjunctival fornix, which can be mechanically enlarged beginning in the first week of life with serial conformers that are changed every 1 to 2 weeks. Persistently inadequate fornices can be enlarged with buccal mucosal grafts and maintained by splinting over conformers. The eyelids are smaller and shrunken, and the palpebral fissures are narrowed. Cilia and meibomian glands may be absent. The medial canthal tendon may be hypoplastic or displaced inferiorly, necessitating a canthopexy. Early reconstruction with meticulous attention to anatomic components and layered repair most adequately restores functional continuity and minimizes the need for secondary procedures.

Reduce Tension Along the Line of Repair by Bringing in Additional Tissue Where It Is Deficient

A number of approaches have been devised to fulfill this principle. Kawamoto and Tessier advocated early use of local interdigitating flaps or Z-plasties, followed by secondary scar revision if necessary, usually with rotation flaps to improve esthetic placement (Figs. 16–1 to 16–3). Initial use of rotation flaps as advocated by van der

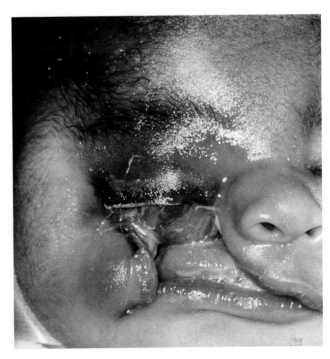

Figure 16–1. Type 4 cleft with defect passing lateral to cupid's bow, between pyriform aperture and infraorbital foramen, to medial third of lower lid. (Photo courtesy of Dr. H. D. Peterson.)

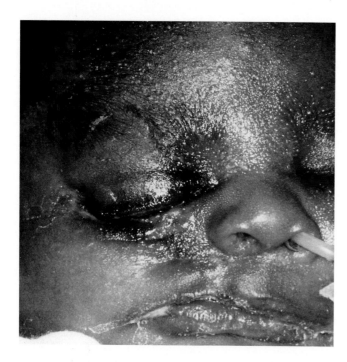

Figure 16–2. Type 4 cleft repaired with local interposition flaps only. (Photo courtesy of Dr. H. D. Peterson.)

Muelen provides for improved placement of scars; however, judicious use of interdigitating flaps within the rotation flap domain may nonetheless be required in order to gain sufficient length along the line of tension of the cleft (Fig. 16–4). Tissue expansion in the future site of rotation flap elevation is also useful in severe cases (Fig. 16–5). Expansion may aid not only by providing increase flap tissue for cleft closure but also by minimizing donor site deformity. All designs necessitate tissue undermining wide enough to impair subsequent growth to some degree.

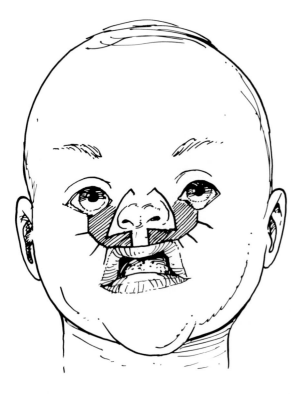

Figure 16–3. Local flaps that may be used in type 4 cleft.

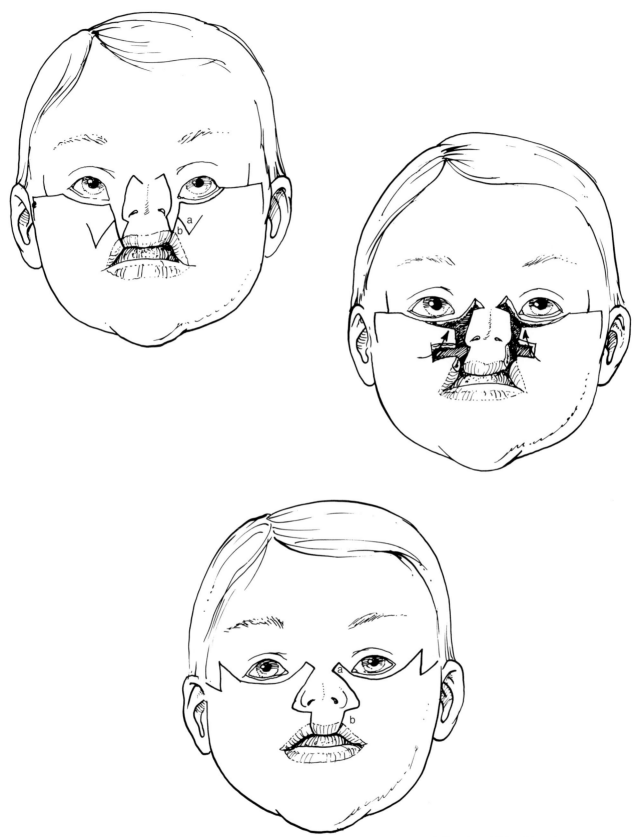

Figure 16–4. Examples of cheek rotation flaps, including integrated local flaps for additional length.

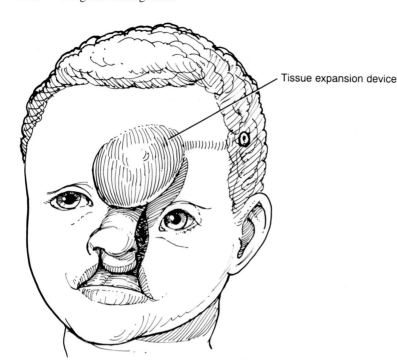

Tissue expansion device

Figure 16–5. Tissue expanders can be used in combination with median forehead flaps or other local flaps to lengthen the nose and increase the alar-canthal distance.

Design Flaps and Incision Placement to Reflect Consideration of Potential Donor Site Morbidity, Final Scar Placement, and Impact of Wide Undermining on Growth and Development

Design incisional flaps allow easier primary or secondary access for correction of associated deformities. They may be required early in treatment, such as at the initial soft tissue repair, or at much later stages of intervention, such as during canthopexy, nasolacrimal extirpation and reconstruction, or bone grafting to the orbit, alveolus, or maxilla. Regardless of timing, careful consideration of incision placement to maximize access and minimize postsurgical deformity is a general surgical principle that remains applicable.

Remember the Importance of Skeletal Support in Soft Tissue Esthetics

Bone grafting to the alveolus, maxilla, orbital rim, orbital floor, and pyriform rim may be required. In the presence of significant bony foundation deficiencies, soft tissue repair done is inadequate for correcting the deformity. Without the appropriate skeletal underpinning, incisions become depressed, shortened, and esthetically unacceptable. Timing should again be dictated by functional, growth, and development concerns. In less severe cases in which growth potential is greatest (albeit reduced), elective bone graft placement of the alveolus, anterior maxilla, and pyriform rim is best done according to the developmental time table of tooth bud eruption, when the cuspid root is one-half to two-thirds formed. Dystopia is corrected by orbital floor and rim grafts on the basis of functional necessity, which is generally greater in normal or microphthalmic but sighted eyes than it is in clinical anophthalmia. In more severe clefts, in which growth potential is severely impaired, early bone grafts have little overall detrimental impact in comparison with the cleft itself, and therefore there is little reason to delay grafting. The extent of grafting capability is restricted practically by availability of suitable bone stock at the calvarial, rib, and iliac crest donor sites. Obviously, the potential impact on donor site growth and esthetics must be considered when sites are selected. Alloplastic materials have no use in children at this time.

CONCLUSION

To the novice and even to the experienced surgeon, complex facial clefts pose challenging and sometimes intimidating problems for treatment planning and reconstruction. This occasionally bewildering array of management issues can be addressed more adequately if a standard set of management principles is followed in diagnosis, planning treatment, and interventional modality selection. The tenets elucidated in this chapter are intended to aid the surgeon in thinking clearly and systematically in the provision of comprehensive care for such challenging patients.

References

1. Antonyshyn O, Gruss JS, Zuker R, Mackinnon SE: Tissue expansion in head and neck reconstruction. Plast Reconstr Surg 1988; 82:58.
2. Argenta LC, Marks MW, Pasyk KA: Advances in tissue expansion. Clin Plast Surg 1985; 12:159.
3. Argenta LC, VanderKolk CA: Tissue expansion in craniofacial surgery. Clin Plast Surg 1987; 14:143.
4. Argenta LC, Watanabe MJ, Grabb WC: The use of tissue expansion in head and neck reconstruction. Ann Plast Surg 1983; 11:31.
5. Bartels RJ, O'Malley JE, Baker JL, Douglas WM: Naso-ocular clefts. Plast Reconstr Surg 1971; 47:351.
6. Boo-Chai K: The oblique facial cleft: A report of 2 cases and a review of 41 cases. Br J Plast Surg 1970; 23:352.
7. David DJ, Moore MH, Cooter RD: Tessier clefts revisited with a third dimension. Cleft Palate J 1989; 26:163.
8. Dey DL: Oblique facial clefts. Plast Reconstr Surg 1973; 52:258.
9. Gunter GS: Nasomaxillary cleft. Plast Reconstr Surg 1963; 32:637.
10. Kawamoto HK Jr: The kaleidoscopic world of rare craniofacial clefts: Order out of chaos (Tessier classification). Clin Plast Surg 1976; 3:529.
11. Kawamoto HK Jr, David DJ: Rare craniofacial clefts. In McCarthy JG (ed): Plastic Surgery, vol 4, pp 2922–2973. Philadelphia: WB Saunders, 1990.
12. Mayou BJ, Fenton OM: Oblique facial clefts caused by amniotic bands. Plast Reconstr Surg 1981; 68:675.
13. McGregor IA: Eyelid reconstruction following subtotal resection of upper or lower lid. Br J Plast Surg 1973; 26:346.
14. Miller SH, Wood AM, Haq MA: Bilateral oro-ocular cleft. Plast Reconstr Surg 1973; 51:590.
15. Morales L: Craniofacial clefts 3–10. In Marchac D (ed): Craniofacial Surgery—Proceedings of the First International Congress of the International Society of Cranio-Maxillo-Facial Surgery, p 254. Berlin: Springer-Verlag, 1985.
16. Ortiz-Monasterio F, Fuente del Campo A, Dinopulos A: Nasal clefts. Ann Plast Surg 1987; 18:377.
17. Resnick JI, Kawamoto HK Jr: Rare craniofacial clefts: Tessier IV clefts. Plast Reconstr Surg 1990; 85:843.
18. Sano S, Tani T, Nishimura Y: Bilateral oblique facial cleft. Ann Plast Surg 1983; 11:434.
19. Shewmake KB, Kawamoto HK Jr: Congenital clefts of the nose: Principles of surgical management. Cleft Palate Craniofac J 1992; 29:531.
20. Tessier P: Anatomical classification of facial, craniofacial and laterofacial clefts. J Maxillofac Surg 1976; 4:69.
21. Thorne CH: Craniofacial clefts. Clin Plast Surg 1993; 20:803.
22. Toth BA, Glafkides MC, Wandel A: The role of tissue expansion in the treatment of atypical facial clefting. Plast Reconstr Surg 1990; 86:119.
23. van der Meulen JC: The use of mucosa lined flap in eyelid reconstruction: A new approach. Plast Reconstr Surg 1982; 70:139.
24. van der Meulen JC: Oblique facial clefts: Pathology, etiology, and reconstruction. Plast Reconstr Surg 1985; 76:212.
25. van der Meulen JC, Mazzola R, Vermey-Keers C, et al: A morphogenetic classification of craniofacial malformations. Plast Reconstr Surg 1983; 71:560.
26. Wilson LF, Musgrave RH, Garrett W, Conklin JE: Reconstruction of oblique facial clefts. Cleft Palate J 1972; 9:109.

Primary Closure of Cleft Lip and Palate

17

Frank E. Åbyholm

The management of children born with cleft lip and palate is best conducted in organized centers staffed by health care providers from multiple disciplines. It is commonly accepted that this approach is most efficacious for the management of all congenital facial malformations, including facial clefts and craniosynostosis.

The Oslo Cleft Center is renowned for its standardized treatment of children with cleft lip and palate, meticulous record keeping, and thorough documentation of the effects of treatment on growth.

This chapter was written to share the author's thoughts on the importance of team management and the surgical techniques for primary lip closure and primary palatal closure, that are currently employed at the Oslo Cleft Center. The chapter is not intended to comprehensively review all surgical approaches of cleft care; rather, it focuses on the procedures that have been performed for decades at the Oslo Cleft Center. Readers interested in this aspect of cleft management should consult other texts that review soft tissue surgery in detail.[1]

PHILOSOPHY AND GENERAL PRINCIPLES

Some factors in cleft lip and palate treatment are of fundamental importance if a satisfactory end result is to be obtained: a team approach, centralization of care and records, the establishment of a long-term treatment plan, and adequate documentation to permit outcome assessment.

Team Approach

A complete cleft lip and palate (CLP) is a severe malformation with direct influence on appearance, mastication, hearing, speech, facial growth, feeding, and breathing. The malformation also has a significant psychological impact on the child and the parents. A cleft palate–craniofacial team must therefore have the expertise necessary to deal with all the problems within these areas. The team should include at least a dentist, a geneticist, an orthodontist, an otolaryngologist, a pediatrician, a plastic surgeon, a prosthodontist, a psychiatrist, a speech pathologist, and a social worker.

Centralization

A cleft palate–craniofacial center should treat an adequate number of cleft patients a year so that all members of the team have experience with problems related to even the rarest clefts. A minimum of approximately 30 new patients with clefts should be treated annually in a center in order for adequate expertise to be gained and maintained. Cleft habilitation should be, never a matter of secondary importance, but a main focus for those involved.

Long-Term Treatment Plan

Overall management of the CLP patient must be evaluated in the context of a team approach. The treatment starts shortly after birth and continues to ages 18 to 20 years.

When the treatment plan has been established, the team members should feel responsible to observe the patient to adulthood. To be involved only in primary repair of clefts does not provide the long-term perspective of the consequences of primary surgery and the timing of the operations. Every surgeon involved in primary cleft treatment should be responsible for observing the long-term effects of surgery, although the outcome may be a humiliating experience. This feedback is an important stimulus to modify and to improve treatment protocols, and without it, cleft care cannot improve.

The complete treatment program reflects the compromises that are required in order to establish priorities between the different members of the team. For example, the speech pathologist would prefer the palate closed as early as possible to secure natural development of speech; the otolaryngologist would also prefer to have the soft palate closed early to improve eustachian tube function; the orthodontist, however, may prefer to delay surgery of the hard palate in the very early period because of the risk of interfering with growth. The operative procedures and the timing of the different operations must therefore be discussed among the different members of the team, and cooperation is essential in establishing a long-term treatment plan. Each patient with a cleft is different, and because of the variables, the long-term treatment plan must be tailored to the individual patient's needs.

It is also necessary for the parents to develop confidence in the team members and in the treatment plan. They must be given adequate information and education to understand the importance of the long-term perspective in cleft habilitation. Knowledge of the risks and benefits of the planned sequential interventions enables the patient and/or parents to make informed decisions. The provider must establish criteria for success and failure, which allow probability estimates to be established for evaluation of outcomes, from both the providers' and the consumer's perspective. A concordance of expectations from the multiple interventions from both the clinician's and the patient's or parents' point of view contributes to overall satisfaction from treatment. Parents naturally prefer to have as much surgery done as early as possible to obtain an optimal result in early childhood. It is therefore important to explain the long-term negative effects that extensive early surgery can cause and that the short-term gains must be weighed against the long-term effects.

Documentation

Standardized long-term documentation at defined times during childhood development provides data concerning facial growth, speech, hearing, dental development, and appearance. Cephalograms, plaster casts of the dental arches, speech recordings, audiograms, and slides or photographs are necessary for analyzing the effects of the different procedures and for comparing the results with other cleft palate–craniofacial centers.

PRIMARY REPAIR OF UNILATERAL COMPLETE CLEFTS

When informed that an infant has been born with a cleft, a team member examines the infant and contacts the parents to provide information, counseling, and education. The family is seen by all team members, and the parents have an opportunity to meet and talk with other parents of children with clefts who are admitted for treatment. If feeding difficulties arise, alternative nursing methods and/or alternative nipples can be demonstrated and practical advice given.

Timing

The optimal time for primary lip repair in (CLP) is controversial. As a general principle, a congenital defect should be corrected as soon as possible after birth. Some surgeons therefore perform the lip operation within the first days after birth. There are, however, good reasons for postponing the surgery: (1) the mortality rate during the first year of life is higher among infants born with CLP than among average newborns, and the majority of deaths among infants with CLP (80% to 85%) occur within

3 months after birth because of coexistent congenital malformations and not because of the CLP defect; (2) at 3 months, the risk of complications from anesthesia is lower and the infant is more able to cope with blood loss and other insults associated with the operation; and (3) the considerable growth that occurs during the 3-month interval makes meticulous repair easier.

The lip and anterior palate are closed at the age of 3 months. No form of presurgical orthodontics is employed to assist the repair. The major reason for this approach is to minimize the total treatment time and intervention. In addition, the efficacy of presurgical orthodontic/orthopedic treatment has not been adequately demonstrated. In view of the large number of operations, treatments, and consultations that CLP patients experience, the number of consultations and the active treatment time should be minimized. Therefore, no active treatment is given before the age of 3 months.

Surgical Procedure

On the operating table, detailed close-up photographs of the cleft are taken, as are impressions of the maxilla (Fig. 17–1). These are part of the permanent records. For closure of the lip, a Millard rotation-advancement procedure is utilized (Fig. 17–2).[2] In complete clefts, closure of the anterior palate with a single-layer vomer flap is performed simultaneously. With this procedure, a nasal floor is constructed from the nostrils into the hard palate (Figs. 17–3, 17–4).

The incisions are marked with Bonnies Blue dye in the usual manner. Local anesthetic (0.5% lidocaine, with 1:50,000 epinephrine) is infiltrated into all layers of both lip segments and under the planned vomer flap and palatal flap. This reduces the bleeding, and blood transfusions are never required. The maximal blood loss that is tolerated is 10% of the child's estimated blood volume.

The incisions for the lip dissection are made to, but not through, the periosteum on the anterior aspect of the maxillary segments. On the lateral side of the cleft, an incision is made in the sulcus to the periosteum. The lateral labial muscle is freed from its abnormal insertion at the pyriform margin and mobilized. The labial muscle is isolated on each side of the cleft and dissected free for at least 5 mm.

The incisions for the vomer flap are made to bone or cartilage, because this dissection is possible only subperiosteally. On the medial side of the lateral segment, the incision follows the border between the oral and nasal mucosa. The oral mucoperiosteum on the hard palate on the cleft side is bluntly undermined. The dissection of the vomer flap is carefully performed over the premaxillary-vomerine suture to avoid tearing the tissue in this area. The cleft side of the premaxilla must also be handled with great care, because it is easy to interfere with the developing tooth buds.

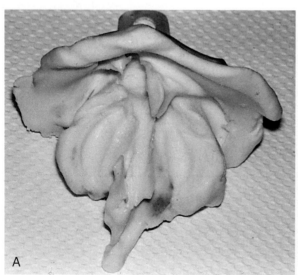
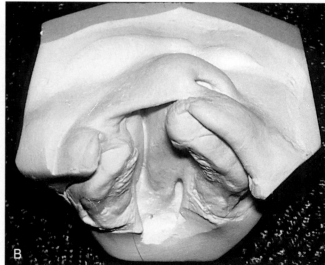

Figure 17–1. Impression of the cleft is taken before the primary lip repair, on the operating table, with the patient under general anesthesia (*A*). A plaster model is made (*B*).

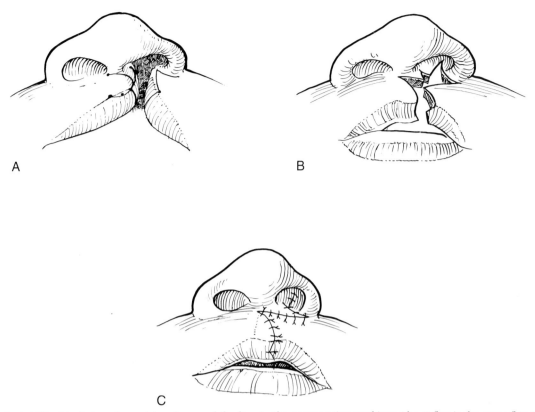

Figure 17–2. A Millard technique is used for closure of the lip. *A,* The preoperative markings (the C flap is the small flap [triangular] at the base of the columella); *B,* the incisions; *C,* closure.

The vomer flap is mobilized sufficiently to allow the flap to be turned, like a book page, across the cleft and sutured beneath the mucoperiosteal palatal flap, raw side against raw side.

The suturing begins posteriorly and moves forward. Either 4–0 or 5–0 polyglactin (Dexon) suture is used. From the anterior part of the palate and forward, the nasal floor is reconstructed by direct everting mattress sutures that connect the anterior part of the vomer flap to the nasal wound edge of the lateral side. This terminates in the nostril sill.

The labial muscle is then reconstructed across the cleft with 4–0 polyglactin sutures (Dexon). The lower third of the labial muscle is directed horizontally, if necessary, by making a horizontal cut between the lower and middle third of the labial muscle.

The skin incision is closed, with 6–0 polypropylene sutures. On the vestibular side of the lip, a Z-plasty is performed to avoid a whistling deformity.

Primary nasal correction is not routinely performed. If a severe alar cartilage deformity is observed when the alar base is brought medially to its normal position, a modified McComb procedure is performed.[3] The skin is dissected free from the alar cartilage on the cleft side, and the alar cartilage is elevated with traction sutures that are looped over bolsters within the vestibule and tied over bolsters on the nasal dorsum (Fig. 17–5). This also raises the nostril rim. Traction on this suture during closure of the anterior nasal floor makes it easier to achieve alar base symmetry.

PRIMARY CLOSURE OF BILATERAL COMPLETE CLEFTS

In bilateral complete clefts, the lip incision is made straight and does not include the C-flap of Millard.[2] The reason for avoiding a C-flap is that the prolabium usually is very small, and including a C-flap on both sides increases scarring. Lengthening of the columella is always performed later in patients with complete bilateral clefts, and a straight-line closure provides the best conditions for a forked-flap procedure.

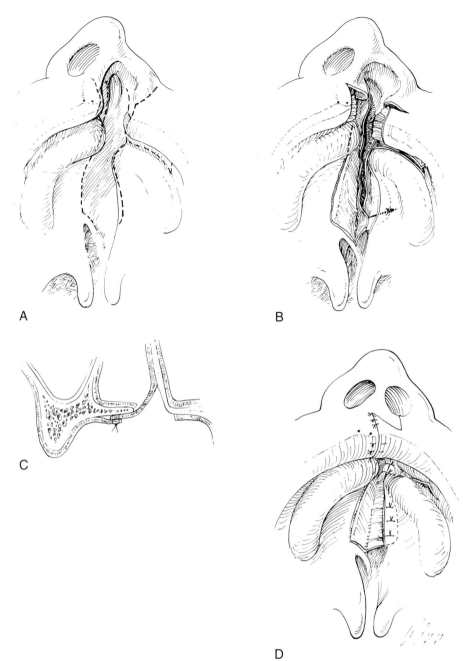

A

B

C

D

Figure 17–3. A vomer flap is used to close the anterior palate. *A,* The incisions are marked with dotted lines. *B,* The vomer flap is dissected free, mobilized, and sutured beneath the mucoperiosteal palatal flap on the cleft side. Inset (*C*) details the insertion of the vomer flap under the soft tissue of the palate. *D,* The closure completed.

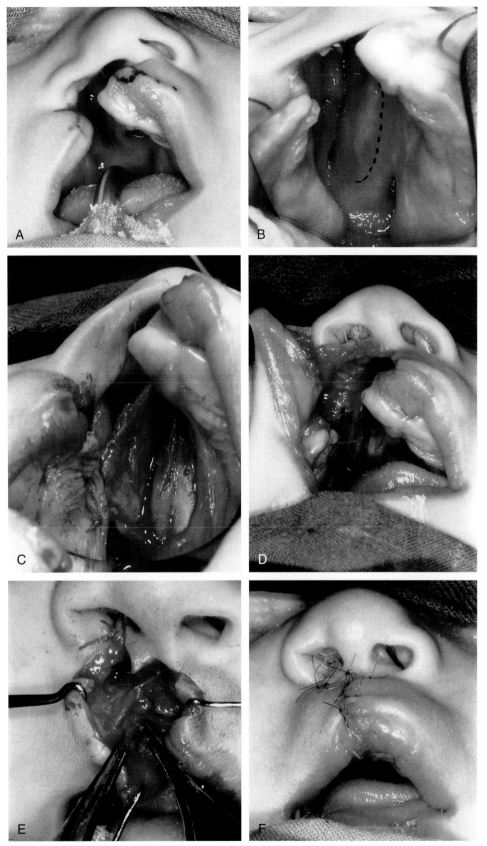

Figure 17–4. *A,* Complete unilateral cleft. *B,* The vomer flap is outlined. *C,* The vomer flap is dissected free and turned over the cleft. The suturing of the vomer flap has started posteriorly (*D*), and the closure of the nasal floor is completed at the nostril sill (*E*). *F,* The labial muscle is sutured. The suturing of the skin and mucosa is completed.

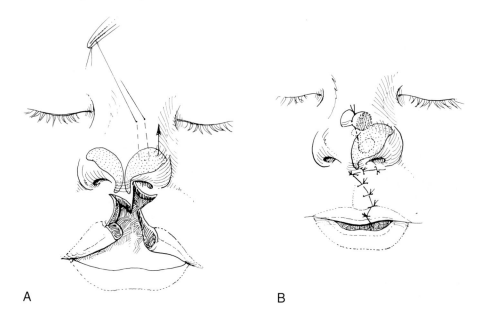

Figure 17-5. In cases with severe deformity of the alar cartilage, a modified McComb procedure is performed. The skin is dissected free from the underlying alar cartilage on the cleft side. The alar cartilage is elevated with traction sutures, which are looped over bolsters within the vestibule (*A*). The sutures are tied over bolsters on the nasal dorsum (*B*).

A   B

The vomer flap is designed as in unilateral clefts, because the procedure is staged with only one side operated at a time. Closure of the opposite side is delayed 5 weeks (Figs. 17-6, 17-7). A two-stage closure is preferable in order to avoid compromising the blood supply to the premaxilla, which is perfused through the posterior septal arteries, running along the sides of the nasal septum.[4] Of 60 patients in whom both sides of bilateral clefts were closed simultaneously with vomer flaps, six developed atrophy of the premaxilla. Such atrophy has not been observed in patients who underwent closure of one side at a time.[5]

Premaxillary setback is never performed even in the most extreme circumstances. Long-term follow-up observation indicates that even in these extreme circumstances, the maxilla ends up in the correct sagittal relationship or in a slightly retruded position.[6]

The primary repair of bilateral clefts is not aimed at a final reconstruction. After primary lip closure, the prolabium increases rapidly in size (Fig. 17-8). The short columella and the flaring nostrils soon become obvious. At the age of 4 years, a columella-lengthening procedure is performed, as described by Millard (Fig. 17-9).[7] This procedure has certain advantages: sufficient donor tissue is available; the old scar can be excised; the labial muscle can be reconstructed; the upper lip can be shortened or lengthened; access to the alar cartilage and the tip of the nose is gained; narrowing of the nostrils is achieved; and the scars remaining in the upper lip are in an unobtrusive position corresponding to the philtral ridges (Fig. 17-10).

A sulcusplasty is commonly required as well. This procedure creates a deep sulcus for the secondary bone grafting procedure, which takes place at the age of 8 to 10 years. The sulcusplasty technique varies, depending on the needs of the patient. The principle is to detach the mucosa from the anterior part of the premaxilla, rotate sufficient mucosa from the side, and suture it high in the sulcus.

The most controversial aspect of this primary repair is the use of a vomer flap to close the anterior hard palate at the time of lip repair. The vomer flap procedure is a one-layer nasal floor reconstruction and seldom results in bone bridging.[8] This procedure differs markedly from the two-layer vomerplasty, which has been reported to produce bony bridges in a high percentage of patients.[9] Bone formation across the cleft at this age is undesirable from growth and orthodontic perspectives, and for these reasons, no primary bone grafting or periostioplasty is performed.[10-12] To eliminate the residual alveolar cleft and to obtain full dental rehabilitation, secondary bone grafting is performed at the age of 8 to 10 years.[8,13,14] There is controversy in the literature regarding the use of a single-layer vomer flap and its effect on maxillary growth.[15-19] In Oslo, this technique has been used for more than 40 years, and thorough growth studies have failed to demonstrate any significant growth disturbance in comparison with the results from other centers in which hard palate closure is delayed. The data

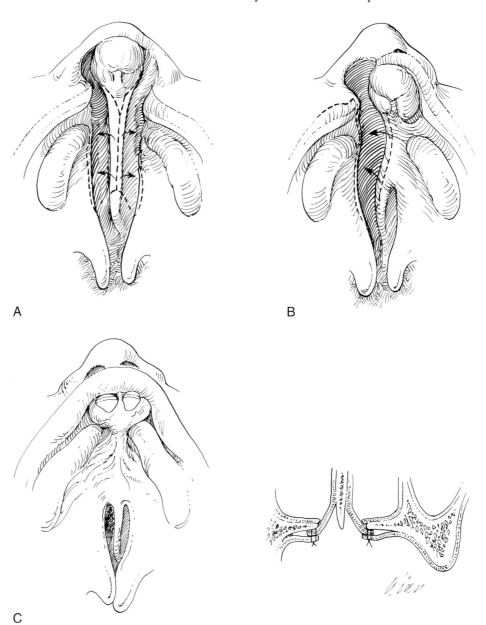

Figure 17–6. In patients with bilateral complete cleft lip and palate, a straight closure of the lip is combined with a vomer flap closure of the hard palate, one side at a time, with an interval of 5 weeks between the operations. The incision is outlined on the left side (*A*). Five weeks later, the right side is closed (*B*). Then the lip and hard palate are closed (*C*).

suggest that maxillary prominence and upper face angulation do not differ between the groups.[6]

The use of a vomer flap provides the advantages of early separation of the oral and nasal cavities without artificial obturators, a low rate of symptomatic fistulas, and an acceptable arch form. A vomer flap also creates a good foundation for alveolar bone grafting in the mixed dentition. This is advantageous, especially in complete bilateral clefts, when a large fistula behind the premaxilla can complicate this procedure and increase the failure rate. The use of a vomer flap may be one of the reasons for the Oslo Cleft Center's high success rate with secondary bone grafting to the alveolar cleft.[13, 14]

POSTERIOR CLEFT PALATE REPAIR

The palatal repair is based on von Langenbeck's principles.[20] The incisions and flap thicknesses are similar, but unlike the von Langenbeck procedure, the oral mucoperiosteal layer as well as the nasal layer is closed.[20] In addition, the levator muscle sling is reconstructed.

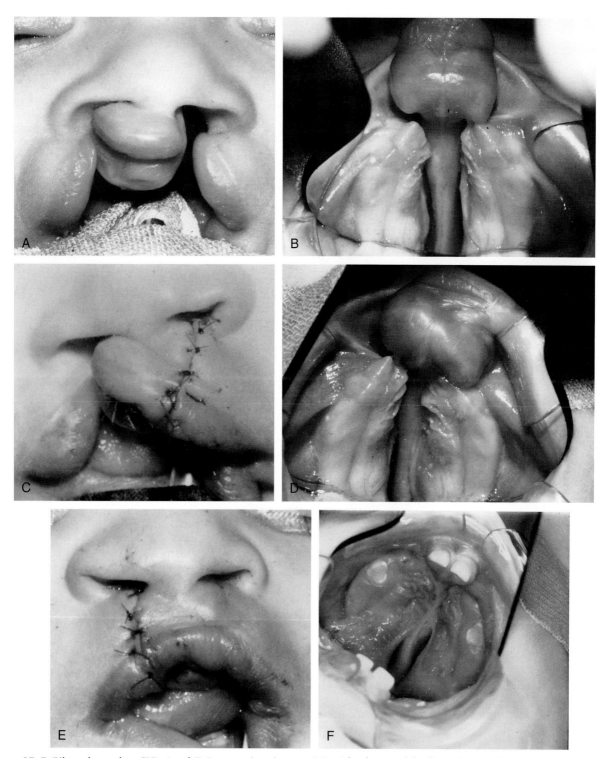

Figure 17–7. Bilateral complete CLP. *A* and *B*, Preoperative pictures. *C*, Straight closure of the lip and vomer flap of anterior palate, left side. *D*, Five weeks later, before closure of the right cleft. *E*, Closure of the right side. *F*, Preoperative view of the palate at the age of 18 months, when the patient was admitted for posterior palatal closure.

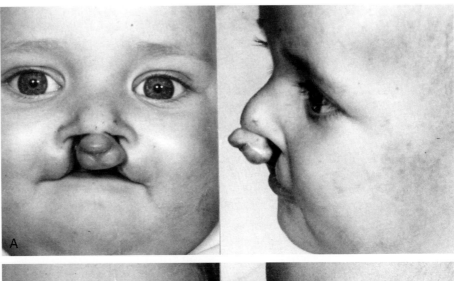

Figure 17–8. The prolabium increases considerably in size after primary lip repair. *A*, Appearance at age 6 months; *B*, appearance at age 11 months. As the child grows, the short columella and the flaring nostrils become obvious. (From Eskeland G, Borchgrevink H, Åbyholm F: Columella lengthening in bilateral cleft lip and palate patients. Scand J Plast Reconstr Surg 1979; 13:430.)

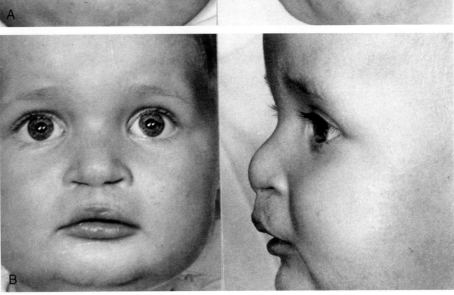

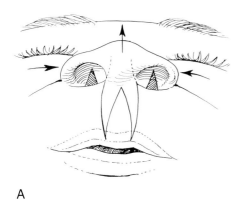

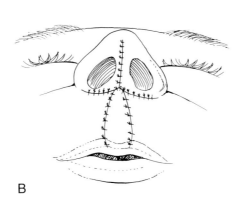

A

B

Figure 17–9. *A* and *B*, The Millard forked flap procedure. The prolabium is reduced to normal size. The old lip scars can be excised, but still there is plenty of tissue available for reconstructing the columella. At the same time, a narrowing of the base of the nose is achieved.

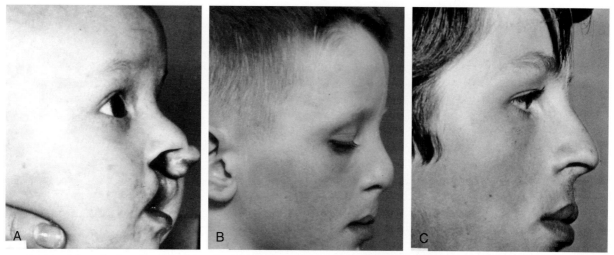

Figure 17–10. Columella lengthening achieved with the forked flap. *A,* Before lip closure. *B,* Appearance at age 9 years, when columella lengthening was performed. *C,* Appearance at 18 years. (From Eskeland G, Borchgrevink H, Åbyholm F: Columella lengthening in bilateral cleft lip and palate patients. Scand J Plast Reconstr Surg 1979; 13:434.)

Timing

Consideration for the timing of palatal repair includes the effect on speech, maxillary growth, and hearing. Until 1968, the palatal closure was performed at 2 to 3 years of age. Since then, closure has been accomplished at 18 months, and impaired growth of the face in association with the earlier repair has not been observed. For speech and hearing considerations, palatal closure at the age of 12 months is currently performed. Short-term growth observation indicates that the effect of lowering the age of palatal closure on facial growth appears minimal.

Surgical Procedure

A self-retaining mouth gag (the Dott gag) is inserted, and the operating field is infiltrated with local anesthetic (0.5% lidocaine) and with epinephrine (1:50,000) to reduce bleeding.

The incisions are made along the cleft at the junction between the oral and nasal mucosa. The dissection begins anteriorly, and the mucoperiosteal flaps are bluntly dissected free from the bony palatal shelfs (Fig. 17–11). The difficult point during the dissection is at the junction between the soft and hard palate, where the mucosa is firmly attached to the bone. Careful dissection of the soft tissue from the bone and definition of the nasal layer allows visualization of the anterior attachment of the levator muscle at the posterior medial edge of the hard palate. The muscle is cut and moved to a posterior position.[21] A lateral longitudinal palatal incision is then made along the alveolar ridge on the borderline between the oral mucoperiosteum and the gingiva on both sides. The incision is carried to bone anteriorly; posterior to the hard palate, however, the incision is superficial through mucosa and submucosa only. The mucoperiosteal flaps are then completely undermined. The neurovascular palatine bundle is identified and is preserved. All connective tissue surrounding the bundles must be removed in order to achieve the necessary mobility of the flaps. In patients with complete clefts, ligation of the neurovascular palatine bundles can lead to a higher frequency of fistula.

Until 1990, the hamulus was routinely fractured to increase flap mobility. Currently, the hamulus is maintained to preserve normal tensor veli palatini muscular relationships.

Suturing is initiated with the nasal layer. The first suture is placed in the soft palate area, where it is easy to approximate the nasal layer without tension before proceeding in an anterior direction. If the cleft is very broad in the anterior part, bilateral vomer flaps can be used in this area to close the nasal layer (Fig. 17–12). The nasal layer is everted with sutures, and the knots are left on the nasal side.

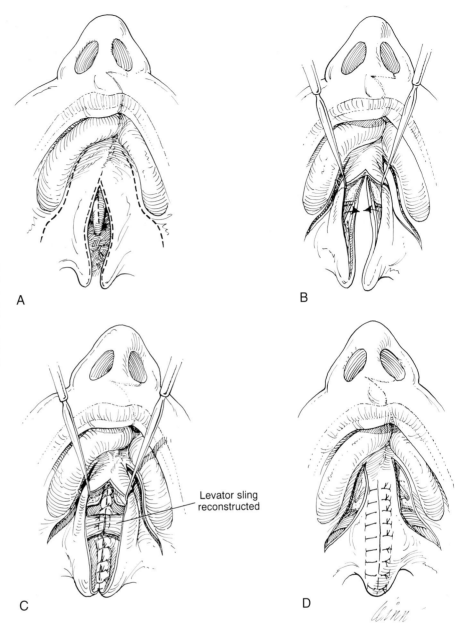

Figure 17–11. The incisions are marked out for a modified von Langenbeck palatal closure (*A*). The levator muscle is defined, cut, and repositioned (*B*). The nasal layer and the levator muscle are sutured separately (*C*). The closure is finished; there is no packing of the lateral wounds (*D*).

Levator sling reconstructed

The levator veli palatini muscle sling is then reconstructed by suturing the two muscles together in the midline with separate sutures. Finally, the oral layer is closed with everting mattress sutures starting anteriorly. In the soft palate, the sutures are full thickness through the velar muscle and mucosa. Absorbable 4–0 polyglactin (Dexon) suture is used.

The lateral incisions are left open for secondary healing, which occurs in 3 to 4 days, and it is never necessary to pack the denuded bone regions.

Prediction of the speech results is not possible merely by examining the pharyngeal anatomy and the velopharyngeal space. There is no indication for combining a primary palate repair with pharyngeal flap or a pharyngoplastic procedure.

This operation has a number of advantages:

1. The method is quite simple, and complications are few.[5]
2. Scarring is minimal, and the scars run in a longitudinal direction.
3. Fistulas, if they occur, are narrow slits, not holes.
4. An anatomic muscle repair is possible.
5. Speech results are comparable with those of push-back techniques.[23]
6. There is only minimal impairment of maxillary growth.[6]

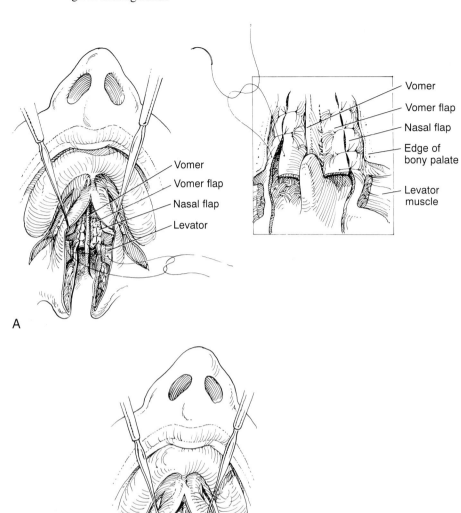

Vomer
Vomer flap
Nasal flap
Levator

Vomer
Vomer flap
Nasal flap
Edge of
bony palate
Levator
muscle

A

B

Nasal layer closed

Figure 17–12. In very broad clefts, a bilateral vomer flap can be used anteriorly to achieve a nasal layer closure (*A,B*).

SUMMARY

For primary cleft management, it is important for a team to select a treatment protocol that remains consistent over a number of years. The agreed sequence of the procedures is maintained and is modified only according to the individual's needs. Introduction of new techniques or altering the timing of procedures should be implemented only after careful consideration. Accurate and standardized documentation, follow-up observation, and evaluation of long-term results are necessary to prove the effectiveness of new procedures and to determine whether the improvement justifies a permanent change of the treatment protocol.

Many different surgical procedures are currently used in primary cleft repair. Every method has some advantages and some negative aspects. When primary cleft lip and palate surgery is planned and performed, it is important to be aware of the secondary problems that will be the consequence of treatment interventions. A long-term treatment plan for addressing these problems should be available by an interactive team approach in which outcome measures are evaluated and developed on a routine basis.

References

1. Millard DR: Cleft Craft. Boston: Little, Brown, 1976.
2. Millard DR: A radical rotation in single harelip. Am J Surg 1958; 95:318.
3. McComb H: Primary correction of unilateral cleft lip nasal deformity: A 10-year review. Plast Reconstr Surg 1985; 75:791.
4. Bøhn A: The course of the premaxillary and maxillary vessels and nerves in cleft jaw. Acta Odont Scand 1963; 21:463.
5. Åbyholm FE, Borchgrevink HC, Eskeland G: Cleft lip and palate in Norway: III. Surgical treatment of CLP patients in Oslo 1954–75. Scand J Plast Reconstr Surg 1981; 15:15.
6. Semb G: Analysis of the Oslo Cleft Lip and Palate Archive: 1991 [Thesis] Oslo, Norway: University of Oslo, Department of Orthodontics, 1992.
7. Millard DR: Columella lengthening by a forked flap. Plast Reconstr Surg 1958; 22:454.
8. Åbyholm FE, Bergland O, Semb G: Secondary bone grafting of alveolar clefts. Scand J Plast Reconstr Surg 1981; 15:127.
9. Prydso U, Holm PCA, Dahl E, Fogh-Andersen P: Bone formation in palatal clefts subsequent to palatovormer-plasty. Scand J Plast Reconstr Surg 1974; 8:73.
10. Friede H, Johanson B: A follow up study of cleft children treated with primary bone grafting: I. Orthodontic aspects. Scand J Plast Reconstr Surg 1974; 8:88.
11. Larson O, Ideberg M, McWilliam J, Nordin K-E: Early bone grafting in unilateral complete cleft lip and palate cases following maxillofacial orthopedics. In Pfeifer G (ed): Craniofacial Abnormalities and Clefts of the Lip, Alveolus and Palate, p 227. New York: Thieme-Verlag, 1991.
12. Hellquist R, Sverdstrom K, Ponten B: A longitudinal study of delayed periostoplasty to the cleft alveolus. Cleft Palate J 1983; 20:277.
13. Bergland O, Semb G, Åbyholm FE: Elimination of the residual alveolar cleft by secondary bone grafting and subsequent orthodontic treatment. Cleft Palate J 1986; 23:175.
14. Bergland O, Semb G, Åbyholm FE, et al: Secondary bone grafting and orthodontic treatment in patients with bilateral complete clefts of the lip and palate. Ann Plast Surg 1986; 17:460.
15. Friede H, Morgan P: Growth of the vomero-premaxillary suture in children with bilateral cleft and palate: A histological and roentgen-cephalometric study. Scand J Plast Reconstr Surg 1976; 10:45.
16. Friede H: The vomero-premaxillary suture—A neglected growth site in mid-facial development of unilateral cleft lip and palate patients. Cleft Palate J 1978; 15:398.
17. Friede H, Johanson B: A follow up study of cleft children treated with vomer flap as part of a three-stage soft tissue surgical procedure: Facial morphology and dental occlusion. Scand J Plast Reconstr Surg 1977; 11:45.
18. Enemark H, Bolund S, Jorgensen I: Evaluation of unilateral cleft lip and palate treatment: Long term results. Cleft Palate J 1990; 27:354.
19. Molsted K: Kraniofacial Morphologi Hos Born med Komplett Unilateral Læbe og Ganespatte [Thesis]. Copenhagen: 1987.
20. von Langenbeck BRK: Operation der angeborenen totalen Spaltung des harten Gaumens nach einer neuen Methods. Deutsche Klinik 1861; 13:231.
21. Kriens OB: Fundamental anatomic findings for an intravelar veloplasty. Cleft Palate J 1970; 7:27.
22. Åbyholm FE, Borchgrevink HC, Eskeland G: Palatal fistulae following cleft palate surgery. Scand J Plast Reconstr Surg 1979; 13:295–300.
23. Myklebust O, Åbyholm FE: Speech results in CLP patients operated on with a von Langenbeck palatal closure. Scand J Plast Reconstr Surg 1989; 23:71.

18

Surgical Management of Velopharyngeal Insufficiency: Pharyngeal Flap and Sphincter Pharyngoplasty

Gerald M. Sloan, William C. Shaw, and Susan E. Downey

VELOPHARYNGEAL INSUFFICIENCY

Velopharyngeal insufficiency (VPI) is the inability to completely occlude the velopharyngeal port during speech. Because of the resultant leakage of air into the nasal cavity, speech has a hypernasal resonance quality. In an attempt to compensate for the hypernasality, misarticulations often develop, further complicating the speech abnormality. That adds an additional layer of complexity to correction of the problem.

The most common cause of congenital VPI and hypernasal speech is a cleft of the secondary palate. Another possible cause is the somewhat confusing entity of submucous cleft palate. The first description of submucous cleft palate is attributed to Roux in 1925.[1] He described a young girl with severe hypernasality and unintelligible speech who had a split in the posterior soft palate and separation of the two sides of the hard palate under an intact mucosa.

Calnan in 1954 described a triad of findings in submucous cleft palate, which is still the most widely accepted definition of this entity: (1) bifid uvula, (2) separation of the soft palate musculature in the midline with intact mucosa, and (3) midline notching in the posterior edge of the hard palate.[2]

In 1972 Weatherley-White and coworkers published a study in which they examined 10,836 school children in the Denver area.[3] They found nine who had submucous cleft palates, an incidence of 1 in 1200. Of particular interest, only one had abnormal speech, and that was corrected by speech therapy without surgery. This study suggested that the incidence of submucous cleft palate was much higher than had previously been appreciated but that most individuals with submucous cleft palate do not have speech abnormalities and do not require surgery or other therapy.

There still is no question that some individuals with submucous cleft palate do have VPI and do require treatment. It is ironic that several studies have shown these patients to have worse speech results following surgery than patients with true cleft palates. Åbyholm reported 47 patients with submucous cleft palate who underwent surgical management at the Oslo, Norway, cleft center.[4] Eleven had undergone previous tonsillectomy and/or adenoidectomy, which might have contributed to their speech problems. Recommended surgery was von Langenbeck or pushback palate repair, including levator muscle repair, plus a superiorly based pharyngeal flap. Better speech results were obtained in patients who underwent surgery before 7 years of age.

In addition to true clefts and submucous cleft palates, other causes of VPI include congenital short palate, congenital large pharynx, paralysis of the soft palate and/or pharyngeal musculature, postsurgical shortening and/or scarring of the soft palate, VPI following adenoidectomy, and functional VPI without identifiable cause.[2,5,6]

Evaluation of hypernasal speech begins with perceptual speech evaluation by a properly trained speech pathologist. When VPI is suspected based on the perceptual speech evaluation, the definitive diagnosis is made by video nasopharyngeal endoscopy.[7,8] This evaluation allows direct observation of the soft palate and the lateral and posterior pharyngeal walls during speech. In the experience of the present authors, it has been striking how often the video nasopharyngeal endoscopy will demonstrate findings that are quite different from what was predicted based on the perceptual speech evaluation. In such cases, endoscopy can help avoid surgery when the appropriate intervention would be speech therapy alone. Unfortunately, many cleft surgeons have not yet fully accepted the important role of endoscopy. Even for those who have, not all patients can be successfully endoscoped, and occasionally a decision regarding surgical intervention is required without benefit of endoscopic findings. Other methods for assessing VPI, which can contribute helpful information in the diagnostic work-up and treatment planning, include pressure-flow measurements, nasometry, cinefluoroscopy of the palate and pharynx, and resting and phonating lateral cephalometric radiographs.

Although nonsurgical management of VPI, such as an obturator or palate prosthesis, can be helpful in some cases, there is general agreement that surgery is the treatment of choice if not otherwise contraindicated in a specific case. Surgical procedures for correction of VPI generally fall into three categories: palatal lengthening and/or muscle repositioning, pharyngeal flaps, and sphincter pharyngoplasties. For the remainder of this chapter it is assumed that we are dealing with residual VPI with an intact palate of proper length. Therefore, the discussion will be confined to pharyngeal flap and sphincter pharyngoplasty.

EVOLUTION OF PHARYNGEAL FLAP SURGERY

The predecessor of the pharyngeal flap was an adhesion of the posterior border of the soft palate to the posterior pharyngeal wall described by Passavant in 1865.[9] Schoenborn initially reported the inferiorly based pharyngeal flap in 1876.[10] By 1886 he had switched to a superiorly based flap from the posterior pharyngeal wall, sutured into the soft palate.[11] In 1924 Rosenthal combined the inferiorly based pharyngeal flap with a modified von Langenbeck palatoplasty, using the two in combination as the primary procedure for all clefts involving the hard and soft palates.[12] This was the first use of the pharyngeal flap as primary treatment for cleft palate.

Padgett popularized the pharyngeal flap in the United States, using the superiorly based flap in cleft palate patients in whom the primary repair had been unsuccessful.[13] Hogan introduced the concept of lateral port control in the design of the pharyngeal flap.[14] Hogan designed a wide, superiorly based pharyngeal flap and lined it with nasal mucosal flaps from the posterior soft palate. As the flaps were sutured in place, the lateral ports were tailored around a 4-mm diameter catheter on either side. He reported restoration of velopharyngeal competence in 91 of 93 patients whose mean age was 16 years, and reported hyponasality lasting more than 6 months in only three patients.

Debate as to the relative advantages and disadvantages of inferiorly and superiorly based pharyngeal flap design has persisted to the present time. To further complicate matters, Kapetansky reported successful results with a third design: bilateral transverse pharyngeal flaps.[15] An S-shaped incision was made in the posterior pharyngeal wall, and two laterally based flaps were elevated. One was used to provide nasal lining and the other to provide oral lining. He believed that basing the flaps laterally would preserve nerve supply, which would both maintain more flap mass and allow preservation of contractile function.

EVOLUTION OF THE SPHINCTER PHARYNGOPLASTY

Contemporary concepts of the pharyngoplasty operation date back to Wilfred Hynes of Sheffield, England, who in 1950 described an operation in which "the salpingopharyngeus muscle and its overlying mucosa" are transplanted bilaterally "upwards and inwards until they lie in a transverse mucosal defect created across the posterior wall of the nasopharynx."[16] His initial report was based on 12 patients with "failed cleft palate." He advocated a two-stage approach. If the palate did not have a residual cleft, the soft palate was divided to allow access to the posterior pharyngeal wall. The salpingopharyngeus muscles were transposed to the posterior pharyngeal wall and overlapped each other in a side-to-side arrangement. At a second operation the palate was repaired and, in some cases, "pushed back" as well. Eight patients had completed the two-stage procedure by the time of the initial report. Hynes described three as showing "dramatic improvement" in speech. The other five had "less marked" improvement, but all could "speak intelligibly to strangers" after completion of surgery.

In his 1953 Hunterian Lecture, Hynes reported 55 patients in whom he had performed the pharyngoplasty operation.[17] By this time he had significantly modified his surgical technique and now advocated much bulkier flaps, including the salpingopharyngeus, palatopharyngeus, and "fibres" of the superior constrictor as well. His illustrations now showed the flaps in an end-to-end arrangement with overlap of their tips, rather than the original side-to-side orientation. He thought that the soft palate, if not cleft, could be "split down the midline without hesitation" to allow exposure of the posterior pharyngeal wall and inset of the flaps in a sufficiently high position. He still believed that the palate should be repaired, and possibly pushed back, at a second operation. However, he acknowledged that in some cases the operation could be done "quite comfortably" by retracting rather than dividing the soft palate. Thirty-six patients had completed their surgical treatment and been followed for at least a year afterwards. Speech was described as "perfect, or almost perfect" in 19 (53%). In another 13 patients (36%) speech had improved to the point that they were "perfectly intelligible though the consonants are weak and some nasal escape is still present." Four patients (11%) showed no speech improvement.

In a 1967 report summarizing his 20-year experience with pharyngoplasty, Hynes emphasized the need for elevating as much muscle bulk as possible with the pharyngoplasty flaps.[18] He still thought it advisable to split an intact soft palate to be able to inset the flaps in the posterior pharyngeal wall, but he now thought it possible to repair a residual palatal cleft at the same surgical procedure. His drawings show both end-to-end and side-by-side patterns of flap inset. Although he did not report actual numbers, he stated that 20% of his pharyngoplasty patients had required further surgical management, such as palatal lengthening, after the completion and healing of the pharyngoplasty.

One year later, in 1968, Miguel Orticochea of Bogota, Colombia, described a similar "dynamic muscle sphincter" operation for cases of VPI.[19] However, Orticochea's approach had several important differences from Hynes'. First, the inset of the flaps was at a much lower level in the posterior pharyngeal wall. Second, Orticochea actually raised a third flap, an inferiorly based flap in the posterior pharyngeal wall, to which he sutured the tips of the posterior tonsillar pillar flaps. Third, Orticochea advocated using the pharyngoplasty procedure in all cleft palate patients, recommending that it be performed 6 months after the initial cleft repair.

In 1977, Jackson and Silverton reported their experience using a modification of the Orticochea pharyngoplasty.[20] The modification was to use a superiorly based midline posterior pharyngeal flap, rather than an inferiorly based flap. They reported having performed the procedure in over 100 cases and presented speech findings in 74 patients who had been followed for at least 1 year. They found speech to be "improved" in 67 (91%), "unchanged" in four (5%), "hyponasal" in three (4%), and "worse" in none.

In 1983 Orticochea updated his experience with his "dynamic muscle sphincter," reporting an experience with 236 cleft patients.[21] There are some unusual aspects of this particular report. Orticochea reported using the dynamic muscle sphincter in all cleft palate patients seen in his clinic since 1958. He divided the patients into four groups, according to the age at which the dynamic muscle sphincter was constructed. In 104 patients the pharyngoplasty was performed at age 2½ years, after palatoplasty without push-back at age 2 years. Another 94 patients had pharyngoplasty between ages 3 and 11 years. The third group, 27 patients, had pharyngoplasty between ages 11 and 18 years, and 11 patients had the surgery, in two stages, as adults between 18 and 32 years of age. The results are somewhat confusing and difficult for the present authors to interpret. Orticochea also advised that "the operation does not produce bleeding. Local anesthesia with constrictor vessels should not be used, because this could produce necrosis of the flaps." The present authors have not found it possible to perform surgery in the posterior pharynx without bleeding, even with the injection of vasoconstrictors, and have never experienced flap necrosis from the injection of local anesthesia with vasoconstrictors in several thousand cases.

A 1984 report by Riski and colleagues recommended modifying the level of insertion of the Orticochea pharyngoplasty.[22] They reviewed a series of 55 patients who underwent Orticochea pharyngoplasty between 1976 and 1982. Patients were evaluated before and after surgery by perceptual judgement of oral-nasal resonance and by lateral radiography. Some of the patients later in the series also underwent pressure-flow studies. Of 29 patients in whom surgical flap insertion was at the height of attempted velopharyngeal contact, 27 (93%) had resolution of hypernasal resonance. On the other hand, only 16 of 26 patients (61%) who had the traditional lower level of flap insertion showed successful resolution of hypernasality. Therefore, these authors concluded that a higher site of flap insertion should be used with the Orticochea pharyngoplasty. They recommended preoperative radiographic assessment to determine the level of attempted velopharyngeal contact, using the first cervical vertebra as a reference point. On the operating table, the first cervical vertebra can be palpated through the posterior pharyngeal wall. That level is then used as a reference point (not a target) for flap insertion.

Moss and associates renewed interest in the modified Hynes pharyngoplasty with their 1987 publication, which analyzed their results in 40 patients.[23] They used end-to-end palatopharyngeus flaps and emphasized suturing these "as high as possible" in the posterior pharyngeal wall. Their patients were evaluated before surgery and at least 6 months postoperatively through perceptual speech evaluation, lateral radiographs, and, "where possible," nasopharyngoscopy. They found that 33 patients had "acceptable" nasal resonance following surgery (normal resonance in 20 and slight hyponasality in 13). Of the seven patients considered to have "unacceptable" results, one was moderately hypernasal, two were slightly hypernasal, and four were moderately hyponasal after pharyngoplasty. In terms of nasal escape, they believed that 38 of 40 patients were "cured," 27 having no escape and 11 having "variable" escape postoperatively. They felt that the two patients who continued to have significant nasal escape after pharyngoplasty should have had different surgical procedures in retrospect. They reported one complication, a "bucket handle" separation of the flaps from the posterior pharyngeal wall. That patient, however, was asymptomatic, had "normal" speech, and did not require reoperation. Thirteen patients had a variety of "side effects," such as catarrh, snoring, nasal obstruction, or difficulty blowing the nose. None of these required reoperation.

Riski and colleagues updated their experience with the sphincter pharyngoplasty in 1992.[24] By this time they had a series of 139 patients. In this report they described their surgical technique as being that of Orticochea in 16 patients prior to April 1978 and a modified Hynes type of procedure in 123 patients after that. In this large series of patients, they found that younger patients had more successful outcomes than older patients. Patients with a circular velopharyngeal closure pattern were more likely to have successful surgical management than those with a coronal closure pattern. Large velopharyngeal gaps were treated as successfully as small ones. The most frequent cause of pharyngoplasty failure was insertion of the flaps below the level of attempted velopharyngeal closure. VPI of varying degrees remained after initial pharyngoplasty in 30 of 139 patients. Surgical revision was undertaken in 16 of the 30 initial "failures." Eight patients (50%) had normal resonance after revision, and eight remained at least mildly hypernasal (in two cases even after a second revision).

INDICATIONS AND TIMING

Before considering pharyngoplasty or pharyngeal flap, the patient undergoes perceptual speech evaluation, video nasopharyngoscopy, and lateral resting and phonating cephalometric radiographs. We have found that nasopharyngoscopy can be successfully performed in almost all patients over the age of 5 years, and in many patients between 3 and 5 years of age. In rare cases we will perform surgery without nasopharyngoscopy when we feel very confident of the diagnosis of VPI based on perceptual speech evaluation, an attempt at nasopharyngoscopy has failed, and we do not feel that a repeat attempt in 6 to 12 months would be more successful.

We believe that surgery should be performed as young as possible once the presence of VPI is confirmed. In mild cases, a finite (usually 3- to 6-month) trial of speech therapy may be warranted before proceeding with surgery. We think that the best speech results following pharyngoplasty or pharyngeal flap surgery are likely to be obtained in the 3- to 8-year age range.

When large tonsils are present, they should be removed at least 1 to 3 months before surgery. Otherwise, it would be difficult or impossible to incise and elevate the flaps. When the adenoid pad extends below the level at which pharyngoplasty flaps would be inserted into the posterior pharyngeal wall, adenoidectomy should be performed prior to pharyngoplasty. Patients and families should be warned that adenoidectomy may worsen the degree of hypernasality during the intervening period between adenoidectomy and pharyngoplasty.

THE AUTHORS' SURGICAL TECHNIQUE FOR SPHINCTER PHARYNGOPLASTY

Our present technique has evolved over the course of 60 operations since 1987. General anesthesia is induced and the patient is positioned supine with the neck slightly extended. The surgeon may sit or stand, depending on individual preference. A mild degree of Trendelenburg position can be helpful in either case. A headlight is worn by the operating surgeon. A Dingman mouth gag is inserted. The posterior tonsillar pillars and the anticipated insertion site in the posterior pharyngeal wall are infiltrated with 1% xylocaine with 1:100,000 epinephrine. The Dingman gag is partially released while the surgeons wait 7 to 10 minutes for the epinephrine to take effect.

To begin the operation, the posterior tonsillar pillar is retracted on one side, using a Hurd retractor, and a vertical incision is made, extending from the level of the upper pole of the tonsil to as low as can safely be reached (Fig. 18–1). A similar incision is made on the other side. Next, the soft palate is retracted as high as possible, using a Goodhew retractor. (An alternative method of soft palate retraction is to pass a red rubber catheter through each nostril, suture the tip of each to the posterior soft palate, pull on the two catheters, and gently clamp them together across the columella to secure the palate in the desired position.) A high transverse incision is then made in the posterior pharyngeal wall arching up from the top of the vertical incision behind each posterior tonsillar pillar and thus connecting the two (Fig. 18–2). This transverse incision is made deep enough to develop a good edge of tissue above and below, to which the pharyngoplasty flaps can subsequently be sutured. Next, the tonsil is retracted with the Hurd retractor, and a vertical incision is made just posterior to the tonsil, first on one side, then the other (Fig. 18–3). These incisions are parallel to and of the same length as the previously made posterior vertical incisions.

Using long right angle scissors and Gerald forceps, the muscle bulk of the posterior tonsillar pillar (palatopharyngeus) is carefully dissected free between the two parallel vertical incisions, leaving the mucosa between the incisions attached to the muscle. An effort must be made to consciously dissect medially from the posterior incision and laterally from the anterior incision to ensure elevating adequate muscle. Otherwise, one can be left with a dishearteningly small amount of muscle in the flap. The muscle is

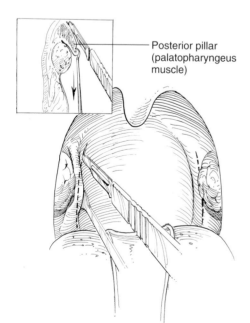

Posterior pillar (palatopharyngeus muscle)

Figure 18–1. An incision is made along the posterior surface of the posterior tonsillar pillar on the patient's right side. The pillar is held in position using a Hurd retractor. An identical incision will then be made on the left side.

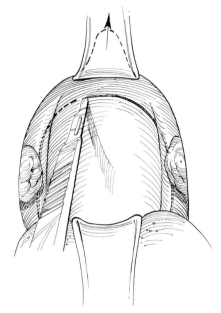

Figure 18–2. A high transverse incision is made across the posterior pharyngeal wall, connecting the previous two incisions. A Goodhew retractor is used to elevate the soft palate.

then dissected free from its deep attachments. The resulting bipedicled flap is retracted, and its inferior attachment is divided with the right angle scissors (Fig. 18–4). An identical muscle flap is elevated on the second side.

The two flaps are sutured to each other, in an end-to-end configuration, with two horizontal mattress sutures of 3–0 or 4–0 polyglactin acid (Fig. 18–5). The flaps are then sutured into the transverse cut in the posterior pharyngeal wall with horizontal mattress sutures of 3–0 or 4–0 polyglactin acid (Fig. 18–6). The size of the resulting port can be tailored by adjusting the position of the flaps. To tighten the port, the flaps can be partially overlapped in a "praying hand" configuration or, in rare cases, the tips of the flaps can be shortened by direct excision.

The sutures in the posterior pharyngeal wall may be very difficult to place, particularly those along the upper cut edge of the recipient site. Our philosophy has been that it is far more preferable to place a few good mattress sutures than to place more numerous flimsy sutures.

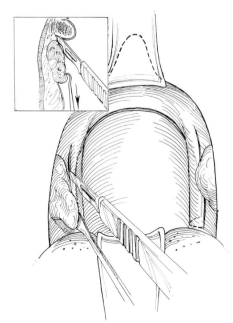

Figure 18–3. An incision is made along the anterior edge of the posterior tonsillar pillar, just posterior to the tonsil, which is retracted using the Hurd retractor. An identical incision is made on both sides.

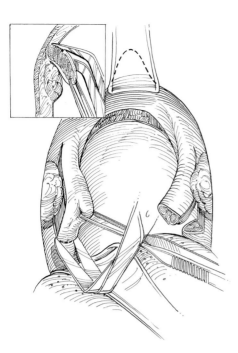

Figure 18–4. The palatopharyngeus muscle bulk has been dissected free using right angled scissors. The inferior attachment of the resulting bipedicled flap is then divided using the same right angled scissors.

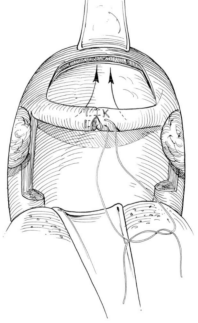

Figure 18–5. The tips of the two flaps are sutured to each other using two horizontal mattress sutures.

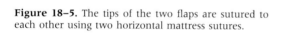

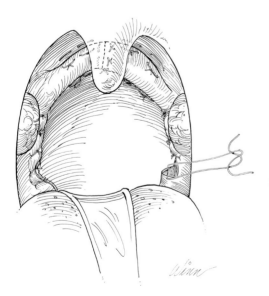

Figure 18–6. The two flaps are sutured into the transverse incision in the posterior pharyngeal wall. When the soft palate retractor is removed, the pharyngoplasty flaps will be above the resting level of the posterior soft palate and uvula.

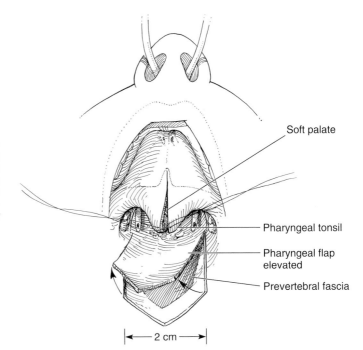

Figure 18–7. The posterior soft palate is divided in the midline. Traction sutures hold the two sides apart. A superiorly based pharyngeal flap is elevated and dissected free from the prevertebral fascia. In most adults and older children, the width of the pharyngeal flap will be two centimeters. The nasal catheters shown in this and the subsequent illustrations help to clarify the anatomy, but are not necessarily used in actual surgery.

Soft palate

Pharyngeal tonsil

Pharyngeal flap elevated

Prevertebral fascia

2 cm

THE AUTHORS' SURGICAL TECHNIQUE FOR PHARYNGEAL FLAP

The positioning and preparation is similar to that for the pharyngoplasty. The soft palate and posterior wall of the pharynx are infiltrated with 1% xylocaine with 1 : 100,000 epinephrine. After allowing time for the epinephrine to take effect, the posterior soft palate is divided in the midline. A traction suture is placed on either side of the soft palate (Fig. 18–7).

A superiorly based flap is incised and elevated on the posterior pharyngeal wall, dissecting in a plane just superficial to the prevertebral fascia (Fig. 18–8). The width of the flap is two-thirds the width of the posterior pharyngeal wall, up to a maximum width of 2 cm. The flap is elevated up to the level at which the dissection plane becomes less clearly defined, which is usually a little above the palpable prominence of the body of the second cervical vertebra.

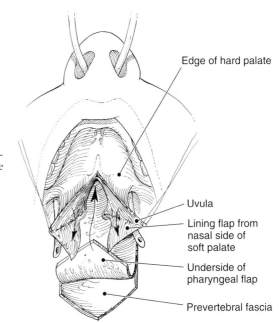

Edge of hard palate

Figure 18–8. A triangular flap is elevated from the nasal surface of each side of the soft palate.

Uvula

Lining flap from nasal side of soft palate

Underside of pharyngeal flap

Prevertebral fascia

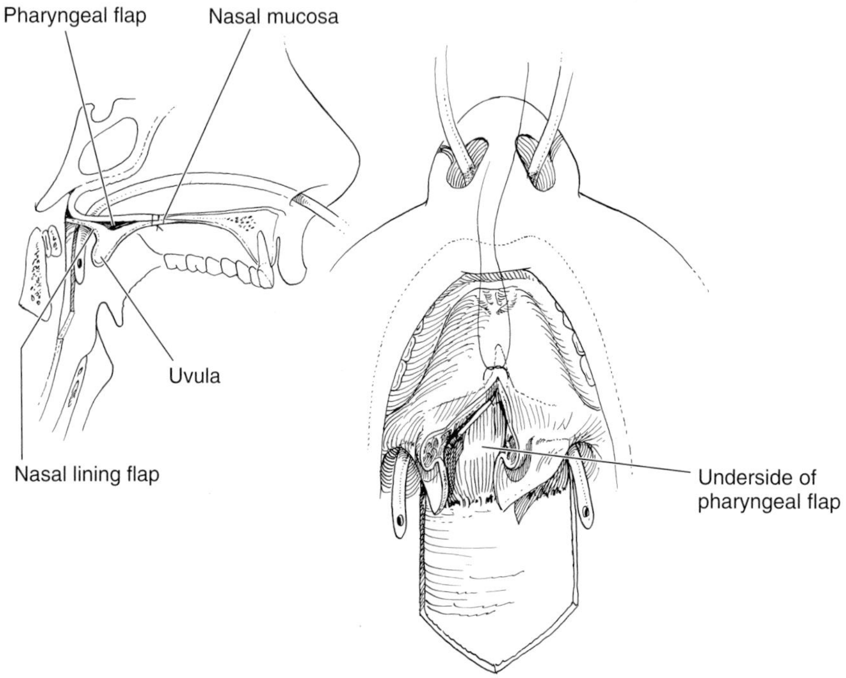

Pharyngeal flap   Nasal mucosa

Uvula

Nasal lining flap

Underside of
pharyngeal flap

Figure 18–9. The tip of the pharyngeal flap is secured to the soft palate with a horizontal mattress suture placed through the raw nasal surface of the palate and tied on the oral surface.

Nasal lining flaps are incised and elevated on either side of the soft palate. These flaps are based posteriorly (Fig. 18–9). The tip of the pharyngeal flap is then secured to the soft palate with one or two full thickness horizontal mattress sutures on either side (Fig. 18–10). The lateral edges of the pharyngeal flap are sutured to the lateral edges of the soft palate nasal lining flaps (Fig. 18–11). Finally, the soft palate is repaired in the midline (Fig. 18–12). The flap donor site is partially or completely closed if feasible. If not, it may be left open to contract and heal.

POSTOPERATIVE COMPLICATIONS

The most frequent complications following pharyngoplasty or pharyngeal flap surgery are nasal obstruction, obstructive sleep apnea, bleeding, flap separation, and undercorrection of VPI. Infections are rare. Most patients develop temporary nasal

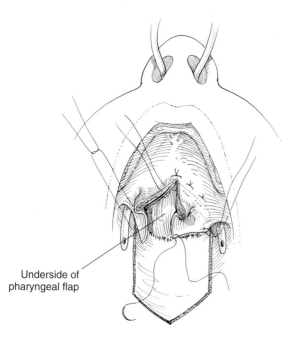

Underside of
pharyngeal flap

Figure 18–10. The lateral edges of the pharyngeal flap are sutured to the lateral edges of the soft palate on each side.

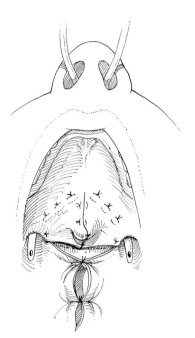

Figure 18–11. The soft palate is repaired in the midline, including the flaps that started on the nasal surface, which are now providing oral lining for the pharyngeal flap. The donor defect in the posterior pharyngeal wall is closed, if feasible.

obstruction as edema increases in the first few hours following surgery. In almost all cases, this resolves after several days to several weeks. However, in rare cases nasal obstruction will persist. If it does not resolve after several months, reoperation to open a larger port or ports may be necessary. Pharyngoplasty flaps can be elevated, repositioned, and sutured back into the posterior pharyngeal wall to produce a larger opening. Pharyngeal flap ports can be incised and resutured.

Symptoms of obstructive sleep apnea (OSA) can include sonorous breathing and observed apneic episodes during sleep, daytime tiredness and sleepiness, and deteriorating school performance. When OSA is suspected, the diagnosis should be confirmed with a formal polysomnographic sleep study. An overnight sleep study is generally preferable to a ''nap'' study. If OSA is confirmed by sleep study, management will vary according to the severity of the findings and how long a time has already passed since surgery. A pulmonary specialist should be consulted. If findings are mild to moderate and the patient presents less than a few months following surgery, conservative management may be appropriate. This may include supplemental oxygen at night. The sleep study should be repeated at 6 months postoperatively, unless a deterioration in symptoms makes an earlier repeat study necessary. If at 6 months postoperatively there is still significant OSA, it is unlikely that this will subsequently resolve, and reoperation to enlarge the port or ports, or the pharyngeal flap, must be considered.

Figure 18–12. The pharyngeal flap is shown, sutured in place, with lining of its underside provided by the soft palate flaps.

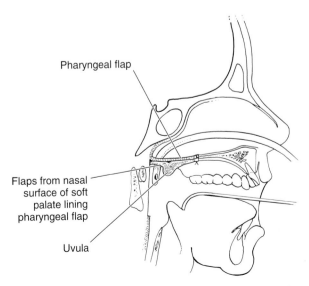

Pharyngeal flap

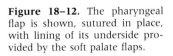

Flaps from nasal surface of soft palate lining pharyngeal flap

Uvula

The true incidence of OSA following pharyngoplasty or pharyngeal flap surgery is not known. In one study Orr and associates identified obstructive sleep apnea by polysomnographic sleep study in 9 of 10 patients, 2 to 3 days following pharyngeal flap surgery. OSA was still present in 2 of the 10 patients 3 months following surgery.[25] We are currently prospectively studying a large group of patients pre-operatively, and at 1 month and 12 months postoperatively, following pharyngoplasty or pharyngeal flap surgery. When that prospective international study is completed, we hope to have a better understanding of the incidence and natural course of OSA following surgical management of VPI.

Bleeding following pharyngoplasty or pharyngeal flap surgery is usually mild and self-limited in the first 12 to 24 hours. Substantial bleeding will require an urgent return to the operating room. In that situation, however, a specific bleeding site may not be identified, but bleeding will usually stop with intraoperative suctioning, irrigation, direct pressure, and topical thrombogenic agents. Packing material, even absorbable agents, might be aspirated following extubation and should not be left in the pharynx.

Partial or complete flap separation can occur, as can a bucket handle type of separation in which the tips of pharyngoplasty flaps remain attached to each other but come apart from the posterior pharyngeal wall. Flap separation will usually cause symptoms such as recurrence of hypernasality, throat irritation, or discomfort. If significantly symptomatic, the flap separation should be corrected surgically. If asymptomatic, a decision may be made to simply observe the situation.

If hypernasality is not improved, or is improved but not adequately corrected following surgery, reoperation to tighten the port or ports must be considered. We usually prefer to wait until about 6 months after the initial surgery. At that time it is often fairly straightforward to elevate the flaps, advance them closer together, and resuture them. Documentation of velopharyngeal anatomy by video nasopharyngeal endoscopy, if at all feasible, is strongly recommended before undertaking such revisional surgery.

THE FUTURE

Pharyngoplasty and pharyngeal flap surgery have never been compared in a prospective randomized study. We have retrospectively compared 30 patients who underwent modified Hynes pharyngoplasty with 30 patients who underwent pharyngeal flap surgery.[26] We found 3 complications (10%) in the pharyngoplasty group and 11 complications (37%) in the pharyngeal flap group ($p < 0.05$). Complications in the pharyngoplasty patients were one partial flap separation, one severe nasal obstruction, and one patient with postoperative sinusitis. In the pharyngeal flap group, three patients had severe nasal obstruction, three had obstructive sleep apnea, two had complete flap separation, two had significant postoperative bleeding (with one requiring reoperation), and one developed aspiration pneumonia. Speech results showed ''normal'' vocal resonance on perceptual speech evaluation by an experienced speech pathologist in 14 (47%) of the pharyngoplasty patients and 7 (23%) of the pharyngeal flap patients. There was a tendency towards hyponasality in the pharyngeal flap patients as opposed to residual hypernasality in the pharyngoplasty patients following surgery.

Surgical revision was required in three (10%) of the sphincter pharyngoplasty patients and in eight (27%) of the pharyngeal flap patients. Among the sphincter pharyngoplasty patients, two underwent revision because of persistent hypernasality and one because of nasal obstruction. All three were successfully managed by minor revision. In the pharyngeal flap group, three revisions were necessary because of persistent hypernasality and five because of nasal obstruction. Three of the patients were successfully managed by minor revision, three by complete division of the flap and conversion to a pharyngoplasty, and two by flap division alone (one of whom first underwent two unsuccessful attempts at minor revision).

In another retrospective study, Pensler and Reich reviewed 10 patients who underwent sphincter pharyngoplasty and 75 who underwent pharyngeal flap surgery.[27] Their review included patients operated on during a period of time exceeding 30 years. They concluded that either operation resulted in improved speech in a majority of patients with VPI. Of interest, the three patients who developed obstructive sleep apnea were all in the pharyngeal flap group.

We are presently in the midst of a 5-year prospective, randomized comparison of pharyngoplasty and pharyngeal flap surgery, being conducted at five centers in the United States and Europe (the University of North Carolina at Chapel Hill, Childrens Hospital Los Angeles, Loma Linda University, Rancho Los Amigos Medical Center, and University Hospital in Oslo, Norway). Patients are being evaluated before and at least twice following surgery by perceptual speech evaluation, video nasopharyngoscopy, nasometry, polysomnographic sleep study, lateral cephalometric radiographs, audiometry, and tympanometry. Surgical techniques are being carefully standardized. When completed around 1997, that study should significantly increase our understanding of both operations and allow an objective comparison between them in terms of speech results, incidence of obstructive sleep apnea, other complications, and rate of reoperation, as well as operating time, length of hospital stay, and financial cost.

References

1. Roux J: Mémoire sur la staphyloraphie, ou Suture du Voile du Palais. Paris: J.S. Chaudé, 1825.
2. Calnan JS: Submucous cleft palate. Br J Plast Surg 1954; 6:264.
3. Weatherley-White RCA, Sakura CY, Brenner LD, et al: Submucous cleft palate: Its incidence, natural history, and indications for treatment. Plast Reconstr Surg 1972; 49:297.
4. Åbyholm FE: Submucous cleft palate. Scand J Plast Reconstr Surg 1976; 10:209.
5. Calnan JS: Permanent nasal escape in speech after adenoidectomy. Br J Plast Surg 1971; 24:197.
6. Calnan JS: Congenital large pharynx. Br J Plast Surg 1971; 24:263.
7. D'Antonio LL, Muntz HR, Marsh JL, et al: Practical application of flexible fiberoptic nasopharyngoscopy for evaluating velopharyngeal function. Plast Reconstr Surg 1988; 82:611.
8. Shprintzen RJ: Evaluating velopharyngeal insufficiency. J Childh Commun Dis 1986; 10:38.
9. Passavant G: Ueber die Beseitigung der naeselden Sprache bei angeborenen Spalten des harten und weichen Gaumens (Gaumensegel, Schlundnacht, und Ruecklagerung des Gaumensegels). Arch Klin Chir 1865; 6:333.
10. Schoenborn K: Ueber eine neue Methode der staphylorrhaphie. Verh Dtsch Ges Chir 1875–1876; 4:235.
11. Schoenborn K: Vorstellung eines falle von Staphyloplastik. Verh Dtsch Ges Chir 1886; 15:57.
12. Rosenthal W: Pathologie und Therapie der Gaumendefekte. Fortschr Zahnheilk 1928; 4:1021.
13. Padgett EC: The repair of cleft palates after unsuccessful operations, with special reference to cases with an extensive loss of palatal tissue. Arch Surg 1930; 20:453.
14. Hogan VM: A clarification of the goals in cleft palate speech and the introduction of the lateral port control (L.P.C.) pharyngeal flap. Cleft Palate J 1973; 10:331.
15. Kapetansky DI: Bilateral transverse pharyngeal flaps for repair of cleft palate. Plast Reconstr Surg 1973; 52:52.
16. Hynes W: Pharyngoplasty by muscle transplantation. Br J Plast Surg 1950; 3:128.
17. Hynes W: The results of pharyngoplasty by muscle transplantation in "failed cleft palate" cases, with special reference to the influence of the pharynx on voice production. Ann R Coll Surg Engl 1953; 13:17.
18. Hynes W: Observations on pharyngoplasty. Br J Plast Surg 1967; 20:244.
19. Orticochea M: Construction of a dynamic muscle sphincter in cleft palates. Plast Reconstr Surg 1968; 41:323.
20. Jackson IT, Silverton JS: The sphincter pharyngoplasty as a secondary procedure in cleft palates. Plast Reconstr Surg 1977; 59:518.
21. Orticochea M: A review of 236 cleft palate patients treated with dynamic muscle sphincter. Plast Reconstr Surg 1983; 71:180.
22. Riski JE, Serafin D, Riefkohl R, et al: A rationale for modifying the site of insertion of the Orticochea pharyngoplasty. Plast Reconstr Surg 1984; 73:882.
23. Moss ALH, Pigott RW, Alberg EH: Hynes pharyngoplasty revisited. Plast Reconstr Surg 1987; 79:346.
24. Riski JE, Ruff GL, Georgiade GS, et al: Evaluation of the sphincter pharyngoplasty. Cleft Palate Craniofac J 1992; 29:254.
25. Orr WC, Levine NS, Buchanan RT: Effect of cleft palate repair and pharyngeal flap surgery on upper airway obstruction during sleep. Plast Reconstr Surg 1987; 80:226.
26. Sloan GM, Reinisch JR, Nichter LS, et al: Surgical management of velopharyngeal insufficiency: Pharyngoplasty vs. pharyngeal flap. Plast Surg Forum 1990; 13:128.
27. Pensler JM, Reich DS: A comparison of speech results after the pharyngeal flap and the dynamic sphincteroplasty procedures. Ann Plast Surg 1991; 26:441.

19

Orthodontic and Surgical Considerations in Bone Grafting in the Cleft Maxilla and Palate

Katherine W. L. Vig, Timothy A. Turvey, and Raymond J. Fonseca

No other therapy for patients with facial clefts has been the source of so much controversy as bone grafting in the cleft maxilla and palate. The introduction of secondary bone grafting of the cleft maxilla and palate, which was pioneered in Europe, was reported in the German literature at the beginning of this century.[1,2] However, it was not until the 1970s that secondary or delayed bone grafting became popular in the United States.

Primary bone grafting in infants, which was introduced in the 1950s, preceded secondary bone grafting by almost 20 years.[3–5] In this early surgical intervention, the cleft alveolus and palate were united by filling the cleft defect with autogenous bone, typically a split-rib graft. This logical and desirable closure of the cleft alveolus came under scrutiny when long-term results indicated that in the infants, who underwent early primary bone grafting, midface deficiency was apparently increased with subsequent craniofacial growth and development.[6–18]

In Europe, neonatal maxillary orthopedics was also adopted in the 1950s as an adjunctive treatment before definitive primary lip repair. This procedure was designed to approximate the segments presurgically, which allowed the surgeon to perform the lip repair more efficiently. The benefits included a shorter operating time, a reduction in the number of dehiscences, and a result that was improved both esthetically and functionally.[19,20] Although many claims were made for the effectiveness of neonatal maxillary orthopedics, the strength of evidence was based on anecdotal case reports, case series, and retrospective studies rather than on more rigorous and carefully designed prospective clinical trials. This was not surprising because the methods of conducting this type of clinical study were not available at a time when primary bone grafting and neonatal maxillary orthopedics were popular clinical interventions. As with all controversies, it was fueled by strong conviction, weak evidence, and imperfect theory. To determine the efficacy of treatment requires strict protocols with well-defined inclusion and exclusion criteria. Because many of the centers engaged in neonatal maxillary orthopedics were also conducting this in conjunction with primary bone grafting, the contributions of each intervention to the multidimensional outcome were difficult to determine or accurately measure.

The current status of presurgical orthopedics is still controversial, but as well-defined and well-designed clinical studies produce evidence that it may be an effective intervention, clinical practice may adopt a more rational approach to infant orthopedics in the future. This would reflect the benefits as a prior probability estimate of the valued outcome, in selected cases.[21]

The purpose of this chapter is to discuss the contemporary issues in the surgical and orthodontic management of the patient for whom bone grafting in the cleft maxilla and palate is recommended. The concerns in alveolar bone grafting include (1) the *age* at which bone grafting should be performed, (2) the *type* and *site* from which the donor bone should be harvested, (3) the *timing* of orthodontic maxillary expansion before or after the bone graft is placed, and (4) the use of osseo-integrated *implants* for prosthetic rehabilitation after placement of the bone graft. Each of these issues is controversial and is discussed. Although primary bone grafting is considered, the emphasis of this chapter is on the efficacy, utility, and technical aspects of secondary bone grafting in patients with bilateral and unilateral clefts of the lip and palate.

CONTEMPORARY TEAM MANAGEMENT OF THE CLEFT MAXILLA AND PALATE

By the end of the 19th century, the role of the prosthodontist was changing to the emerging concept of a functional occlusal relationship of the dentofacial complex. One of the earliest team collaborations in the management of patients with clefts resulted from the interaction of Harvold,[22] an orthodontist, and Bohn,[23] a prosthodontist, who collaborated on the decision to reposition the maxillary segments by expansion and retention. This was to preserve the dentition and manage the mutilated cleft maxilla more conservatively. This pioneering, collaborative approach to the management of patients with clefts was innovative at a time when surgical repair was performed by general surgeons,[24] and it resulted in a more rational approach; the concept of multiple specialists working together in the planning and treatment aspects of interdisciplinary treatment has been adopted by contemporary cleft/craniofacial teams.[25]

In 1943, the establishment of the American Cleft Palate Association fostered the approach of team care. As an advocate for the patients and the parents of infants with clefts and craniofacial anomalies, this organization currently has a membership of over 2500 professionals representing more than 20 disciplines, such as medicine, dentistry, speech pathology, and basic science. These specialties are coordinated in a team approach in the management of patients with cleft and craniofacial anomalies. The mission of the organization is to foster the acquisition and dissemination of knowledge concerning growth, development, diagnosis, and treatment of individuals with those anomalies, as well as fostering communication and cooperation among disciplines.

The interdisciplinary management of patients by the cleft/craniofacial team requires an interactive approach to the timing and sequencing of treatment interventions and the reporting of results in a more standardized and comparable way. A lack of this approach has resulted in problems when alternative methods and their outcomes are compared.[26]

The surgeon and orthodontist traditionally have been involved in primary bone grafting, especially when it involves presurgical maxillary orthopedics. The rationale for the early attempts of presurgical orthopedic techniques relates to the expectation of producing a narrow cleft between well-aligned segments. Surgical repair could then be accomplished more easily, and the chances of success (in terms of reduction in wound dehiscence) would be greater than when the segments were displaced with a wide intervening cleft. It would be logical to restore the integrity of the alveolus at an early age, on the basis of the premise that normal growth and development of the midface and the presence of bone in the cleft site would promote eruption of the primary dentition into the cleft. Advocates speculated on the ability of the restored continuity of the maxilla to allow normal midfacial development with the forward and downward growth vector of the nasal septum.

Primary Bone Grafting

According to when the alveolar bone graft is placed, the accepted terminology[27] for primary osteoplasty is a "combination of soft tissue closure of lip and cleft alveolus with a concomitant bone grafting in infancy."[28] Primary bone grafting coincides with surgical repair of the lip and therefore occurs during infancy, although its effect is not appreciated fully until growth and development of the maxilla are complete.

Early results[19, 20] in the 1950s gained popularity because of the advantages associated with this technique, including prevention of maxillary arch collapse and normal development of the craniofacial complex. Migration of teeth into the grafted area was observed. In bilateral clefts of the palate, stabilization of the mobile premaxilla was achieved. Although enthusiasm for this approach continued for the next decade, comparisons between patients who had undergone primary bone grafting and those who had not indicated that early bone grafting compromised growth of the midface and resulted in a higher incidence of malocclusion. These negative reports[29, 30] caused many centers to discontinue primary bone grafting.[31, 32] Operator differences, the effect of subperiosteal undermining, and length of follow-up observation of the treated patients resulted in a disparity of findings. A few centers continued to support the benefits of primary bone grafting.[33] They concluded that primary bone grafting provided stabilization of the maxilla in the infants with bilateral clefts, restoration of the continuity of the alveolar arch, and the opportunity for eruption of the primary canine through the graft. They also considered support for the alar base as an additional benefit, and because palatal closure was facilitated, an improvement in speech could be expected.

Later reports[29] confirmed inhibition of maxillary growth, causing many centers to abandon primary bone grafting in favor of delaying bone grafting. Koberg[27] reviewed the history of bone grafting and, from reports available in the literature, concluded that severe maxillary deformity predictably resulted from primary bone grafting.

Despite the lapse of almost 50 years, with ample opportunity to evaluate the consequences of primary bone grafting, the controversy continues; the procedure is still performed in a few centers in the United States and Europe.[34]

Periosteoplasty was introduced as an alternative to primary bone grafting.[35] The advantage of this ''boneless bone graft'' was that continuity of the maxillary segments was established by local periosteal flaps with the intention of promoting bone formation in the cleft site. After completion of this procedure in infants, bone formation was reported in the cleft with no apparent adverse effects on facial growth.[36] However, perioplasty is not accepted widely, although the results have been reasonably successful.

Neonatal Maxillary Orthopedics

Presurgical orthopedics[19,20] was developed and popularized in Great Britain by a prosthodontist and orthodontist. The role of maxillary orthopedics therefore was evaluated by orthodontic criteria, including craniofacial growth and development and the effect of this early intervention on the dentoalveolar component of the occlusion. The involvement of orthodontists in this early treatment was assessed on the basis of the results when the dentition was established rather than the ease with which the surgeon could perform the primary surgical repair. The literature is replete with studies that, unfortunately, are confounded by the use of different orthopedic devices, various surgical techniques, and nonuniform timing of these interventions. These reports suggest that neonatal maxillary orthopedics may have a deleterious effect on growth of the midface.[31] However, because primary bone grafting was frequently an integral part of the procedure, the results may reflect an inevitable bias.

The enthusiasm for presurgical orthopedics and primary bone grafting was disrupted by Pruzansky,[37] an orthodontist, in his classic dissent from presurgical orthopedics and bone grafting for infants with cleft lip and palate. It was perhaps unfortunate that presurgical orthopedics was embraced so enthusiastically by the proponents of primary bone grafting as the panacea by which surgical problems would be eliminated, clefts would fuse without additional intervention, and feeding problems in the affected infant would be eradicated.[19] These unrealistic expectations justifiably were challenged,[37,38] and the result was the abandonment of both procedures before any well-designed clinical studies were done to test the efficacy of each treatment intervention independently.

As a result of inadequate evidence, clinicians (especially orthodontists) had diverse opinions concerning the benefits of presurgical orthopedics. These opinions were related to interference with craniofacial growth of the midface and dentoalveolar attributes such as the prevalence of dental crossbites. As an alternative to maxillary orthopedics, surgeons have closed wide clefts with lip adhesions[39] before definitive lip repair. Lip adhesions may be indicated sequentially in infants with a grossly displaced premaxilla in bilateral clefts to avoid dehiscence at the wound site. The selection of patients who might benefit from repositioning of the premaxilla before surgical repair is an issue in which the orthodontist should defer to the surgeon's judgment. Despite the continuing controversy in the literature concerning the benefit of neonatal maxillary orthopedics, the ease of surgical closure prevails in the decision-making process. With the demise of presurgical orthopedics and primary bone grafting, there was a need to restore the cleft alveolus and provide bone into which the permanent canine could erupt. Secondary bone grafting has gained increasing popularity since the mid-1970s. It currently is considered an integral part of contemporary cleft palate rehabilitation.

THE RATIONALE FOR BONE GRAFTING THE CLEFT MAXILLA

Formerly, rehabilitation of the maxillary dentition in patients with cleft lip and/or cleft palate depended on the expertise of the prosthodontist in the replacement of both teeth and in closing the cleft. In the late 19th century, surgical correction of the cleft became the treatment of choice; the effective surgical closure of the palate was accomplished by von Langenbeck.[40] Closure of the defect was often traumatic as the surgeon attempted to position the cleft margins with inadequate tissue, which resulted in collapse of the segments and subsequent distortions of future growth and development of the maxillary complex. To correct the three-dimensional maxillary deficiency that commonly occurred after closure of the cleft, the prosthodontist was often involved in construction of an overdenture. Thus the era of the orthodontist and prosthodontist working as a team came into existence in the 1940s with Harvold and Bohn.[22] The importance of bone reconstruction of cleft defects and preservation of the permanent dentition was recognized by Axhausen as a critical but unmet possibility of cleft repair.[41] The challenge to the prosthetic therapy was the surgical technique of Boyne and Sands,[42, 43] in which providing continuity of the maxilla and palate by grafting bone into the cleft site at an appropriate time eliminated the need for prosthetic replacement. The repair of the residual cleft without significant growth disturbance was a major advance in the surgical/orthodontic management of the cleft maxilla and virtually eliminated the role of the prosthodontist in the rehabilitation of patients with clefts. This contemporary management of the cleft maxilla is predicated on the close collaboration of the surgeon and orthodontist on the team in the context of a closely coordinated and problem-oriented approach of the team members. The challenge of prosthodontic rehabilitation was met by the surgical techniques that eliminated the need for prosthetic replacement by providing continuity of the cleft alveolus.

Secondary Bone Grafting

By definition, secondary or delayed alveolar bone grafting is performed after primary lip repair.[42, 43]

Early Secondary Bone Grafting (2–5 Years of Age)

This typically is performed during the primary dentition period (age range, 2–5 years). According to advocates of this relatively early timing of grafting, the bony support for the future eruption of the lateral permanent incisor is an important consideration in the periodontal health of this tooth adjacent to the cleft site. However, many of the issues affecting growth and development of the midface in primary bone grafting are also considerations when early timing of secondary alveolar bone grafts is recommended.

Intermediate or Secondary Bone Grafting (6–15 Years of Age)

Contemporary opinion is that this is the optimal time for alveolar bone grafting. Bone is provided for the eruption of the permanent canine into the cleft site; this has the added advantage of including alveolar bone with the eruptive process. Minimal interference in midfacial growth and development can be expected.

Late Secondary Bone Grafting (Adolescence to Adulthood)

Reconstruction in the skeletally mature patient with a cleft does not involve the same requirements as in younger patients. The need for a graft material to allow eruption of teeth through the graft into the dental arch is obviated, and replacement of missing teeth by implants is a consideration, especially in the nongrowing patient.

The rationale for bone grafting the cleft maxilla and palate is the elimination of the residual cleft with continuity of the alveolar ridge and maxilla while preserving the natural dentition. The benefits include the following:

1. Bone is provided into which the unerupted teeth may erupt and/or the orthodontic repositioning may occur (Fig. 19–1*A,B*). The optimal timing and sequencing of the bone graft relates to the position of the unerupted teeth adjacent to the cleft and the development of the dentition. The bone graft procedure requires appropriate planning and orthodontic preparation, if the developing teeth adjacent to the cleft are to have adequate bone into which they can erupt. Ideally, unerupted teeth should have about one third to one half of the root developed at the time of graft placement. Bone grafts resorb to the level of crestal bone supporting the teeth adjacent to the cleft. Therefore, the bone graft should not be delayed until complete eruption of the dentition, nor should orthodontic preparation, with the potential to move roots into the cleft, commence before the bone graft is performed. Once periodontal defects occur, as happens when teeth erupt and/or are moved into cleft defects, they cannot be significantly

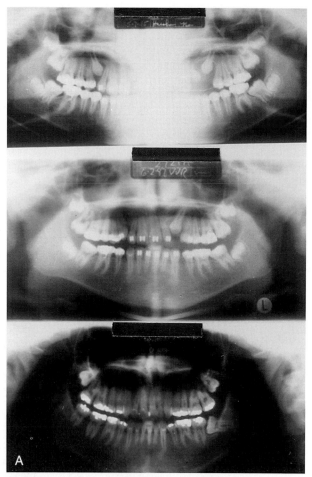

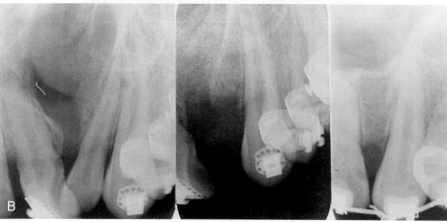

Figure 19–1. *A,* Series of radiographs demonstrating bone graft placement and eruption/orthodontic movement of teeth into the bone graft with preservation of the entire dentition. *B,* Series of radiographs demonstrating bone graft placement and orthodontic movement of teeth into the bone graft. This demonstrates the contemporary goal of cleft management: to avoid dental prostheses.

improved. In addition, delaying the bone graft until complete eruption of the dentition increases the risk of external root resorption.

2. At the time of the surgical placement of the bone graft in the alveolus, patent oronasal fistulas either in the palate or in the nasolabial vestibule may be closed. This is achieved by a three-layered closure technique with the grafted bone sandwiched between the two soft tissue planes. The size and location of fistulas should not be a consideration in the decision to place a graft. Most of the time, local soft tissue can be used to close these defects. Rarely is it necessary to use distant donor sources such as the tongue (Figs. 19–2A,B and 19–3A,B). There is hardly ever a need to stage closure of multiple fistulas, but this depends on their locations. These fistulas commonly create problems with reflux more than with speech. Many children with clefts do not complain of oral-nasal reflux because they are accustomed to functioning with this condition and do not realize that reflux is abnormal. In some instances, oral-nasal fistulas are a novelty to young children, and they do not desire closure because of their acceptance and notoriety among peers. The effects of reflux on the health of the oral and nasal mucosa and the periodontium are considerations for closing these fistulas. As a general rule, fistulas anterior to premolars have little consequence on speech, but posterior fistulas may contribute to nasality and abnormal speech resonance. To determine the contribution of these fistulas to altered speech, they can be temporarily obturated with Vaseline gauze, chewing gum, or soft wax.

3. Support and elevation of the alar base on the affected side from the grafted bone in the alveolar defect contributes to restoration of nasal and lip symmetry. By constructing a nasal rim, which is symmetric with the opposite side, the nasal base and even the tip are supported (Fig. 19–4A,B). This contribution to esthetics may be subtle in some instances and more dramatic in others. However, it is critical to achieve this support before definitive rhinoplasty and/or definitive lip revision if optimal results are

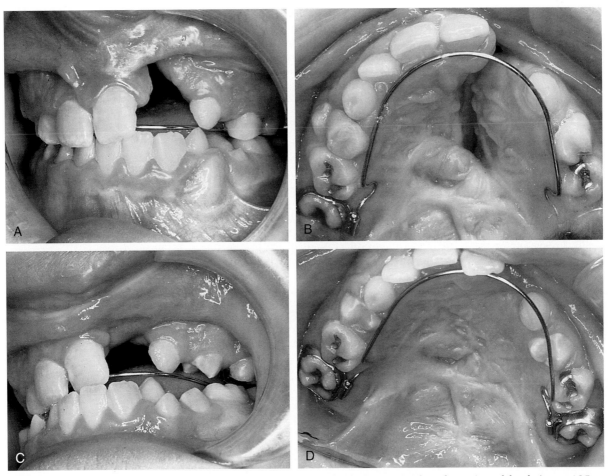

Figure 19–2. Large buccal and palatal defect (*A,B*, preoperative) closed with bone graft and rotation of local tissues (*C,D*, postoperative). (From Turvey TA, Vig K, Moriarty J, Hoke J: Delayed bone grafting in the cleft maxilla and palate: A retrospective multidisciplinary analysis. Am J Orthod 1984; 86[3]:247.)

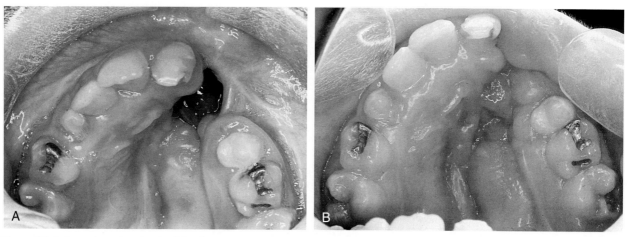

Figure 19–3. Large buccal and palatal fistulas (*A*, preoperative) closed with bone graft and rotation of local tissues (*B*, postoperative).

to be obtained. Without appropriate skeletal support, soft tissue revisions always fall short of their potential.[44]

4. Providing continuity of the alveolar ridge even if teeth are missing provides the restorative dentist with support for a more esthetic and hygienic prosthetic replacement. However, it is unrealistic for a non–dental-bearing bone graft to maintain the height and width of the adjacent ridge. To do this, the ridge must be subjected to the functional demands of a tooth. In the contemporary setting, the placement of endosseous dental implants into a bone graft not only is possible but is gaining acceptance as the standard of care; many practitioners believe that this alternative is far superior to constructing a conventional bridge. The problems encountered in placing endosseous implants in patients with clefts who have previously undergone bone grafting relate to bone resorption. The amount of resorption is associated with the length of time between placement of the bone graft and insertion of the implant. If bone grafts are not subjected to the functional demands of a tooth root, they inevitably resorb, both vertically and transversely, and therefore it is critical for the clinicians planning treatment to know how the bone graft will be utilized so that an endosseous implant can be placed at the optimal time (Fig. 19–5*A,B*). Currently, there are many unanswered questions about placement of implants in bone grafts of patients with clefts.[45, 46] Experience gained in the future should provide some insight into the optimal timing of placement of endosseous implants, the type of implant to be used, the ideal bone graft consistency, and the technique of implant placement into bone grafts of the cleft maxilla and palate.

5. In repaired bilateral clefts of the lip and palate, the placement of grafts bilaterally into the cleft defects stabilizes the premaxilla while providing bone into which the adjacent unerupted teeth may erupt. However, before a bone graft is placed, it is critically important for the teeth of the premaxillary segment to be positioned in an atraumatic occlusal relationship. If the premaxilla is continually subjected to traumatic

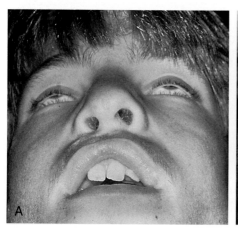
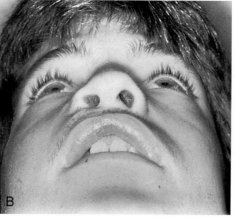

Figure 19–4. *A*, Preoperative photograph demonstrating nasal and lip deformities associated with unilateral cleft lip and palate. *B*, After bone grafting. Notice the improved support for the nose and lip; also, the nasal tip on the cleft side has been improved by the support that the bone graft provides to the nasal base. (From Turvey TA, Vig K, Moriarty J, Hoke J: Delayed bone grafting in the cleft maxilla and palate: A retrospective multidisciplinary analysis. Am J Orthod 1984; 86[3]:249.)

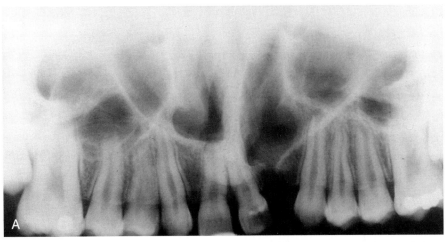
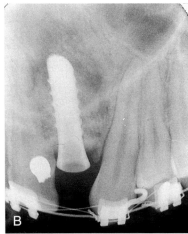

Figure 19–5. *A,B,* Examples of endosseous implants placed into bone grafts in clefts. (Courtesy of Dr. M. Farmand, Erlangen, Germany.)

occlusal forces postsurgically, union and healing of the bone graft does not occur. This underscores the importance of the cooperative efforts between the surgeon and orthodontist in bone grafting the cleft maxilla and palate.

Today, most cleft palate teams appreciate the benefits derived from delayed bone grafting and have adopted the procedure for their patient populations. However, there are certain unrealistic expectations and misconceptions about bone grafts. A successful bone graft is a vital unit that responds to its environment and functional demands. It is *unrealistic* to expect a bone graft to prevent maxillary arch collapse, especially when significant palatal and labial scars are present. Maintaining arch form is probably an unreasonable goal of bone grafting the cleft maxilla and palate.

CURRENT CONTROVERSIES

The three contemporary controversies relate to

1. The timing of surgery for the placement of the alveolar bone graft.
2. The type of bone for the alveolar bone graft and the selection of the donor site.
3. The sequencing of orthodontic expansion to correct the transverse discrepancy before or after the surgical procedure of alveolar bone grafting.

In resolving controversies, evidence is necessary to accept or refute the different alternatives. Clearly, in order to recommend one alternative over another, clinicians need evidence that the outcome of one procedure is more beneficial than the outcome of the alternative. There is a hierarchical approach to evidence-based information: whether this information was obtained from an anecdotal case report, a case series, a cohort study, a retrospective study, or a randomized prospective controlled clinical trial, as discussed in Chapter 30. Until the methods for clinical research are more widely adopted and evidence-based medicine is espoused by clinicians in resolving the risks, costs, and benefits of alternative treatment strategies, there will continue to be controversy as to which approach is the best. Certainly there is merit to all the current alternative approaches, and all provide satisfactory outcomes, or they would not continue to be practiced. Clinicians believe that their method of treatment is the most appropriate for their patients and therefore continue to practice their preferred procedure.

PRINCIPLES OF BONE GRAFTING THE CLEFT MAXILLA AND PALATE

Patient Selection

Most patients with clefts of the maxilla and palate are candidates for placement of a bone graft. There are very few medical contraindications to this procedure. However, it is important to coordinate this aspect of care with orthodontic treatment. An important reason for bone grafting is to preserve the permanent dentition without periodontal defects and to preclude the need for a prosthesis. This can be accomplished in most instances if the graft is placed at an appropriate time: before the eruption of the permanent dentition adjacent to the cleft. Bergland and associates'[47] finding of a decline in the success rate of bone grafting when the graft is placed after the eruption of the secondary dentition is similar to that of others. Patients older than 25 years should be carefully counseled about wound dehiscence, infection, necrosis, and sequestration, because these complications occur with greater frequency in this population. The effects of chronic inflammation on soft tissues, as occurs with fistulas and periodontal disease, can be detrimental to bone graft revascularization, and the longer these effects are in existence, the worse is the prognosis for the bone graft.

Timing and Sequencing

An important goal of bone grafting the cleft maxilla and palate is preservation of the permanent dentition without periodontal defects and without the need for prosthetic rehabilitation. In meeting this goal, it is critical to place the graft at an appropriate time: before the eruption of the permanent teeth adjacent to the cleft. In many instances, this precedes the eruption of the permanent cuspid (ages 6–8 years). In other instances, when eruption of the central or lateral incisor is in question, the age at grafting may be reduced to 4 to 6 years. After eruption of the permanent dentition, the success of bone grafting the cleft maxilla and palate decreases, and so the optimal time to place the graft should be guided by the prognosis of the teeth adjacent to the cleft.

Once a periodontal defect is present, as occurs when teeth erupt into nonrepaired cleft sites, the loss of supporting tissues is apparently permanent, and these tissues cannot be restored by grafting bone into the defect. Bone grafts tend to resorb to the height of the crestal bone at the cleft margin, although as teeth erupt, they bring supporting bone with them, if they erupt into bone and not into an unrepaired cleft site. Therefore, the timing of this procedure is best determined by stage of dental development, not by age. Ideally, the graft should be placed when root development is one-third to one-half developed and before the crown emerges. When a bone graft is placed into cleft sites after the eruption of the permanent dentition, there is an increased risk of damaging the roots of adjacent teeth and initiating external resorption.

Orthodontic preparation is helpful and sometimes necessary before bone graft placement. If orthodontic treatment is undertaken before bone grafting, it is important to avoid moving teeth into the cleft site. Although it may be tempting to align and rotate incisors adjacent to the cleft before bone graft placement, it is always prudent to determine the existing bone support when the proposed movement of the crowns and roots of the teeth is considered.

The need for orthodontic and/or orthopedic expansion before bone grafting continues to be an area of controversy. Advocates of expanding before bone grafting contend that once the graft is placed and matures, the palatal suture is fused, and resistance to expansion increases. In some instances, there is resistance that may necessitate surgical assistance to achieve appropriate arch width later in life. Slow expansion initiated 6 weeks after graft placement has the potential of stimulating immature bone, which may enhance bone graft survival. Expanding the arch before bone grafting facilitates surgery by creating more space for placement of the graft and also increases the size of the cleft defect. This then requires more soft tissue dissection to achieve adequate closure and also increases the amount of bone to be grafted. The dilemma of the timing of arch expansion and the decision to expand must be made on the merits of each case.

Current opinion favors bone grafting when patients are 8 to 11 years old, with presurgical orthodontic treatment to correct the transverse discrepancy;[47–50] this provides an operational guideline, although individual variability of dental development may revise the timing for the bone graft. Each patient should therefore be evaluated for individual needs, and the timing of the bone graft can be determined best by the patient's dental development rather than by chronologic age. Clinical studies reported in the literature are almost exclusively retrospective in design,[48–53] and ethical constraints in examining the grafted site have limited the criteria of success and failure to the development of measurements from clinical examination and radiographic appearance.

The optimal time for grafting patients with clefts has been revised to coincide more closely with the eruption of the lateral incisor, especially if it is on the distal side of the cleft (Fig. 19–6A,B,C,D). However, Bergland and associates[47] reported retrospective data with strict protocols on a series of more than 350 patients, and they concluded that elimination of the residual alveolar cleft with the use of cancellous bone grafts before eruption of the permanent canine tooth promoted consolidation of the supporting bone in the cleft site and eliminated the need for bridgework in young adults. In a smaller series, it was also found that placing the graft before eruption of the canine tooth provided periodontal benefits (Fig. 19–7A,B).[48] Other researchers[51]

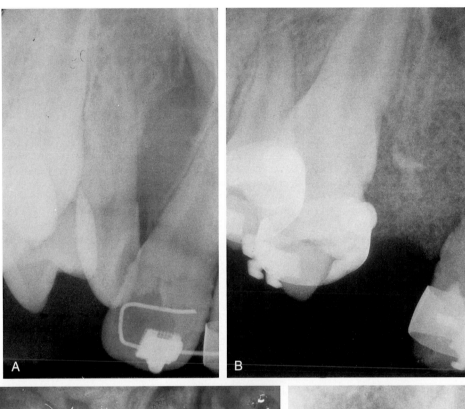

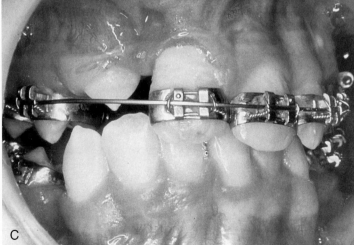

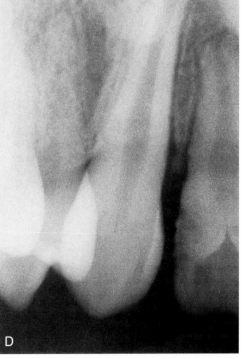

Figure 19–6. *A*, Periapical radiograph illustrating the maxillary lateral incisor on distal side of the cleft with minimal bone on mesial aspect of the root. *B*, Autogenous iliac crest cancellous bone graft has been placed with extraction of the peg-shaped, hypoplastic lateral incisor. *C*, Intraoral photograph of the permanent canine erupting through the bone graft. *D*, Periapical radiograph of the canine adjacent to the hypoplastic maxillary central incisor. (From Vig KWL, Fonseca RJ, Turvey TA: Bone grafting of the cleft maxilla. *In* Bardach J, Morris HL [eds]: Multidisciplinary Management of Cleft Lip and Palate, pp 543–549. Philadelphia: WB Saunders, 1990.)

have also examined the periodontal status after surgery and have found an improvement postoperatively.

The timing of bone grafting should be related to root development of the unerupted canine, which should be approximately one quarter to two thirds complete at the time of bone grafting. At this stage in root development, there is apparently an accelerated eruption.[52,53] In an attempt to define the most appropriate timing of the secondary bone grafting, a comparison was made among three groups of patients who had received bone grafts.[54] The three groups each had a sample size of approximately 100, and the mean ages were 9.6 years (range, 5–14), 13.5 years (range, 11–15), and 20.9 years (range, 16–38). No periodontal defects were found in the youngest group, although periodontal defects were present in the oldest group, in which there was also an increased incidence of fistulas.

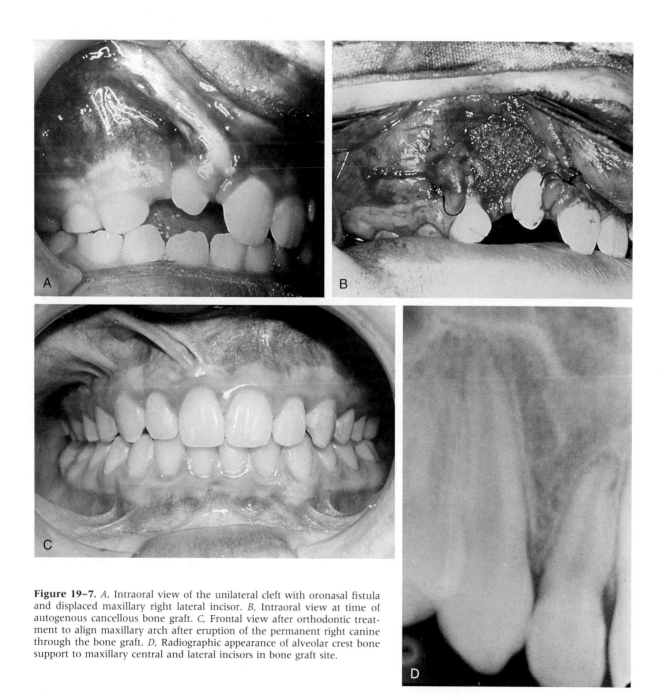

Figure 19–7. *A,* Intraoral view of the unilateral cleft with oronasal fistula and displaced maxillary right lateral incisor. *B,* Intraoral view at time of autogenous cancellous bone graft. *C,* Frontal view after orthodontic treatment to align maxillary arch after eruption of the permanent right canine through the bone graft. *D,* Radiographic appearance of alveolar crest bone support to maxillary central and lateral incisors in bone graft site.

Type of Grafting Material

Just as the timing of secondary alveolar bone grafting is controversial, so are the type of graft material and the donor site. Several types of bone grafting materials are currently used, although autogenous bone is considered the most effective. Allogeneic bone is used in some centers, but there are some contraindications to the use of this type of bone. Alloplastic materials prevent eruption of teeth and therefore are not used in children.

Documented clinical studies indicate that autogenous cancellous bone is the preferred and most successful grafting material. From the surgeon's perspective the most popular donor site has been the iliac crest, although the morbidity associated with harvesting cancellous bone from the hip has resulted in alternative sites. The calvaria has been considered a viable alternative from which particulate cancellous bone may be harvested.[55, 56] The advantage of autogenous bone is the active osteogenic capability that it brings to the recipient site and the appropriate architecture that may facilitate eruption of teeth and/or orthodontic tooth movement. After the rapid incorporation of bone into the cleft alveolus, migration of teeth into the cleft allows the unerupted canine to replace a missing lateral incisor (see Fig. 19–3). The stabilization of the premaxilla in patients with bilateral cleft lip and palate (while providing bone for the eruption of the canines adjacent to the permanent central incisors) allows continuity of the dental arch bilaterally. At the time of bone grafting, the mobile premaxilla may also be repositioned vertically to correct the maxillary occlusal plane differentially (Fig. 19–8A,B,C,D).

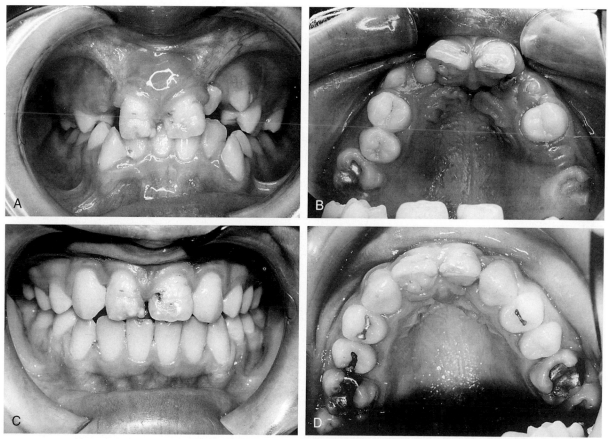

Figure 19–8. *A,* Bilateral complete cleft lip and palate. Note hypoplastic incisors and displaced lateral incisor. *B,* Palatolabial view to show oronasal fistula. Clinically, the premaxillary segment was mobile. *C,* Frontal view after bilateral bone grafts and eruption of the canines through the iliac crest cancellous alveolar bone grafts. Alignment and closure of space by orthodontic treatment before restorative treatment to hypoplastic central incisors. *D,* Palatal view to illustrate closure of palatal fistula. The premaxillary segment is firm and stable after the bilateral alveolar bone grafts at 9 years of age. (From Vig KWL: Timing of alveolar bone grafting: An orthodontist's viewpoint. Prob Plast Reconstr Surg 1992; 2[1]:66.)

Autogenous Bone Grafts

The timing of autogenous bone grafts depends not only on the root development of the permanent canine but also on the donor site. It is generally agreed that cancellous particulate bone is the preferred graft in the maxillary alveolus. Experiences in primary bone grafting with split rib grafts and corticocancellous blocks resulted in future problems with the eruption of teeth through the graft and were considered to compromise maxillary growth.

Iliac Crest

The ilium has been recognized as the preferred donor site for harvesting large amounts of cancellous bone, even in young children. This preferred source of cancellous bone is not free of complications. Discomfort from the recipient site in the maxillary alveolus may be minimal, but the patient, regardless of age, may have difficulty in walking during the week after discharge from the hospital. However, this still remains the primary source of bone, from both the orthodontist's perspective and the perspective of many surgeons. If the orthodontist has corrected the transverse maxillary discrepancy preoperatively (Fig. 19–9), there is typically an increase in the size of the cleft to be grafted. This also may increase the size of an existing oral-nasal fistula, and clinical judgment (based on the collaboration of the orthodontist with the surgeon) is essential for determining the feasibility of expansion before the grafting procedure. Soft tissue closure with excessive undermining at the time of alveolar bone grafting to cover the widened cleft site may compromise the grafted unilateral or bilateral alveolar clefts. For this reason, placing the cancellous bone graft before orthodontic expansion may be the preferred sequence of events in selected cases. This often is done when the patient is 6 or 7 years of age, to provide support for the erupting lateral incisor. The grafted area is responsive to orthodontic expansion, which may be instituted within 1 month after the graft is placed to take advantage of the reactive osteogenic potential of the graft to tension placed across the cleft site.

Cranial Bone

Calvarial bone dust has been used by neurosurgeons for reconstruction of skull defects,[57] but its application as a donor site for alveolar cleft grafts was not popularized until the 1980s.[55,58] Cranial bone provides a convenient source of donor cancellous bone, and there is also less pain during the postsurgical recovery period. There is a potentially higher risk and possible morbidity because of the close proximity to the brain, and there is also more cortical bone in relation to cancellous bone in cranial bone grafts than in those harvested from the ilium. The orthodontist therefore may find that small spicules dehisce during movement of the teeth into the grafted site. From

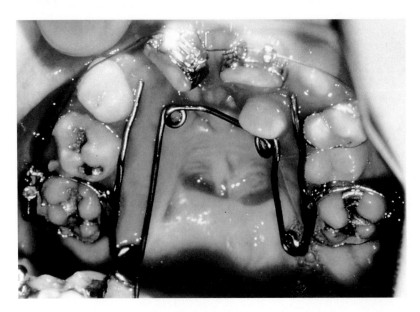

Figure 19–9. Intraoral palatal view of quadhelix appliance for transverse expansion before alveolar bone graft.

the orthodontist's perspective, consolidation of bone into the cleft defect is of considerable importance when teeth are moved into the grafted site. Cranial bone grafts may provide less cancellous bone in some children; thus this may not be an adequate alternative donor site in some children. Therefore, cranial bone graft use depends on the timing of the graft, the size of the defect, and the amount of available cancellous bone.

Mandibular Symphysis

Controversy concerning the use of endochondral versus intramembranous bone has become an issue in choosing the donor site for cancellous bone. An alternative site from which to harvest membrane bone is the mandibular symphysis. Intraoral access to the donor site avoids scarring and morbidity postoperatively. However, the amount of bone that is available depends on the timing of the bone graft and the age of the patient. When early secondary bone grafting is contemplated, the surgeon must avoid the unerupted mandibular canine, and the bone available to harvest may be limited.[59] The proximity of the mandibular incisor roots and of the mental nerve also entails potential risks when symphyseal cancellous bone is harvested from the mandible. The claim that intramembranous bone maintains more of its original volume than endochondral bone is an attractive concept but not easily substantiated.[60] Likewise, the more rapid revascularization of membranous bone from experimental studies endorses intramembranous bone as an attractive choice.[61]

Allogeneic Bone Grafts

Eliminating a second surgical site reduces potential morbidity, which is important from the patient's perspective when allogeneic bone grafts are advocated. However, the ability of allogeneic bone to produce results comparable with those produced by autogenous bone is still equivocal. Studies have shown convincing evidence of the eruption of the canine through freeze-dried bone[62–64] and also the response of the graft to moving the teeth orthodontically into the graft. Because allogeneic bone grafts rely on osteoinduction for new bone formation, revascularization of the graft is slower and less responsive than when autogenous cancellous bone is used; the latter has the ability to mount a viable cellular response at the recipient site. Allogenic bone grafts therefore provide a scaffold from which new bone develops from subperiosteal and endosteal sources.

This is important for an orthodontist working in a team whose preference may be allogeneic bone for alveolar bone grafts. The timing of orthodontic movement of teeth into the grafted site should be delayed for at least 3 months postoperatively. This is logical if the biologic process is one in which bone substitution must be induced through migration of peripheral bone-generating sources. The type of bone (cortical or cancellous), the physical size of the graft material (powder, chips, or blocks), and the mineral content of the bone (undecalcified, surface decalcified, or totally decalcified) all may influence the ultimate success or failure of an allogeneic bone graft. Therefore, allogeneic bone may be considered as an alternative graft material in secondary alveolar cleft grafting.[65–67]

Disadvantages of Allogeneic Bone Grafts

The devastating complication of transmission of disease from donor to the host is theoretically possible but is prevented by careful bone banking procedures and donor screening.[68,69] The risk of transmission of human immunodeficiency virus (HIV) is much less than 1:1,000,000 if careful bone banking procedures are followed.[68]

Infection at the recipient site secondary to a contaminated specimen is possible. The bone is cultured an average of six times at the bone bank.[69] This measure, coupled with adherence to aseptic technique and watertight nasal closure before bone graft placement, should limit recipient site infections.

Host incompatibility and rejection of the allogeneic graft are also possible; however, properly treated allogeneic bone possesses minimal antigenicity and does not elicit the rejection phenomenon.[68–72] If the nonvital allogeneic graft does become contaminated and infected, the entire graft often is lost. With autogenous bone grafts, usually only part of the infected graft is lost. Small sequestra of the allogeneic bone graft are exfoliated from the graft site for the first 3 months after surgery.[73,74] This is a normal process and does not reflect infection.

Allogeneic bone has a longer incorporation phase than autogenous bone. Therefore, the postoperative initiation of orthodontic treatment is delayed (>3 months vs. 1 month with autogenous grafts).[75] Allogeneic bone should not be used in bilateral clefts or wide unilateral clefts. These clefts have a decreased blood supply to the graft, which increase the risk of failure. In such cases, grafting should be performed with autogeneous bone. Use of allogeneic bone should be reserved for first-time operated unilateral clefts in 9- to 11-year-old patients, after the majority of maxillary growth is achieved and before eruption of the canine tooth.[47]

Use of Fresh Autogenous Particulate Cancellous Bone

The use of fresh autogenous bone for grafting has been claimed to provide the best chances of success with clefts of the maxilla and palate. Autogenous bone contains osteogenic cells and this is the major advantage of its use. In view of the fact that most clefts have impaired vascularity because of scars from previous surgery, the use of fresh autogenous bone is the most predictable choice of bone graft material.

It has been demonstrated that particulate cancellous bone responds most favorably to the odontogenic demands of this part of the maxilla and palate. Corticocancellous bone blocks have been successfully used in the cleft maxilla and palate, but dental eruption has been impaired. Similarly, rib grafts and cortical bone blocks have also been used, but these too may impair the eruption of teeth. The optimal size of the bone particles is considered to be 5 mm, and as Marx[76] suggested, the particles must be densely packed into the defect for optimal transference of osteogenic cells.

Although many bone donor sources are available for use, the ilium is the most commonly used site because of the predictable quantities of cancellous bone, the ease of procurement, the concealed scar, and little morbidity. The cranium is another excellent cancellous bone donor site, but it is not as predictable as the ilium.[77–79] Harvesting bone from the cranium requires more operating time and has minimal morbidity when the operator is experienced, but the potential for morbidity is greater. The tibia is an excellent source of cancellous bone, but the residual scar is obvious, and the potential to fracture this weight-bearing bone postoperatively is another consideration. If the primary purpose of the bone graft is to support an endosseous dental implant, the use of a corticocancellous block graft wedged into the defect may be considered.[45] Which type of graft is best to use when implants are placed into clefts is an area for future research.

PREPARATION OF THE BONE GRAFT DONOR SITE

A principle of bone graft donor site preparation is to completely expose the bone margins on either side of the defect. It is not necessary to expose the cancellous layer on the proximal and distal segments, as is necessary with bone grafting of some other defects. Therefore, rotary instrumentation of the bone margins is not necessary.

Removal of Teeth

Supernumerary teeth and/or malformed permanent teeth are commonly present in the cleft sites (Fig. 19–10). These teeth should be removed, unless they can be used to facilitate arch preparation. This decision must be made in conjunction with the orthodontist. Removal at the time of the bone graft is preferable and can almost always be accomplished without jeopardizing the graft site preparation. The only time they are removed before the bone graft is when it is determined that their removal will leave mucosal defects in the area of the graft. For most children with clefts, even the simplest dentoalveolar procedures are aversive, and it is preferable to have these done in one operation.

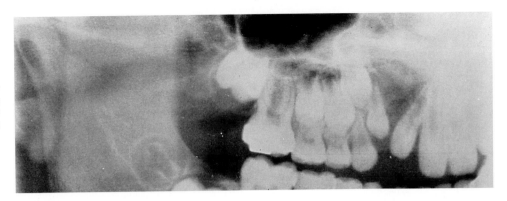

Figure 19-10. Radiograph showing supernumerary lateral incisor in the path of eruption of the permanent canine. This incisor was removed at the time of the alveolar bone graft.

Closure of the Bone Graft Site

There are multiple areas adjacent to clefts into which soft tissues can be rotated and/or advanced to cover the bone graft site. As a general rule, proximal tissues should always be used before more distant sources are considered. The adjacent gingival tissues, palatal tissues, and buccal mucosa are excellent tissue sources for consideration of closure over bone graft recipient sites (see Fig. 11-17).

SURGICAL MANAGEMENT OF THE CLEFT ALVEOLUS

Bone Grafting the Cleft Maxilla and Palate

Surgical Technique

Nasotracheal intubation is preferably through the nostril on the noncleft side because it removes all obstructions from the surgical field. If nasotracheal intubation is not possible, the oral route, although less desirable, can be used. If the oral route is used, the endotracheal tube can be sutured to the mandibular anterior teeth to remove it from the immediate surgical area and to secure its position. Occasionally, a mouth gag is helpful in positioning the endotracheal tube and in gaining access to the palatal tissues, but it may also be cumbersome.

The surgical field, including the buccal, palatal, and nasal tissue, is injected with local anesthesia and epinephrine (1:100,000). Sterile preparation of the surgical field is then performed.

Incision Design

The procedure begins by incision of the fixed gingival tissues from the cleft margin and around the adjacent teeth so that they are preserved. These tissues are reflected back on themselves and sutured to expose the crestal alveolar bone (Fig. 19-11). The tissues lining the cleft margins are then incised from the alveolus superiorly to the depth of the mucobuccal fold, where there is normally a buccal fistula. The incision continues around the margins of the fistula, but the depth of the circumferential part of the incision is shallower than the marginal incision, because there is no periosteum (Fig. 19-12). This incision is made on both sides of the cleft. A full-thickness flap is then developed, beginning from the alveolar crest, superiorly to the height of the buccal fistula. Care is taken when this flap is elevated so that thin bone overlying the adjacent tooth root is not damaged. If bone is elevated and roots become exposed or damaged, periodontal defects will occur and/or external resorption may result. Superiorly, at the circumferential part of the buccal fistula, the tissues are undermined sufficiently to permit the mucosal surface to be turned in toward the center of the fistula and elevated into the nasal cavity. The tissues lining the cleft must also be reflected from the palatal mucosa; this can be done by incising the tissues, through the cleft from the buccal side. This flap is then elevated in a subperiosteal plane, and the bone margins of the cleft are exposed to the level of the nasal cavity (Fig. 19-13A).

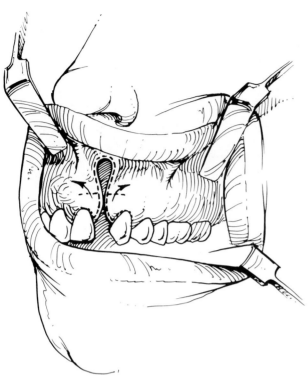

Figure 19–11. Outline of incision to prepare the cleft site for bone grafting. The fixed gingival tissues are preserved and sutured back.

Closure of the tissues lining the cleft is accomplished with resorbable sutures on a small cutting needle. A mattress suture technique with the knots tied on the nasal side assists in establishing a watertight seal (Fig. 19–13*B*). Access to suturing in this confined area is facilitated by the use of a Castroviejo needle holder. If the fistula continues posteriorly on the palate, it is sometimes helpful and necessary to pass a traction suture through the nasal floor to the posterior palatal tissue to seal the posterior nasal floor. This is facilitated by bending a straight needle to the appropriate curved contour, passing it through the fistula, and retrieving it on the palate (Fig. 19–14*A,B,C*). Sometimes it is necessary to mobilize the palatal tissues to achieve

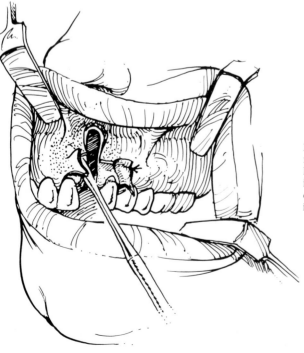

Figure 19–12. The incisions are made through periosteum on the lateral sides of the cleft, preserving the fixed gingiva. The circumference tissues must also be incised.

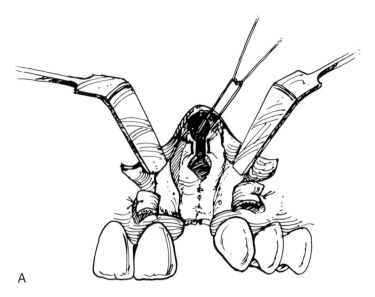

Figure 19–13. *A,* The tissues lining the cleft are elevated to the nasal cavity to construct a floor. *B,* Closure of the nasal lining is accomplished with a horizontal mattress suture to evert the edges toward the nasal side.

A

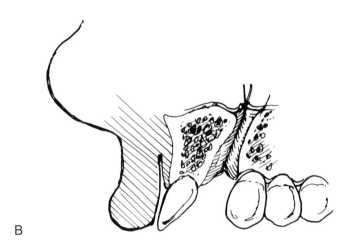

B

adequate palatal coverage. In such instances, an incision made from the molar region, approximately 5 mm from the gingival margin and parallel to the dental plane, can be extended to the cleft. The flap is then elevated in a subperiosteal plane and rotated medially and anteriorly to achieve coverage (Fig. 19–15*A,B*). An alternative is to elevate the palatal tissue from the first molar forward to the cleft area. A relaxing incision at the first molar area is then made to allow the flap to be advanced to cover the palatal defect. The relaxing incision should not extend to the greater palatine vessels, and the vessels should be included in the flap (Fig. 19–16*A,B*).

Placement of the Bone Graft

The anterior and posterior bone margins of the cleft should be completely stripped of all soft tissues. The lateral surface of the maxilla on either side of the cleft is exposed, and the hypoplasia of the bone margins is always apparent from the alveolus superiorly to the pyriform rim. Autogenous particulate cancellous bone is densely packed into the entire cleft defect. The success of this type of bone graft is enhanced by transferring osteogenic cells; this is facilitated by tightly condensing the graft. The bone must extend from the pyriform rim to at least the alveolar crest height of the bone in the region (Fig. 19–17). Because bone margins of clefts are always hypoplastic, bone should be grafted over the margins. A strip of cortical bone can also be used at the pyriform fossa to construct a pyriform rim. In older patients, this is normally secured with screws (Fig. 19–18); in younger patients (less than 10 years), it is normally placed into the defect and retained by the soft tissues (Fig. 19–19).

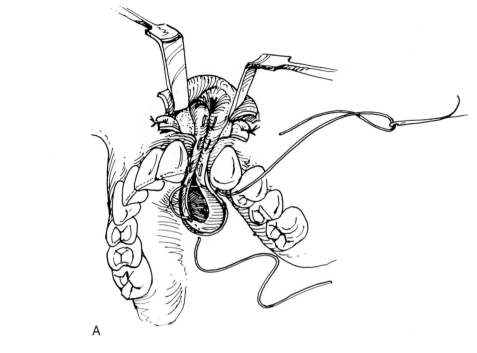

A

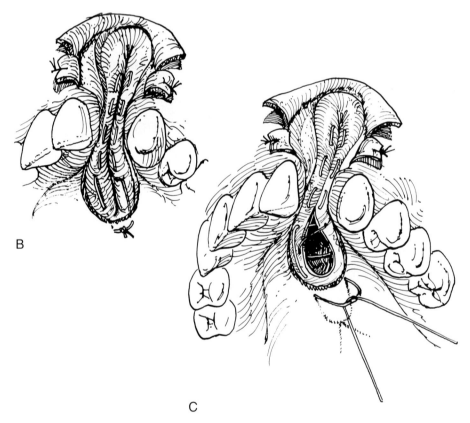

B

C

Figure 19–14. *A,B,C,* Sometimes it is helpful and necessary to pass a traction suture through the reconstructed nasal floor and the posterior palatal tissues in order to pull the reconstructed floor posteriorly to form a seal.

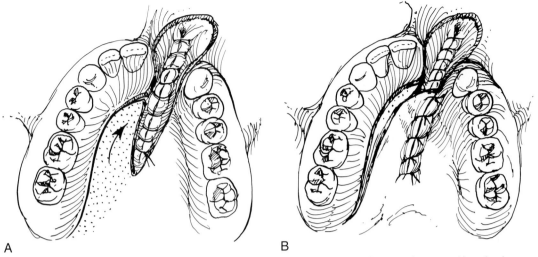

Figure 19–15. *A,B,* A full-thickness palatal flap is elevated and rotated medially and anteriorly to provide palatal coverage.

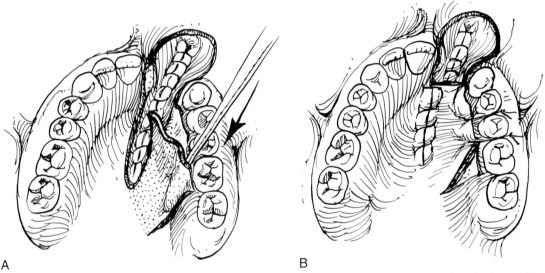

Figure 19–16. *A,* A full-thickness flap is elevated from the teeth, and a vertical relaxing incision is placed at the first molar region to allow the flap to advance. *B,* The defect is left to granulate.

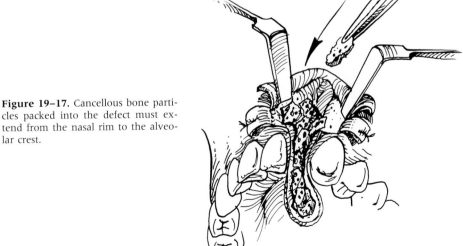

Figure 19–17. Cancellous bone particles packed into the defect must extend from the nasal rim to the alveolar crest.

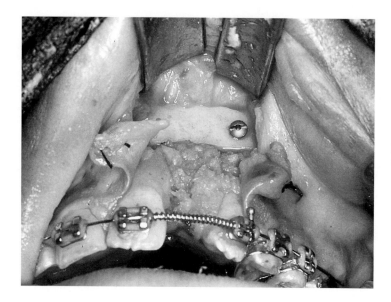

Figure 19–18. Cortical bone graft to construct a nasal rim is secured with a screw in older patients.

Closure

Closure of the buccal side of the bone graft almost always requires the addition of more tissue to the area. A variety of flaps can be used for this purpose, but each has its own indications and potential pitfalls.

Buccal Mucosal Flaps

Tissues can be rotated from the buccal mucosa or can be advanced from the buccal mucosa to cover the grafted bone. A rotational flap is the most predictable way of adding tissue to the cleft area with minimal tension. The flap is normally anteriorly based and incised to the level of the submucosa but above the periosteum.[80] The base of the flap must be adequately undermined to permit the necessary 90° rotation (Fig. 19–20). As with all pedicled flaps, the base must be broad enough and deep enough to

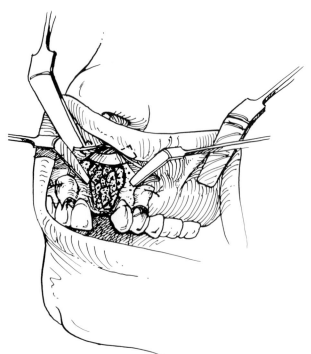

Figure 19–19. In children, the cortical graft is only placed and held by the soft tissues.

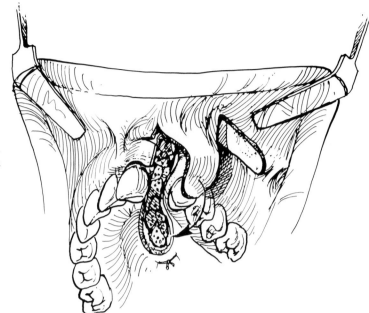

Figure 19–20. A buccal mucosal flap is elevated, maintaining a wide and thick anterior base. The flap is then rotated to cover the defect.

ensure perfusion of the tip. In general, the base should be at least one third the length of the flap. Once elevated and rotated, the tip of the flap is sutured to the palatal tissue with resorbable material. The base of the flap is also secured with sutures to the mucosa, adjacent to the cleft.

The fixed gingival tissues are preserved, and returning them to their original position is important for periodontal considerations. The mucosa of the flap in the area where the fixed gingival tissues have been elevated should be de-epithelialized. This is done with a No. 15 scalpel by shaving this area of the flap (Fig. 19–21A). The fixed gingival flaps are released on either side and sutured together over the flap. They can also be further secured to the palatal tissues (Fig. 19–21B). Occasionally, the edges of

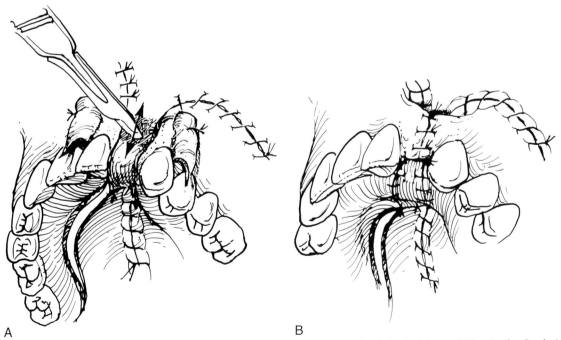

A   B

Figure 19–21. A, The rotated flap is then de-epithelialized in the areas where the fixed gingival flaps will lie. B, The fixed gingiva is then secured to the flap and around the margins of the teeth.

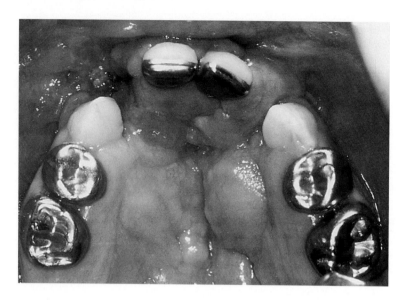

Figure 19–22. Photograph of mucosal flap around cuspid that requires a palatal graft.

the fixed gingival tissues cannot be stretched enough to allow primary closure. When this occurs, the adjacent fixed gingiva is not undermined further; rather, the two edges are secured to the flap and the dehiscence is left. If necessary, a palatal graft can be placed later in life (Fig. 19–22).

The major advantage of rotational mucosal flaps are that they allow more tissue to be added to the region of the cleft. This is especially important because an adequate volume of bone must be transferred to the cleft. Unless more soft tissue is added, tension-free closure of the mucosa over the grafted bone is impossible.

Another advantage of the rotational mucosal flap is that it requires no periosteal stripping. Such stripping is detrimental to further growth, and it is an important consideration in young children. The disadvantage of the rotational mucosal flap is that it transfers loose buccal mucosa to the dental supporting area of the alveolus. Some clinicians believe that this impedes the eruption of permanent teeth. Although that is possible, it has not been problematic in the second author's experience, nor has the use of this flap increased the need to surgically uncover teeth in the area.

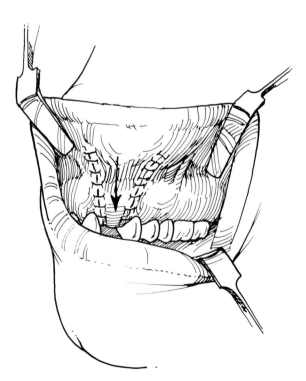

Figure 19–23. A broadly based mucosal flap can be advanced over the bone graft.

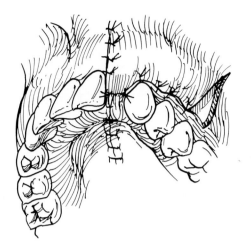

Figure 19–24. A sliding buccal gingival flap is elevated from around the teeth and advanced forward, leaving the posterior defect to granulate.

Advancement Buccal Mucosal Flap

This simple flap design can also be employed to cover the bone graft site, when there is minimal need for additional tissue to cover the cleft. It has a broad base in the lip, is undermined, and is advanced to cover the bone graft (Fig. 19–23). There is always tension on the closure when this flap design is used, and dehiscence is likely. In addition, it reduces the depth of the sulcus and may shorten the vermilion of the donor site area. Indications for using this flap are limited to situations in which the need for additional soft tissue over the bone graft is minimal.

Sliding Buccal Gingival Flap

This design is probably the most commonly used to cover bone grafts of the cleft maxilla and palate. It requires elevation of a full-thickness flap from around the crowns of the teeth on the lateral segment of the maxilla. The flap usually extends to at least the first molar, where a vertical release is placed (Fig. 19–24). The lateral aspect of the maxilla on this side of the cleft is stripped, and the full-thickness flap is advanced to cover the bone graft. The major advantage of this flap is that it advances tissue into the cleft region, and the fixed gingival tissues remain on the dental-bearing part of the maxilla. The major disadvantage is that it strips the lateral maxilla of its periosteum and leaves a defect posteriorly. The effect of this scarring on further growth is a consideration, especially when the flap is used in younger children.

SPECIAL CONSIDERATIONS FOR BILATERAL CLEFTS

The principles and steps involved in bone grafting bilateral clefts are identical to those in unilateral clefts. There is little reason to stage this procedure, because it can always be performed in one operation. The major differences in managing the bilateral condition include more operating time, and occasionally the mucosa of the vomer must be elevated to facilitate nasal floor construction. When this is done, it is necessary to extend the bone graft to the vomer and then develop enough soft tissue to cover it. This often requires elevation and rotation of palatal flaps toward the midline (Fig. 19–25). If this is done, the buccal flap must be attached to these flaps (Fig. 19–26A,B). Sometimes a bipedicled buccal mucosal flap[81] can be developed and transposed over the entire buccal and palatal defect (Fig. 19–27A). The flap is less likely to dehisce and/or necrose at the midpalatal region than are multiple flaps joining at the same place (see Fig. 19–27B). The disadvantage of this flap is that it may shorten the buccal vestibule.

It is rarely necessary to reposition the premaxilla simultaneously with the bone graft. This need occasionally arises when the premaxilla is vertically overerupted. Under normal circumstances, orthodontic treatment without surgery can almost always resolve

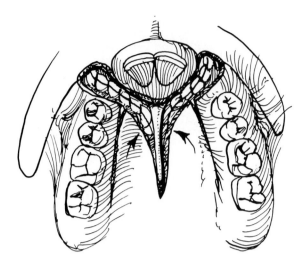

Figure 19–25. Sometimes palatal flaps must be elevated and mobilized toward the midline to close the palatal defects.

situations in which the premaxilla is forward or palatally inclined. Sometimes staging the osteotomy and the bone graft is necessary, especially if there are soft tissue deficiencies that necessitate excessive stripping.

When a premaxillary osteotomy and repositioning are undertaken, it is crucial to design the flaps so that the premaxilla remains perfused. In the bilateral cleft, the blood supply is from the nasal septal vessels, and adequate mucosa must be left attached to the premaxilla to ensure survival. If a bone graft is simultaneously performed, the nasal floor is constructed as usual. The premaxilla is either mobilized through a midline incision in the buccal mucosa to facilitate separation from the septum and vomer or separated from the palatal side and fractured forward (Fig. 19–28). Large buccal pedicles must be detached, and occasionally a piece of the nasal septum must be resected to allow for adequate superior repositioning (Fig. 19–29).

COMPLICATIONS

Major complications of bone grafting the cleft maxilla and palate, such as massive dehiscence, tissue necrosis, and infection, are uncommon. Minor complications, such as small wound dehiscence and sequestration, occur occasionally but, when handled expeditiously and conservatively, seldom compromise the result. All patients undergoing this procedure are administered prophylactic antibiotics (cephalosporin) to minimize the risks of infection and steroids to control swelling. The frequency of complications associated with bone grafting the cleft maxilla and palate appear age-related.

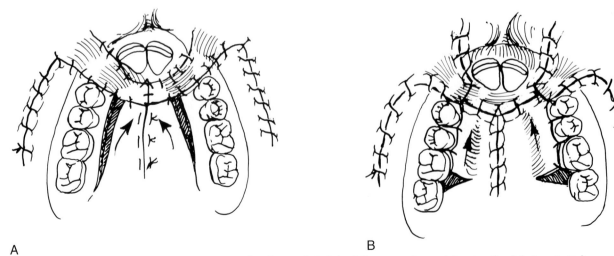

A   B

Figure 19–26. *A,* Palatal flaps are elevated and rotated. *B,* Palatal flaps are advanced, leaving the defect posteriorly.

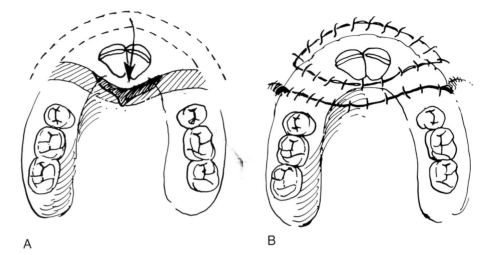

Figure 19–27. *A,* Bipedicled or bucket-handle mucosal flap described by Egyedi.[81] *B,* The flap is elevated and placed over the cleft defect.

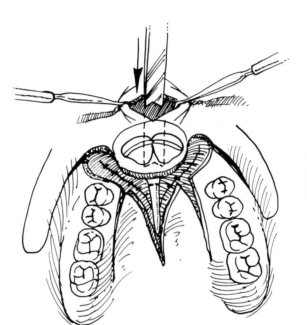

Figure 19–28. Separation of premaxilla with osteotome placed buccally to separate the nasal septum and the vomer.

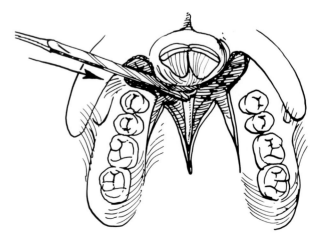

Figure 19–29. Osteotome placed through the cleft to separate the vomer.

Seldom do major complications occur in children, when the bone graft is placed before eruption of the permanent dentition. In patients older than 25 years, the complication rate and failure of the bone graft are considerable.

When wound dehiscence occurs on the oral surface, it is usually identified within the first postsurgical week. Minimal débridement with frequent irrigation and covering with petroleum jelly–impregnated gauze almost always resolve the condition with minimal loss of bone. When massive wound dehiscence and exposure of the graft occurs, the wound is treated similarly, but more extensive débridement of bone may be necessary. Attempting primary closure over the exposed bone is not indicated, because the wound is contaminated and the exposed bone is almost always avascular.

When wound dehiscence occurs on the nasal surface, it is more difficult to detect initially, because adequate visualization is not always possible, especially in children. In time, a distinct odor is detectable, and any dead bone that has migrated to the surface can usually be removed with forceps.

Radical débridement is rarely indicated, and usually this means complete failure of the bone graft. Although some patients and parents are inconvenienced by the conservative approach of irrigation and packing, this alternative results in better long-term graft survival than does the surgeon's debriding the area.

CHOICE OF PROCESS AND OUTCOME MEASURES

The methodologic approach to outcome assessment has been elaborated in Chapter 29. The different perspectives brought to an evaluation of treatment for facial clefts and the levels at which treatment outcomes are measured are important in identifying appropriate outcomes. The use of utilities as a scale by which to measure the desirability of treatment and its consequences may provide clinicans with information from which treatment decisions and results, in terms of the providers' and consumers' expectations of treatment, may be evaluated. There is an obvious need to compare the relative benefits of treatment with the appropriate method and select the best alternative for management.

In the evaluation of treatment alternatives, the rigors of contemporary clinical trial design have not been considered. Chapter 30 describes and applies measurement parameters and the design of clinical trials in detail. The reader should consult this chapter for methods of meaningful appraisal of care, including the effectiveness of treatment, the cost, and the burden of care imposed on the patient and family.

When multiple specialists are managing the care of patients within a team approach, precision in terminology is essential. Moyers[82] translated Aristotle into contemporary English: "It is the mark of an educated man to demand that degree of precision in the treatment of a subject which the nature of the subject allows. To accept mere guesses from a mathematician is as bad as expecting positive proof of a politician."

FUTURE PERSPECTIVES

An international symposium was held in 1984 to address the complex issues of early treatment of cleft lip and palate.[64] Two issues were discussed by a team of experts in the field. First, has early orthopedic treatment stood the test of time alone or as an ancillary measure? The consensus was that this treatment was valuable as an ancillary measure; the influence on subsequent maxillary growth was inconclusive because the contribution of other surgical procedures to the result could not be clearly defined. Second, is primary bone grafting still desirable as a means of stabilization, or is intermediate bone grafting a preferable alternative? Long-term results of primary bone grafting were not considered to be satisfactory; the success of the procedure was considered to be operator-sensitive and depend on the surgical technique used. In contrast, bone grafting during the mixed dentition period was considered to have a high rate of success, especially if autogenous bone was used and covered with alveolar mucosa.

The continuing interest in neonatal maxillary orthopedics and bone grafting is proof that these unresolved issues require further discussion. The controversy will, however, remain unresolved until clinical studies have been designed to provide unequivocal data on the utility and efficacy of these treatments. The problem with undertaking randomized controlled clinical trials in the climate of uncertainty provokes ethical considerations. This dilemma has been addressed by several centers, and an intercenter collaboration with a well-designed prospective clinical trial has been suggested. However, such studies are expensive, and any treatment started in infants necessitates long-term evaluation at adolescence.

Data from the international symposium on early treatment of cleft lip and palate[63] also were analyzed by an orthodontist for facial growth and development.[83] Early repair of the alveolar cleft with primary bone grafting affected both vertical and anteroposterior growth of the maxilla, confirming earlier reports on the deleterious effects of early alveolar bone grafts. The timing of secondary alveolar grafts from the orthodontist's perspective relates to the presence of teeth adjacent to the cleft site and the need for maxillary expansion. Solutions to unresolved clinical controversies rely on unequivocal evidence, and the strength of evidence relies on a hierarchic approach.[84] Randomization of alternative treatments prospectively avoids bias in the sample selection, although ethical issues in clinical trials result in practical constraints (Chapter 29). However, this is still the most appropriate modeling strategy available.[85]

The timing of orthodontic treatment in conjunction with bone grafting, particularly maxillary expansion before or after bone grafting, would be an interesting intercenter study, if designed prospectively with strict protocols involving inclusion and exclusion criteria. Likewise, criteria for success and failure should be established a priori in clinical trials in which alternative treatments are evaluated in a risk/benefit cost analysis. To provide evidence, instead of controversial opinion, on the timing of alveolar bone grafting from the orthodontist's perspective, methods for conducting clinical trials are now available. These results would provide reliable and valid information to resolve the controversies surrounding individual preference of alternative treatments.

Future trends in health care policy in the United States may mandate that when more than one alternative treatment exists, clinicians should be prepared to provide prior probability estimates for expected outcomes in order for the patient to make an informed decision. The timing for secondary alveolar bone grafts is no exception; successful results have been achieved with contradictory strategies for maxillary expansion before and after surgery. Policymakers have urged researchers to gather information to define health outcomes more definitively and to develop consensual practice standards.

Clinicians in the future will be expected to reconcile the variability among patient responses and preferences to avoid doctrinairian approaches to clinical problems.[86] From the viewpoint of an orthodontist, the timing of alveolar bone grafting reflects the bias of issues pertaining to growth and development of the craniofacial complex. However, although it is generally agreed that facial growth is a complex process, the intrinsic potential for midfacial growth cannot be quantified easily. Biologic variability and the superimposed pathogenesis of clefting further confounds the issue when clinicians attempt to discriminate the effects of treatment from the intrinsic growth deficit of the midface. The yardstick that the orthodontist uses reflects bias in preferred outcome measurements of success and failure, and these measurements should be viewed, not in isolation, but as part of the fabric of team management.

Case 1: K.B.

A 7-year-old boy with a unilateral cleft lip and cleft palate was referred for management. A patent oral-nasal fistula was present, as were ectopically erupting incisors. The lateral incision was present on the medial side of the cleft, and no teeth were in the eruption pathway of the permanent cuspid. The arch width was adequate, and although there was anterior collapse of the segments, there was enough room to perform the surgery.

Diploic cranial bone was harvested from the right parietal region, and small cortical chips were mixed to supplement this bone and were transferred to the cleft. No teeth were removed before or during surgery. The buccal mucosa was rotated to cover the graft. Two weeks after surgery, a few cortical sequestrae surfaced and were easily retrieved from the oral side. Irrigation with saline for a week helped resolve the situation. Healing and graft maturation were otherwise uneventful.

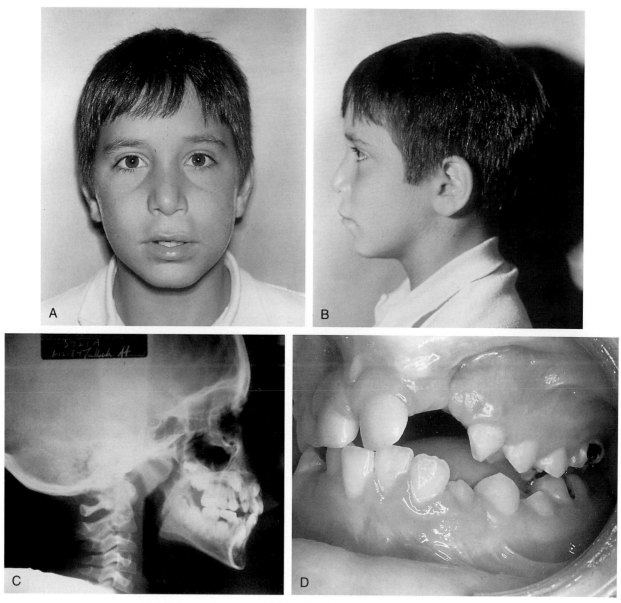

Figure 19–30.

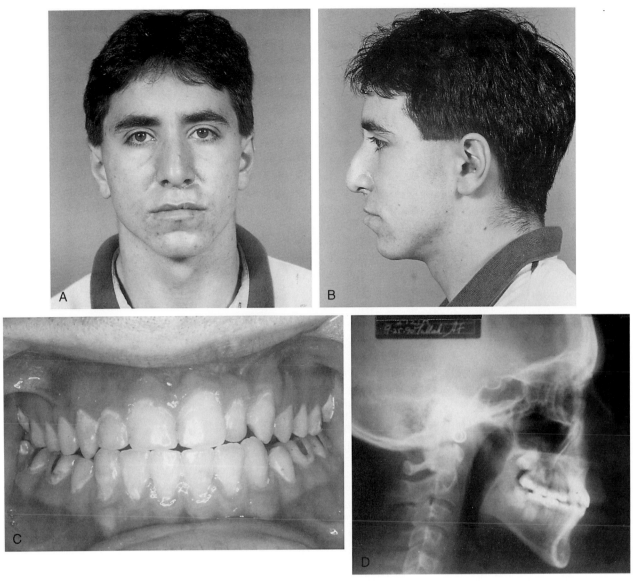

Figure 19–31.

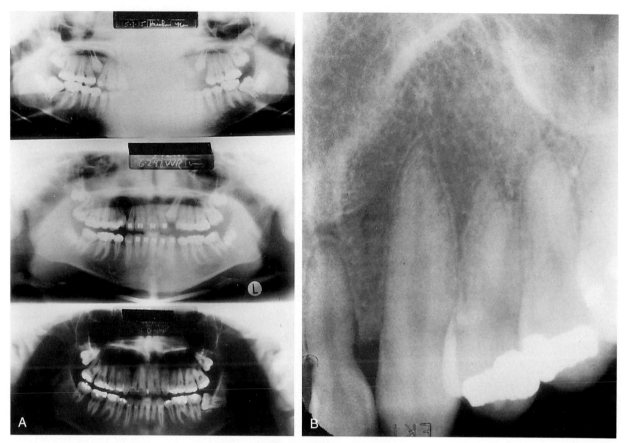

Figure 19-32.

Orthodontic alignment was initiated several months after surgery. Definitive orthodontic treatment was delayed until age 12, at which time the cuspid erupted through the graft and the mucosal flap. The patient underwent debanding at age 14. At age 18, he returned for removal of his wisdom teeth. No other lip and/or nasal revision was desired by the patient; he was happy with the result.

This case illustrates the long-term benefits (10 years after surgery) of bone graft to the cleft maxilla and palate at a developmentally appropriate time. No presurgical orthodontic treatment was given, and the complete dentition was salvaged. Presurgical orthodontic alignment was not undertaken because the arch was wide enough to permit the surgery and because incisor alignment had the potential for causing periodontal problems (Figs. 19-30 to 19-32).

Case 2: N.H.

A 10-year-old girl with a unilateral cleft lip and cleft palate had previously undergone primary lip and palate repair. At this time, she was interested in pursuing orthodontic improvement of her dentition.

Examination indicated 180° rotation of the left central incisor, adjacent to the cleft. In addition, bilateral crossbite and an anterior open bite were noted. A buccal fistula was present in the depth of the mucobuccal fold. Good palatal movement was identified, and normal closure of the velopharyngeal mechanism was noted. Radiographs confirmed the extension of the cleft distal to the central incisor with the lateral incisor and a supernumerary tooth positioned in the lateral segment. The teeth were in the eruption pathway of the cuspid.

An iliac cancellous bone graft was performed before orthodontic treatment. A mucosal flap was rotated to cover the graft. The lateral incisor and supernumerary tooth were extracted at the time of surgery to facilitate eruption of the cuspid.

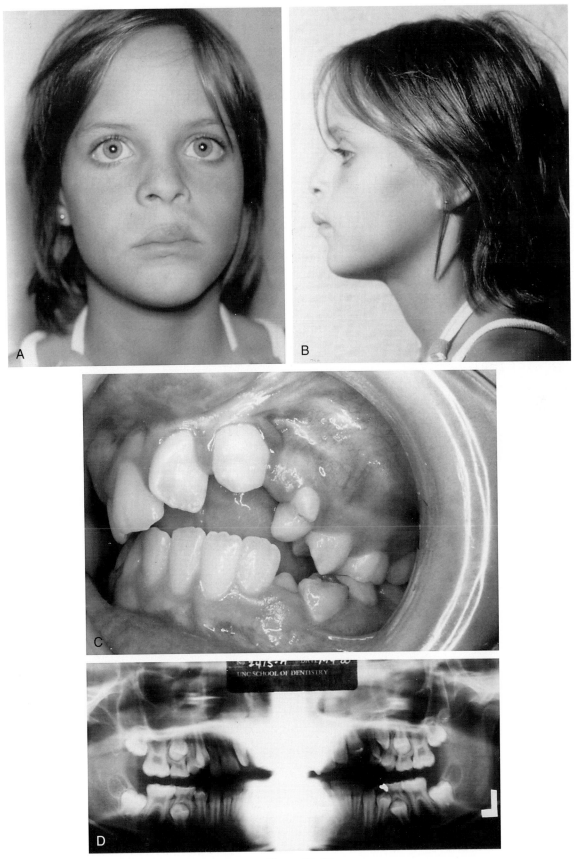

Figure 19–33.

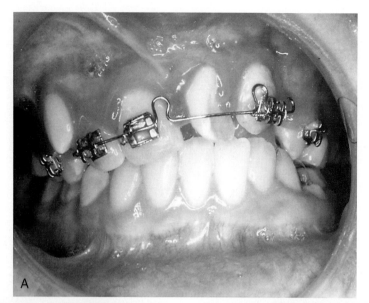

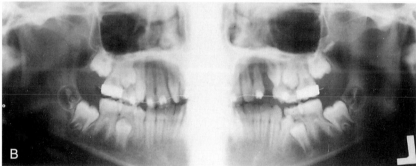

Figure 19–34.

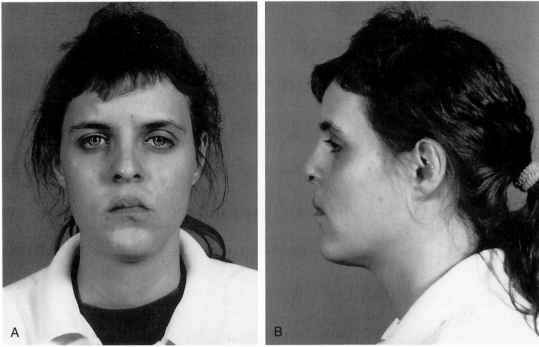

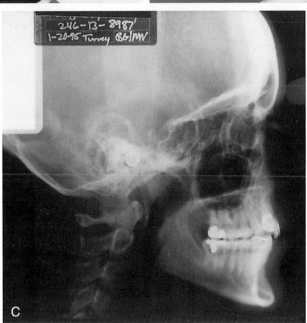

Figure 19–35.

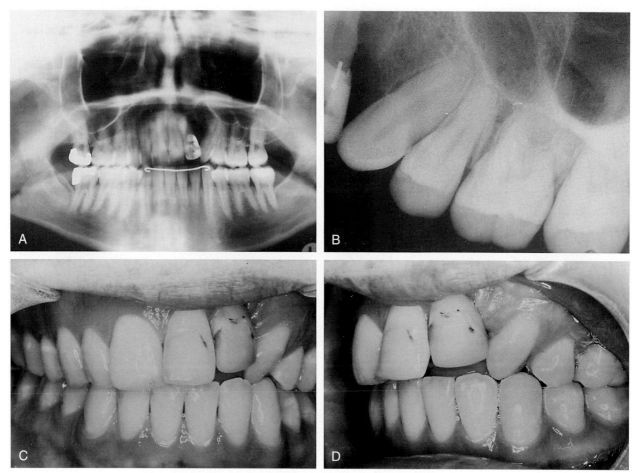

Figure 19–36.

Presurgical orthodontic movement was not attempted because of the potential for creating periodontal problems if the root of the central incisor were inadvertently moved into the cleft. Within 1 month of surgery, orthodontic treatment was begun with the intention of rotating the incisor, expanding the arch, and leveling, while maintaining space for the cuspid. These goals were accomplished within 18 months, and retainers were placed. At age 13, definitive orthodontic treatment was begun. By age 15, the patient had lost interest in completing treatment. At this time, the cuspid had erupted through the graft and was positioned adjacent to the central incisor.

This case illustrates the long-term benefit (15 years after surgery) of bone graft placement, even in patients who lose interest in completing orthodontic treatment. Orthodontic alignment was delayed until after the bone graft was placed, in order to prevent periodontal defects. The lateral incisor and supernumerary teeth were extracted at the time of the graft to permit the eruption of the cuspid, and the cuspid was advanced through the graft adjacent to the central incisor. Although the occlusion is less than ideal, the sound periodontal condition without the need for prostheses, closure of the fistula, and support for the lip and nose justify bone graft placement (Figs. 19–33 to 19–36).

Case 3: L.S.

An 8-year-old girl with a repaired bilateral cleft lip and cleft palate was referred for treatment. She had undergone primary lip and palate closure and columella lengthening earlier in life and was now ready to initiate preliminary orthodontic treatment. Examination revealed a grossly overerupted premaxilla with the maxillary incisors contacting

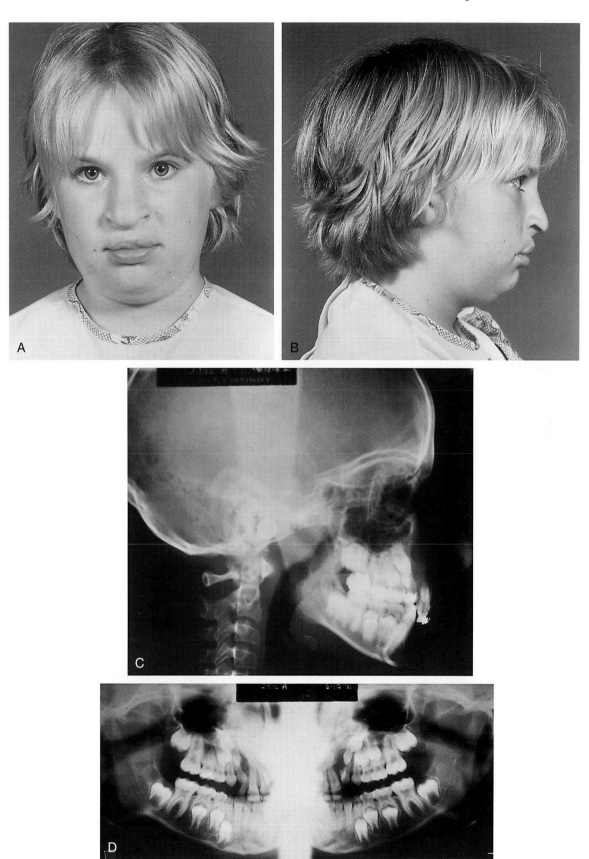

Figure 19–37.

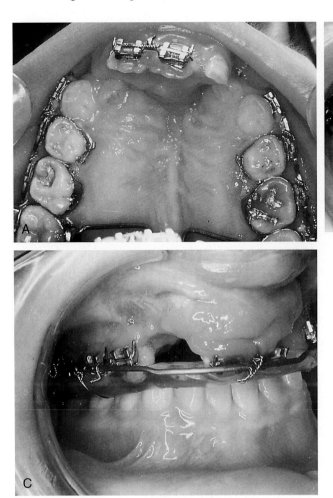

Figure 19–38.

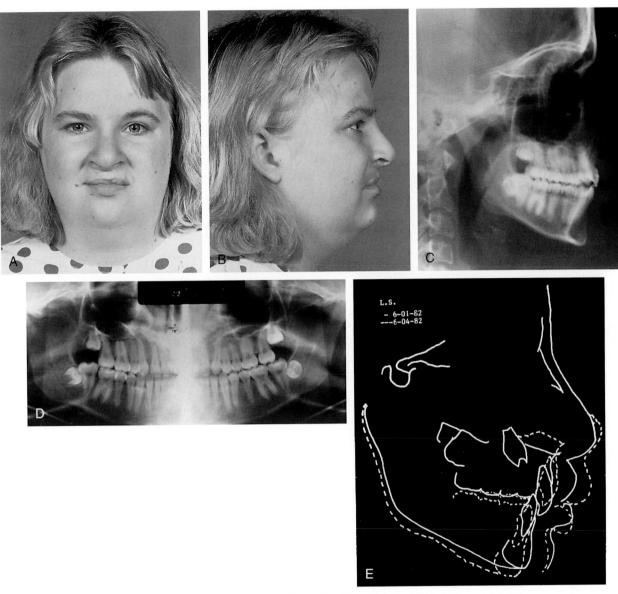

Figure 19-39.

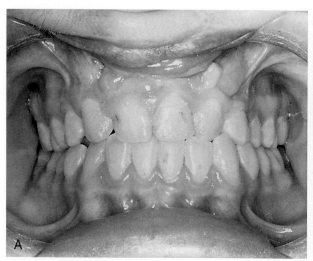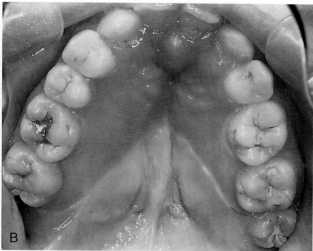

Figure 19-40.

the mandibular alveolus when the posterior teeth were occluding. The molar relationship was Class II, and the arch width was adequate to accommodate the width of the premaxilla. Buccal and palatal fistulas were present, and the premaxilla was freely mobile. Multiple supernumerary teeth were identified in the cleft area, as were developing permanent cuspids. There was adequate function of the velopharyngeal mechanism.

Previous experiences with similar conditions suggested that the position of the premaxilla was beyond orthodontic and/or orthopedic correction. Feasibility model surgery indicated that the premaxilla could be positioned superiorly and the incisors could be leveled with the posterior segments. There was adequate arch width so that orthodontic expansion before surgery was not necessary. Cuspid substitution for the lateral incisors was the anticipated plan, and so the unerupted lateral incisors and supernumerary teeth in the cleft were removed at the time of surgery.

Orthodontic appliances were placed with segmental arch wires on each of the three maxillary units. Molar bands with headgear tubes were used so that a 0.036 auxiliary wire could be placed during surgery to help stabilize the premaxillary segment with the two posterior maxillary segments. The surgery was executed as described in the text. Bone was harvested from the ilium and grafted to the defects, and mucosa was rotated from the cheek to cover the grafted bone. An occlusal index was also used during surgery to help maintain the position of the premaxilla.

After surgery, healing occurred uneventfully. Clinical and cephalometric examinations confirmed nasal tip elevation with this procedure as well as improved nasal base and upper lip support.

Continued alignment of incisors after surgery was accomplished, and the patient underwent debanding and placement of retainers. Definitive orthodontic treatment commenced at age 13 and was completed by age 15. Records at age 18 (10 years after bone grafting) indicate maintenance of the vertical position of the premaxilla and detailing of the occlusion with cuspid substitution for the lateral incisors. All buccal and palatal fistulas were closed, and there was good periodontal support for all teeth and adequate nasal support. Although lip and nasal revisions could benefit appearance, the patient was not interested (Figs. 19-37 to 19-40).

Case 4: S.A.

A 7-year-old girl had previously undergone primary lip and palate closure and, as a separate procedure, columella lengthening. She initiated orthodontic consultation for alignment before bone grafting. Extreme malposition of the premaxilla and central incisor and collapse of the lateral segment were noted. Patent buccal and palatal fistulas were also present. The palate was short and scarred, but it moved well, as did the lateral pharyngeal walls. Velopharyngeal inadequacy was noted.

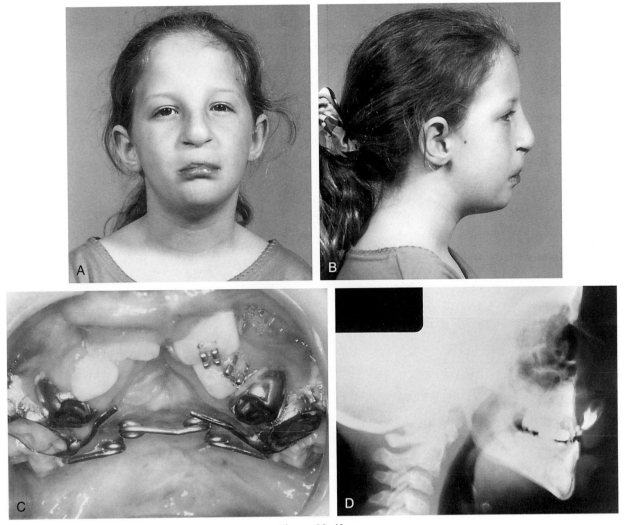

Figure 19–41.

A plan was developed and included presurgical expansion of the lateral segments with a W-arch. The extreme palatal position of the central incisors precluded placement of orthodontic appliances, and therefore surgical alteration of the position of the premaxilla was necessary. Because of the complexity of this surgical movement, the concern for vascularity of the segment, and the paucity of adequate soft tissue, the decision was to stage the osteotomy and bone grafting procedures.

The osteotomy was conducted through a vertical vestibular incision to separate the vomerine and nasal septal attachments. Another mucosal incision on one side of the vomer allowed adequate mobilization with an osteotome and repositioning of the premaxilla. Wires were placed on the maxillary incisors, and these wires were stabilized to an 0.036 auxiliary wire, which was inserted into the first molar headgear tubes. An acrylic splint was also placed to ensure minimal occlusal trauma to the premaxilla. Healing occurred uneventfully, and orthodontic treatment resumed 5 weeks after surgery. Also noted was improvement of upper lip and nasal support.

The bone graft was performed 6 months after the osteotomy. Because of the amount of bone necessary and the lack of adequate skull thickness, the ilium was the donor source for the bone grafts. Simultaneously, all fistulas were closed, buccal mucosal flaps were rotated to cover the bone grafts bilaterally, and a superiorly based posterior pharyngeal flap was inserted into the soft palate. Healing was uneventful, and with the assistance of speech therapy, speech improved. Orthodontic appliances remained for another 4 months. The patient has undergone debanding and is currently awaiting the

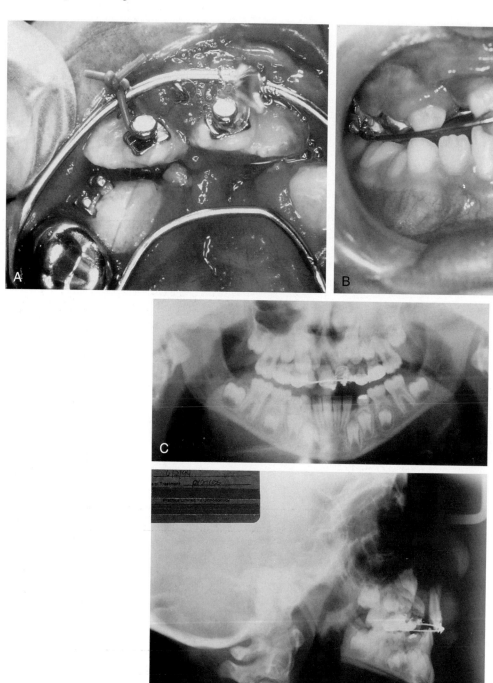

Figure 19–42.

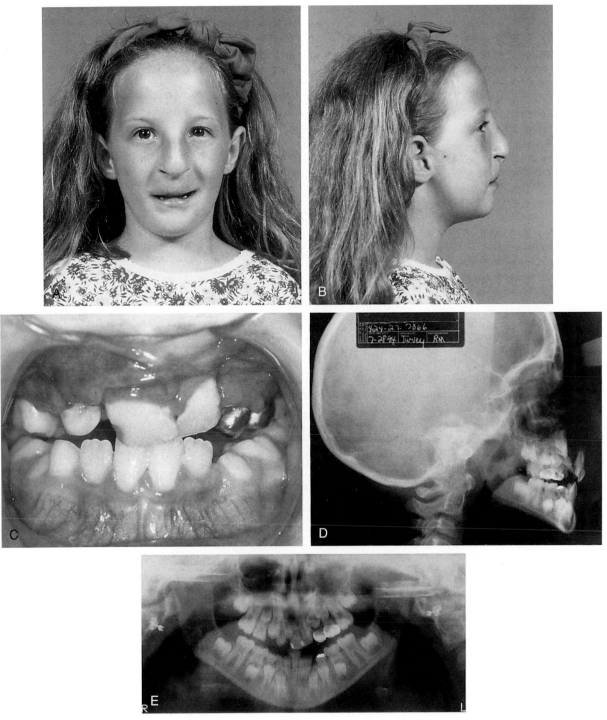

Figure 19–43.

eruption of the permanent dentition before definitive treatment commences. Complete correction of the lateral crossbite was not possible, and it is anticipated that orthognathic surgery will be necessary in the future to assist orthodontic treatment.

This difficult case illustrates the importance of a comprehensive team approach to rendering care. Timing and sequencing of orthodontic, speech therapy, and surgery are highlighted in this case report.

The authors acknowledge Dr. David Sarver for the orthodontic treatment of this patient (Figs. 19–41 to 19–43).

References

1. Lexer E: Die Verwendung der freien Knochenplastik nebst Versuchen über Gelenkversteifung und Gelenktransplantation. 1908; Arch F Klin Chir 36:939–954.
2. Drachter R: Die Gaumenplalte und derer operative. Behandung Dtsch Chir 1914; 131:1–89.
3. Schmid E: Die Annaherung der Kieferstumpfe bei Lippen-Kiefer. Gaumensplaten: Ihre schadlichen Folgen und Vermeidung. Forschr Keifer Gesichtschir 1955; 1:168.
4. Nordin KE, Johansen B: Freie Knochentransplantation bei Defekten im Alveolarkamm nach Kieferorthopadischer Einstellung der Maxilla bei Lippenkiefer-Gaumenspalten. Forschr Keifer Gesichtschir 1955; 1:37.
5. Schrudde J, Stellmach R: Primarie osteoplastik und Kieferbogenformung bei Lippen-Kiefer-Gaumenspaltung. Forschr. Kiefer und Gesichtschirurgie, Stuttgart, 1959.
6. Schuchard K: Primary bone grafting in clefts of lip, alveolus and palate. In Gibson T (ed): Modern Trends in Plastic Surgery, vol 2. London: Butterworths, 1966.
7. Brauer RO, Cronin Thd, Reaves EL: Early maxillary orthopedics, orthodontia, and alveolar bone grafting in complete clefts of the palate. Plast Reconstr Surg 1962; 29:625.
8. Davies D: The radical repair of cleft palate deformities. Cleft Palate J 1970; 7:550.
9. Fujino H: Primary osteoplasty in cleft lip, alveolus and palate patients. Chicago-Cine Symposium (I) Hare-Lip and Cleft Palate, p 87. 1972.
10. Georgiade NG, Pickrell KL, Quinn GW: Varying concepts in bone grafting of alveolar palate defects. Cleft Palate J 1964; 1:43.
11. Harle F: Die Zeitwahl der Osteoplastik bei Lippen-Kiefer-Gaumenspalten. Freiburg: Habil-Schrift, Med Fakultat, 1971.
12. Johanson B, Ohlsson A: Bone grafting and dental orthopedics in primary and secondary cases of cleft lip and palate. Acta Chir Scand 1961; 122:112.
13. Kriens O: Primary osteoplasty in patients with clefts of lip, alveolus and palate. Acta Otorhinolaryngol Belg 1968; 22:687.
14. Longacre JJ: Diskussion zum Vortrag von R. Stellmach: Modern procedures in uni- and bilateral clefts of the lip, alveolus and hard palate with respect to primary osteoplasty. In Schuchardt K (ed): Treatment of Patients with Clefts of Lip, Alveolus, and Palate: 2nd Hamburg International Symposium, July 6–8, 1964. Stuttgart: Thieme, 1966.
15. Lynch JB, Lewis SR, Blocker RG Jr.: Maxillary bone grafts in cleft palate patients. Plast Reconstr Surg 1966; 37:91.
16. Manchester WM: Discussion of the lecture from A. Rehrmann, W. Koberg and H. Koch: Long term postoperative results of primary and secondary bone grafting in complete clefts of lip and palate. First International Congress on Cleft Palate, Houston, 1969. Cleft Palate J 1970; 7:206.
17. Pickrell KG, Quinn R, Massengill, K: Primary bone grafting of the maxilla in clefts of the lip and palate: A four-year study. Plast Reconstr Surg 1968; 41:438.
18. Schuchard K: Primary bone grafting in clefts of lip, alveolus and palate. In Gibson T (ed): Modern Trends in Plastic Surgery, vol 2. London: Butterworths, 1966.
19. Burston WR: The early orthodontic treatment of cleft palate conditions. Trans Br Soc Orthod Dent Practit 1958; 9:41.
20. McNeil CK: Orthodontic procedures in the treatment of congenital cleft palate. Dent Rec 1950; 70:126.
21. Vig KWL: Timing of alveolar bone grafting: An orthodontist's viewpoint. Prob Plast Reconstr Surg 1992; 2:58–72.
22. Harvold E: Observations on the development of the upper jaw by hare lip and cleft palate. Odontol Tidskr 1947; 55:289.
23. Bohn A: Retention construction following Harvold's method of repositioning of the maxillary complex in cleft palate cases. Trans Eur Orthod Soc 1951; pp 219–221.
24. Semb G: Analysis of the Oslo Cleft Lip and Palate Archive: Long term dentofacial development [Thesis]. Oslo, Norway: University of Oslo, 1991.
25. Vig KWL: Parameters for evaluation and treatment of patients with cleft lip/palate or other craniofacial anomalies. Cleft Palate Craniofac J 1993; 30(22, Suppl).
26. Dalston RM, Marsh JL, Vig KWL, et al: Minimal standards for reporting the results of surgery on patients with cleft lip, palate or both: A proposal. Cleft Palate 1988; 25:3–7.
27. Koberg WR: Present view on bone grafting in cleft palate: A review of the literature. J Maxillofac Surg 1973; 1:185.
28. Nylen B: Surgery of the alveolar cleft. Plast Reconstr Surg 1966; 37:42–46.
29. Friede H, Johanson B: A follow up study of cleft children treated with primary bone grafting: Orthodontic aspects. Scand J Plast Reconstr Surg Hand Surg 1974; 8:88.
30. Robertson NR, Jolley A: Effects of early bone grafting in complete clefts of the lip and palate. Plast Reconstr Surg 1968; 42:414.
31. Jolleys A, Robertson NR: A study of the effects of early bone grafting in complete clefts of the lip and palate: Five year study. Br J Plast Surg 1972; 25:229.
32. Rehrmann AH: The effect of early bone grafting on the growth of the upper jaw in cleft lip and palate children: A computer evaluation. Minerva Chir 1971; 26:874.
33. Nylen B. Korloff B, Arnander C, et al: Primary, early bone grafting in complete clefts of the lip and palate. Scand J Plast Reconstr Surg Hand Surg 1974; 8:79–87.
34. Rosenstein SW, Monroe CW, Kernahan DA, et al: The case for early bone grafting in cleft lip and cleft palate. Plast Reconstr Surg 1983; 70:297.
35. Skoog T: Repair of the cleft maxilla using periosteal flaps. Panminerva Med 1967; 9:405.
36. Hellquist R, Ponten B: The influence of infant perioplasty on facial growth and dental occlusion from five to eight years of age in cases of complete unilateral cleft lip and palate. Scand J Plast Reconstr Surg Hand Surg 1979; 13:305.
37. Pruzansky S: Presurgical orthopedics and bone grafting for infants with cleft lip and palate: A dissent. Cleft Palate J 1964; 1:164–187.

38. Glass D: The early management of bilateral cleft lip and palate. Br J Plast Surg 1970; 23:130.
39. Randall P: A lip adhesion operation in cleft lip surgery. Plast Reconstr Surg 1965; 35:371.
40. von Langenbeck B: Operation der angeborenen totalen Spalttung des harten Gaumens nach einer neuen Methode. Dtsch Klin 1861; 8:231.
41. Axhausen W: The osteogenic phases of regeneration of bone. J Bone Joint Surg Am 1956; 38:593.
42. Boyne PJ, Sands NR: Secondary bone grafting of residual alveolar and palatal clefts. J Oral Maxillofac Surg 1972; 30:87.
43. Boyne PJ, Sands NR: Combined orthodontic-surgical management of residual palato-alveolar cleft defect. Am J Orthod 1976; 70:20.
44. Borchgrevink HH: Secondary bone grafting of alveolar clefts, part III: The influence on the secondary lip and nose deformities. Fourth International Congress on Cleft Palate and Related Craniofacial Anomalies, 1981; p 184.
45. Verdi FJ: Use of Branemark implant in the cleft palate patient. Cleft Palate-Craniofacial J 1991; 28:301.
46. Farmand M: Enossale implantate bei der kieferosteoplastik. In Schwamzer N (ed): Fortschritt der Kiefer und Gesichts Chirurgie Band XXXVIII, pp 112–114. Stuttgart: Thieme, 1993.
47. Bergland O, Semb G, Åbyholm FE: Elimination of the residual alveolar cleft by secondary bone grafting and subsequent orthodontic treatment. Cleft Palate J 1986; 23:175–205.
48. Turvey TA, Vig K, Moriarty J, et al: Delayed bone grafting in the cleft maxilla and palate: A retrospective multidisciplinary analysis. Am J Orthod Dentofac Orthop 1984; 86:243–256.
49. Vig KWL, Turvey TA: Orthodontic-surgical interaction in the management of cleft lip and palate. Clin Plast Surg 1985; 12:735.
50. Vig KWL, Fonseca RJ, Turvey TA: Bone grafting of the cleft maxilla. In Bardach J, Morris H (eds): Multidisciplinary Management of Cleft Lip and Palate, pp 543–550. Philadelphia: WB Saunders, 1990.
51. Johanson B, Ohlsson A, Friede H, et al: A follow up study of cleft lip and palate patients treated with orthodontics, secondary bone grafting and prosthetic rehabilitation. Scand J Plast Reconstr Surg Hand Surg 1974; 8:121–135.
52. Waite DE, Kersten RB: Residual alveolar and palatal clefts. In Bell WH, Proffit WR, White RP (eds): Surgical Correction of Dentofacial Deformities, pp 1329–1367. Philadelphia: WB Saunders, 1980.
53. Troxell JB, Fonseca RJ, Osborn DB: A retrospective study of alveolar cleft grafting. J Oral Maxillofac Surg 1982; 40:721–725.
54. Sindet-Pedersen S, Enemark H: Comparative study of secondary and late secondary bone-grafting in patients with residual cleft defects: Short term evaluation. Int J Oral Maxillofac Surg 1985; 43:389–398.
55. Wolfe SA, Berkowitz S: The use of cranial bone grafts in the closure of alveolar and anterior palatal clefts. Plast Reconstr Surg 1983; 72:659.
56. Wolfe SA, Price GW, Stuzin JM, et al: Alveolar and anterior palatal clefts. In McCarthy JG (ed): Plastic Surgery, vol 4, pp 2753–2770. Philadelphia: WB Saunders, 1990.
57. Shehadi SI: Skull reconstruction with bone dust. Br J Plast Surg 1970; 23:227.
58. Harsha BC, Turvey TA, Powers SK: The use of autogenous cranial bone grafts in maxillofacial surgery: A prelminary report. J Oral Maxillofac Surg 1986; 44:11.
59. Sinder-Pedersen S, Enemark H: Reconstruction of alveolar clefts with mandibular or iliac crest bone grafts: A comparative study. J Oral Maxillofac Surg 1990; 48:554–558.
60. Zins JE, Whittaker LA: Membranous vs. endochondral bone autografts: Implications for craniofacial reconstruction. Surg Forum 1979; 30:521.
61. Kusiak JK, Zins JE, Whittaker LA: The revascularization of membranous bone. Plast Reconstr Surg 1985; 76:510.
62. Maxson BB, Baxter SD, Vig KWL, et al: Allogeneic bone for secondary alveolar cleft osteoplasty. J Oral Maxillofac Surg 1990; 48:933–941.
63. Kraut RA: The use of allogeneic bone for alveolar cleft grafting. Oral Surg Oral Med Oral Pathol 1987; 64:278.
64. Hotz M: Concluding remarks. In Hotz M, Gnoinski W, Perko M (eds): Early Treatment of Cleft Lip and Palate, pp 269–270. Toronto, Ontario, Canada: Hans Huber, 1986.
65. Fonseca RJ, Clark PJ, Burkes EJ, et al: Revascularization and healing of onlay particulate autogenous bone grafts in primates. J Oral Surg 1980; 38:572.
66. Fonseca RJ, Nelson JF, Clark PJ, et al: Revascularization and healing of onlay particulate allogeneic bone grafts in primates. J Oral Maxillofac Surg 1983; 41:153.
67. Frost DE, Fonseca RJ, Burkes EJ: Healing of interpositional allogeneic lyophilized bone grafts following total maxillary osteotomy. J Oral Maxillofac Surg 1982; 40:776.
68. Bright RW, Friedlander GE, Sell KW: Tissue banking: The United States Navy Tissue Bank. Milit Med 1977; 142:503.
69. Marx RE, Kline SN, Johnson RP, et al: The use of freeze-dried allogeneic bone in oral and maxillofacial surgery. J Oral Surg 1981; 39:264.
70. Marble HB: Hemografts of freeze-dried bone in cystic defects of the jaws: A survey of ninety-one cases. Oral Surg Oral Med Oral Pathol 1968; 26:118.
71. Schaberg SJ, Petri WH, Gregory EW, et al: A comparison of freeze-dried allogeneic and fresh autologous vascularized rib grafts in dog radial discontinuity defects. J Oral Maxillofac Surg 1985; 43:932.
72. Wolford LM, Epker BN: The use of freeze-dried bone as a biologic crib for ridge augmentation: A preliminary report. Oral Surg 1977; 43:499.
73. Maxson BB, Baxter S, Vig KWL, et al: Allogeneic bone for secondary alveolar cleft osteoplasty. J Oral Maxillofac Surg 1990; 48:933–941.
74. Nique T, Fonseca RJ, Upton LG, et al: Particulate allogeneic bone grafts into maxillary alveolar clefts in humans: A preliminary report. J Oral Maxillofac Surg 1987; 45:386.
75. Vig KWL, Fonseca RJ, Turvey TA: Bone grafting of the cleft maxilla. In Bardach J, Morris HL (eds): Multidisciplinary Management of Cleft Lip and Palate, p 543. Philadelphia: WB Saunders, 1990.
76. Marx RE: Philosophy and particulars of autogenous bone grafting. Oral Maxillofac Surg Clin North Am 1993; 5:599–612.

77. Wolfe SA, Berkowitz SB: The use of cranial bone grafts in the closure of alveolar and anterior palatal defects. Plast Reconstr Surg 1983; 72:659.
78. Tessier P: Autogenous bone grafts taken from the calvarium [*sic*] for facial and craniofacial applications. Clin Plast Surg 1982; 9:531.
79. Harsha B, Turvey TA, Powers SK: Use of autogenous cranial bone grafts in maxillofacial surgery: A preliminary report. J. Oral Maxillofac Surg 1986; 44:11–15.
80. Burian F: Chirurgie der Lippen-und Gaumenspalten. Berlin: VEB Verlag, 1963.
81. Egyedi P: The bucket-handle flap for closing fistulae around the premaxilla. J Oral Maxillofac Surg 1976; 4:214–216.
82. Dixon A, Sarnat BG (eds): *In* Summary and Discussion (Session IV) Normal and Abnormal Bone Growth: Basic and Clinical Research, vol 187, pp 485–490. New York: AR Liss 1985.
83. Ross RB: An overview of treatment and facial growth. Cleft Palate J 1987; 24:71.
84. Shaw WC: Risk benefit appraisal in orthodontics. *In* Moorrees CFA, Van der Linden FPGM (eds): Orthodontics: Evaluation and Future, pp 63–81. Alphen aan den Rijn, The Netherlands: Samson Stafleu, 1988.
85. Vig KWL: The application of risk assessment to severity of dental malocclusion and craniofacial anomalies. *In* Bader JD (ed): Risk Assessment in Dentistry: Proceedings of the NIH Sponsored Symposium. Chapel Hill: University of North Carolina Press, 1990.
86. Vig KWL: Orthodontic considerations applied to craniofacial dysmorphology. Cleft Palate J 1990; 27:141–145.

20

Maxillary Advancement and Contouring in the Presence of Cleft Lip and Palate

Timothy A. Turvey, Katherine W. L. Vig, and Raymond J. Fonseca

Midface deficiency is common with facial clefting disorders, especially those affecting the palate. Cleft palate surgery leaves areas of denuded palatal bone to granulate, and the consequent scarring may result in underdevelopment and deformation of the maxilla. A major problem associated with maxillary deficiency and facial clefts is the residual scarring from previous surgery and its interference with maxillary advancement. Maxillary advancement in the presence of facial clefts and its effect on function constitute the focus of this chapter.

FREQUENCY OF MIDFACE DEFICIENCY

Most patients with congenital clefts affecting the nose, maxilla, and/or palate have some expression of midface deficiency. Class III malocclusion is only one indicator of midface deficiency, and its absence does not preclude the diagnosis. Midface deficiency may be manifested in the paranasal, nasal, infraorbital, and zygomatic regions, as well as at the occlusal level.[1] Considering the ubiquitous observation of paranasal deficiency in patients with cleft lip and palate and of hypoplasia of cleft margins in patients with other facial clefts, the actual frequency of midface deficiency in the presence of repaired facial clefts may approach 100%.

Ross estimated that midface deficiency and class III malocclusion necessitating skeletal surgery occur in approximately 25% of patients with repaired unilateral cleft lip and/or cleft palate.[2] In this study and many others, Class III malocclusion has been used as the major indicator of midface deficiency; thus the accuracy of the reported incidence of midface deficiency in facial clefts is questionable.[2-6] The percentage of patients expressing midface deficiency with isolated cleft palate, isolated cleft lip, bilateral cleft lip and palate, and incomplete clefts of the lip and/or palate is unknown, as is the incidence of midface deficiency in other facial clefting disorders. To establish a true incidence of midface deficiency in facial clefts, the criteria must include anthropometric, skeletal, and occlusal characteristics.[7,8]

Maxillary deficiency adversely affects functions beyond the problems of malocclusion, including nasal breathing, nasal drainage, speech, hearing, and olfaction.[9-13] It may also contribute to exorbitism and eyelid inadequacy. Cosmetically, maxillary deficiency and deformation are major contributors to the stigma of cleft lip and palate. Lack of normal cheek contour, nasolabial imbalance, lack of nasal tip, and lack of upper lip support contribute to this appearance. Even if the esthetic components of the cleft lip and/or nose are repaired and soft tissue landmarks matched perfectly, the deficiency and deformity of supporting skeletal tissues result in the "cleft appearance."

ETIOLOGY

The etiology of midface deficiency in facial clefts is unknown. The lack of class III malocclusion in unrepaired clefts suggests that the surgical procedures to correct cleft lip and palate, not the cleft itself, are causes of the condition.[14-16] However, these observations are based on occlusal and cephalometric findings, and the other diagnostic features of midface deficiency have not been considered. In almost all instances of maxillary deficiency secondary to facial clefting disorders, the maxilla is not merely repositioned but is also deformed. Although this observation offers nothing to resolve the etiology of midface deficiency in facial clefting disorders (deformation as well as retropositioning may be secondary to the effect of previous surgery), it has significant clinical implications. If optimal esthetic results are to be achieved, repositioning the maxilla alone is inadequate. Contouring the maxilla to improve form and to achieve symmetry and adequate projection is critical for achieving maximal improvement.

Historically, midface deficiency in the cleft population was ignored, and dental compensations by orthodontic treatment were employed to improve the occlusion. Only the most severely affected were offered surgical correction, and usually that was limited to posterior movement of the mandible.[17] Not only did this surgical approach fail to address the problem of midface deficiency, it often resulted in additional facial imbalance and occasionally in functional problems such as snoring and obstructive sleep apnea. As surgical techniques to advance the midface evolved, patients with clefts benefited substantially, both esthetically and functionally.[18-22]

MAXILLARY ADVANCEMENT

Complications

Maxillary advancement in the presence of repaired cleft palate is more difficult and complex than in the noncleft population. Problems such as infection, soft tissue and bone necrosis, loss of teeth, delayed healing, and relapse occur with greater frequency in patients with clefts who undergo this surgery.[23-30] Impairment of the vascularity and scarring from previous surgery are the major causes of these problems (Fig. 20–1). The intrinsic nature of the cleft, its effect on bone and soft tissue perfusion, and the influence of these variables on osteotomy healing require further study. The patient's

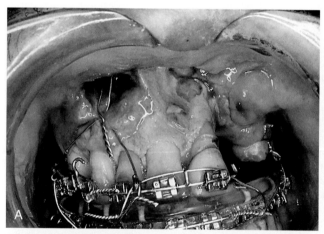
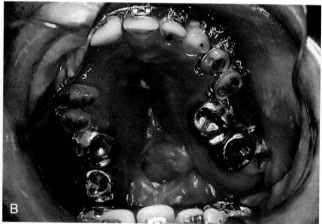
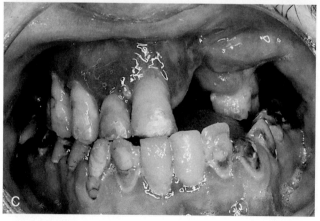

Figure 20–1. *A,* Three weeks before this picture was taken, a patient with unilateral cleft lip and palate underwent LeFort I advancement via the downfracture approach. The most likely explanation for the dehiscence and necrosis is the palatal scarring secondary to previous island flap palatal procedures. A more difficult but safer procedure would have been to leave an anterior pedicle during the surgery rather than using a circumvestibular incision and downfracturing the maxilla, as was done. *B,* Palatal view in the same patient before surgery, demonstrating dental arch constriction secondary to severe palatal scarring. *C,* The final outcome after treatment, which consisted of frequent irrigation and covering with petroleum jelly–coated gauze. One maxillary incisor and some alveolar bone were lost.

age at surgery and tobacco use are other variables to be considered. Complications that occur with midface advancement surgery in the cleft population occur more commonly in patients over 20 years of age. The impairment of the vascularity, compounded by the effects of chronic inflammation on the mucosa from oral-nasal reflux and/or smoking, contributes to the problem and may be the explanation for this observation in this population.

Stability

Stability of maxillary advancement in the noncleft population is typical, but in the presence of a repaired cleft palate, maxillary advancement may be unstable, regardless of the method of fixation (plates or wires).[20, 31–34] For many patients with clefts, several operations to repair the lip and palate precede maxillary advancement. In general, the more surgery undertaken before midface advancement, the greater the likelihood of complications associated with the surgery, including instability. The number of previous surgical procedures is not as important as the nature and extent of mucoperiosteal elevation and the resulting scar. Scarring related to cleft lip/palate repair has been linked to relapse, but palatal scarring and quality of palatal tissue are the most important considerations for predicting difficulty with surgery and relapse associated with midface advancement. Specific surgical procedures, such as pharyngo-plasty, increase the likelihood of instability in this population because of more extensive palatal scarring that results from the surgery. The tightness and quality of tissue of the upper lip are other important variables related to postsurgical relapse.

The age at which surgery to repair the lip and especially the palate is undertaken is related to the extent of the deformity. The younger the patient when the palate is repaired, the greater the risk of growth disturbance. However, if the hard palate closure is delayed past school age, incomplete bone bridging may occur across the cleft defect, and this may complicate later maxillary advancement surgery.

Velopharyngeal Considerations

Many patients with cleft palate have impaired velopharyngeal function. An effect of midface advancement is to displace the palate forward, farther from the posterior pharyngeal wall. When this occurs, the velopharyngeal mechanism may not be able to compensate as it does in the noncleft population.[35] When compensation is not possible, hypernasality results. After maxillary advancement in the presence of a repaired cleft palate, even when complete velopharyngeal adequacy is present, deterioration of the function of the velopharyngeal mechanism may occur.[35–39] Turvey, Frost, and Warren, using aerodynamic studies to calculate velopharyngeal orifice size, described three responses of the velopharyngeal apparatus in repaired cleft palate patients after maxillary advancement[36]: (1) no change in the velopharyngeal orifice size, (2) initial increase in the velopharyngeal orifice size with progressive decrease and improvement of function over 6 months after surgery, and (3) an increase in the velopharyngeal orifice size without adequate improvement over time after surgery (Fig. 20–2). In a sample of 25 patients with repaired cleft palate who underwent midface advancement, Watzke and associates noted deterioration of the velopharyngeal function in 25% of the patients who had complete adequacy of the velopharyngeal mechanism initially.[37] It is notable that in one patient with adequate function of the velopharyngeal mechanism who underwent minimal maxillary advancement (less than 4 mm), speech became hypernasal after surgery, to the extent that a pharyngeal flap was necessary to restore adequacy. There was no association between the amount of maxillary advancement and the development of velopharyngeal inadequacy in this study. Interestingly, in the patients who had posterior pharyngeal flaps and did not have complete velopharyngeal adequacy before midface advancement, velopharyngeal function improved after surgery. It is postulated that changing the dynamics of the velopharyngeal mechanism by stretching the palate and pharyngeal flap favorably altered the mechanics in these patients.

Dalston, Turvey, and Warren reported lack of predictability of velopharyngeal function after maxillary advancement in patients with repaired cleft palate, according to speech, rhinomanometric measurements, airflow data, and nasopharyngeal endoscopic

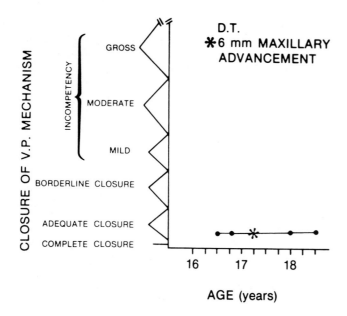

A

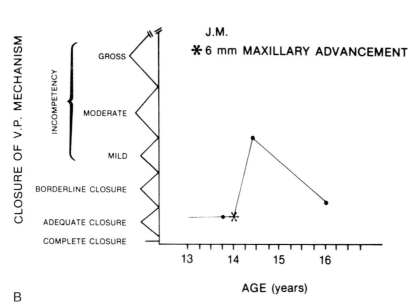

B

Figure 20–2. Three patterns of changes in the velopharyngeal sphincter after maxillary advancement. *A*, Adequacy before and after surgery. *B*, Adequacy before surgery, followed by deterioration after surgery. Gradual improvement of the sphincter with time was observed. *C*, Adequacy before surgery, followed by deterioration without improvement. A pharyngoplasty was performed, and there was return of adequacy.

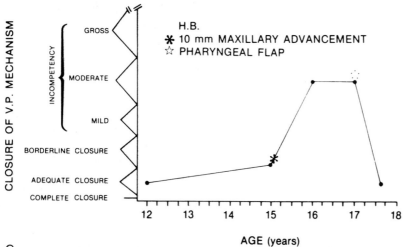

C

findings.[38] This highlights the variability of response of the velopharyngeal sphincter to maxillary advancement and the unpredictability of velopharyngeal compensation in the cleft population. These findings underscore the need to warn all patients with repaired cleft palate of the possibility that velopharyngeal inadequacy could develop after midface advancement (see Chapter 11).

Because speech changes in patients with repaired cleft palate after midface advancement are not predictable, pharyngeal flap surgery should not be undertaken prophylactically. Some authors have suggested placing or lengthening a pharyngeal flap simultaneously with maxillary advancement, but there is no evidence that this is beneficial or necessary for speech.[40] Combining these procedures places the airway at risk and introduces more scarring. Because the maxilla is prone to relapse in patients with clefts, additional scarring from pharyngoplasty and/or posterior pharyngeal flap is undesirable and may lead to greater instability. In addition, performing this surgery before midface advancement increases the difficulty of nasotracheal intubation and increases healing risks and the risk of instability.

If hypernasality occurs after midface advancement, a posterior pharyngeal flap should be delayed at least 6 months and preferably 1 year. The velopharyngeal mechanism is capable of adaptation, and at least 6 months should be allowed for this process to occur. In addition, healing of the maxilla and consolidation of bone grafts should occur before more scar tissue is introduced. In patients in whom velopharyngeal inadequacy develops and who cannot tolerate the hypernasality, a temporary speech appliance may be constructed (see Chapter 13). This makes postsurgical orthodontic treatment awkward; for some patients, however, it is beneficial and necessary to allow them to return to their normal daily routines (Fig. 20–3).

Timing of Bone Graft and Maxillary Advancement

Since the mid-1970s, bone grafting the maxillary and palatal cleft defects before the eruption of the permanent dentition has become standard.[41–45] This procedure, when delayed until approximately age 6 to 8 years, has not increased the incidence of maxillary deficiency, which did increase when the grafting was done as a primary procedure.[46,47] In adult and adolescent patients with clefts who have not undergone bone grafting, buccal and palatal oral-nasal fistulas are common. Nasal rim support and tip support are deficient or absent on the affected side. Teeth in the line of the cleft may be absent or ectopically positioned, and periodontal support for teeth adjacent to the cleft is deficient. Although some of these problems may be managed at the time of maxillary advancement, the advantages of bone grafting at an earlier age are

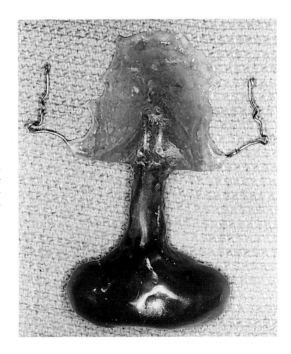

Figure 20–3. Example of a speech appliance used after maxillary advancement in a patient in whom speech became hypernasal. The appliance required frequent adjustments to permit orthodontic detailing of the occlusion.

considerable. The benefits of bone grafting during childhood strongly outweigh those of delaying the bone graft until the time of maxillary advancement, inasmuch as the major benefits cannot be completely appreciated if the graft is delayed (see Chapter 19, on bone grafting). Delaying the placement of the bone graft in an age-appropriate child with midface deficiency who will eventually require midface advancement later in life should be discouraged. Loss of permanent teeth and/or periodontal support is irreversible, and these teeth and support cannot be recaptured if bone grafts are placed later in life. Once permanent teeth erupt in the cleft area, without adequate supporting tissue, the crestal level of bone cannot be improved by bone grafting. There is greater success and predictability with bone grafting during the mixed-dentition stage than after complete eruption of the permanent teeth.[43] Finally, maxillary advancement is technically easier and associated with less morbidity in a patient with a cleft who has previously undergone bone grafting than in one who has not.[44]

Orthodontic Considerations

Oral hygiene instructions, periodontal treatment (if necessary), and prosthetic consultation should be initiated before presurgical orthodontic preparation. The decision to extract teeth is based on arch length requirements (spacing and crowding), incisor angulation, and periodontal health.

In general, dental compensations are removed from the respective arches by flaring the mandibular incisors and uprighting the maxillary incisors. It is safer and technically easier for the surgeon to avoid multiple (more than two) dento-osseous segments in the presence of a repaired cleft palate when maxillary advancement is performed. Consideration of the amount of palatal scarring and its effect on perfusion and healing is critical in deciding the feasibility of surgically segmenting the maxilla. An equally important consideration is the presence of dental compensations, because these may result in instability and poor periodontal health. Therefore, the surgeon and orthodontist must decide the safest and most stable movements on an individual basis.

Achieving transverse stability of the maxillary dental arch remains the greatest orthodontic and surgical challenge in patients with repaired cleft palate. Regardless of orthodontic, orthopedic, and/or surgical expansion, palatal scarring has such an overbearing effect that permanent transverse retention is often required after treatment. It is prudent to orthodontically expand the dental arch within reason but to avoid significant arch expansion, because this will not be maintainable over the long term.[48, 49] If significant transverse deficiency is present, the surgical option to widen the arch must be carefully assessed in consideration of the long-term benefit. In some instances, it may be prudent to accept posterior crossbite in patients with clefts rather than risk necrosis of bone and soft tissue.

If vertical steps are present in the maxillary arch, segmental leveling is accomplished before surgery. The maxillary segments can be leveled at surgery by interdental cuts at the planned site. Surgical vertical movement allows avoidance of extrusive and intrusive orthodontic mechanics and may provide better long-term stability. If the surgeon is to conduct an interdental osteotomy safely, the orthodontist must provide adequate interdental space. This requires divergence of the roots at the proposed site (Fig. 20–4). It is much more important for adequate space to be present between the root apices than at the crowns.

As with preparation for any orthognathic surgery, large rectangular arch wires with soldered lugs should be wired to the orthodontic bands and brackets before surgery in order to facilitate intermaxillary fixation. Because maxillary advancement in the cleft patient is usually accomplished with forces exceeding those needed in the noncleft population, it is helpful to band the maxillary cuspids as well as the molars. If transverse correction is necessary, bands placed on the teeth adjacent to the proposed interdental osteotomy site are also helpful. Bonded appliances do not withstand forces as well and are commonly lost during segmental cleft surgery. If the maxilla is to be moved in more than one piece, molar headgear tubes placed bilaterally facilitate placement of an auxiliary wire at the time of surgery. This wire is constructed from the mock surgical models, and its purpose is to unitize and retain the maxillary segments during surgery and the postoperative period. Additional positional support of the maxillary segment is afforded by the occlusal splint and intermaxillary fixation (Fig. 20–5).

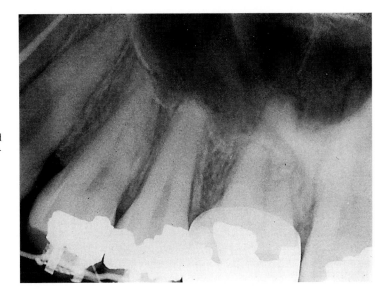

Figure 20–4. To facilitate interdental osteotomies and avoid damage, roots at the proposed sites (cuspid-premolar) should be parallel or divergent.

Intubation

Because maxillary advancement requires the intraoperative establishment of occlusion and the application of intermaxillary fixation, nasal endotracheal intubation is necessary. For most patients with repaired cleft lip and palate, this is possible and can be accomplished with care.[50–52] A vasoconstrictor should be applied to the nasal mucosa. Nasal septal deviation and turbinate enlargement are common in this population, and preintubation inspection of the nose identifies the more patent nostril. Nasal mucosal scars and scarring from previous vomer flaps can also interfere with tube insertion. The more patent nostril should be selected for endotracheal tube insertion, and sometimes this is the nostril on the cleft side. When possible, endotracheal tube insertion through the nonaffected side is preferable, in order to facilitate surgical reconstruction of the floor of the nose. On occasion, forceful dilation of the nasal passage with a small finger is necessary before tube insertion.

When a pharyngeal flap is present, a fiberoptic endoscope can be used to guide the endotracheal tube through the nasopharyngeal ports. An alternative is to pass a small suction catheter through the nose and posterior velopharyngeal ports into the nasopharynx. The endotracheal tube can then be guided by passing it over the smaller catheter (Fig. 20–6). Tracheostomy is not necessary and should be avoided even if the

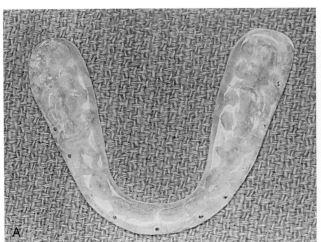

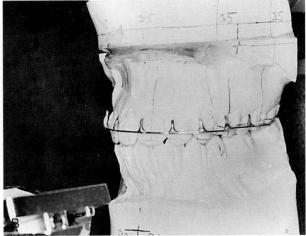

Figure 20–5. *A*, An acrylic occlusal splint is constructed from mock surgery models to index the planned occlusion. *B*, The .036 auxiliary orthodontic wire is inserted into molar headgear tubes and further secured to several brackets in the arch. This wire unitizes the maxillary arch when segmental surgery is performed and retains the segments during the postsurgical phase.

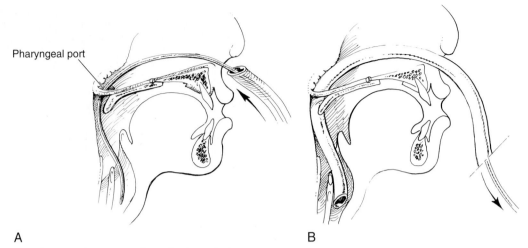

Pharyngeal port

A   B

Figure 20–6. *A* and *B*, A catheter, passed nasally through the velopharyngeal ports, serves to guide the nasoendotracheal tube past the pharyngeal flap.

pharyngeal flap must be removed. Rarely is it necessary to remove the flap in order to insert a nasoendotracheal tube, and in this unlikely circumstance, replacement of the pharyngeal flap is optional and dependent on speech needs *after* surgery.

Intraoperative and Postoperative Management

The intraoral route is always used for this type of surgery. In spite of the usual routine preparation with a sterilizing soap, tooth brushing, and chlorhexidine rinses, the surgical environment remains contaminated. Penicillin G is the most efficacious antibiotic against organisms in the oral cavity and is routinely administered except in patients allergic to penicillin, in which case erythromycin or a cephalosporin is administered. When bone is harvested from a distant site such as the cranium and/or ilium, the use of a cephalosporin is preferred because of its superior protection against *Staphylococcus.*

Steroids are administered to minimize swelling. The medications (both steroids and antibiotics) are administered shortly after intubation and before the surgery begins. The steroids are discontinued after 24 hours. When bone grafts are placed, antibiotics are continued for 10 days. When these medications are appropriately used, infection and swelling can be minimized.

TECHNIQUE FOR MAXILLARY ADVANCEMENT IN PATIENTS WITH UNILATERAL CLEFT PALATE WHO HAVE NOT UNDERGONE BONE GRAFTING

This technique was presented at the meeting of the American Cleft Palate Association in Denver in 1982. The principles of the surgery have not changed since then; however, the technique now includes bone plates and screws to stabilize the segments and bone grafts.[53]

Designing the Osteotomy

The exact design of the midface advancement osteotomy is limited only by the surgeon's imagination and should be determined by the patient's esthetic needs. Some surgeons have successfully employed LeFort II and III osteotomies for patients with cleft palate and midface deficiency.[54] The techniques described in this chapter are confined to lower level osteotomies only. For higher level osteotomies, consult Chapters 21 and 26.

Incision

The initial step in maxillary advancement is exposing the surgical field. For most patients with unilateral cleft lip and cleft palate, a circumvestibular incision is placed high in the mucobuccal fold, especially at the zygomatic buttress region to ensure an adequate vascular pedicle (Fig. 20–7). The incision is made through the mucosa to the periosteum and proceeds anteriorly through the oral-nasal fistula. The entire lateral maxillary wall to the level of the infraorbital rim is exposed. The nerve exiting the infraorbital foramen is identified, dissected, and protected. If the zygomatic prominence is to be advanced or augmented, the dissection includes this region as well. Dissection over the zygomatic prominence requires elevation of the periosteum, which is tightly bound and in contact with the fat pad. From the zygomatic buttress, the dissection is tunneled posteriorly to the pterygoid region.

The nasal mucosa is elevated from the lateral nasal walls, floor of the nose, and nasal crest of the maxilla. On the repaired cleft side, this elevation is difficult because the scar requires sharp dissection, which can be accomplished more easily at the time of downfracture. The bone asymmetry at the pyriform region can be appreciated, as can the deviation of the anterior nasal spine away from the cleft side. The configuration of the lateral maxillary wall in normal persons is usually convex. In the cleft population, the configuration is concave suggesting that the maxilla is deficient and dysmorphic (Fig. 20–8).

The attached gingival tissues surrounding the teeth at the cleft margins are always preserved. These tissues are incised and sutured back on themselves, especially when the segments are to be repositioned so that the cleft becomes smaller.

Procedure

When the maxilla is advanced in the presence of a repaired cleft palate, the lateral maxillary osteotomies are designed according to the patient's needs. If the infraorbital and/or zygomatic regions are deficient, the osteotomy may extend to include these regions (Fig. 20–9).

Figure 20–7. A circumvestibular incision is used when LeFort I downfracture is performed. The incision is made high on the zygomatic maxillary buttress to ensure adequate perfusion to the anterior maxilla. Note that the attached gingiva around the teeth on both sides of the cleft is reflected and preserved. The remaining tissue lining the cleft walls will be incised and reflected palatally or buccally, depending on where it is needed for closure (see Fig. 20–22B).

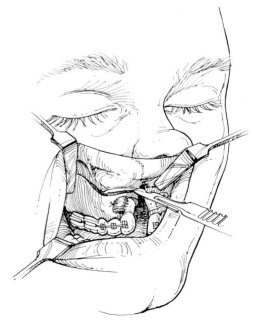

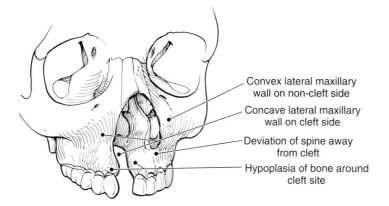

Convex lateral maxillary wall on non-cleft side

Concave lateral maxillary wall on cleft side

Deviation of spine away from cleft

Hypoplasia of bone around cleft site

Figure 20–8. The typical skeletal anatomy observed in a unilateral cleft lip and palate condition. Notice the asymmetry and hypoplasia of the pyriform region, the deviation of the nasal spine, and the concave lateral wall of the maxilla.

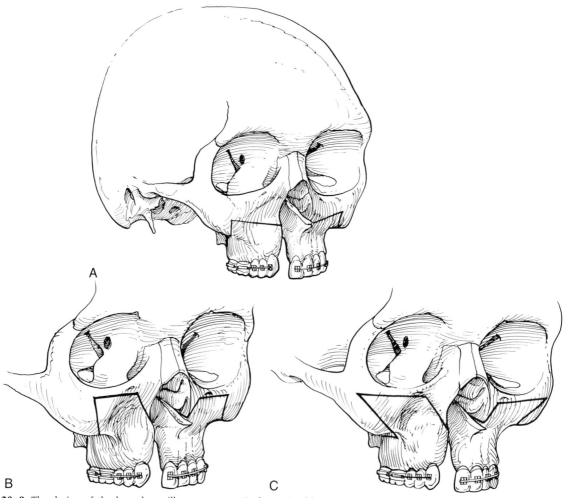

Figure 20–9. The design of the lateral maxillary osteotomy is determined by the patient's esthetic needs. *A,* The classical low-level cut. *B,* A higher level cut approaching the infraorbital rims. *C,* A modification used when enhancement of the cheek prominence is desired. When options *B* and *C* are utilized, there is risk of fracturing these buttresses because the bone is thin. Repair is possible with microplates.

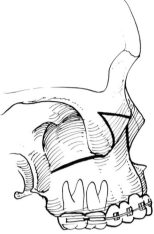

Figure 20–10. Regardless of which lateral wall osteotomy is performed, a vertical step at the zygomatic maxillary buttress is always employed because this is a key bone graft site. The osteotomy along the posterior lateral maxillary wall tapers inferiorly toward the pterygoid plate to minimize the risk of damaging the internal maxillary vessels. The osteotomy should be at least 5 mm above the root apices in order to minimize the risk of devitalizing teeth.

Usually the lateral maxillary osteotomy includes a vertical step at the zygomatic buttress and a high-level lateral wall cut just under the infraorbital nerve. If the zygomatic prominence is to be advanced, the osteotomy can be directed farther superiorly and posteriorly to accomplish this. At the pyriform region, the osteotomy is below the inferior turbinate, and so the cut tapers inferiorly in the anterior region to minimize the risk to the nasolacrimal canal.

The osteotomy posterior to the zygomaticomaxillary buttress is directed inferiorly to reduce the risks of bleeding at the pterygomaxillary juncture (Fig. 20–10). Once this is done bilaterally, the nasal septum is released with an osteotome. The lateral nasal walls are then cut with a thin osteotome, which is directed inferiorly and posteriorly. The osteotome is tapped through the thin lateral nasal wall until the perpendicular portion of the palatine bone is reached. At this point, resistance is much greater, and the osteotome is tapped partially through this area of resistance. The greater palatine artery and vein course through the posterior medial maxillary wall, and hemorrhage can occur at this step (Fig. 20–11). Should this occur, the operation proceeds quickly to the downfracture stage.

The final step is separating the pterygoid plate from the maxilla, and this is normally done under direct vision with a curved osteotome (Fig. 20–12). Once the maxilla is downfractured, direct visualization and management of the bleeding is possible. As with all maxillary surgery, the blood pressure must be controlled (systolic pressure, 90 mm Hg), the head should be elevated and vasoconstrictors should be injected into the area before surgery.

Figure 20–11. A small osteotome is tapped through the lateral nasal wall posteriorly toward the perpendicular part of the palatal bone. At this point, the resistance increases because this part of the lateral nasal wall thickens. The greater palatine neurovascular bundle descends through this region and is at risk.

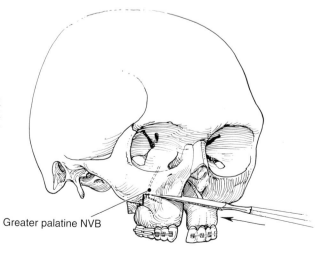

Greater palatine NVB

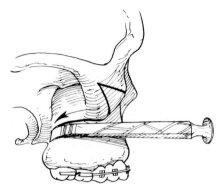

Figure 20–12. A curved osteotome is used to separate the pterygoid plate from the maxilla. The tip of the osteotome should be palpable from the palatal side.

Mobilization

The next step in the surgery is to mobilize the maxilla. The cleft maxilla requires greater force and offers more resistance to downfracturing than the noncleft maxilla. The difficulty encountered is attributable to the scarring along the nasal floor and pterygoid region. Thickened palatine bone may also be encountered and may necessitate additional cutting with an osteotome from the lateral nasal approach and from the posterior junction of the maxilla and pterygoid plate.

When the maxilla is downfractured, severing and elevation of the scar along the nasal floor under direct visualization is possible (Fig. 20–13). This, combined with forward traction from mobilizers, facilitates displacement and advancement of the maxilla (Fig. 20–14A,B). This is a critical aspect of the surgery, and adequate time must be spent stretching the scarred tissues to permit passive placement of the maxillary segments in the planned position. Downfracturing the cleft maxilla allows the scarred nasal mucosa to be elevated, but this maneuver eliminates a potential source of perfusion. In most patients with unilateral cleft lip and cleft palate, it does not result in adverse effects on healing. For patients who have previously undergone an island palatal flap repair or who have palatal scarring beyond the ordinary, avoidance of downfracturing and maintenance of an anterior buccal pedicle may be prudent when the maxilla is advanced. In this circumstance, blood perfusion through the scarred palatal tissues is reduced and may not be adequate for revascularization and healing of the maxilla (Fig. 20–15).

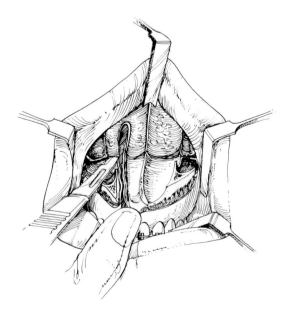

Figure 20–13. Scarring along the entire palate is tethering and must be cut sharply.

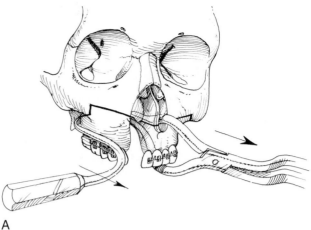

A

Figure 20–14. *A,* Disimpaction forceps are used to pull the maxilla forward, severing the posterior attachments of the maxilla. *B,* Mobilizers are inserted along the posterior maxillary walls and are used to displace the maxilla forward. They must be kept low and placed posteriorly in the pterygomaxillary region to avoid damage to the lateral maxillary walls.

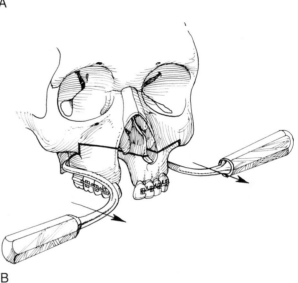

B

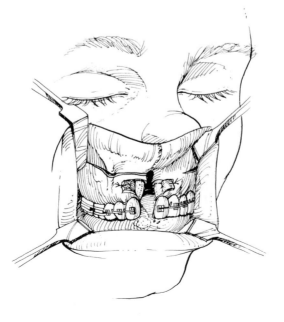

Figure 20–15. An alternative to the circumvestibular incision used in maxillary advancement is to leave an anterior pedicle. If this approach is used, the maxilla cannot be downfractured. This makes maxillary advancement more difficult, but an additional source of perfusion to the maxilla is preserved. This design should be used when there is excessive palatal scarring, as occurs when island palatal flaps have been used in previous palate repair.

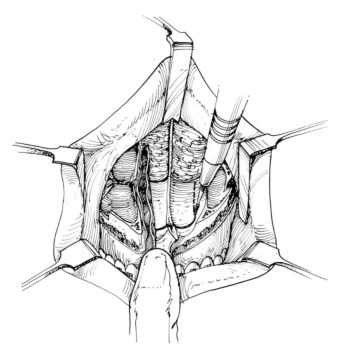

Figure 20–16. When the maxilla is segmented, a palatal island of bone is formed. This facilitates expansion by dispersing resulting tension from the stretch of the soft tissue across the entire palate and by reducing the size of the bone defects.

Segmenting the Maxilla

After cleft palate repair, bone bridging across the palate is variable. Sometimes the maxilla mobilizes in one piece, and sometimes it moves in two segments. If the planned movement requires segmenting the maxilla, the palatal floor is cut to free it from the alveolar portion of the maxilla bilaterally. The bone cleft is reopened on the affected side and another osteotomy parallel to the cleft is placed along the lateral aspect of the nasal floor on the nonaffected side. These are joined by a third osteotomy across the nasal floor just posterior to the nasopalatine canal (Fig. 20–16). Interdental cuts are then placed at the planned sites and are connected to the nasal floor cuts. The interdental osteotomies are initially scored on the buccal surface of the alveolus at the desired interdental region with a small fissure bur. A thin osteotome is then used to complete the cuts to the palate (Fig. 20–17). If the maxilla is expanded, the soft tissues of the palate are partially released from the nasal floor segment to facilitate the movement. This maneuver is done bilaterally to evenly

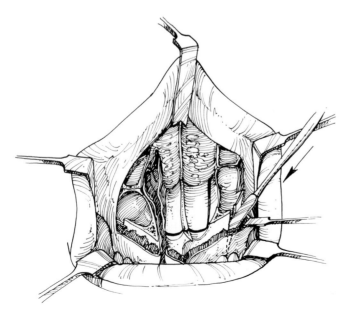

Figure 20–17. A small fissure bur is used to score the bone at the interdental site. A straight, thin osteotome is then used to complete the separation through the alveolus.

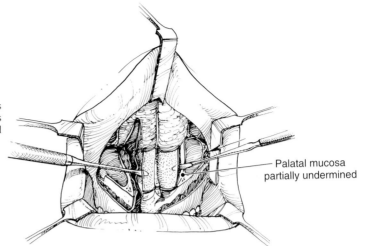

Figure 20–18. The palatal mucosa on the bone island is partially elevated through the osteotomy site. This relaxes the soft tissues to facilitate expansion. The bone island maintains soft tissue attachment in the midline.

Palatal mucosa partially undermined

distribute the soft tissue tension resulting from the expansion (Fig. 20–18). Sometimes additional parallel osteotomy cuts are placed along the nasal floor to facilitate expansion[55] (Fig. 20–19). Tissue is never released from the dento-osseous segments, because such release would eliminate a source of perfusion. Small nasal floor bone defects are then grafted and are more likely to heal than one large defect would if the osteotomy were placed in the midline or just unilaterally. The midline of the palate is always avoided during a segmental osteotomy because the bone is thickest and the soft tissue is always thin and likely to tear or perforate.[49]

Once the osseous surgery is completed, but before the maxilla is repositioned, the soft tissues of the floor of the nose are repaired with resorbable sutures. It is usually possible to reapproximate the nasal lining by relaxing the mucosa from the lateral nasal wall and the nasal septum (Fig. 20–20). If large tissue defects are present, they are left to granulate, but every attempt should be made to cover the osteotomy defects when bone has been grafted.

If the cleft maxillary and palatal defect has not previously been bone grafted, it is always repaired with a bone graft at the time of maxillary advancement. This requires both nasal and oral tissue covering. As with the preparation of any bone graft recipient

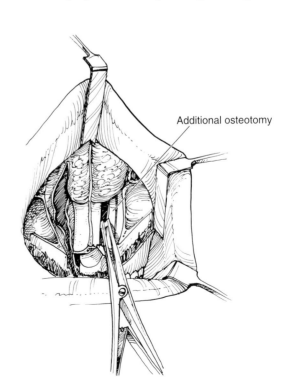

Additional osteotomy

Figure 20–19. When extensive expansion is necessary, several parallel palatal osteotomies may be used, and the palatal spreader facilitates separation.

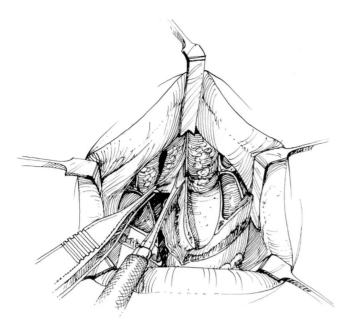

Figure 20–20. The nasal mucosa is relaxed from the lateral nasal wall and from the nasal septum to allow primary closure of the nasal floor, if possible.

site, the osseous margins of the cleft must be stripped of the soft tissue lining. Because the nasal floor is repaired primarily, as described earlier, the oral coverage comes from the tissues lining the cleft. With the maxilla mobilized, visualization and access into the cleft area is facilitated. The tissue lining the cleft defect is dissected in the subperiosteal plane and reflected toward the palate and the buccal side of the cleft (Fig. 20–21). If bone grafting the cleft is a goal of surgery as well as advancement, it is critical to expose the entire cleft site in the superiosteal plane. If the intended movement of the maxilla includes closing the cleft space, closure of the oral mucosa should precede placing the segments into the splint. The soft tissues can be thick and may prevent the segments from being adequately positioned. When this occurs, the tissues should be trimmed as needed. The tissues are then sutured on both the palatal (when necessary) and buccal sides (Fig. 20–22*A,B*).

Once the maxilla is adequately mobilized, it is placed in the planned occlusal position, and intermaxillary fixation is applied. If two-jaw surgery is performed, an interim splint is used to relate the maxilla to the intact mandible. The maxilla, wired into the splint and wired to the mandible, is then rotated superiorly to make contact with the stable bone superiorly. Vertical landmarks should be checked to ensure that the maxilla has been adequately advanced and not just rotated inferiorly. Inferior maxillary movements, especially when the mandible is not simultaneously mobilized,

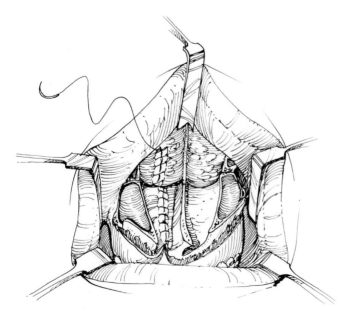

Figure 20–21. The mucosa lining the cleft alveolar region is elevated from the nasal side and pushed orally, where it is sutured on both the palatal and buccal sides. The bone edges of the cleft must be adequately exposed for successful reconstruction. The nasal mucosa is also closed primarily.

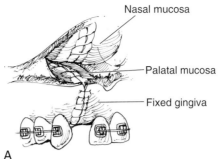

Nasal mucosa

Palatal mucosa

Fixed gingiva

A

Figure 20–22. *A,* Buccal view, demonstrating the tissues lining the cleft elevated, pushed orally and sutured on the oral side. *B,* Deeper view into the cleft, demonstrating the closure of oral and nasal tissues and the pocket for the bone graft.

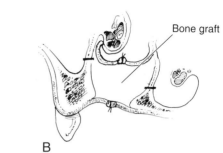

Bone graft

B

are highly unstable and should be avoided because they can lead to relapse.[56,57] The maxilla is then secured to stable bone along the osteotomy by either wire or plate osteosynthesis. Plate stabilization is always used in patients with clefts even if wires are initially applied, because the added rigidity may improve stability in this population. Additional wire and/or screws may be used to help maintain the position of bone grafts.

The bone defects along the anterior and posterior lateral walls, at the zygomaticomaxillary buttress, and at the base of the nose are examined. The maxilla is then stabilized with bone plates (Fig. 20–23). Bone grafts are wedged into the defects to facilitate bone healing and to buttress the position of the maxilla. Sometimes it is necessary to stack several pieces of bone because of the size of the defect. The bone grafts can be secured with either wire or screws to prevent dislocation into the sinus (Fig. 20–24*A,B*). The pterygomaxillary juncture is usually not grafted because often the pterygoid plates fracture and provide no support for the bone grafts. In addition, bone grafts placed at this region cannot be secured and depend, at best, on wedging to maintain their position.

Figure 20–23. The advanced maxilla is occluded into the splint and platted into position.

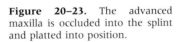

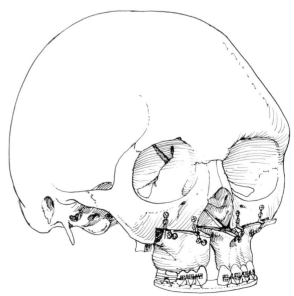

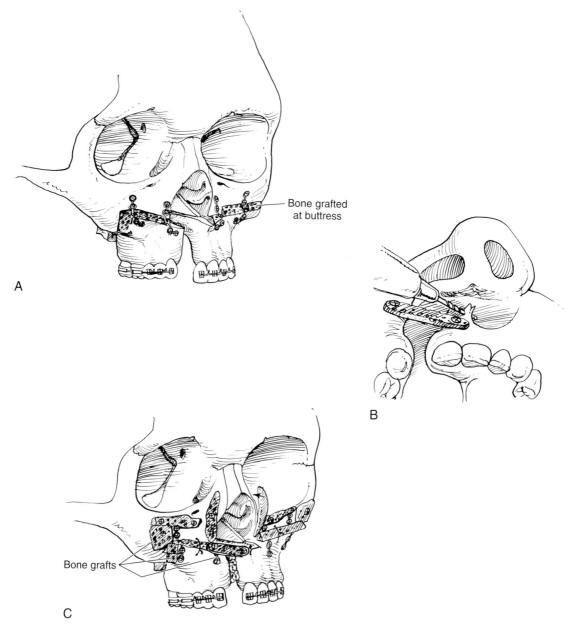

Bone grafted
at buttress

A

B

Bone grafts

C

Figure 20–24. *A,* and *B,* Split-thickness cranial bone grafts are wedged into the osteotomy defects and are used to contour areas of skeletal deficiency. They are also used to construct a pyriform aperture. *C,* Onlay bone grafts are positioned and secured with screws. Wires are occasionally necessary to prevent displacement of the inlayed bone grafts into the sinus.

With the segments held in the occlusal splint, the cleft defect is packed with cancellous bone, harvested from either the cranium or the ilium. It is important to condense this grafted bone and to be certain that it extends to at least the crestal level of bone on either side of the cleft. Overpacking the bone graft is advised, to ensure adequacy of osteogenic cells and because it is predictable that the grafted bone will resorb to the pre-existing level of the alveolar bone on either side of the cleft.[42] The thickness of the reconstructed ridge will thin with time and, especially when osseointegrated implants are anticipated at a later date, the thickness of the entire alveolus must be reconstructed.

Many patients with repaired clefts benefit from additional onlay bone grafts to highlight the prominence of the zygoma, the inferior orbital rims, or the lateral nasal regions. If the cleft involves the pyriform area, an onlay bone graft is placed over the cancellous graft to provide additional support for the base of the nose, for the columella, and for the upper lip. All onlay or contour grafts are secured with small bone screws to prevent displacement and to facilitate revascularization. When the inferior orbital rim is grafted, the graft must be contoured to prevent impingement of the infraorbital nerve.

For interpositional bone grafting, it appears to make little difference which autogenous bone donor source (ilium or cranium) is utilized. For onlay or contour grafts, cranial bone provides greater long-term survival. The reason for this is its cortical density and the rich haversian system, which enhances early revascularization of cranial bone.[58]

TECHNIQUE FOR MAXILLARY ADVANCEMENT IN PATIENTS WITH UNILATERAL CLEFT PALATE WHO HAVE PREVIOUSLY UNDERGONE BONE GRAFTING

In the patient who has previously undergone bone grafting the osteotomy technique is identical to that for the patient who has not undergone bone grafting, but the surgery is much simpler, is less time consuming, and is associated with less morbidity. The oral-nasal fistula has previously been closed and the cleft has been grafted, and so the procedure is more similar to the conventional LeFort I downfracture. If the orthodontist has been able to achieve arch compatibility and has been able to move teeth into the grafted bone, the maxilla is repositioned in one piece. If multiple maxillary segments are indicated, the previous bone graft site may be used for an interdental osteotomy, and healing occurs normally, providing that the palatal soft tissues are protected.

The maxilla is repositioned and secured as described earlier. The area of the previously placed bone graft is almost always hypoplastic at the pyriform region. An onlay graft may be placed to aid in improving the symmetry of the nasal base. Sometimes the maxilla fractures at the bone graft site during the mobilization process. This is usually not problematic because a splint and the orthodontic arch wire lend support to control the position of the segments, and healing occurs uneventfully. Contour grafts are placed appropriately, and the soft tissues are closed as described later.

Lip Closure

Hardly any circumstances justify opening the cutaneous lip simultaneously with maxillary advancement. Swelling that occurs with maxillary advancement distorts the soft tissue landmarks and makes accurate approximation of lip tissues difficult. In addition, the support for the upper lip changes as bone and bone grafts remodel after maxillary advancement. This ongoing process stabilizes at about 9 months to 1 year after surgery, and lip revision can better be accomplished at that time.

Layered closure of the circumvestibular incision should be done as usual. The musculoperiosteal layer is first secured with absorbable sutures, and the lip is brought forward as the sutures are tied. Care should be taken to reconstruct the transverse nasalis muscle.[59] Sometimes a hole drilled through the anterior nasal spine facilitates the placement and securing of sutures to achieve this goal (Fig. 20–25A).

The mucosa is usually closed in a V-Y manner, being advanced to the anterior portion of the lip (Fig. 20–25B). This method maintains the vermilion fullness and improves the prominence of the philtral columns. Closure can also be done asymmetrically, depending on the specific needs.

TECHNIQUE FOR MAXILLARY ADVANCEMENT IN THE PATIENT WITH BILATERAL CLEFT LIP AND CLEFT PALATE

Advancing the maxilla in the presence of a bilateral cleft palate is more than twice as difficult as in the presence of unilateral cleft palate. Understanding the perfusion differences between unilateral and bilateral cleft malformations and the perfusion alterations occurring after osteotomies is critical to understanding the necessity for the altered soft tissue flap designed.[60–63]

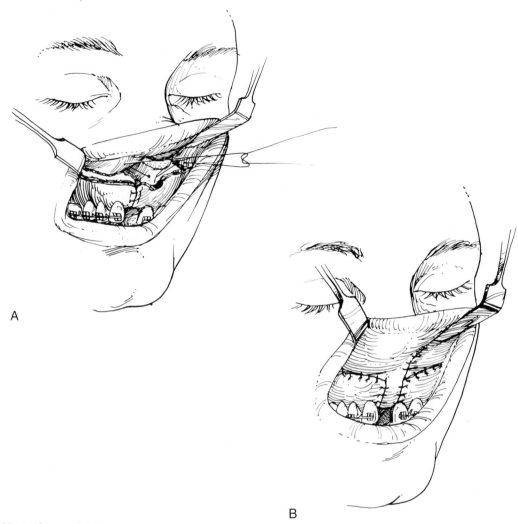

Figure 20–25. *A,* Closure of the lip is accomplished in two layers: a musculoperiosteal layer and the mucosa. The transverse portion of the nasalis muscle is secured medially by suturing it through a hole drilled at the nasal spine. *B,* The mucosa is then closed in a Y pattern, with tissue advanced toward the midline.

In the cleft and noncleft situations, once the maxillary osteotomy is performed and the segments are mobilized, endosteal blood supplies are interrupted. Perfusion of the segments then becomes totally dependent on the mucoperiosteal source. In the unilateral cleft maxilla and palate, the blood supply from the posterior and lateral pharyngeal regions, as well as the contributions from the greater palatine vessels, perfuses the downfractured maxilla. In the bilaterally cleft maxilla and palate, the lateral segments are dependent on vascularity from the posterior and lateral pharynx and the greater palatine artery. The premaxilla of the bilateral cleft is dependent on perfusion from the nasal septum, the vomer, and the mucosa covering these surfaces. When an osteotomy is performed in the presence of a bilateral cleft, the premaxilla must be treated separately, and its blood supply must be protected during maxillary advancement. This can be done only by preserving buccal mucosal pedicles on the premaxilla. In the bilateral cleft, if the mucosa overlying the maxillary segments has been united with previous surgeries and the fistulas are closed but no bone graft has been placed, it is too risky to attempt maxillary advancement by downfracturing the maxilla. Soft tissues heal by scarring, and scarring is an area of reduced perfusion. Relying on scars to maintain adequate blood flow to the premaxilla is ill-advised. If the bilateral cleft has been previously bone grafted, the premaxilla has an endosteal blood source from the lateral segments. Bone does not heal by scarring and so perfusion into the premaxilla should be adequate if the bone grafts have healed well. Downfracturing the bilateral cleft maxilla, once it has been bone grafted, is a consideration, but it still remains

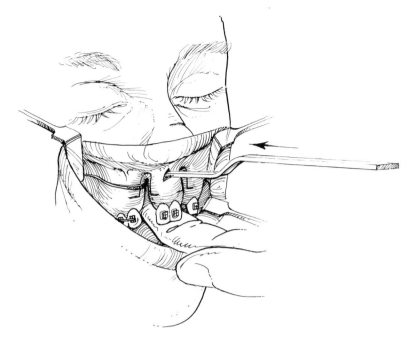

Figure 20–26. Incisions outlined for maxillary advancement and simultaneous bone grafting in the bilateral cleft lip and palate. The anterior pedicles provide perfusion for the premaxilla.

hazardous. The authors believe that an anterior pedicle should always remain, to ensure the survival of the premaxilla.

Incisions

Horizontal incisions high in the mucobuccal fold are used to approach both lateral maxillary walls. The incisions begin at the zygomaticomaxillary buttress and terminate at the anterior extent of the lateral segment (usually at the cuspid region). In most patients, oral-nasal fistulas are present bilaterally in the mucobuccal fold, and the incision should circumscribe the fistulas. The fixed gingival tissues should be preserved as the cleft margins are exposed and prepared for bone grafting.

The flap is elevated superiorly to expose the entire lateral maxillary wall from the pyriform rim to the zygomaticomaxillary buttress. Posteriorly, the dissection is tunneled to the pterygoid region. A vertical incision is placed high in the midline of the mucobuccal fold of the upper lip to access the separation of the premaxilla from the nasal septum (Fig. 20–26). This separation may also be accomplished from the palatal side or transnasally, and therefore the midline incision is not always necessary (Fig. 20–27).

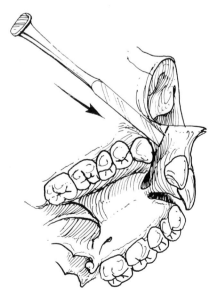

Figure 20–27. The premaxilla can also be separated from the septum and vomer through the cleft site once the mucosa has been reflected.

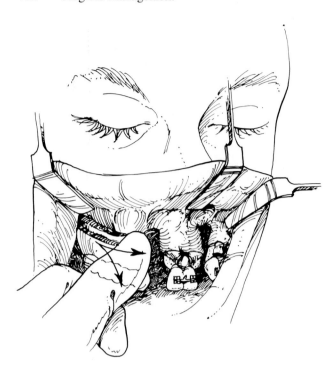

Figure 20–28. The lateral maxillary segments are mobilized by medial and inferior forces.

Osteotomy

Vertical landmarks are scribed on the maxilla anteriorly at the pyriform region and at the zygomaticomaxillary buttress region. The lateral maxillary wall is then cut. The design of the osteotomy is dependent on the patient's esthetic needs. The nasal septum may be released along its entire length through the vertical incision placed at the midline of the premaxilla. The lateral nasal walls are separated with a thin osteotome introduced from the pyriform region.

Mobilization

Mobilization is begun by infracturing the lateral segments with digital pressure. This is commonly met with resistance, and the palatine bone may require greater separation with an osteotome. In addition, the scar along the nasal floor secondary to previous palatal repair must be separated. This is facilitated by a combination of infracturing toward the midline and downfracturing (Fig. 20–28). Alternating between downfracturing and advancing forces applied from the pterygomaxillary region is commonly necessary to achieve the desired mobilization (Fig. 20–29). The premaxillary segment usually mobilizes without difficulty but remains pedicled anteriorly to the labial mucosa. On occasion, an osteotome must inserted through the cleft region to separate the vomerine attachment to the premaxilla. This is done after the mucosa is incised and elevated.

Closing the Bilateral Clefts

Once all three segments are mobilized, reconstruction of the nasal floor is begun with the segments distracted. The tissues from the lateral nasal wall and vomer are elevated and sutured to seal the nasal cavity. Then the tissues lining the clefts are carefully elevated and mobilized inferiorly toward the oral cavity. The edges are sutured on the oral surface both palatally and buccally (Fig. 20–30). Care must be taken to preserve the buccally pedicled flaps perfusing the premaxilla while the bone graft recipient sites are prepared bilaterally. The segments are then placed in the splint, and a previously constructed orthodontic wire is inserted into buccal headgear tubes placed on the first molar bands. The premaxillary teeth are also wire-ligated to this auxiliary wire to provide additional support to the premaxilla (Fig. 20–31).

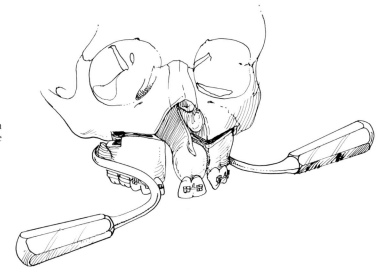

Figure 20–29. Anterior displacement of the maxilla can be accomplished with mobilizers placed between the maxilla and pterygoid plates.

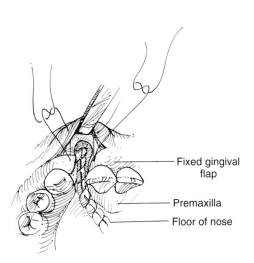

Fixed gingival flap

Premaxilla

Floor of nose

Figure 20–30. The nasal floor is constructed with tissue lining the cleft, which are mobilized superiorly and sutured.

Figure 20–31. The occlusal splint is used for the three maxillary segments. An auxiliary orthodontic wire is inserted into the molar headgear tubes and further secured to several teeth in each segment.

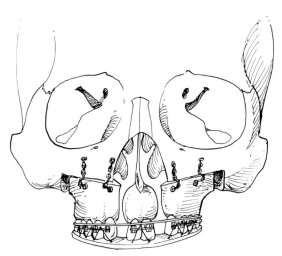

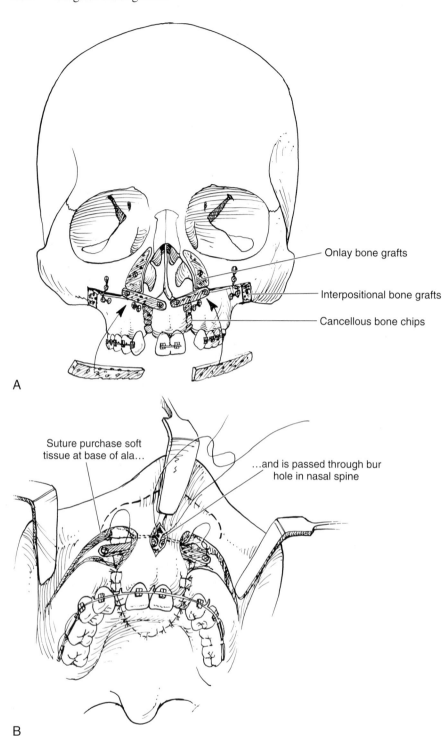

Onlay bone grafts

Interpositional bone grafts

Cancellous bone chips

A

Suture purchase soft
tissue at base of ala...

...and is passed through bur
hole in nasal spine

B

Figure 20–32. *A* and *B*, The premaxilla is secured by bone grafts, which are used to construct the inferior pyriform rim. These grafts are tunneled under the buccal flaps and screwed to the nasal spine anteriorly and to the lateral maxilla posteriorly.

Bone Grafts

Intermaxillary fixation is applied, and the complex is rotated closed. The maxilla is then secured with four plates on the lateral maxillary segments. The lateral and posterior maxillary wall defects are bone grafted, as has been described previously for the unilateral cleft (see Fig. 22–24C). The clefts are packed densely with cancellous bone bilaterally. Next, the alar rim is reconstructed by securing cortical bone grafts from the lateral maxillary segments to the anterior nasal spine region on the premaxilla bilaterally. Meticulous dissection of a subperiosteal pocket high on the premaxilla is necessary to cover the grafts (Fig. 20–32A). These bone grafts are held in place with bone screws and provide additional stability to the premaxilla. They are critical for

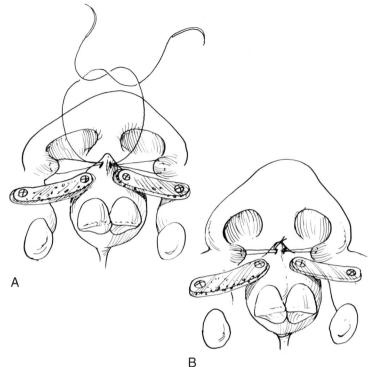

Figure 20–33. *A* and *B,* To assist in securing the nasalis muscle, a hole is drilled through the nasal spine and the suture is passed through the hole and tied.

improving the projection and support of the columella, lip, nasal base, and nasal tip (Fig. 20–32*B*). Contour bone grafts are then placed and secured in areas requiring greater projection.

Closure

The midline incision over the premaxilla is closed in one layer with resorbable sutures. The lateral incisions are closed in two layers (a musculoperiosteal layer and a separate mucosal layer). If alar width is to be narrowed, a suture passed from the alar base can be tunneled under the flap and tied through a hole drilled through the bone graft to the premaxilla (Figs. 20–33, 20–34). Sometimes buccal mucosal flaps are

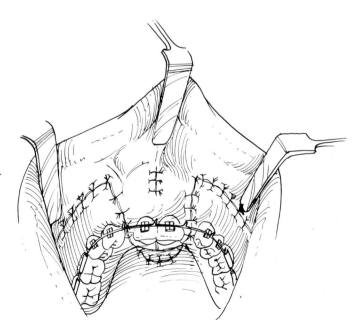

Figure 20–34. All mucosal flaps are closed primarily.

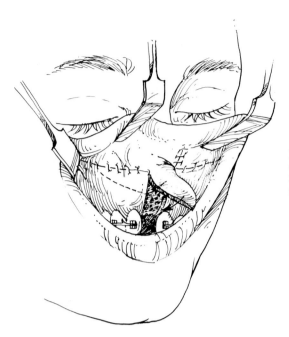

Figure 20–35. When additional mucosa is required for covering the grafted maxilla, anteriorly based mucosal flaps are rotated and sutured into place.

necessary to close the palatal region. If necessary, they are rotated 90° and attached to the palate (Figs. 20–35, 20–36).

Because of the length of the flaps, the tips occasionally necrose and bone grafts sequestrate. Repairing the residual midpalatal oral-nasal fistula may necessitate additional surgery.

Sequencing and Timing of Surgery

One of the major dilemmas facing clinicians who treat patients with cleft palate and maxillary deficiency is deciding the optimal timing of surgery. Residual facial growth

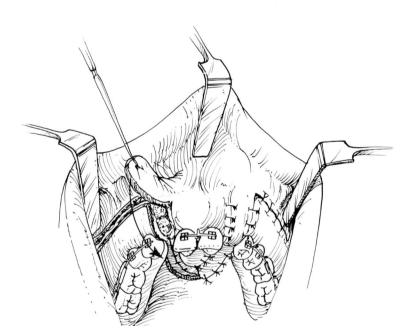

Figure 20–36. Bilateral anteriorly based mucosal flaps are rotated to cover defects.

is the major concern. Mandibular growth lags behind that of the maxilla, and substantial postpubertal mandibular growth may cause relapse. From a biologic viewpoint, it is better to delay surgery until complete maturation; however, such delay sometimes overlooks the patient's psychosocial interests, and herein lies the dilemma. Peer pressure and concerns of physical attractiveness peak at adolescence. If surgery can improve appearance and reduce psychosocial trauma, it is justified, even if the consequence is additional surgery (if relapse occurs) later in life (see Chapter 17).[64-66]

CASE HISTORIES

Case 1

A 31-year-old man with a repaired unilateral cleft lip and cleft palate (Fig. 20–37) presented for comprehensive treatment focusing on improving appearance and occlusion. He had previously undergone lip and palatal closure and, as a teenager, lip revision and comprehensive orthodontic treatment. In addition, he had received extensive speech therapy, but surgery to reposition the jaws was never undertaken.

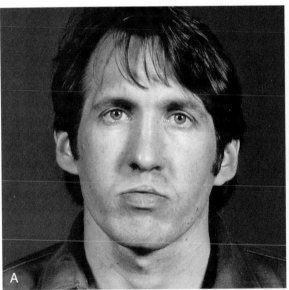
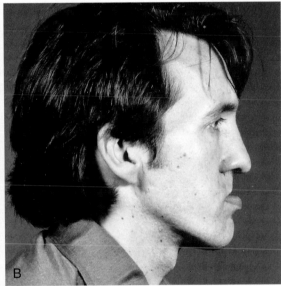
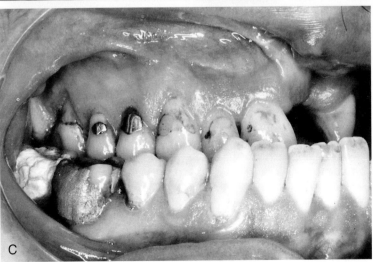

Figure 20–37. Preoperative facial (*A*, *B*) and occlusion (*C*) views.

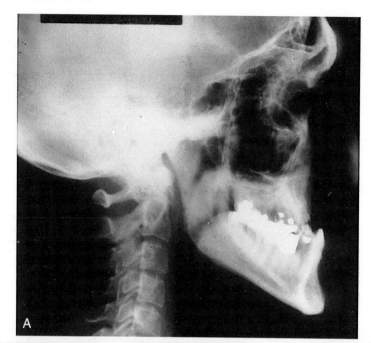

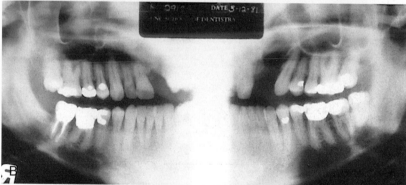

Figure 20–38. Lateral cephalometric (*A*) and panoramic (*B*) radiographs before treatment. Notice the overclosed vertical dimension and the missing central and lateral incisors on the cleft side.

The facial examination confirmed midfacial deficiency. There was a minimal component of vertical facial deficiency and the freeway space was normal. The occlusion was class III, and a lateral incisor on the cleft side was missing (Fig. 20–38). Several teeth had extensive decay, and the maxillary anterior teeth were stained from tobacco use. An oral-nasal fistula was also present and was symptomatic. The soft palate and lateral pharyngeal walls moved well, and the velopharyngeal mechanism was marginally adequate. Mild hypernasality was present with sibilant distortions, which were consistent with the malocclusion.

Periodontal and general dental treatments were initiated. Once the oral health was improved, orthodontic banding ensued. The presurgical goal of orthodontics was to level and align the arches independently. An additional goal was to narrow the mandibular arch and widen the maxillary arch. No attempt at maxillary expansion was undertaken.

Eighteen months later, when the patient was 32, a maxillary advancement was performed with a complete circumvestibular incision and the LeFort I downfracture approach (Fig. 20–39). The maxilla was advanced in two pieces because there was no bone continuity across the hard palate. The oral-nasal fistula was repaired by a three-layer closure, which included the nasal mucosa, the bone graft, and rotation of oral mucosa to cover the grafted bone. Fresh autogenous cancellous bone harvested from the ilium was condensed into the cleft along its entirety from the anterior alveolar region to the posterior margin of the hard palate. In the alveolar region, bone

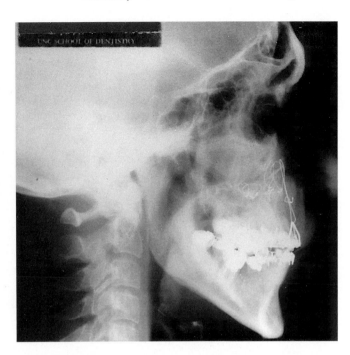

Figure 20–39. The patient underwent surgery at age 32. Immediate postoperative lateral cephalometric radiograph demonstrates maxillary advancement with osseous wires, skeletal wires, and intermaxillary fixation. Autogenous bone grafts were placed in all osseous defects.

was packed inferiorly to the level of the alveolar bone supporting the adjacent teeth. The maxilla was advanced and stabilized with the use of intermaxillary fixation and four osseous wires. Corticocancellous blocks were cut and wedged into the lateral maxillary wall defects. Their positions were secured with osseous wires. Additional onlay bone grafts were placed along the lateral maxillary walls. A cortical bone graft was suspended from the anterior nasal spine to the lateral aspect of the pyriform area on the cleft side to construct a nasal rim and to improve the symmetry of the maxillary skeleton.

Four weeks after surgery, an infection was noted along the lateral maxilla on the cleft side. A sequestrum was removed, and the wound was irrigated frequently and packed. After 8 weeks of intermaxillary fixation and another 4 weeks of elastic traction, the patient returned to orthodontic care. Eighteen months after surgery, another bone sequestrum necessitated removal from the floor of the nose. By this time, there was good healing of all maxillary segments, and orthodontic care had been completed (Fig. 20–40).

Prosthetic treatment commenced at this time, and an eight-unit bridge was placed anteriorly with a pontic to substitute for the missing lateral incisor. Colored acrylic was used to disguise the alveolar ridge defect that resulted from bone graft resorption and sequestration at the reconstructed alveolar region.

Hypernasal speech was apparent immediately after surgery. Although it improved, it was still present 1 year after surgery. It did not interfere with speech intelligibility, and the patient resumed his career as a literature instructor. He elected not to undergo pharyngoplasty.

Twelve years after surgery, the position of the maxilla was maintained, as was the esthetic and occlusal changes (Fig. 20–41). The oral-nasal fistula remained closed, but the esthetics of the cleft area were compromised by bone resorption. Grafted bone always resorbs to the height of the bone adjacent to the cleft margins, and it always thins if not supported by a tooth or an implant. Dental neglect claimed its toll, as evidenced by multiple missing teeth and periapical lesions (Fig. 20–42). A prosthesis was required for this patient because of missing teeth; prosthetic devices require continuous lifetime maintenance, which is time consuming and costly. By contemporary standards, a prosthesis should be avoided when possible.

Factors complicating the surgical phase of treatment included the patient's age and smoking. Both of these variables are linked to increased complications from this surgery.

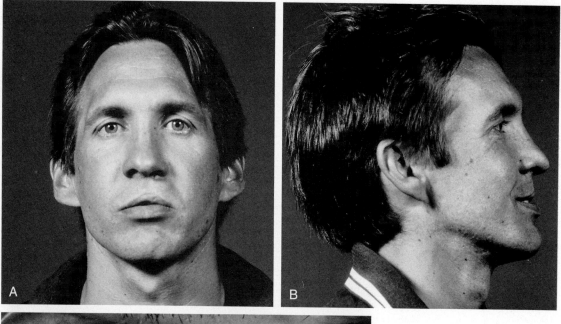

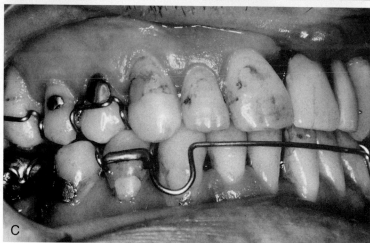

Figure 20–40. Facial (*A, B*) and occlusion (*C*) views 18 months after surgery. Notice the improved nasolabial support and class I occlusion.

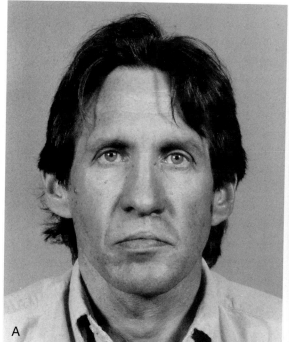

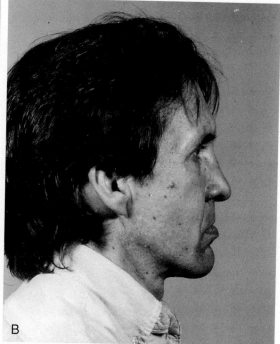

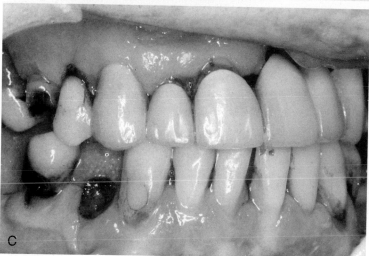

Figure 20–41. Facial (*A, B*) and occlusion (*C*) views 12 years postoperatively; the facial features remain improved. The anterior occlusion has been restored with an eight-unit bridge.

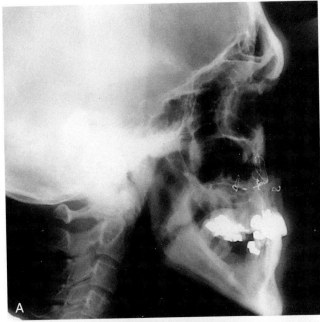

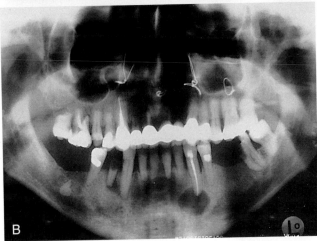

Figure 20–42. Lateral cephalometric (*A*) and panoramic (*B*) radiographs 12 years postoperatively indicate excellent skeletal and dental stability. Inadequate postoperative dental care has taken its toll on the dentition.

Case 2

A 12-year-old boy with a repaired unilateral cleft lip and cleft palate presented for treatment (Fig. 20–43). Multiple previous operations were performed to close and revise the lip and nose, to close the palate, and to place a pharyngeal flap.

Maxillary deficiency and overclosure of the vertical dimension were noted, as was a patent oral-nasal fistula and class III malocclusion (Fig. 20–44). Speech was not hypernasal, but sibilant distortions were noted and thought to be consistent with the malocclusion. The velopharyngeal mechanism had good movement and competent function with a pharyngeal flap in place.

Orthodontic treatment was initiated, and the presurgical goal was to eliminate dental compensations so that the maxilla could be advanced and widened.

A decision to proceed with surgery at age 13 was made by the patient and parents. They were advised of the potential for relapse because of growth but decided to proceed with surgery nonetheless, believing that the esthetic improvement would benefit the patient's acceptance in a new school environment.

Nasotracheal intubation was performed as described earlier in this chapter and was not problematic. A LeFort I osteotomy via circumvestibular incision and downfracture in two pieces was performed (Fig. 20–45). The maxilla was advanced and widened,

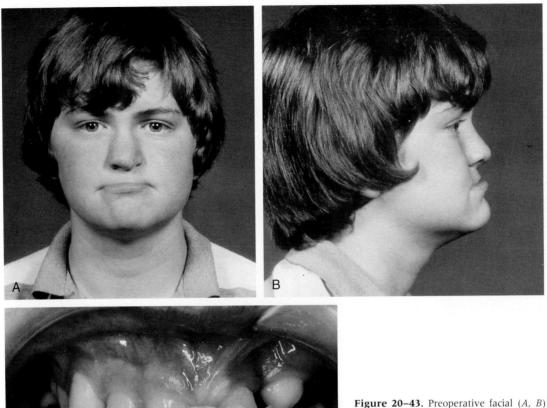

Figure 20–43. Preoperative facial (*A, B*) and occlusion (*C*) views at age 12.

and the oral-nasal fistula was simultaneously closed. The bone of the palate was sectioned free, and the tissues pedicled to the bone island were undermined to facilitate widening of the maxillary arch. The nasal mucosa and the oral mucosa were closed primarily.

The pharyngeal flap and palatal mucosa were scarred and required stretching in order to advance the maxilla the required amount. The bone defects along the lateral maxilla were repaired with iliac corticocancellous grafts and secured with osseous wires. The palatal and alveolar defects were repaired with cancellous bone. An auxiliary arch wire was placed on the maxillary orthodontic appliance at surgery to retain the maxillary segments. Intermaxillary fixation was applied for 8 weeks (Fig. 20–46). A year after surgery, the orthodontic appliances were removed and retainers were placed. A composite bridge was placed when the patient was 17 to replace the missing lateral incisor, and a permanent prosthesis was later fabricated.

Ten years after surgery, the crossbite had returned to the cleft side, and the reconstructed alveolus had narrowed. The alveolar ridge narrowed because it lacked supporting dental structures. Progressive mandibular growth, not loss of maxillary projection, is the cause of the occlusal relapse (Figs. 20–47, 20–48). Additional treatment would be necessary to improve this situation. The patient was content with the result and refused all additional offerings, including lip and nasal revisions. Interestingly, he indicated that he would pursue treatment again at the same age because of the positive changes appreciated, even knowing that a better result may have been obtained if surgery were delayed several years.

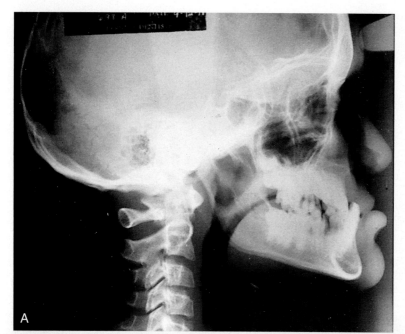

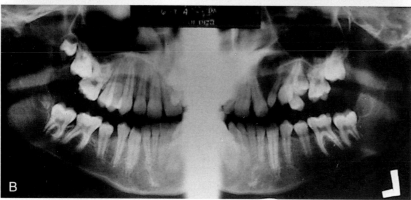

Figure 20–44. Preoperative cephalometric (*A*) and panoramic (*B*) radiographs. The tooth in the cleft was removed, but all others were preserved.

Figure 20–45. The patient underwent surgery at age 13. Immediate postoperative cephalometric radiograph demonstrates maxillary advancement, interosseus and suspension wires, and intermaxillary fixation. Bone grafts were wedged into all bone defects.

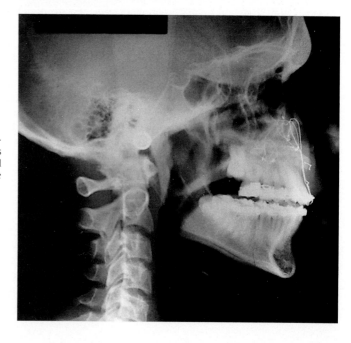

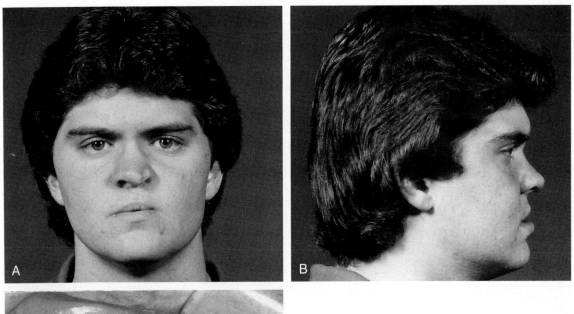

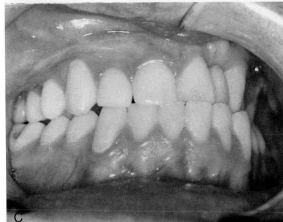

Figure 20–46. Facial (*A, B*) and occlusal (*C*) views when the patient was 16.

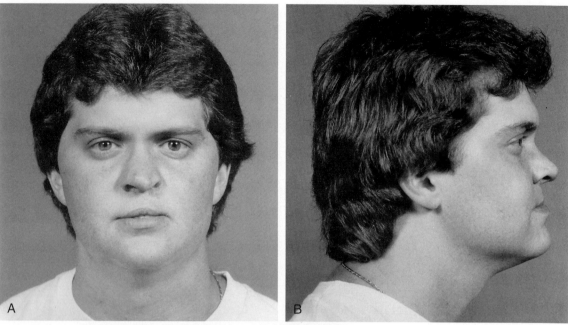

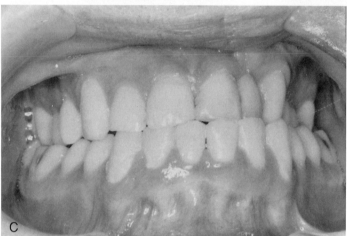

Figure 20–47. Facial (*A, B*) and occlusion (*C*) views at age 24, 10 years after surgery. Maintenance of midfacial projection and upper lip support is good. Cross bite on the left has returned.

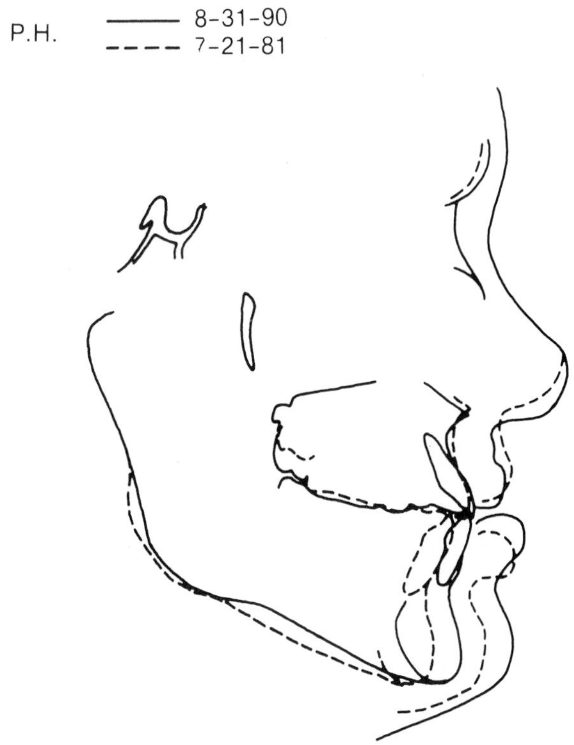

P.H. ——— 8-31-90
      - - - - 7-21-81

Figure 20-48. Superimposition cephalometric tracing demonstrating continued mandibular and nasal growth between the ages of 15 and 24 years. Note that the position of the maxilla has not undergone relapse. Dental compensation by mandibular incisor uprighting and maxillary incisor flaring has occurred.

The patient's best biologic interest (delaying maxillary advancement until completion of growth) is not always consistent with psychosocial concerns. If patients and parents understand that additional treatment, including surgery, may be necessary if the correction is outgrown, there is little reason to deny early maxillary advancement.

In the treatment outcome of this patient in comparison with that of the previous patient, there were no postsurgical complications (other than growth). The lack of postsurgical complications is partially attributed to the young age at which surgery was undertaken and no tobacco use.

Case 3

A 15-year-old boy had previously undergone lip and palate closure, multiple lip and nasal revisions, placement of a pharyngeal flap, and an attempted bone graft from the cranium before transferring from another center (Figs. 20-49, 20-50). At age 8, he underwent a repeated bone graft from the ilium with successful results. Preliminary orthodontic intervention was initiated to align and widen the maxillary arch shortly after the bone graft. Permanent teeth were guided into the bone graft, and the space for the missing lateral incisor was closed. Definitive orthodontic treatment was delayed until age 14. No attempt was made to camouflage the class III malocclusion, and the arches were coordinated for maxillary advancement via circumvestibular incision and downfracture.

Maxillary advancement and a bone graft from the cranium were undertaken at age 15 (Figs. 20-51, 20-52). The decision to proceed with surgery was left to the patient, and he and his parents realized the potential to outgrow the correction. Nasotracheal intubation around the pharyngeal flap was accomplished as described in the text. The surgery was enhanced by the previously placed bone graft in that operating time and blood loss were reduced. The bone graft donor site was the left parietal region, because the right side had been used several years before. The maxilla was stabilized with bone plates, and bone grafts were placed into the lateral wall defects. Additional cortical onlay grafts were placed to highlight the cheeks and to contour the paranasal regions. The pyriform rim was also constructed with a bone graft suspended from the anterior nasal spine to the lateral maxillary wall. These grafts were secured with screws.

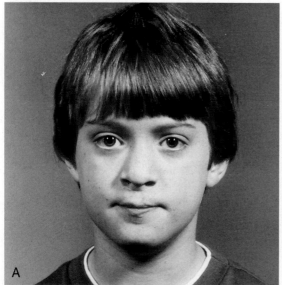
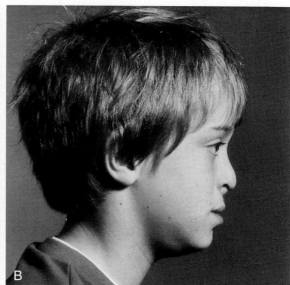
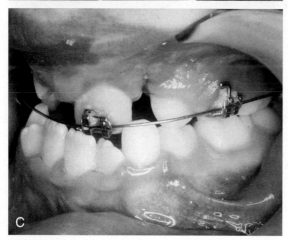

Figure 20–49. Facial (*A, B*) and occlusion (*C*) views at age 8 after failed bone graft.

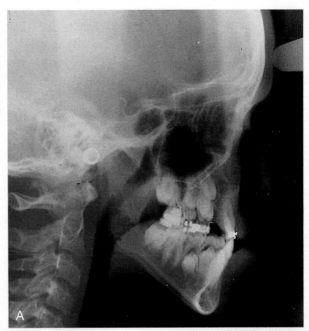

Figure 20–50. Lateral cephalometric (*A*) and panoramic (*B*) radiographs at age 8, before the second bone graft.

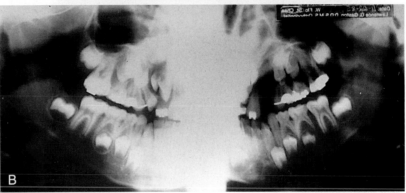

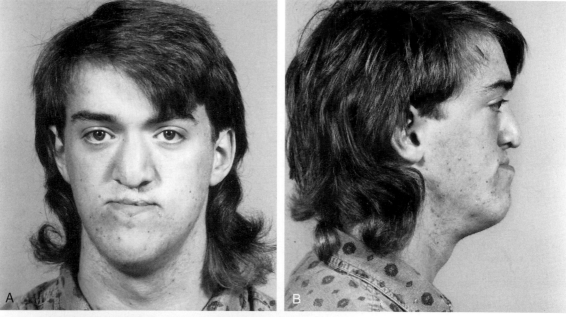

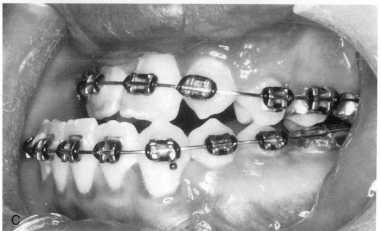

Figure 20–51. Preoperative facial (*A, B*) and occlusion (*C*) views at age 15.

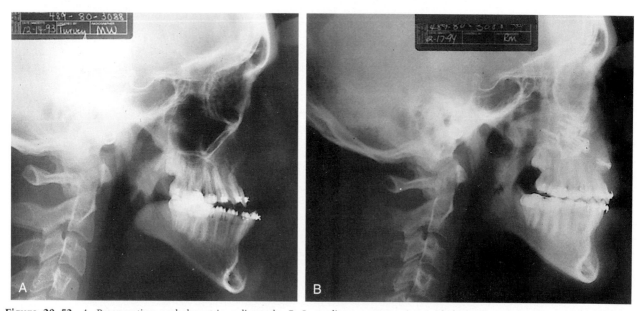

Figure 20–52. *A,* Preoperative cephalometric radiograph. *B,* Immediate postoperative cephalometric radiograph. Notice the screw securing the cranial bone graft used to construct the pyriform rim.

Intermaxillary fixation was removed, and heavy elastic bands were used to control the occlusion after surgery. Orthodontic treatment resumed after 6 weeks and was completed within 4 months.

Velopharyngeal function was unchanged after surgery; however, the sibilant distortions and articulation errors improved. No prosthetic treatment was required, because the bone graft facilitated preservation of the natural dentition and orthodontic treatment was able to advance the posterior teeth to close the space at the cleft site (Figs. 20–53, 20–54). Final lip and nasal revisions are awaited.

This case illustrates contemporary treatment of cleft lip and cleft palate with the goals of placing a bone graft during the mixed dentition and eliminating the need for a prosthesis. Even though an initial bone graft was not successful, a second one was successfully placed at an age-appropriate time, and this allowed adequate arch development with good periodontal support. Enabling the patient and parents to participate in the timing of surgery is important and allows the patient to feel in control.

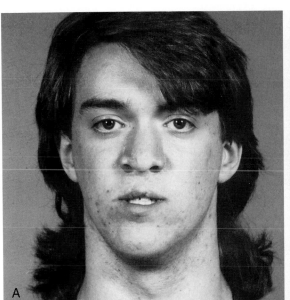
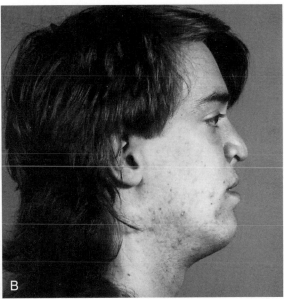
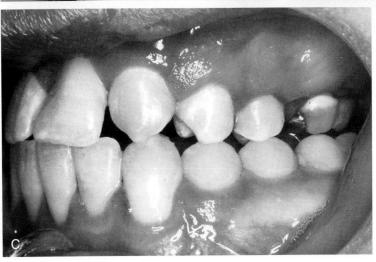

Figure 20–53. Facial (*A, B*) and occlusion (*C*) views 1 year after surgery.

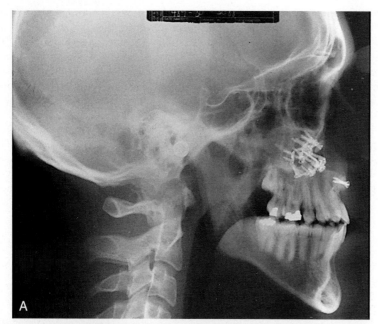

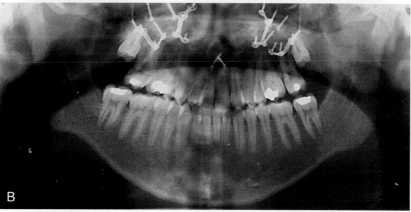

Figure 20-54. Lateral cephalometric (*A*) and panoramic (*B*) radiographs 1 year after surgery. Notice good periodontal support and the lack of prosthetics.

Case 4

A 13-year-old girl had undergone isolated cleft palate repair at age 18 months and pharyngeal flap surgery at age 6 years (Fig. 20–55). A class III malocclusion developed (Fig. 20–56), and orthodontic treatment was initiated after the eruption of the permanent dentition. From the outset, maxillary advancement was planned, and the presurgical goals of orthodontic treatment were to level, align, and coordinate the arches.

The facial examination demonstrated complete midface deficiency, including deficiencies of the orbits and nose. Mild prognathism and retrogenia were noted. The initial surgical plan included LeFort III osteotomy, cranial bone grafts, mandibular setback, and a genioplasty. Before surgery, the patient and family decided upon LeFort I–level advancement and onlay bone grafts combined with mandibular surgery as an alternative.

Nasoendotracheal intubation as described in the text was accomplished without injuring the pharyngeal flap. A LeFort I downfracture via a circumvestibular incision, bilateral sagittal osteotomies of the mandibular ramus, and a genioplasty were performed (Fig. 20–57). Mobilization of the maxilla was difficult and required stripping and incising the palatal scar. Once the maxilla was mobilized, the pharyngeal flap was stretched without difficulty. Cranial bone grafts were wedged into the lateral maxillary defects, and bone plates were placed to stabilize the position of the maxilla. Contour

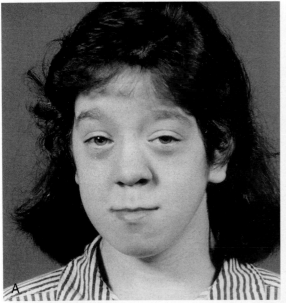
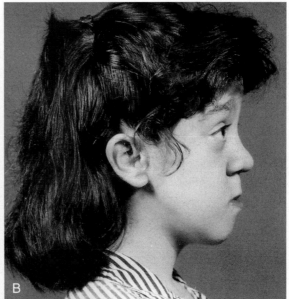
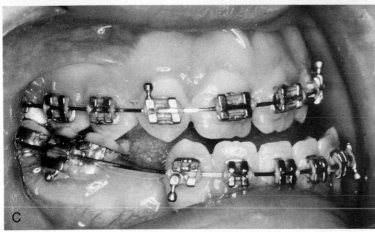

Figure 20–55. Preoperative facial (*A*, *B*) and occlusion (*C*) views of a 19-year-old with a repaired cleft palate and midface deficiency affecting the orbits, nose, and zygoma as well as the occlusion (class III).

Figure 20–56. Preoperative lateral cephalometric radiograph confirms midface deficiency. Notice the flaring of the mandibular incisors, which was necessary to create enough space in the arch.

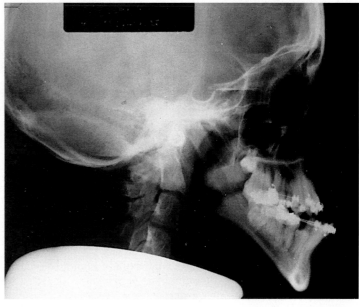

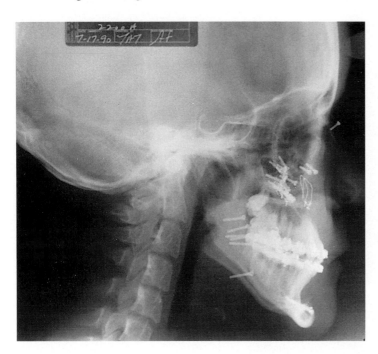

Figure 20–57. The patient underwent surgery at age 15. A maxillary advancement and downgrafting were performed at the LeFort I level, as were mandibular sagittal osteotomies and a genioplasty. Split cranial bone grafts were used interpositionally and to contour the nose orbits and cheeks. All contour grafts were secured with screws, as were the sagittal osteotomies and genioplasty. Notice the improved relationship of the mandibular incisors to the chin.

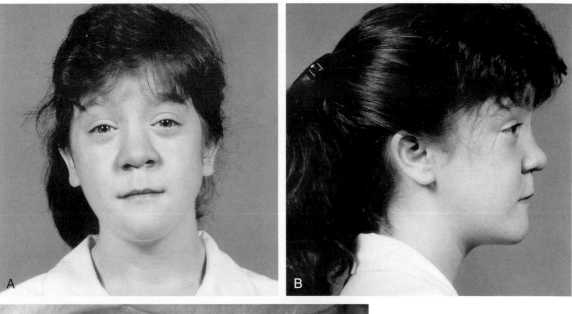

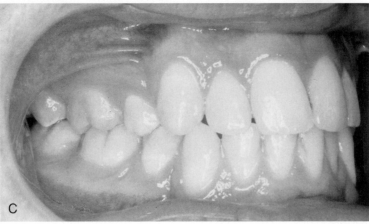

Figure 20–58. Facial (*A, B*) and occlusion (*C*) views 1 year after surgery; improved facial balance and a class I occlusion are obvious.

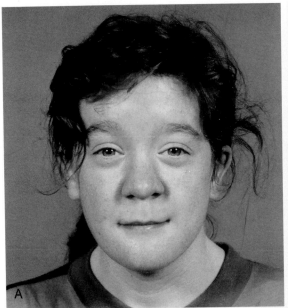
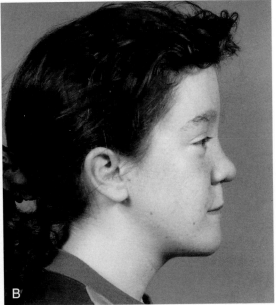
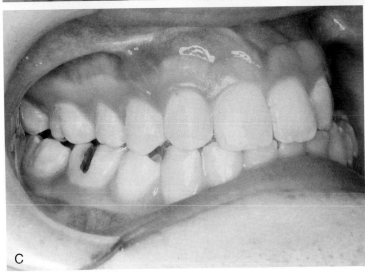

Figure 20–59. *A* to *C,* Five years after surgery, at age 20, maintenance of the esthetic change is observed. There has been some transverse occlusal changes attributed to the lack of retainer wear. Notice the lack of mandibular incisal recrowding. It is possible that altering the chin lip balance by augmentation genioplasty contributed to this observation?

bone grafts were onlayed to highlight the cheeks, the lateral orbital and inferior orbital rims, the paranasal regions, and the nasal bridge. The transnasal route was used to augment the nasal bridge; however, all other grafts were placed transorally. All contour grafts were stabilized with screws placed transorally except the nasal bridge, which required a stab over the nasal dorsum. The sagittal osteotomy and genioplasty were stabilized with transorally placed screws.

Eight weeks after surgery, the patient resumed orthodontic care. Speech was unchanged, and no additional speech therapy was required. Orthodontic treatment continued for 6 months, and debanding was accomplished (Fig. 20–58). Five years after surgery, facial projection and balance were maintained (Figs. 20–59, 20–60). Minimally remodeled cranial bone grafts maintained their contour on the orbital rims, nasal bridge, and cheeks. Relapse of posterior crossbite occurred, and this demonstrates a major frustration in the orthodontic treatment of patients with cleft palate.

This case highlights the use of cranial bone to contour the face, combined with maxillary advancement and mandibular surgery to achieve a desirable occlusal and esthetic result. Unlike other bone sources, cranial bone, when appropriately stabilized with screws, maintains its volume and resorbs minimally. The likely explanations for this observation include the dense cortical consistency of this bone in relation to other donor sources and the rich haversion network that enhances revascularization.[58]

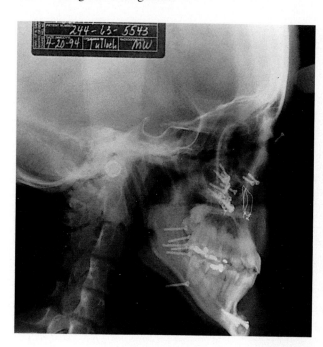

Figure 20–60. Five-year postoperative cephalometric radiograph confirms stability.

Case 5

A 23-year-old man with a repaired bilateral cleft lip and cleft palate presented for improvement of the condition. He had undergone multiple operations to close the lip and palate and to elongate the columella. No bone grafts had been attempted. Speech was grossly nasal, and he had sibilant distortions that were consistent with the malocclusion.

Examination revealed severe maxillary deficiency, a freely movable premaxilla that was overerupted, and multiple oral-nasal fistulas, including two buccal and one midpalatal (Figs. 20–61, 20–62).

A treatment plan consisting of orthodontics, surgery, and prosthetics was developed. Because of the poor periodontal support for the maxillary cuspids, they were removed bilaterally. The presurgical goal of orthodontics was to align and level the three maxillary segments independently. In the mandibular arch, the preoperative goal was to align, level, and decompensate the arch by flaring the anterior teeth.

At surgery, the maxilla was advanced in three pieces (Figs. 20–63, 20–64). An anterior buccal pedicle remained to perfuse the premaxilla, and although this made the operation more difficult, it was necessary to ensure survival of the premaxilla. The bone clefts were prepared on either side for bone grafting. Bone was grafted from the ilium into all surgical defects along the lateral walls of the maxilla. Cancellous bone was grafted into the cleft defects, and long buccal mucosal flaps were rotated bilaterally and joined in the midline to close over the bone grafts and to close the midpalatal defect. Osseous wire fixation was used to hold the bone segments and to support the corticocancellous grafts in the lateral maxillary walls. Intermaxillary fixation was applied for 8 weeks.

After surgery, a midpalatal dehiscence occurred, where the two buccal flaps joined and bone sequestered through the defect. This was treated with irrigation and gauze packing. Hypernasality persisted, as did oral-nasal reflux, but the patient was not concerned and refused further surgery. Once orthodontic detailing was completed, prosthetic management was initiated.

The premaxilla stabilized, and the anterior teeth were able to be used as abutments. A fixed bridge was fabricated from first molar to first molar.

Seven years after surgery, the patient remained pleased with the outcome (Fig. 20–65). Although he could have benefited from additional treatment to improve velopharyngeal function and to close the palatal fistula, he was not concerned. He continued to obturate the midpalatal fistula with gauze each day.

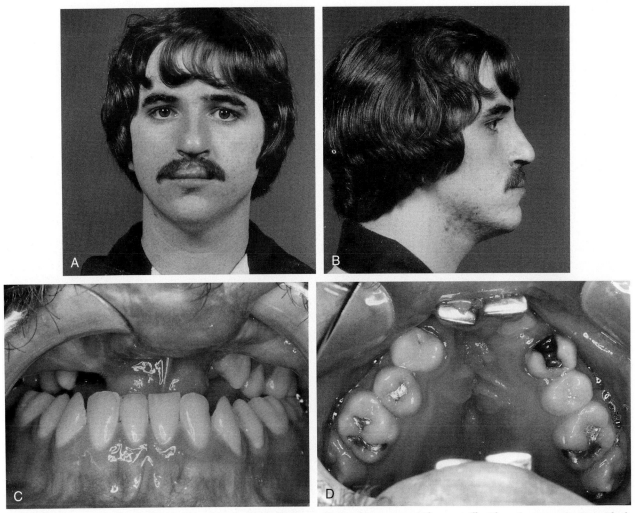

Figure 20–61. Preoperative facial (*A, B*) and occlusal (*C, D*) views. Notice the overerupted premaxilla. There is no continuity with the lateral segments.

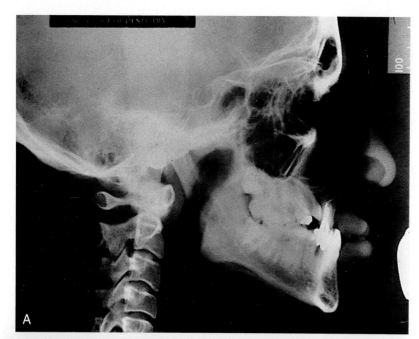

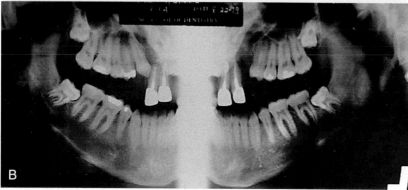

Figure 20–62. Lateral cephalometric (*A*) and panoramic (*B*) radiographs demonstrating severe maxillary deficiency and an upright and overerupted premaxilla.

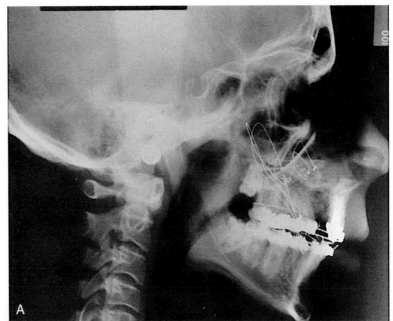

A

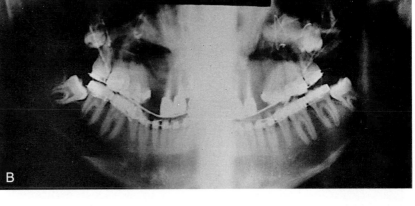

B

Figure 20–63. The patient underwent surgery at age 23. Lateral cephalometric (*A*) and panoramic (*B*) radiographs indicate maxillary advancement in three pieces and leveling of the premaxilla with the lateral segments. Bone grafting with direct osseous and suspension wiring was used, as was intermaxillary fixation.

—9/18/80
--9/29/80

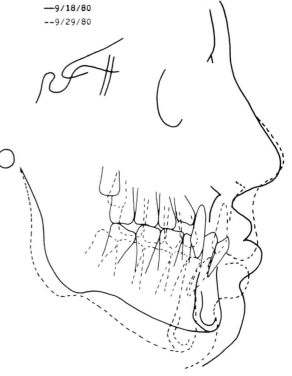

Figure 20–64. Superimposition lateral cephalometric tracing demonstrating the skeletal changes at surgery.

489

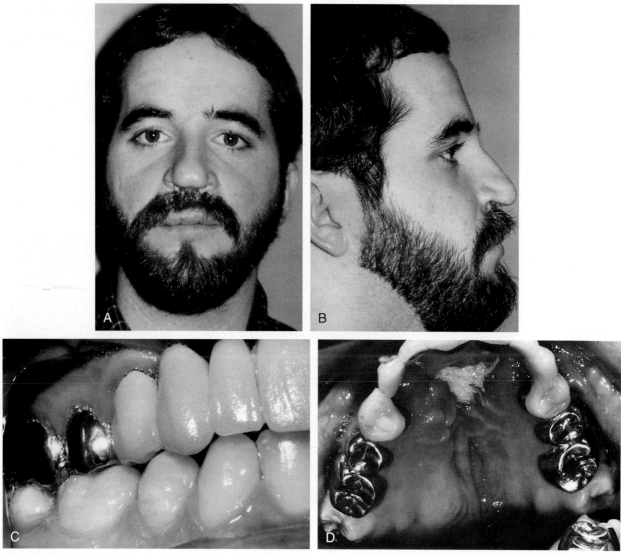

Figure 20–65. Facial (*A, B*) and occlusion (*C, D*) views 7 years after surgery; there has been maintenance of the surgical changes. An eight-unit fixed prosthesis was constructed. Notice the packing in the midpalatal fistula. The patient elected this rather than surgical closure.

This case illustrates many of the difficulties in managing the adult patient with a bilateral cleft. Had bone grafts been placed at an age-appropriate time, the premature loss of teeth may have been avoided, prosthetic needs may have been minimized or completely eliminated, and a better chance of maintaining closure of the oral-nasal fistulas may have been realized. The midpalatal fistula is particularly problematic in bilateral clefts undergoing maxillary advancement. Staged procedures, sometimes with the use of distant tissue transfers, are necessary.

Case 6

A 19-year-old woman with a repaired bilateral cleft lip and cleft palate presented for comprehensive treatment. In the past, she had undergone bilateral lip closure, which was facilitated by amputation of the premaxilla (Figs. 20–66, 20–67). Palate closure had been delayed until age 7.

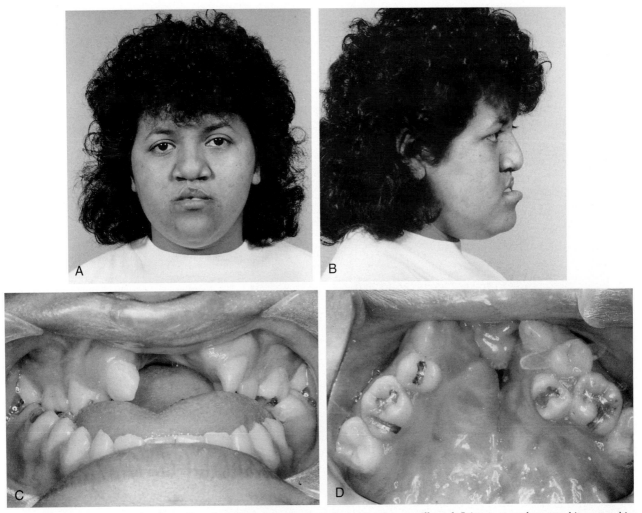

Figure 20–66. Preoperative facial (*A*, *B*) and occlusion (*C*, *D*) views demonstrating maxillary deficiency, complete crossbite, open bite, and amputation of the premaxilla. Notice the palatal fistula.

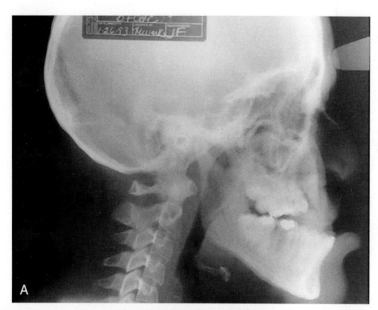

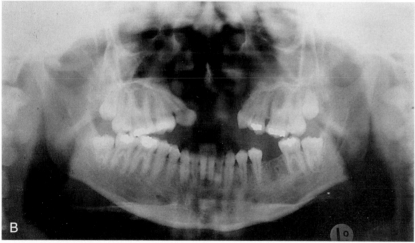

Figure 20–67. Lateral cephalometric (*A*) and panoramic (*B*) views confirming midface deficiency, overclosure of the facial vertical dimension, retrogenia, and open bite and divergent occlusal planes.

Examination confirmed severe maxillary deficiency and overclosure of the vertical dimension. The palatal tissues were severely scarred, the maxillary arch was collapsed, and the occlusal plane was divergent. A midpalatal fistula was present, and all the maxillary anterior teeth were missing. Speech was hypernasal, with sibilant distortions consistent with the malocclusion.

These complex problems necessitated the involvement of multiple disciplines; however, limited finances and family support precluded all care except surgery.

Maxillary advancement, bone graft reconstruction of the premaxilla from the ilium, mandibular setback, and genioplasty were performed simultaneously, and all segments were rigidly secured with either bone plates or screws (Fig. 20–68). The left and right sides of the maxilla had no continuity, and the scarred palatal tissues limited the transverse movements. Anteriorly based buccal mucosal flaps were rotated bilaterally to cover the bone grafted to the premaxilla.

Two weeks after surgery, a dehiscence of the rotated buccal flaps and sequestration of the anterior bone graft were noted. Irrigation and packing for another 6 weeks were required as additional bone sequestered. By 6 months after surgery, the bone segments were well consolidated, but all that remained of the reconstructed premaxilla were two corticocancellous struts, which reconstructed the inferior part of the pyriform rim. A palatal defect that was larger than the original defect persisted (Fig. 20–69).

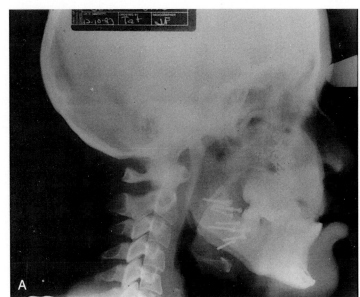

Figure 20–68. Cephalometric (*A*) and panoramic (*B*) radiographs taken after surgery. The patient underwent surgery at age 19. It consisted of a maxillary advancement, bilateral sagittal mandibular osteotomies, and a genioplasty. Iliac bone grafts were used to stabilize the maxilla and to reconstruct the premaxilla. Bone plates and screws were used to stabilize the segments.

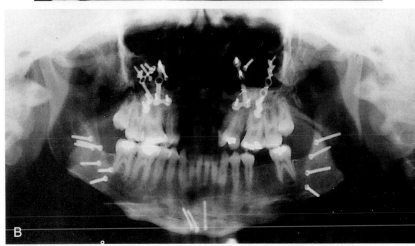

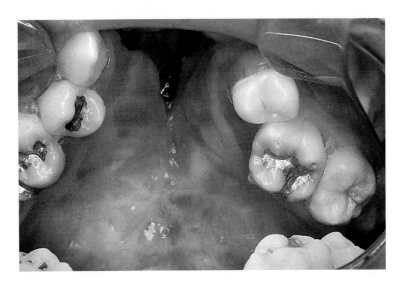

Figure 20–69. After surgery, the midpalatal fistula reopened and resulted in an even larger defect.

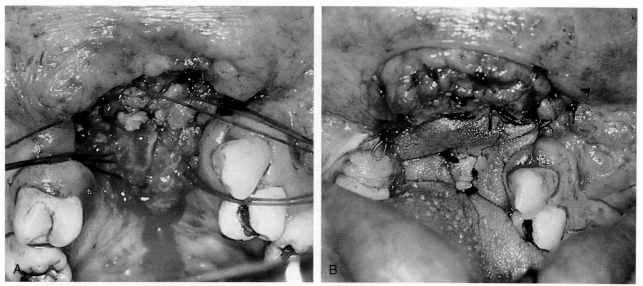

Figure 20–70. Turnover flaps were used to create a surface on the nasal side (*A*), and a tongue flap was used to provide oral coverage to close the residual oral-nasal fistula (*B*).

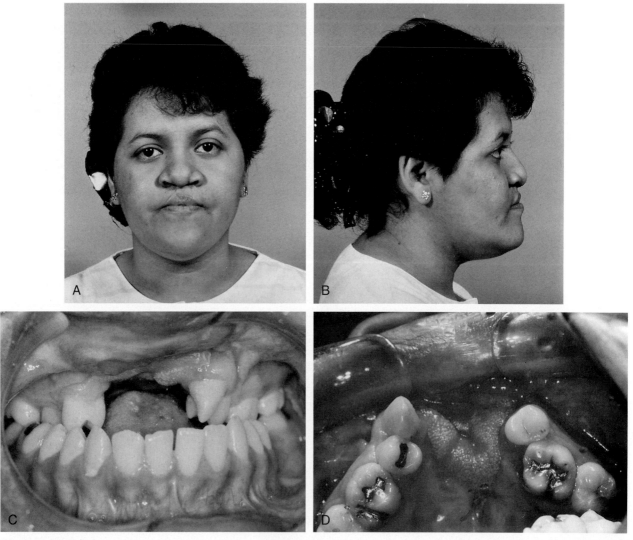

Figure 20–71. Facial (*A, B*) and occlusion (*C, D*) views 18 months after the initial operation. Notice complete obturation of the palatal fistula with the tongue flap. The bite has been closed, but elimination of the crossbite was not possible because of the palatal tissue deficiencies. Orthodontic correction was not possible, and prosthetics is not completed. Without bone graft reconstruction of the premaxilla, prosthetic options are limited to removable partial dentures.

An anteriorly based tongue flap was used to cover the palatal defect (Fig. 20–70). Although this was successful in closing the fistula, the prosthetic possibilities were limited to removable partial dentures, because there was inadequate bone to support implants or even a conventional bridge (Fig. 20–71). The lip and nasal support and facial balance have improved, but the patient did not complete care.

This case illustrates several frustrations in dealing with adult patients with clefts:

1. Amputation of tissues in cleft patients should be avoided because the tissues are almost always needed later for reconstruction.

2. Procedures that can be reliably performed during childhood or adolescence, specifically bone grafts, should be performed at age-appropriate intervals, because these procedures may not always be successful in adulthood.

3. Excessive scarring limits the amount of osseous movements.

4. Limited funding and limited access to comprehensive team care limit the results.

5. Many of these procedures are more difficult for adults than for children to endure, and adults are less likely to complete care.

Case 7

An 8-year-old girl had previously undergone bilateral lip adhesions, definitive lip repair, and, at 18 months, columella lengthening and palatal repair. At age 3 years, a pharyngeal flap was placed, and another lip revision and columella lengthening were performed. At 8, the patient underwent bone grafting from the cranium to the cleft maxilla and palate bilaterally (Fig. 20–72). At this time, the patient had a class III malocclusion (Fig. 20–73), caused primarily by maxillary deficiency. Before bone grafting, no interceptive orthodontic treatment was undertaken, and because of extreme skeletal disharmony, a decision was made not to attempt orthodontic correction. The grafts were placed to provide support for unerupted teeth and the teeth adjacent to the cleft, to close the oral-nasal fistulas, to construct a continuous and intact maxillary arch, and to improve the support for the lip and the nose.

Six months after graft placement, preliminary arch alignment was undertaken. The discrepancy between the maxilla and the mandible worsened as mandibular growth progressed, and comprehensive orthodontic treatment was delayed until age 13.

The presurgical goal of orthodontics was to level and align both dental arches independently (Figs. 20–74, 20–75). In the maxillary arch, the left cuspid had erupted through the bone graft and was advanced to substitute for the missing lateral incisor. The incisors were uprighted, space was closed, and the arch required some minor dental expansion. In the mandibular arch, the incisors were flared and leveled.

The facial configuration was consistent with maxillary deficiency extending to the infraorbital rims from the zygomatic prominence to the paranasal regions bilaterally. Greater deficiency was noted on the left. The maxilla was also vertically deficient, as was the lower third of the face. This accentuated the prognathic appearance. Retrogenia was also present.

Speech assessment indicated sibilant distortions related to the malocclusion and dialect. The soft palate was scarred, but it and the lateral pharyngeal walls moved well and functioned well with the pharyngeal flap in place. There was no evidence of hypernasality. Palatal scarring was present but not of great concern.

When the patient was 15½, a high-level LeFort I osteotomy was performed, and an anterior pedicle was left on the premaxilla to provide adequate perfusion, even though the previously placed bone grafts were successful (Fig. 20–76). The bone grafts were visualized along the nasal floor and pyriform rim, and the quality of the bone was indistinguishable from that of adjacent host bone. The maxilla advanced easily and in one piece. Asymmetry and contour differences of the midfacial skeleton were observed; greater deficiencies on the left were noted.

Split cranial bone grafts were used to fill all osteotomy defects by securely wedging them into place. When wedging was not possible, the grafts were further secured with wires or screws to prevent displacement into the sinus. Other bone grafts were used to contour the cheeks, infraorbital regions, and paranasal regions. These grafts were also secured with bone screws to minimize displacement and to enhance revascularization and survival.

Text continued on page 500

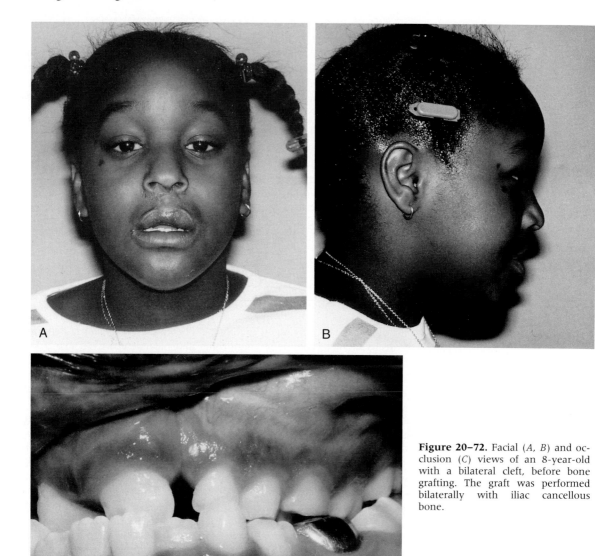

Figure 20–72. Facial (*A, B*) and occlusion (*C*) views of an 8-year-old with a bilateral cleft, before bone grafting. The graft was performed bilaterally with iliac cancellous bone.

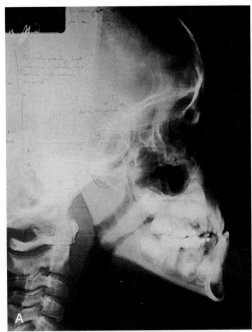

Figure 20–73. Lateral cephalometric (*A*) and panoramic (*B*) radiographs demonstrating maxillary deficiency, anterior crossbite, a small tooth in the cleft on the left, and absence of a lateral incisor on the right. The small incisor was preserved on the left.

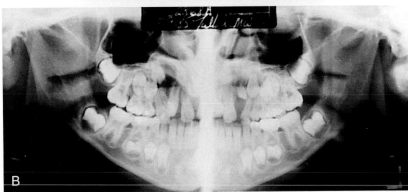

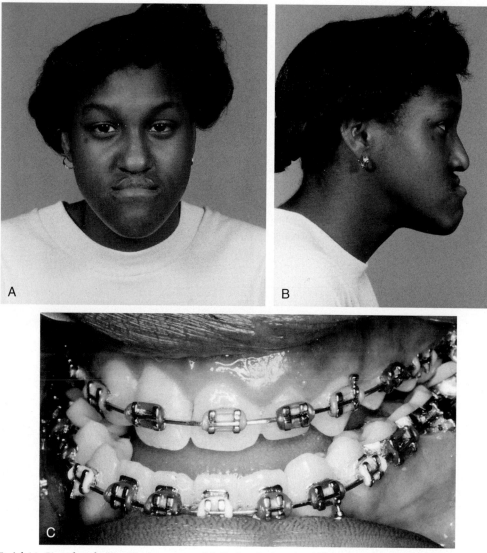

Figure 20–74. Facial (*A, B*) and occlusion (*C*) views at age 14. Notice the increased discrepancy between the maxilla and mandible and the worsening class III malocclusion. The small incisor and cuspid on the left have erupted into the graft. The cuspid on the right has been advanced adjacent to the central incisor.

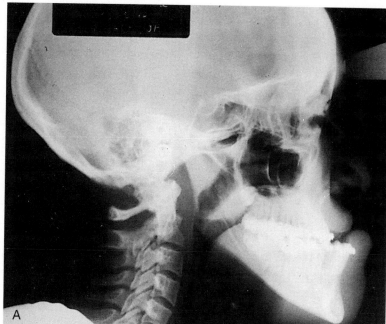

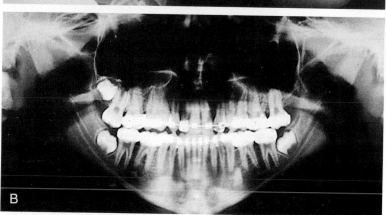

Figure 20–75. Lateral cephalometric (*A*) and panoramic (*B*) radiographs demonstrating maxillary deficiency, mandibular prognathism, and retrogenia. Notice the eruption of the permanent teeth and the periodontal health, especially of the teeth adjacent to the cleft.

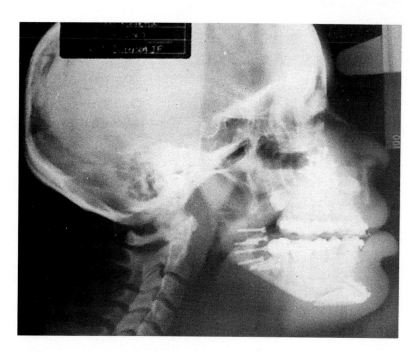

Figure 20–76. At age 15, the patient underwent maxillary advancement in one piece, mandibular setback, and a genioplasty. Cranial bone was used interpositionally on the maxilla and was also onlayed to contour the cheeks and paranasal regions. Stabilization was achieved with bone plates and screws.

Bilateral sagittal osteotomies of the mandible were simultaneously performed to facilitate posterior movement. An appropriate amount of buccal cortex was excised bilaterally from the distal segments to minimize the displacement of the proximal segment. By reducing displacement of the proximal segment, stability of the mandibular and maxillar positions is enhanced. Four 2-mm screws were used to secure the ramus on each side.

A genioplasty was also performed to effect anterior and inferior movement. The pedicled bone flap was secured with three screws.

An acrylic splint and intermaxillary fixation were placed for 1 week, and then elastic guidance continued for another 6 weeks while the patient functioned into the splint. Once the occlusal splint was removed, orthodontic treatment continued for 6 more months. After debanding, orthodontic retention continued with the use of removable appliances.

Two and one-half years after surgery, the patient (aged 18) demonstrated a favorable esthetic and functional result (Figs. 20–77, 20–78). Rhinoplasty and lip revision could have enhanced the result, but the patient was content and not interested in these procedures at that time. There was no need for prosthetic treatment, inasmuch as bone grafting successfully provided adequate support to enable the orthodontist to develop the maxillary arch without spaces.

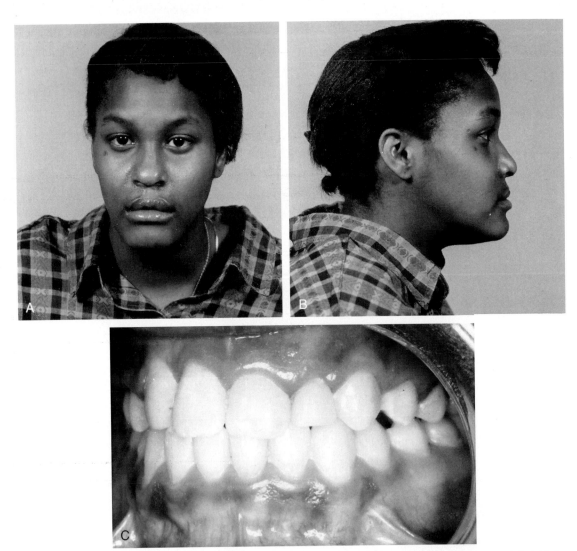

Figure 20–77. Facial (*A, B*) and occlusion (*C*) views at age 18, 2½ years after surgery, demonstrating improved facial balance and a class I occlusion. No soft tissue revisions or rhinoplasty have been performed, but these procedures could enhance the result. Currently, the patient is delighted and does not want to pursue these options.

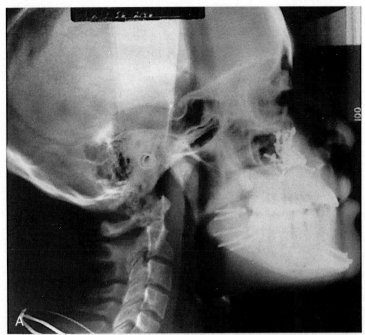

Figure 20–78. Lateral cephalometric (*A*) and panoramic (*B*) radiographs taken 2½ years after surgery, documenting stability and sound periodontal support for all teeth.

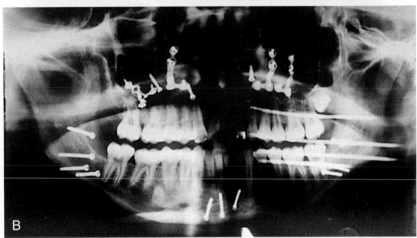

References

1. Stella JP, Chaisresoahurnpon N, Epker BN: Diagnostic Criteria for Midface Deficiency in Cleft Lip and Palate Patients. Program of the 50th annual meeting of the American Cleft Palate–Craniofacial Association (Abstract 182, p 69), Pittsburgh, May 1993.
2. Ross RB: Treatment variables affecting facial growth in complete unilateral cleft lip and palate. Cleft Palate J 1987; 24(1):1–77.
3. Bardach J: The influence of cleft repair on facial growth. Cleft Palate J 1990; 27(1):76–78.
4. Vargervik K: Orthodontic treatment of cleft patients: Characteristics of growth and development/treatment principles. *In* Bardach J, Morris H (eds): Multidisciplinary Management of Cleft Lip and Palate, pp 642–648. Philadelphia: WB Saunders, 1990.
5. Semb G: A study of facial growth in patients with unilateral cleft lip and palate treated by the Oslo CLP team. Cleft Palate Craniofac J 1991; 28(1):1–21.
6. Shaw WC, Dahl E, Asher-McDade C, et al: A six-center international study of treatment outcome in patients with clefts of the lip and palate: Part 5. General discussion and conclusions. Cleft Palate Craniofac J 1992; 29:413–418.
7. Farkas LG, Sohm P, Kolar JC, et al: Inclinations of the facial profile: Art versus reality. Plast Reconstr Surg 1985; 75:509.
8. Farkas LG: Anthropometrics of the Head and Face in Medicine. New York: Elsevier, 1981.
9. Warren DW, Duany LF, Fischer ND: Nasal pathway resistance in normal and cleft lip and palate subjects. Cleft Palate J 1969; 6:134–140.
10. Watson RM, Warren DW, Fisher ND: Nasal resistance, skeletal classification, and mouth breathing in orthodontic patients. Am J Orthod 1968; 54:367–379.
11. Gotfried HF, Thumfast WF: Pre- and postoperative middle ear function and muscle activity of the soft palate after total maxillary osteotomy in cleft patients. J Craniomaxillofac Surg 1987; 16:64.

12. DeReyter F, Diefendorf AO: Hearing sensitivity and measurements of middle ear and eustachian tube function after maxillary osteotomy with advancement surgery. J Oral Surg 1980; 38:343.

13. Baddour HM, Watson J, Erwin BJ, et al: Tympanometric changes after total maxillary osteotomy. J Oral Surg 1981; 39:336.

14. Mars M, Houston WJB: A preliminary study of facial growth and morphology in unoperated male unilateral cleft lip and palate subjects over 13 years of age. Cleft Palate J 1990; 27(1):7–10.

15. Mestre J, DeJesus J, Subtelney D: Unoperated oral cleft maturation. Am J Orthod 1960; 30:78–85.

16. Ortiz-Monasterio F, Rebeil AS, Valderrama M, Cruz R: Cephalometric measurements on adult patients with non-operated cleft palates. Plast Reconstr Surg 1959; 24:53–61.

17. Dingman RD, Dodenhoff TG: Surgical correction of mandibular deformities. In Grabb WE, Rosenstein SW, Bzoch DR (eds): Cleft Lip and Palate, pp 449–514. Boston: Little, Brown, 1971.

18. Wassmund, Lehrbuck: Der Praktischen Chirurgie Des Mund Und Der Kiefer. Leipzig: Barth, 1939.

19. Auxhausen G: Technik Und Ergebnisse Der Lippenplastik. Leipzig: Thieme, 1941.

20. Obwegeser H: Presentation on Oral and Maxillofacial Surgery. Walter Reed Army Medical Center, June 1966.

21. Obwegeser H: Surgical correction of maxillary deformities. In Grabb WE, Rosensteine SW, Bzoch DR (eds): Cleft Lip and Palate, p 515. Boston: Little, Brown, 1971.

22. Obwegeser H: Surgical correction of small or retrodisplaced maxillae: The dish face deformity. Plast Reconstr Surg 1969; 43:351.

23. Banks P: The surgical anatomy of secondary cleft lip and palate deformity and its significance in reconstruction. Br J Oral Surg 1983; 21:78.

24. Wilmar K: On LeFort I osteotomy. Scand Plast Reconstr Surg 1974, Suppl 12.

25. Braun TW, Sotereanos GC: Orthognathic and secondary cleft reconstruction of adolescent patients with cleft palate. J Oral Surg 1980; 38:425.

26. Tideman H, Stoelinga P, Gallia L: LeFort I advancement with segmental palatal osteotomies in patients with cleft palates. J Oral Surg 1980; 38:196.

27. Westbrook MT, West RA: Simultaneous maxillary advancement and closure of bilateral alveolar clefts and oronasal fistulas. J Oral Maxillofac Surg 1983; 41:260.

28. West RA: Treatment of secondary cleft deformities: Orthognathic surgery. In Peterson LJ, Indresano TA, Marciani RD, Roser SM (eds): Principles of Oral and Maxillofacial Surgery. Philadelphia: JB Lippincott, 1992.

29. Poole MD, Robinson PP, Vunn ME: Maxillary advancement in cleft palate patients. A modification of the LeFort I osteotomy and preliminary results. J Maxillofac Surg 1986; 14:123.

30. Freichofer HPM: Latitude and limitations of midface movements. Br J Oral Maxillofac Surg 1984; 22:393.

31. Posnick JC, Ewing MP: Skeletal stability after LeFort I maxillary advancement in patients with unilateral cleft lip and palate. Plast Reconstr Surg 1980; 85(5):706–710.

32. Stoelinga PJ, v.d. Vijver HR, Leenen RJ, et al: The prevention of relapse after maxillary osteotomies in cleft palate patients. J Craniomaxillofac Surg 1987; 15(6):326–331.

33. Teuscher U, Sailer HF: Stability of LeFort I osteotomy in class III cases with retropositioned maxillae. J Maxillofac Surg 1982; 10:80.

34. Garrison BT, Lapp TH, Bussard DA: The stability of LeFort I maxillary osteotomies in patients with simultaneous alveolar cleft bone grafts. J Oral Maxillofac Surg 1987; 45:761.

35. Mason A, Turvey TA, Warren DW: Speech considerations with maxillary advancement procedures. J Oral Surg 1980; 38:752.

36. Turvey TA, Frost D: Maxillary Advancement and Velopharyngeal Function in the Presence of Cleft Palate. Abstract of presentations at the 38th annual meeting of the American Cleft Palate Association, Lancaster, PA, May 1980.

37. Watzke I, Turvey TA, Warren D, Dalston R: Alterations in velopharyngeal function after maxillary advancement in cleft palate patients. J Oral Maxillofac Surg 1990; 48:685–689.

38. Dalston R, Turvey TA: Prognosticating Resonance Effects of Orthognathic Surgery. Program of the 50th annual meeting of the American Cleft Palate–Craniofacial Association (Abstract 156), Pittsburgh, May 1993.

39. Schwarz C, Gruner E: Logopaedic findings following advancement of the maxilla. J Maxillofac Surg 1976; 4:40.

40. Ruberg RL, Randall P, Whitaker LA: Preservation of a posterior pharyngeal flap during maxillary advancement. Plast Reconstr Surg 1976; 57:335.

41. Boyne PJ, Sands NR: Secondary bone grafting of residual alveolar and palatal defects. J Oral Surg 1982; 30:87–92.

42. Turvey TA, Vig KW, Moriarty J, Hoke J: Delayed bone grafting in the cleft maxilla and palate: A retrospective multidisciplinary analysis. Am J Orthod 1984; 86:244–256.

43. Åbyholm FE, Bargland O, Semb G: Secondary bone grafting of alveolar clefts. Scand J Plast Reconstr Surg 1981; 15:127–140.

44. Turvey TA, Tejera TJ, Tulloch C: Maxillary Advancement in Clefts: A Comparison Between Previously bone grafted and Simultaneously Bone Graft Repaired Patients. Abstract of the annual meeting of the American Association of Oral and Maxillofacial Surgeons, 1995, Toronto.

45. Enemark H, Sindet-Pedersen S, Bundgaard M: Long-term results after secondary bone grafting of alveolar clefts. J Oral Maxillofac Surg 1987; 45:913–918.

46. Robertson NRE, Jolleys A: Effects of early bone grafting in complete clefts of lip and palate. Reconstr Surg 1968; 42:414–421.

47. Jolleys A, Robertson NRE: A study of the effects of early bone grafting on complete clefts of the lip and palate—Five year study. Br J Plast Surg 1972; 25:229–237.

48. Phillips C, Medland WH, Fields HW, et al: Stability of surgical maxillary expansion. Adult Orthod Orthognath Surg 1992; 7:139–146.

49. Turvey TA: Maxillary expansion: A surgical technique based on anatomical considerations. J Maxillofac Surg 1985; 13:51–58.
50. Bell CNA, MacIntyre DR, Ross JW, et al: Pharyngoplasty: A hazard for nasotracheal intubation. Br J Oral Maxillofac Surg 1986; 24:212–216.
51. Becker DW, Bass CB, Williams VL: An aid to nasotracheal intubation in orthognathic surgery. Cleft Palate Craniofac J 1993; 30:350.
52. Kopp VJ, Rosenfeld MH, Turvey TA: Nasotracheal intubation in the presence of a pharyngeal flap. Accepted for Publication in Anesthesiology, in press.
53. Turvey TA: Maxillary Advancement, Closure of Oral Nasal Fistulas and Simultaneous Bone Graft Reconstruction of the Alveolus and Palate in Unilateral Cleft Deformities. Program of the 39th annual meeting of the American Cleft Palate Association, p 27. Denver: 1982.
54. Henderson D, Jackson TT: Nasomaxillary hypoplasia—The LeFort II osteotomy. Br J Oral Surg 1973; 11:77.
55. Krekmanov VL, Kahnberg KE: Transverse surgical correction of the maxilla. A modified procedure. J Craniomaxillofac Surg 1990; 18:332–334.
56. Proffit WR, Phillips C, Previtt JW, Turvey TA: Stability after surgical-orthodontic correction of skeletal class III malocclusion: II. Maxillary advancement. Int J Adult Orthognath Surg 1991; 6:7–18.
57. Obwegeser JA: Osteosynthesis in using biodegradable poly-p-Dioxanon (PDS II) in LeFort I osteotomy without postoperative intermaxillary fixation. J Craniomaxillofac Surg 1994; 22:129–137.
58. Marx RE: Philosophy and particulars of autogenous bone grafting. Oral Maxillofac Surg Clin North Am 1993; 5:599–613.
59. Schendel S, Delaire J: Functional musculoskeletal correction of secondary unilateral cleft lip deformities: Combined lip-nose correction and LeFort I osteotomy. J Maxillofac Surg 1981; 9:108–116.
60. Maher WP: Distribution of palatal and other arteries in cleft and non-cleft human palates. Cleft Palate J 1977; 14:1.
61. Bell WH, Fonseca RJ, Kennedy JW, Levy BM: Revascularization after total maxillary osteotomy. J Oral Surg 1975; 33:253–260.
62. Nelson RL, Path MG, Ogle RG, et al: Quantitation of blood flow after LeFort I osteotomy. J Oral Surg 1977; 35:10.
63. Drommer R: Selective arteriographic studies prior to LeFort osteotomy in patients with cleft lip and palate. J Maxillofac Surg 1979; 7:264.
64. Tobiasen JM: Psychosocial correlates of congenital facial clefts: A conceptualization and model. Cleft Palate J 1984; 21(3):131–139.
65. Tobiasen JM: Discussion of emotional and behavioral reaction to facially deformed patients before and after craniofacial surgery. Plast Reconstr Surg 1988; 77:409–410.
66. Tobiasen JM: Psychosocial adjustment to cleft lip and palate. In Bardach J, Morris HL (eds): Multidisciplinary Management of Cleft Lip and Palate, pp 820–825. Philadelphia: WB Saunders, 1990.

21

End-Stage Reconstruction in the Complex Cleft Lip/Palate Patient

Larry M. Wolford and David A. Cottrell

Patients with cleft lip and palate malformations that have been partially or completely repaired may present in adolescence or early adulthood with malocclusions; maxillomandibular skeletal alignment discrepancies; missing, deformed, or malpositioned dental units; residual oronasal fistulas; and alveolar clefts. In addition, deformities of the adjacent hard and soft tissue structures result in nasal and lip defects, midface hypoplasia, and other defects. Diagnostic and treatment considerations also include nasal airway obstruction, speech disorders (i.e., velopharyngeal incompetence, articulation disorder), and psychosocial problems. The focus of this chapter is predominantly functional and esthetic considerations for the end-stage reconstruction of the complex cleft. Discussion includes diagnosis and treatment sequencing, specific surgical procedures, as well as the effects of surgery on soft tissue changes and growth if performed during adolescence.

NATURE OF THE DEFORMITY

Jaw growth in the unrepaired cleft lip and palate population is generally favorable,[1-6] with probably no significant difference in the distribution of vertical deformities or class I, II, or III skeletal jaw relationships, when compared with the noncleft population, except that posterior crossbite may be more common. Most growth aberrations seen in the cleft population result from surgical repairs and/or other types of management. These include deformities affecting the jaws, alveolus, dentition, and associated soft tissue structures. Following is a list of procedures commonly performed during childhood and their potential effects on facial growth.

1. Repair of cleft lip: Repair affects anterior maxillary alveolar morphology but does not significantly effect other changes in the craniofacial complex.[7-11] The morphologic disturbance is probably related to the extent of tissue undermining.

2. Repair of alveolar cleft: When performed primarily (within the first 2 years), maxillary growth inhibition is the usual response. Several authors have reported early and intermediate repairs, using specific techniques, that may have less unfavorable effect on craniofacial growth.[12-16]

3. Repair of hard and soft cleft palate: The usual response following these procedures is a decrease in the posterior vertical maxillary height; the anteroposterior (AP) development of the teeth and alveolar process and maxillary transverse growth and basal maxillary length may be affected.[17-19] Periosteal stripping at the time of surgery and the resulting scar are the most likely reasons for this response.

4. Pharyngeal flap: Pharyngeal flaps have a profound effect on facial growth and development, decreasing the AP and transverse growth, and in many cases increasing the vertical component of growth.[20] It is postulated that the increased vertical maxillary growth occurs because of altered breathing patterns and a mouth-open posture.

5. Repair of cleft lip, alveolus, and palate: Complete repair of the cleft lip/palate may result in severe maxillary retrusion and a significant clockwise rotation of the maxilla.[7]

6. Orthognathic surgery: Surgery arrests AP growth of the maxilla and may affect further vertical and transverse growth in the patient. Patients grow predominantly vertically following surgery.[21]

Patients with clefts may have missing permanent teeth, deformed teeth, or supernumerary teeth in the cleft area. Some reach adolescence or adulthood with unrepaired oronasal fistulas and alveolar clefts, even though the primary cleft lip and/or palate has been repaired. The primary repairs may have untoward effects on subsequent maxillary growth in the AP, transverse, and vertical dimension. The mandible may also exhibit an abnormal growth vector or pathologic growth characteristics unrelated to the cleft deformity.[19] This may include conditions such as condylar hyperplasia, condylar resorption, internal derangement of the temporomandibular joint, and others. The severity of the residual deformities of the repaired lip and nose may also contribute to functional and esthetic concerns. As a result of all these factors, moderate to severe deformities of the jaws can develop, affecting not only the basal bone and alveolus, but also the alignment and position of the primary and permanent teeth. Anterior and posterior crossbite, midface hypoplasia, vertical and transverse maxillary deficiency, residual nasal defects, and speech problems are often the consequences observed in this population. The resultant deformities can create major functional, esthetic, and psychosocial problems.

With cleft lip and palate, a number of coexisting problems may require specific attention. Each problem area is addressed and treatment considerations presented. In general, end-stage reconstruction is considered when patients are in late adolescence or early adulthood. The treatment is commonly delayed until this time because of growth factors.

TREATMENT SEQUENCING IN THE PATIENT WITH END-STAGE CLEFT

In adolescent and adult patients with clefts, it is usually best to correct the underlying dental, maxillary, mandibular, and infraorbital deformities prior to other cosmetic and functional repairs. This allows the overlying soft tissues to adjust to the altered skeletal and dento-osseous structures. For predictable results, external nasal reconstruction and lip revisions are preferably done as a secondary procedure. However, simultaneous orthognathic surgery, lip revisions, and major rhinoplasty surgery can be performed in selected patients with unilateral clefts. When performing simultaneous orthognathic and nasal procedures in the patient with a unilateral cleft, a nasoendotracheal tube is usually required for the orthognathic surgical portion. Orthognathic surgery, using rigid fixation, is performed initially. The endotracheal tube is then changed to the oral position, and the nasal/lip and/or rhinoplasty procedures are completed. In the patient with a bilateral cleft, particularly one with coexisting alveolar clefts, it is imperative to stage the lip-nose and external rhinoplasty procedures separately from the orthognathic procedures, so that the vascular supply to the anterior portion of the maxilla (premaxilla) is not jeopardized. The premaxilla is vascularized through the nasolabial vessels from the septum, columella, and the upper lip.[22] Major lip-nose revisions in the bilateral cleft, if done simultaneously with the alveolar cleft grafting and orthognathic surgery, may result in avascular necrosis of the premaxilla.

Orthognathic surgical sequencing follows a specific order to improve the predictability of the procedures. Mandibular osteotomies with rigid fixation are completed first. This is followed by maxillary surgery with rigid fixation, including closure of oronasal fistulas and grafting of the alveolar clefts. Rigid fixation is mandatory if rhinoplastic procedures are simultaneously performed. After completion of the orthognathic surgery, the nasoendotracheal tube is removed and an oral endotracheal tube inserted to maintain the airway while the rhinoplasty procedure is performed. A tracheostomy is rarely indicated or necessary in any of these cases.

MAXILLARY DEFORMITIES

Although the details regarding orthognathic surgery in patients with clefts are discussed elsewhere in this book, the indications for some surgical modifications are highlighted.

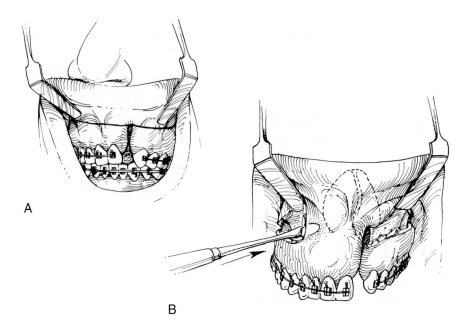

Figure 21–1. *A*, A circumvestibular incision can be used if there is adequate blood supply to the maxillary segments through the palatal tissues. The incision begins posterior to the zygomatic buttress and extends anterior and across to the buttress on the opposite side. The buttress area incisions can be curved superiorly. In the alveolar cleft and oronasal fistula area, the incision is generally directed toward the superior portion of the fistula. *B*, When vascular compromise to the maxilla exists, it may necessitate the maintenance of a buccal pedicle. Through two horizontal posterior incisions, access to the nasal septum is obtained by either a vertical midline incision or a tunneling approach beneath the labial flap.

Oronasal Fistulas and Alveolar Clefts

Oronasal fistulas are frequently closed and alveolar clefts bone grafted prior to eruption of the permanent teeth into the cleft area and prior to orthognathic surgery. However, if the alveolar graft can be delayed until orthognathic surgery is performed so as not to jeopardize tooth eruption or periodontal health of the teeth, the orthognathic surgery and alveolar cleft grafting can be performed in one operation. This eliminates untoward effects on growth and vascular supply that may be created by the alveolar cleft grafting and associated soft tissues procedures, when they are performed in a younger patient.

Maxillary Viability

Of importance in maxillary orthognathic surgery in patients with clefts is the evaluation for significant vascular compromise to the maxillary palatal tissue and dental alveolus, particularly if additional segmental maxillary surgery is planned. This is difficult to precisely determine, but the number of previous surgeries; presence of soft tissue scarring, fibrosis, or blanching; and analysis of previous operative reports are helpful in quantifying the vascular supply. Arteriography may be indicated in questionable cases to determine blood flow to the maxilla. If there is no significant vascular compromise in the unilateral cleft, the traditional circumvestibular incision can be used (Fig. 21–1A). If there is significant vascular compromise, labial soft tissue pedicle flaps to the anterior segments may be necessary to assure vascularity and viability to these segments, particularly if the maxilla is segmentalized (Fig. 21–1B).

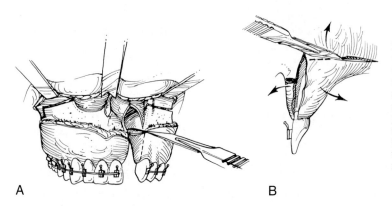

Figure 21–2. *A*, A horizontal incision is made parallel to the palatal plane through the mucoperiosteum on the lateral nasal wall, as well as on the septal side of the palate. A vertical incision is made in the cleft area on both the greater and the lesser segment. The incision is located to incorporate enough tissue on the palatal flap side to assure adequate tension-free closure of the palatal soft tissue wall. *B*, The position of the flaps on the greater segment and the direction of elevation and mobilization are demonstrated. Minimal reflection of tissue is necessary.

Figure 21–3. *A,* Elevation of tissue flaps off the lateral nasal wall and nasal septum is performed. The flaps are brought together and stitched with resorbable sutures. *B,* Horizontal mattress sutures are used to create closure of the palatal flaps, achieving a water-tight closure.

A

B

An anterior soft tissue pedicle to the premaxilla is necessary in the bilateral cleft to maintain vascularity and viability to the premaxilla (see Fig. 21–7*A*).

Unilateral Cleft Soft Tissue Flaps

In the unilateral cleft with vascular compromise, an anterior pedicle can be maintained on the anterior portion of the greater segment (see Fig. 21–1*B*). Two horizontal incisions are made posteriorly. On the greater segment side, the incision is generally extended from the cuspid to the zygomatic buttress. On the lesser segment, the incision usually extends from the medial portion of the oronasal fistula/alveolar cleft area to the zygomatic buttress area. Either a tunneling approach through the horizontal incisions or a small vertical midline incision can be used to reach the nasal septum. Flap designs for closure of oronasal fistulas in the alveolar cleft area (Fig. 21–2) incorporate the tissues lining the cleft to provide closure of the three soft tissue walls (i.e., palatal, nasal, and buccal). This allows maximal efficient use of these tissues to close the palatal and nasal floor of the alveolar cleft, while minimizing reflection of tissue from the bony segments. Following completion of the osteotomies and mobilization of the maxilla, the soft tissue nasal and palatal walls are closed, usually prior to stabilization of the maxilla. This facilitates access to the tissue flaps (Fig. 21–3). Rigid stabilization and grafting of the maxilla and bone grafting of the alveolar cleft are then completed (Fig. 21–4). The labial aspect of the oronasal fistula can be closed with a direct local flap, particularly when the cleft is very narrow or decreased in size, by moving the greater and lesser segments together (Fig. 21–5). When inadequate tissues are available for direct closure, a trapezoid lip flap (Fig. 21–6) (preferred by the

Figure 21–4. *A,* A maxillary step osteotomy is utilized in the maxilla. The step area provides an additional place to bone graft and maximize the maxillary stability. The osteotomies are carried back to the pterygoid plates, and the pterygoid plates are separated with a thin, curved osteotome. This area can also be used for grafting as long as the pterygoid plate remains intact. *B,* The maxilla is advanced, downgrafted, and stabilized with bone plates, occlusal splint if necessary, and appropriate grafting. The authors prefer the use of porous block hydroxyapatite for grafting the orthognathic defects. Cancellous bone is preferred for the alveolar graft area.

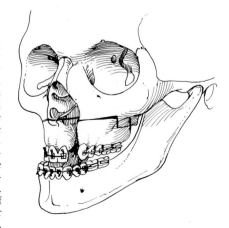

A

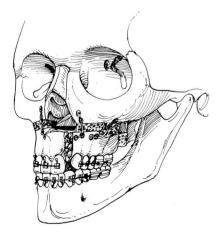

B

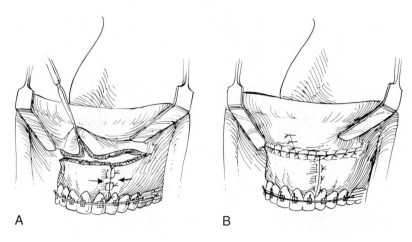

Figure 21–5. *A,* If the segments are advanced to close the cleft area, usually direct closure with the labial flaps is accomplished. *B,* Closure of the circumvestibular incision with a V-Y closure helps maintain thickness of the upper lip and vermilion. The labial aspect of the incision line is elevated to help provide the vertical closure, and then the traditional closure is continued and completed.

authors) or a rotational flap can be used. The trapezoid lip flap provides an excellent base width-to-length ratio and is easy to advance to cover the bone graft at the completion of the osseous surgery.

Bilateral Cleft Soft Tissue Flaps

In bilateral alveolar clefts, the surgical design generally dictates maintaining an anterior pedicle to the premaxilla. Access to the lateral maxillary walls is accomplished through bilateral horizontal vestibular incisions extending from the medial margin of the labial aspect of the oronasal fistula and carried posteriorly, curving upward at the zygomatic buttress area (Fig. 21–7A). The premaxilla is pedicled to the upper lip so that the blood supply is maintained (Fig. 21–7B–E). This allows closure of at least two soft tissue walls (the nasal floor and the palatal aspect), using the tissue lining the cleft. Following completion of the maxillary osteotomies (Fig. 21–8A) and mobilization, the palatal and nasal flaps are closed. Closure of the palatal aspect of the bilateral cleft is the most difficult and technique-sensitive of all of the flap procedures. The palatal tissue of the premaxilla is mobilized very carefully to help close the palatal soft tissue defect. These flaps receive their blood supply from the upper lip, through the premaxilla. If the segments are moved together, decreasing the width of the clefts, the labial sides may also be directly closed (Fig. 21–9A). Otherwise, the labial side is closed with the trapezoid lip flap (Fig. 21–9B) or a rotational flap.[23]

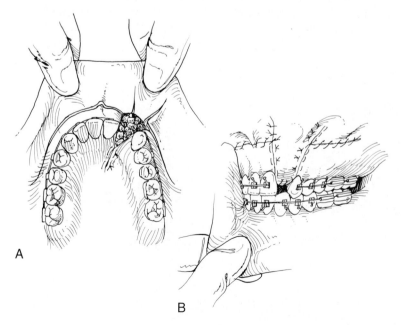

Figure 21–6. *A,* A trapezoid flap may be indicated to close the labial side if a wide soft tissue defect is present. Two divergent incisions are made out into the lip from the vestibular incision area. *B,* The flap is undermined to the level of the orbicularis oris muscle, and then advanced over the cleft area to attach to the palatal flaps. The base/length ratio of this flap design is very good.

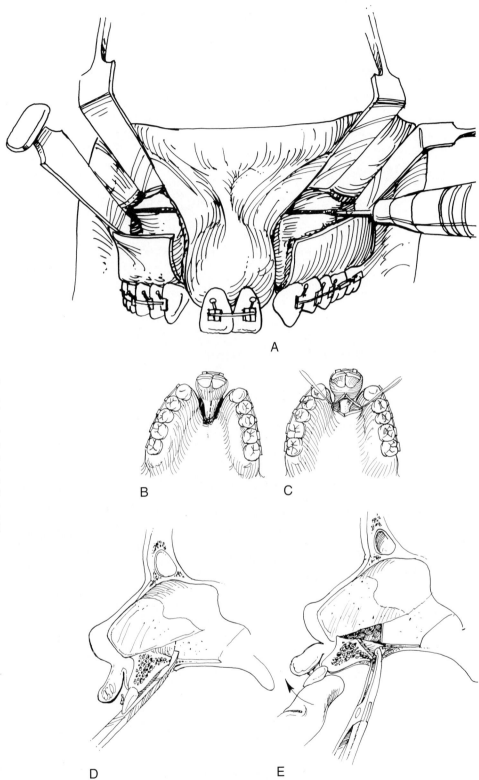

Figure 21–7. *A,* In the patient with a bilateral cleft, bilateral posterior horizontal incisions are made, beginning at the oral-nasal fistula area and extending behind and upward over the zygomatic buttress. An anterior pedicle is maintained on the premaxilla. The vertical incisions in the cleft area are made similarly to those made for the unilateral cleft to provide closure of the nasal floor and palate, but with minimal reflection of tissue from the premaxilla. *B, C,* and *D,* The premaxilla is mobilized by cutting vertically through the vomer portion of the septum and rotating anteriorly, separating it from the cartilaginous septum. *E,* Areas of the vomer or cartilaginous septum may require removal if they are interfering with the movement and repositioning of the premaxilla.

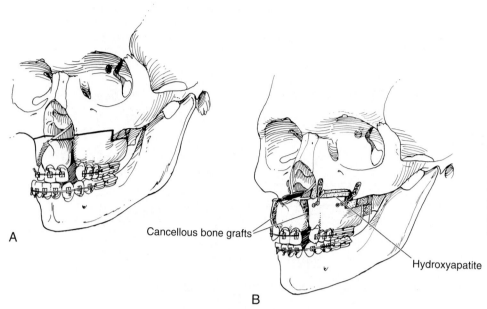

Cancellous bone grafts

Hydroxyapatite

A

B

Figure 21–8. *A,* A lateral view of the osteotomy design is seen for the patient with a bilateral cleft. The maxillary step osteotomy technique provides an additional area for grafting in the maxillary step. *B,* The maxilla has been advanced and stabilized with bone plates and porous block hydroxyapatite or bone grafts. Cancellous bone grafts are placed in the bilateral cleft areas.

Osteotomy Design and Stabilization

With orthognathic procedures on unilateral or bilateral cleft deformities, the maxillary step osteotomy is used (see Figs. 21–4 and 21–8).[24] The maxillary step osteotomy permits more accurate determination of advancement and vertical repositioning of the maxilla. The step area also provides an additional area to bone graft to maximize AP stability.

Decreasing the size of the cleft area by advancing the maxilla on the cleft side (i.e., placing the cleft side into a class II cuspid relationship when the lateral incisor is missing) eliminates the need for a bridge in the cleft area and decreases the volume of bone required to graft the alveolar defect. The result is improved graft maintenance, with fewer periodontal defects. In addition, maxillary expansion is minimized when the cuspids are advanced into a class II position. However, the required additional advancement of the maxilla on the cleft side creates a greater challenge for adequate mobilization and stabilization of the maxilla. In addition, some patients may be at greater risk of developing velopharyngeal inadequacy with the additional advancement.

The stabilization of maxillary osteotomies in patients with clefts is more difficult than in the noncleft patient. Specific steps are incorporated into the procedure to minimize relapse. Adequate mobilization must be achieved with minimal tension on the maxilla when placed in the new position. Four bone plates are used to stabilize the

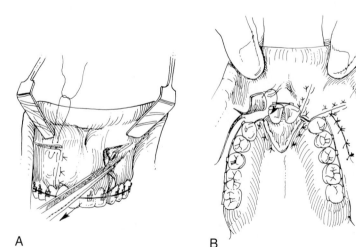

A

B

Figure 21–9. *A,* The segments were moved together and direct closure of the labial flaps is accomplished. *B,* Lateral trapezoid flaps may be necessary to close the labial soft tissue defect. The palatal flaps are usually closed before application of rigid fixation.

maxilla. Each plate is secured with a minimum of four bone screws, two above and two below the osteotomy line (see Figs. 21–4*B*, 21–8*B*). Bone grafting or insertion of an alloplast may be necessary to fill osseous defects. The authors prefer the use of porous block hydroxyapatite (PBHA) (Interpore 200, Interpore International, Irvine, California) to provide and maintain vertical, AP, and transverse stability of the maxilla.[25, 26, 27] The PBHA functions as a matrix for bone and soft tissue ingrowth. Stability has been favorable when the material is used in conjunction with rigid fixation, as described earlier. Wardrop and Wolford reported similar stability in cleft and noncleft patients undergoing maxillary advancements and/or downgrafting when rigid fixation and PBHA were used.[25] In bilateral clefts, it is frequently difficult to attach a bone plate on the premaxillary segment because of (1) decreased bone structure; (2) necessity of limiting soft tissue stripping; and (3) location of tooth roots. Stabilization of the premaxillary segment using an occlusal splint or other methods may be necessary. Autogenous cancellous bone grafting in the alveolar cleft is indicated if the teeth are to be orthodontically moved into the cleft or if eruption of teeth through the cleft is anticipated. Otherwise, portions of cortical bone can be used. PBHA should *not* be used to graft alveolar clefts because of the common incidence of infection and loss of the graft. This should not be confused with the favorable stability and healing properties of using this material in the maxillary osteotomy sites, even those communicating with the maxillary sinus. Granular hydroxyapatite (HA) can be used for esthetic reasons in alveolar clefts, but it will not provide bone growth through the cleft area and should not be used if orthodontic movements or tooth eruption into the cleft are anticipated. Mixing granular HA and cancellous bone provides a well-healed graft with less loss of bone height, but it likewise prevents tooth movement and eruption through it. The authors do not recommend the use of freeze-dried bone for alveolar cleft grafting because of experiences with a high rate of infection, poor revascularization, excessive resorption, extrusion of bone particles, and other complications.

Transverse Expansion

Often, the cleft maxilla is narrow and may require surgical expansion. There are three soft tissue techniques that may be employed to permit the surgical expansion of the maxilla, yet maintain a viable blood supply to the segments. These include vomer flaps, split-thickness palatal flap, and midpalatal incision.

Vomer Flaps

The palatal tissue is incised directly over the vomerian base in an AP direction. The mucoperiosteum is then reflected off the vomer, either unilaterally or bilaterally, to allow expansion of the maxilla (Fig. 21–10). The residual palatal defect is left to heal

Figure 21–10. A vomer flap is prepared by (*A*) incising directly over the vomer in either unilateral or bilateral clefts and then (*B*) reflecting the mucoperiosteum off of the vomer to allow expansion. Illustrated here is the unilateral cleft. The *arrows* indicate the direction of expansion of the lesser segment.

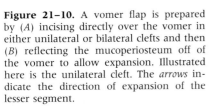

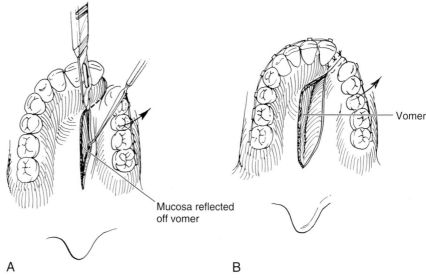

Mucosa reflected off vomer

Vomer

A

B

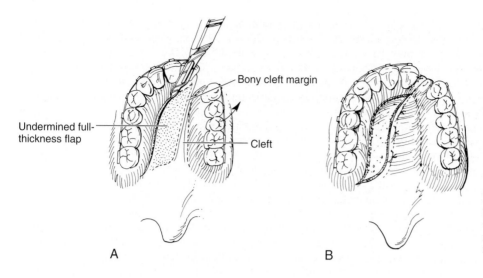

Figure 21–11. *A*, Demonstrated is the split-thickness palatal flap from the greater segment on the unilateral cleft and dissecting over to and then through the mucoperiosteum at the margin of the bony cleft. Preservation of the anterior branches of the palatal vessels with the greater segment is important for maintaining good viability. For small expansions, a full-thickness flap may be utilized, particularly if the vascularity to the maxilla is very good. *B*, Holes can be placed adjacent to the margin of the palatal bone and the edge of the split thickness flap sutured to the bony margin to help prevent the development of oronasal fistulas.

by secondary intention. When properly performed, this flap does not violate the separation between the nasal and oral cavity. This approach may impose some limitations on the amount of maxillary advancement achievable.

Split-Thickness Palatal Flap

A palatal incision is made over the lateral aspect of the palatal bone, on one side of the cleft. A split-thickness dissection of the mucosa to the bony cleft margin is performed. This allows expansion of the maxilla with soft tissue coverage over the expanded palatal area and helps prevent oronasal fistula development (Fig. 21–11*A*). It is best to make the incision on the side with the largest bony shelf. If needed, the lateral flap margin can be sutured to the palatal shelf through holes placed in the bony margin along the cleft (Fig. 21–11*B*). This is a delicate technique, but it is effective when large expansions are performed. Careful design and extreme care must be employed so that the split-thickness flap and osseous segments maintain viability.

Midpalatal Incision

The palatal midline is incised directly into the nasal cavity, and the maxilla is expanded. This creates an oronasal fistula (Fig. 21–12). The fistula must then be closed secondarily after completion of the healing of the maxilla. As a secondary procedure, mobilization of palatal flaps or the use of a tongue flap is indicated to close the residual fistula. This technique is most appropriate in patients with fibrotic palatal tissue and vascular compromise.

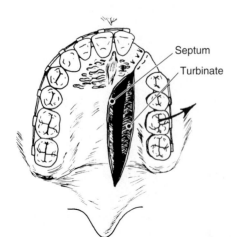

Figure 21–12. Patients having significant fibrosis of the palatal tissues, and requiring a major expansion, may benefit from the creation of an oronasal fistula. This is done by incising into the nasal cavity along the midline of the palate. As a secondary procedure, the fistula is closed with palatal flaps, tongue flaps, or other techniques.

Alar Base Cinch Suture and V-Y Lip Closure

Maxillary surgery, particularly advancement, affects the morphologic characteristics of the nose for three reasons: (1) the periosteum and perinasal musculatures are reflected from the bone in the perinasal area and the relaxation of these tissues allows the alar bases to widen; (2) the postsurgical edema causes further widening of the alar base structures during healing; and (3) anterior repositioning of the supportive osseous structures widens the alar bases. The nasal changes that occur with maxillary advancement include increased alar base width, increased nares width, and increased rotation and projection of the nasal tip. Inadequate management of the soft tissues during closure of the maxillary vestibular incisions contributes to shortening of the upper lip and AP thinning of the upper lip.

After stabilization of the maxilla and prior to closure of the maxillary vestibular incisions, the alar base cinch suture is placed intraorally through the perinasal musculature and the fibro-adipose tissue of the alar base on one side of the nose. Then, in figure-eight fashion, it is passed through the perinasal musculature and fibro-adipose tissue of the opposite alar base (Fig. 21–13). The technique works well when the alar widths are symmetric. Direct control of the alar bases is achievable by tightening the suture. In the presence of alar base asymmetry, an independent suture is passed through each nasal ala and attached to the septum or to a hole drilled through the anterior nasal spine. This permits independent control of each alar base. This is usually necessary in the unilateral cleft. The preferred suture material is 2–0 PDS, because it maintains strength through the initial healing phase, but it subsequently resorbs. Nonresorbable suture material can be used with the added risk of infection and/or long-term discomfort. The advantages of the alar base cinch suture are as follows: (1) it controls the alar base width, (2) it minimizes the vertical shortening of the lip, and (3) it maintains a greater anteroposterior thickness of the upper lip. Guymon and associates reported on the effects of the alar cinch suture and V-Y closure of the vestibular incision for maxillary osteotomies. The data revealed that when the suture was used, the alar base expanded an average 3.5% of the amount of original alar base width.[28] In a matched sample of patients with the same spatial movements of the maxilla, but without the suture, the alar base width increased 10.8% of the original width. A V-Y closure of the circumvestibular incision (if used instead of maintaining anterior soft tissue pedicles) also improves upper lip esthetics by increasing the amount of vermilion exposed and thus maintaining lip thickness (see Fig. 21–5).

Lip/Nose Changes With Maxillary Advancement

With maxillary advancement, the soft tissue response in the patient with a cleft is more favorable than response of soft tissues in noncleft groups. Studies by Kawauchi and coworkers compared the effects of a 5-mm maxillary advancement on the soft

Figure 21–13. *A* and *B,* The alar base cinch suture is made through an intraoral approach by passing a 2–0 suture through the fibroadipose tissue of one alar base to the fibroadipose tissue of the opposite alar base in a figure-eight pattern. Individual attachment of sutures from each alar base to the anterior nasal spine area or to the septum may be necessary in asymmetric cases.

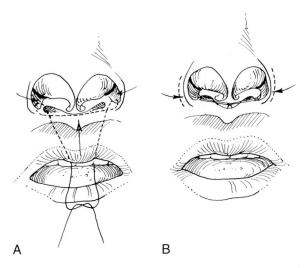

A   B

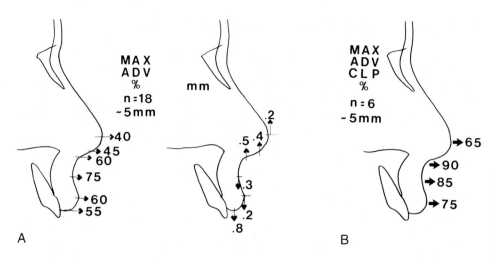

Figure 21–14. *A,* Soft tissue changes are seen relative to maxillary advancement of 5 mm in noncleft patients. On the left, the percentage of horizontal soft tissue change correlates to the amount of dento-osseous advancement. On the right, the vertical changes are measured in millimeters. No vertical movements of the maxilla were done in this group of patients. *B,* The horizontal soft tissue changes are observed with a 5 mm advancement in patients with clefts. There is a greater soft tissue/hard tissue change in this group. Most likely, this is the result of fibrosis in the lip from previous lip repairs.

tissues in cleft and noncleft patients (Fig. 21–14*A, B*).[29, 30] The difference in soft tissue change between the two groups is most likely the result of the significant scarring and fibrosis in the repaired cleft lip. This results in less thinning of the upper lip in the cleft group. The nasal tip is advanced further forward in the cleft group, and this is the result of the pre-existing lack of support in the nose of the patient with a cleft. With the support to the alar bases being increased, the nasal tip advances further than in the noncleft group.

Effects of Maxillary Osteotomies in Growing Patients With Clefts

Correction of vertical maxillary excess (VME) in noncleft adolescents results in decreased AP growth of the maxilla but continued vertical growth until maturation.[31–33] Friehofer demonstrated decreased AP growth of the maxilla following maxillary advancement in patients with clefts.[34] Wolford and associates reported that orthognathic surgery in the growing patient with clefts had untoward effects, with postsurgical decreases in vertical, AP, and transverse maxillary growth.[21] In this study, maxillary osteotomies and alveolar cleft bone grafting were performed simultaneously. Whether the maxillary osteotomies or alveolar cleft bone grafting, or both, caused the deficiency in growth was not determined. The facial growth vector in many of the cases changed from a down and forward vector to a vertical and posterior rotational vector. SNA decreased in angulation because the nasofrontal growth proceeded, whereas maxillary growth did not. Previous studies demonstrated relatively normal vertical growth with reduced AP growth of the maxilla in noncleft after maxillary surgery. Therefore, alveolar cleft bone grafting and associated soft tissue procedures may play a role in decreasing the vertical growth of the alveolus and further decreased AP growth of the maxilla.[31–33] Ross observed that repair of the alveolus by bone grafting in patients under 9 years resulted in reduced AP maxillary growth. Repair in patients under 10 years resulted in decreased vertical maxillary growth.[14] Semb claimed that alveolar cleft bone grafting, even in patients as young as 8 years, had no adverse effect on AP or vertical growth.[13] Other findings in Wolford and associates' study include a fairly consistent increase in maxillary incisor angulation and a tendency for the occlusion to develop into a class III relationship. Pre-existing pharyngeal flaps further alter maxillary growth following osteotomies by causing a greater decrease in SNA angulation but increased vertical growth. Maxillary osteotomies in patients with clefts are most predictable following completion of growth, and this should be used selectively in growing patients. Indications for maxillary osteotomies in the growing patient may include the following: (1) significant functional deformity, (2) significant esthetic deformity, and/or (3) significant psychosocial problems associated with the deformity.

INFRAORBITAL HYPOPLASIA

In the severe expression of maxillary deficient cleft deformities, there may also be hypoplasia of the infraorbital and zygomatic malar eminence areas. When these deficiencies are present, they can be improved by augmentation. Choices of techniques include, modified LeFort III (zygomaticomaxillary) osteotomies, zygomatico-orbital osteotomies, or augmentation with grafting materials such as cranial bone, HA, hard tissue replacement (HTR) alloplast, and other materials. The augmentation can be done at the same time as the orthognathic surgery or as a secondary procedure.

NASAL AIRWAY OBSTRUCTION

Nasal airway obstruction is common in patients with clefts and may be caused by one or more of the following: (1) deviated nasal septum or other types of septal deformities or pathology; (2) hypertrophied turbinates (real or relative); (3) nasal polyps, or other pathology; (4) posterior choanae deficiencies; (5) hypertrophied adenoid tissues and/or tonsils that may be obliterating the nasal pharynx or posterior choanae; (6) narrow and/or decreased size of nares (luminal valve) or intranasal strictures, and (7) presence of a pharyngeal flap. Management of nasal airway obstruction is an important adjunctive aspect of providing optimal care of the patient with a cleft.

Nasal Septal Deviation

Nasal septal deformities can contribute to three common problems: (1) esthetic deformity such as nasal tip deviation, particularly in the patient with a unilateral cleft; (2) nasal airway obstruction; and (3) sinus problems created by blockage of the normal sinus drainage system (Fig. 21–15). In unilateral cleft lip/palate, the base of the septum is usually deviated toward the noncleft side and the dorsal portion toward the cleft side. Bone spurs can also develop and contribute to nasal obstruction. In bilateral palatal clefts, the septum is usually centered, but it may be increased in width, particularly in the vomerian portion.

Septoplasty may be indicated for correcting these functional and esthetic problems. The nasal septum is approached by one of three methods: (1) subnasal approach with access through the LeFort I down-fracture procedure (see Fig. 21–17);[35] (2) intranasal approach, which is the traditional technique used in septal rhinoplasty; and (3) external rhinoplasty technique, which approaches the septum by separating the upper and lower lateral cartilages and reaching the septum from the superior and anterior direction. Through the subnasal approach, the septoplasty is performed at the same time as the LeFort I osteotomy. The subnasal approach provides optimal access to the cartilaginous septum, as well as the vomer and perpendicular plate of the ethmoid bone. If anterior soft tissue pedicles are maintained, the subnasal approach does not provide adequate access, so one of the other techniques can be used. The deformed septal cartilage and bone can be corrected by employing the technique the surgeon feels

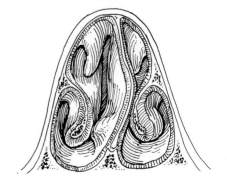

Figure 21–15. Nasal septal deviation can cause blockage of the nasal airway (left side). On the right, a bone spur is present at the inferior base of the septum and also can block the airway. Treatment usually requires septoplasty, with removal of bone spurs or other pathology.

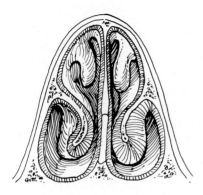

Figure 21–16. Hypertrophy of the turbinates can create nasal airway obstruction. Treatment generally involves partial turbinectomies.

appropriate. Intranasal suturing and/or splints can be used to readapt the mucoperiosteum and mucoperichondrium into proper position to decrease the incidence of hematoma and maintain straightness and thinness of the septum.

Inferior Turbinate Hyperplasia

The inferior turbinates can be enlarged and can cause nasal airway obstruction (Fig. 21–16) for the following reasons: (1) bony enlargement; (2) hyperplastic mucosa and submucosal tissue; and (3) vasomotor changes. Patients with cleft deformities can have nasal airway obstruction secondary to absolute or relative enlargement of the turbinates. Transverse deficiency of the nasal cavity or a deviated nasal septum may make normal-sized turbinates appear large. Partial or complete turbinectomies may be indicated in these patients, as well as in those with absolute turbinate hyperplasia, to improve the functional nasal airway. Turbinectomies may be necessary in superior repositioning of the maxilla to eliminate bony interferences with the turbinates, although in cleft patients, vertical maxillary excess is uncommon.

Turbinectomies can be directly performed through the subnasal (Fig. 21–17) approach following the maxillary downfracture. An incision is made through the nasal mucoperiosteum along the entire length of the nasal floor. This exposes the entire inferior turbinate, including its most posterior extent. Submucous, partial, or complete resection of the soft and hard tissues can be performed as deemed necessary by the surgeon. Partial resection of the turbinate can be coupled with out-fracturing (into the sinus) of the remaining portion of the turbinate, particularly when the transverse dimension of the nose is narrow. Suturing the out-fractured turbinate to the medial sinus wall will be helpful in maintaining stability of the out-fracture procedure. If the out-fractured turbinates are not stabilized in a lateral position by suturing, splinting, or packing, relapse may be significant and may result in partial reobstruction.

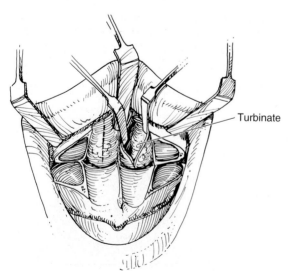

Turbinate

Figure 21–17. The subnasal approach provides excellent access to the turbinates. By incising the nasal mucoperiosteum, direct access to the turbinate along its entire length is gained. The same approach also provides access to the nasal septum so that a septoplasty can be done from this subnasal approach. The same approach can be used to gain access for removal of adenoid tissue in the superior nasopharyngeal area.

Adenoid Hypertrophy

Hypertrophied adenoids that extend into the nasopharynx or in the posterior choanal area can cause nasal airway obstruction. Adenoid tissue can be approached directly through the subnasal incision (as with the turbinectomies and septoplasty), or by the more routine oropharyngeal approach. The subnasal approach allows direct visualization at the superior aspect of the posterior pharyngeal and choanal area. Adenoid curettes can be used to clear the area of obstructive adenoid mass. The more traditional oral approach to the pharyngeal adenoid tissue can be used to remove tissue located lower on the pharyngeal wall. Before adenoidectomy, the patient should have a speech evaluation. The adenoid mass sometimes contributes to velopharyngeal function, and its removal could potentially lead to velopharyngeal inadequacy. Preoperative evaluation involves nonphonating and phonating (E or S sounds) lateral cephalometric radiographs, nasopharyngoscopy, cinefluoroscopy, and speech evaluation.

Maxillary Sinus Pathology

Maxillary sinus disease can exist in the patient with a cleft and can be caused by blockage of the sinus ostium by a deviated nasal septum, turbinate hyperplasia, polyps, allergies, chronic sinusitis, mucous retention cysts, and other forms of sinus pathology. Decreased nasopharyngeal drainage because of a pharyngeal flap may also increase the likelihood of sinusitis. With orthognathic surgery, pre-existing maxillary sinus problems usually improve or remain the same. Pathology that may be present in the sinuses prior to surgery can be addressed at the time of maxillary surgery. The subnasal approach allows the surgeon to remove mucous retention cysts or polyps, irrigate and débride sinus infections, remove diseased tissues, and other procedures. A nasal septoplasty and/or partial turbinectomy to eliminate nasal airway obstruction may also improve sinus function by eliminating obstruction of the ostium and improving the sinus drainage system. Iatrogenic antrostomies often result from maxillary orthognathic procedures, which may improve drainage. Surgical nasal antrostomies may be necessary in some cases to further improve drainage and to allow irrigation of the sinuses.

Nasal Polyps

Occasionally, nasal polyps cause nasal airway obstruction in the cleft population. These can be removed by either direct intranasal approach or through the subnasal approach when the turbinectomies and nasal septoplasty are being done.

MANDIBULAR DEFORMITIES

Ross has observed subtle differences in mandibular morphology in patients with clefts, but the size of the mandibular basal bone appears genetically determined.[19] The majority of patients exhibit relatively normal AP mandibular growth. Silva Filho and coworkers have demonstrated that mandibular morphology and spatial position are inherent, and not greatly influenced by cleft lip/plate repair.[7] Transverse, vertical, and AP deficiencies in the development of the maxilla may affect the dental and alveolar morphology of the mandible. Other functional and environmental factors may also influence mandibular growth and morphology.

Specific procedures may be indicated for the mandible to correct associated deformities. In general, the authors prefer to correct the mandibular deformity with mandibular ramus sagittal split osteotomies, using rigid fixation with the bicortical screw technique.[36] Additional procedures that may be indicated in the mandible include subapical osteotomies, body osteotomies, and genioplasty procedures. If active excessive growth of the mandible occurs either unilaterally or bilaterally, and it is anticipated that the growth may continue beyond maturation, a high condylectomy may be necessary to arrest the abnormal growth. It has been demonstrated by Wolford and coworkers that condylectomy stops subsequent mandibular growth on the treated sides.[37]

VELOPHARYNGEAL INSUFFICIENCY AND MAXILLARY ADVANCEMENT

Maxillary advancement generally increases the anteroposterior dimensions of the nasopharynx, resulting in an increased distance for the soft palate to move during velopharyngeal closure.[38] Most patients have sufficient compensatory reserve to ensure normal velopharyngeal closure. Persistent hypernasality following maxillary advancement in the noncleft population is extremely rare, but it can occur when there are accompanying defects such as occult submucous cleft, muscle disorders (myotonia), or other abnormalities present. Although noncleft patients without pre-existing speech disorders rarely benefit from a speech evaluation, patients with repaired cleft palates are at risk for velopharyngeal insufficiency, and preoperative evaluation may be warranted. The compensatory ability of a patient with a cleft following maxillary advancement may be impaired as a result of scarring, a shortened hard and soft palate, relatively increased nasopharynx depth, improperly positioned musculature, muscular atrophy, and perhaps an already extended compensatory system.

Schendel and coworkers investigated the static velopharyngeal mechanism before and after surgery in cleft and noncleft groups using lateral cephalograms.[39] Results in noncleft patients demonstrated soft palate lengthening of 50% of the amount the maxilla advanced at the posterior nasal spine. In the patients with clefts, the soft palate lengthened by only 40% of the maxillary advancement. In addition, it was determined that if pharyngeal depth was divided by soft palate length, a ratio of greater than 1.0 indicated possible velopharyngeal incompetence. Therefore, gross predictions of the associated changes occurring in the soft palate and the likelihood of velopharyngeal competence may be possible. However, variables such as Passavant ridge adaptive capacity, adenoid tissue, and variations in soft palate movement make predictions less reliable.

A thorough speech evaluation assessing speech adaptability, nasal resonance, and static and dynamic function (phonating cephalogram, cinefluoroscopy, nasopharyngoscopy) may help identify borderline velopharyngeal insufficiency not otherwise apparent, and may indicate the potential for hypernasal speech following surgery. If velopharyngeal insufficiency occurs, a pharyngeal flap, palatoplasty, a posterior pharyngeal wall augmentation, or a prosthesis may be needed to correct the problem. Delaying the surgical procedure for 6 to 12 months is advisable because speech compensations often occur, resulting in normal speech without treatment, and flap procedures before maxillary healing is complete can lead to relapse.

PRE-EXISTING PHARYNGEAL FLAPS AND MAXILLARY ADVANCEMENT

Pre-existing pharyngeal flaps must be managed appropriately to maintain an adequate airway and to allow advancement of the maxilla. The problems encountered with pre-existing pharyngeal flaps are as follows: (1) difficulty in the nasal intubation of the patient; (2) potential postsurgical airway concerns, particularly if intermaxillary fixation is used and the pharyngeal flap is a wide obliterating type of flap; (3) decreased ability to mobilize and stabilize the advanced maxilla.

Airway Management

Nasal intubation can usually be accomplished by passing the nasoendotracheal tube through one of the oronasal portals. Placing a finger through the portal and guiding the tube through is usually quick and simple (Fig. 21–18). The intubation is then completed in the usual manner. Fiberoptic endoscopy is another technique to pass the tube through the portals. If the portals are too small to pass the endotracheal tube, an oral airway can be maintained while a right-angled hemostat is used to dilate the portal. If this technique is unsuccessful, surgical enlargement may be necessary.

Postoperative airway management is of concern in a patient with a pharyngeal flap. With appropriate rigid fixation, no intermaxillary fixation (IMF) is required, and an adequate oral airway can be maintained. Nasopharyngeal airways can also be placed

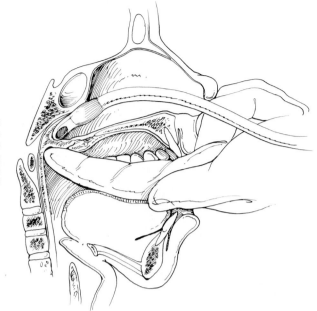

Figure 21–18. Intubation can be accomplished by passing a nasoendotracheal tube through one of the oral-nasal portals. Placing a fingertip up through the portal and guiding the tube through is usually quick and simple.

through the oronasal portals to assist nasal breathing. If the surgeon uses techniques requiring IMF, a bite opening splint to create an oral airway may be of benefit. Tracheostomy can be used, but it is rarely indicated or necessary.

Maxillary Mobilization

Pharyngeal flaps offer resistance to mobilization of the maxilla and also cause tension on the repositioned maxilla following surgery. If the maxilla is being expanded or downgrafted, usually no alteration of the pharyngeal flap is necessary. If the maxilla is being advanced, one of the following methods to manage the flap may be required to assist in the mobilization and stabilization of the maxilla.

1. Lengthen the flap by stretching. This may be effective for short advancements (<3–4 mm) but may be contraindicated for large advancements (>4 mm) because of the soft tissue tension that would displace the maxilla posteriorly postsurgically.

2. Resect the flap. This is simple but will result in hypernasal speech, requiring a secondary pharyngeal flap procedure.

3. Undermine and lengthen the pharyngeal flap. Parallel vertical incisions are made adjacent to the flap superiorly through the oronasal portals. A horizontal incision at the base of the pharyngeal flap joins the two vertical incisions. The flap is then undermined in a superior direction to increase the length of the pharyngeal flap without having to sever it (Fig. 21–19A,B,C). This maneuver reduces soft tissue tension on the advanced and repositioned maxilla and improves the overall stability. Generally, this facilitates mobilization and stabilization of the maxilla while maintaining the adequacy of the velopharyngeal mechanism.

EXTERNAL LIP/NOSE DEFORMITY

In many patients with clefts, unilateral or bilateral, upper lip and nasal deformities may exist. The nasal deformities involve the septum as well as the external nasal bones, upper and lower lateral cartilages, adjacent supporting bony structures, and overlying soft tissues. After lip repair in the unilateral cleft lip/palate, the anterior nasal spine remains deviated toward the noncleft side, and the alar cartilage are also distorted. Often the nares have an oblong shape with less support of the ala on the cleft side. Columellar length is usually shorter on the cleft side and slanted toward the noncleft side. The nasal dome is usually deviated away from the cleft side because

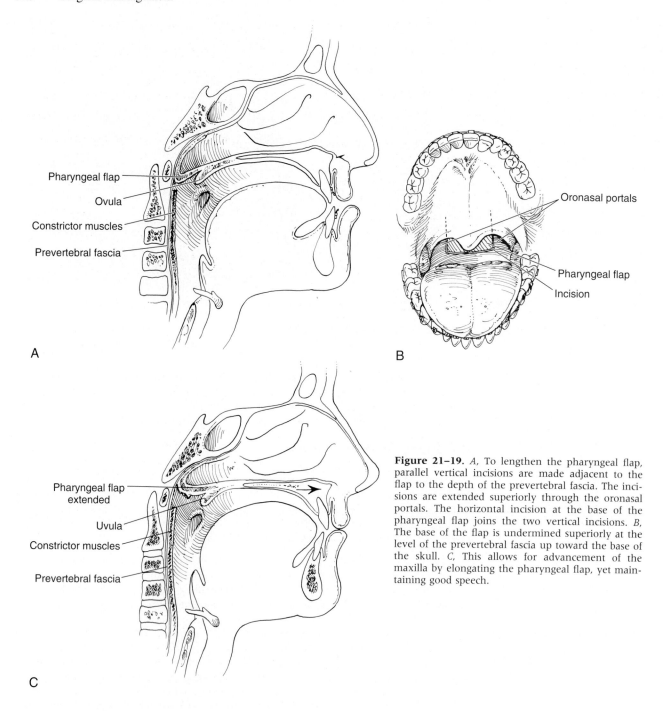

Figure 21–19. *A,* To lengthen the pharyngeal flap, parallel vertical incisions are made adjacent to the flap to the depth of the prevertebral fascia. The incisions are extended superiorly through the oronasal portals. The horizontal incision at the base of the pharyngeal flap joins the two vertical incisions. *B,* The base of the flap is undermined superiorly at the level of the prevertebral fascia up toward the base of the skull. *C,* This allows for advancement of the maxilla by elongating the pharyngeal flap, yet maintaining good speech.

the noncleft dome is often elevated and more prominent. The anterior dorsal septum most often leans toward the cleft side. In the previously repaired bilateral lip deformity, residual nasal defects include a severely shortened columella, wide and poorly projecting nasal tip, asymmetries, poorly supported ala, and oblong nares, with an underdeveloped anterior nasal spine and poor premaxillary support to the nose.

Residual esthetic and functional deformities of the upper lip can exist. Lip scars, asymmetries, vertical excess or deficiency, horizontal deficiency (tight lip), muscle malalignment, and functional and cosmetic defects in the vermilion and/or lip area are commonly seen in repaired unilateral cleft lip cases. Bilateral cases include the above but also have unique residual defects including philtrum abnormalities, vermilion deficiency, and buccal sulcus abnormalities.

At the end-stage reconstruction, corrective rhinoplasty and nasal tip reconstruction, as well as lip revisions (including Abbé flaps), are ideally done secondarily.

Lip / Nose Revisions

Because repositioning the maxilla and mandible changes the appearance and function of the nose, performing the lip/nose reconstruction secondarily allows reassessment of the structures following orthognathic surgery. In addition, in patients with compromised vascularity to the maxilla, it is best to delay the lip/nose reconstruction, particularly in the bilateral cleft, so that maximal blood supply to the premaxilla is maintained.

External rhinoplasty provides the best access to reconstruct the bony, cartilaginous, and soft tissue structures of the cleft patient's nose. Autogenous or banked cartilage grafts can be used to provide strength and support to the columella, ala, nasal tip and dorsum. In addition, cranial bone can be used for nasal augmentation, or other tissues, both autogenous or alloplastic, can be substituted. Autogenous cartilage grafts can be harvested from areas such as the ear, nasal septum, or rib, depending on availability, volume, and strength requirements. Rib cartilage can be advantageous because of the large volumes available and its excellent strength.

Tip reconstruction is commonly necessary to increase projection, rotation, and tip definition, which are usually deficient. Patients with bilateral clefts often require columella lengthening, which is accomplished using special soft tissue approaches such as the fork flaps, rotational flaps, V-Y advancements, and Z-plasty procedures. Nasal septoplasty is commonly necessary to reconstruct the nose, and this is usually approached during the orthognathic surgical procedure or secondarily with lip/nose revisions. The cartilage from the septum can be applied to the nasal reconstruction (i.e., columella grafting, shield graft, build-up or lower lateral cartilage on deformed sides). Deferring the septoplasty at the time of orthognathic surgery and delaying it until definitive nasal reconstruction is done may save the patient a second cartilage donor site in some cases. An alternative is to bank the cartilage at the time of orthognathic surgery against the lateral maxilla or mandible.

Cleft lip reconstruction may include scar revision, orbicularis oris muscle reconstruction, lengthening or shortening of lip structures, reconstruction of the vermilion, or correction of other functional and esthetic concerns. Occasionally, tissue transfer procedures (e.g., Abbé-Eshlander flaps) may be necessary. When performed at the same time as the nasal reconstruction, careful soft tissue incision design is important so that vascular supply to the flaps is not compromised. Vertical suspension of the orbicularis oris muscle may be necessary in some cases to prevent the lip from lengthening excessively, particularly if the lip is long initially. Meticulous soft tissue management will yield the best results.

CASE PRESENTATIONS

Case 1

A 16-year-old patient was born with a unilateral right cleft lip and palate, which were repaired in infancy and early childhood. He presented with (1) vertical and anteroposterior maxillary deficiency, (2) right maxillary oronasal fistula and alveolar cleft, and (3) class III occlusion (Figs. 21–20A–E, 21–21A). Treatment included (1) presurgical orthodontics to align the maxilla segmentally and to align and level the mandibular arch; (2) surgery, which included (a) maxillary advancement on the left side of 5 mm and downgraft 4 mm to place the patient into a class I cuspid-molar relationship, (b) advancement of the right maxilla (lesser segment) 12 mm and downgraft 7 mm, with the right cuspid advanced into a class II occlusal relationship (see Fig. 21–21B), and (c) closure of oronasal fistula and bone graft alveolar cleft; (3) postsurgical orthodontics; and (4) secondary lip-nose revision and rhinoplasty.

Advancing the cuspid into a class II relationship, allowing it to function as the lateral incisor, makes the alveolar cleft quite small and eliminates the necessity for a bridge to replace the lateral incisor. The bone defects for the maxillary osteotomies were grafted with PBHA, and the alveolar cleft was grafted with a cancellous bone from the iliac crest. Bone plates were used to stabilize the maxilla in its new position.

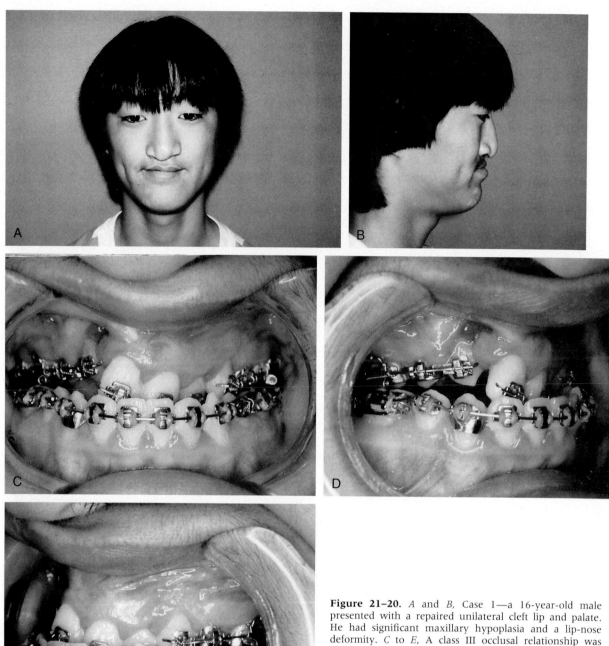

Figure 21–20. *A* and *B,* Case 1—a 16-year-old male presented with a repaired unilateral cleft lip and palate. He had significant maxillary hypoplasia and a lip-nose deformity. *C* to *E,* A class III occlusal relationship was present with missing maxillary lateral incisors.

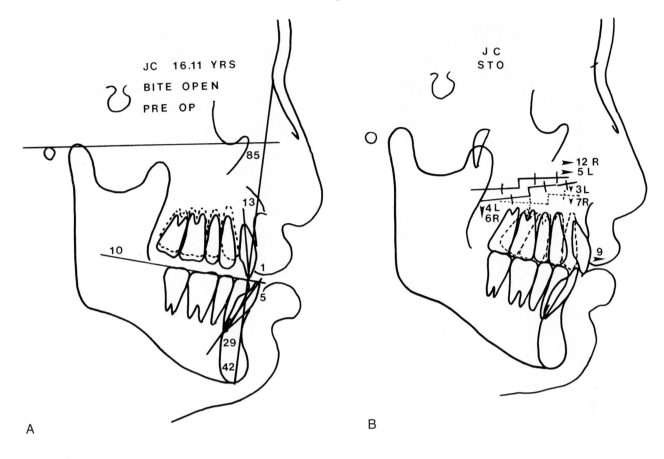

A

B

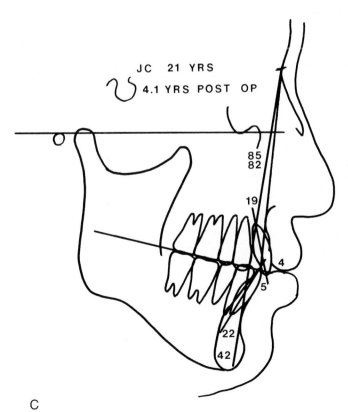

C

Figure 21–21. A, Case 1: cephalometric analysis demonstrates significant AP maxillary deficiency. B, The surgical treatment objective tracing demonstrates the planned corrective surgery on the maxilla. The right side will be advanced 7 mm and the left side 3 mm. The maxillary incisors were to be advanced 10 mm at the incisor tips. The maxilla also was downgrafted 7 mm on the right side and 3 mm on the left side. C, Postsurgical cephalometric changes are observed.

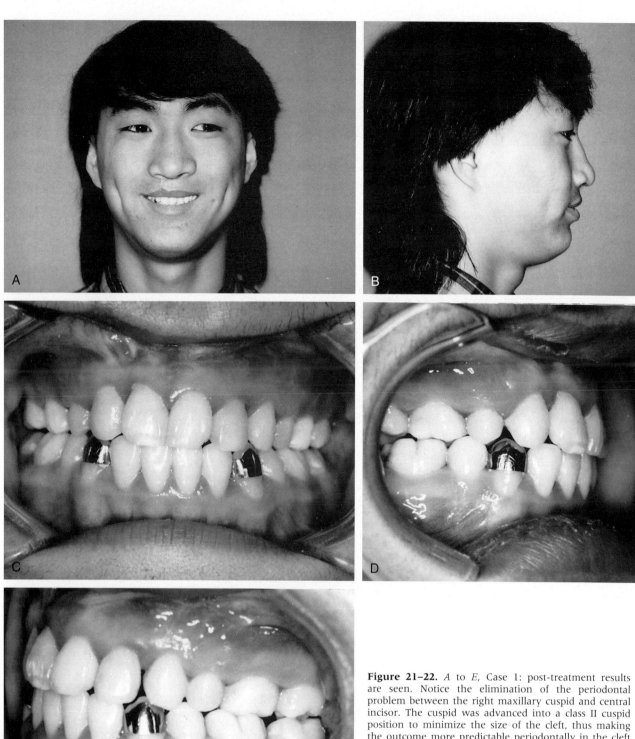

Figure 21–22. *A* to *E*, Case 1: post-treatment results are seen. Notice the elimination of the periodontal problem between the right maxillary cuspid and central incisor. The cuspid was advanced into a class II cuspid position to minimize the size of the cleft, thus making the outcome more predictable periodontally in the cleft area, as well as eliminating the need for a prosthetic replacement of the lateral incisor.

After treatment, good alignment of the maxilla and mandible was achieved with good nasal projection (Figs. 21–22A–E, 21–21C). A class I cuspid-molar relationship was established on the left side and a class II cuspid-molar relationship on the right side, as a result of advancing the right cuspid into the lateral incisor position. Notice the good periodontal results in the area of the cleft.

Case 2

A 16-year-old male was born with a unilateral right cleft lip and palate; the lip was repaired at 2½ months of age and the palate at 4 years. A pharyngeal flap was performed at 6 years of age. His diagnosis at 16 years of age included (1) severe maxillary hypoplasia, (2) maxillary right oronasal fistula and alveolar cleft, (3) mandibular prognathism, (4) active bilateral condylar hyperplasia, (5) retrogenia, (6) anterior vertical mandibular excess, (7) class III occlusion with severe anterior and bilateral posterior crossbite, (8) nasal airway obstruction, and (9) significant lip-nose deformity (Figs. 21–23A–E, 21–24A). Speech quality was good except for an articulation disorder related to his severe malocclusion. The treatment plan included the following: (1) presurgical orthodontics to align the maxillary teeth in three segments; (2) surgery, including (a) maxillary osteotomies to advance the maxilla 7 mm, (b) mandible set-back of 10 mm, (c) bilateral condylectomies to arrest disproportionate mandibular growth, and (d) augmentation genioplasty of 6 mm (see Fig. 21–24B); and (3) postsurgical orthodontics.

The maxilla was stabilized with bone plates and PBHA grafting. The alveolar cleft was grafted with cancellous bone from the iliac crest. The mandible was stabilized with bone screws. The patient had a superiorly based posterior pharyngeal flap, which required undermining and extension to allow passive advancement of the maxilla, yet maintain velopharyngeal competence. The patient was maintained in a bilateral posterior crossbite. It was elected to do this because of the gross transverse maxillary deficiency, severe scarring that existed on the palate, and the lack of vascularity to the maxilla. Six months later, a second procedure was performed, which included an external rhinoplasty with extensive tip work (recontouring and positioning lower lateral cartilages, cartilage grafts including the columella) and a lip revision. Completion of treatment provided a stable functional jaw relationship, improved nasal airway, normal speech, and a good esthetic result for this patient (Figs. 21–25A–F, 21–24C).

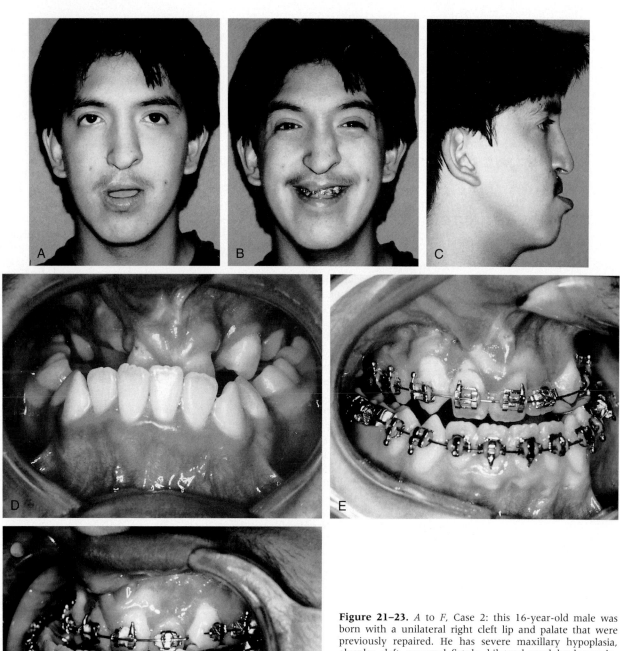

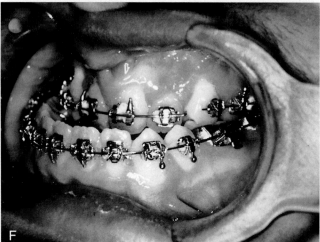

Figure 21–23. *A* to *F*, Case 2: this 16-year-old male was born with a unilateral right cleft lip and palate that were previously repaired. He has severe maxillary hypoplasia, alveolar cleft, oronasal fistula, bilateral condylar hyperplasia, mandibular prognathism, and anteroposterior microgenia. He has a class III malocclusion with severe anterior and posterior crossbites.

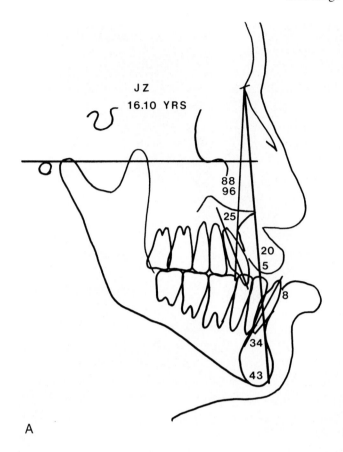

A

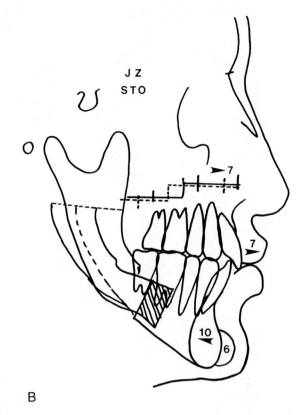

B

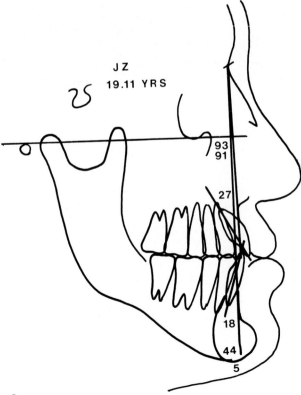

C

Figure 21–24. *A*, Cephalometric analysis demonstrates the severe musculoskeletal deformity. *B*, The surgical treatment objective tracing illustrates the intended surgical procedures to correct the problem, which also includes bilateral high mandibular condylectomies to arrest the disproportionate growth. *C*, Post-treatment cephalometric analysis shows the achievement of good facial harmony with no further mandibular growth.

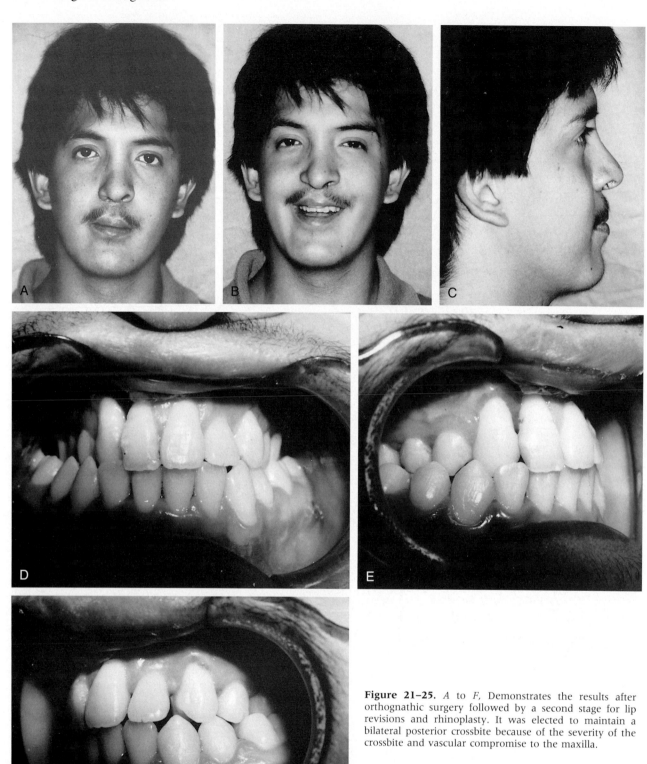

Figure 21–25. *A* to *F,* Demonstrates the results after orthognathic surgery followed by a second stage for lip revisions and rhinoplasty. It was elected to maintain a bilateral posterior crossbite because of the severity of the crossbite and vascular compromise to the maxilla.

Case 3

A 17-year-old male was born with a bilateral cleft lip and palate. Primary repairs were done in infancy and early childhood. Oronasal fistulas had been closed at age 8 years. Speech was normal. His diagnosis included (1) maxillary hypoplasia, (2) severe lip-nose deformity, (3) discontinuity of the orbicularis oris muscle, and (4) missing maxillary lateral incisors (Figs. 21–26*A–F*, 21–27*A*). The treatment plan included (1)

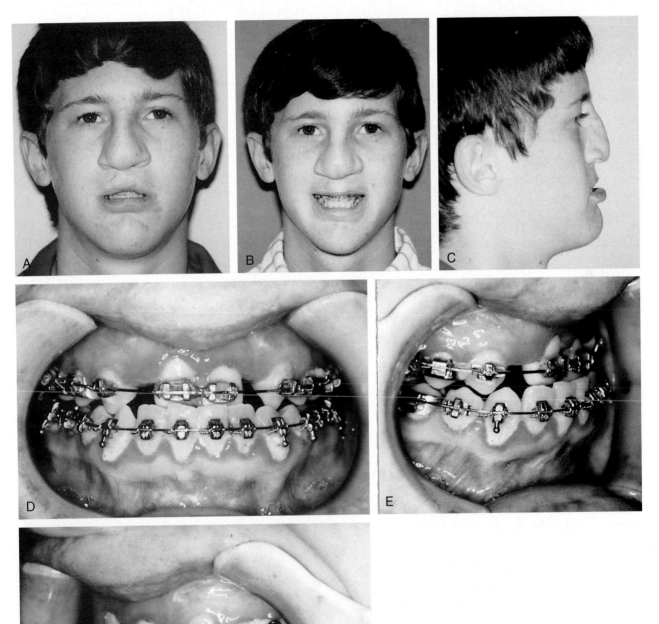

Figure 21–26. *A* to *F*, Case 3: this 17-year-old male presented with a repaired bilateral cleft lip and palate. He was diagnosed as having maxillary hypoplasia, missing maxillary lateral incisors, and severe lip-nose deformity.

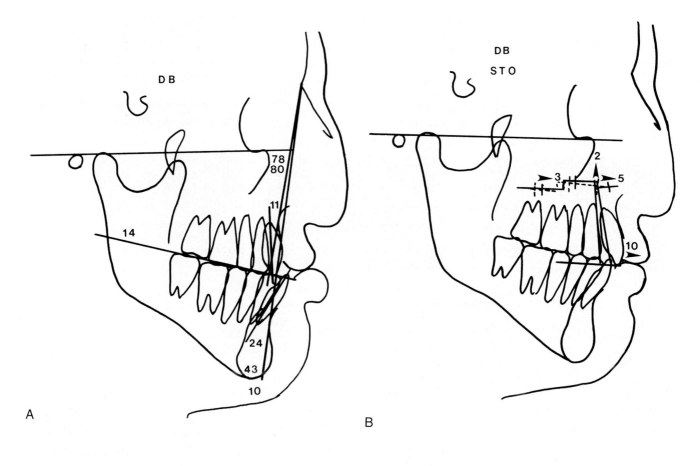

A

B

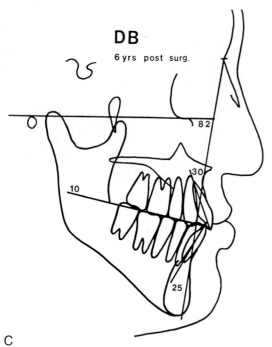

C

Figure 21–27. *A,* Cephalometric analysis demonstrates the AP maxillary deficiency. *B,* The surgical treatment objective includes maxillary advancement of 10 mm at the incisor tip with maxillary expansion and creation of space to replace the missing lateral incisors. The alveolar cleft areas were grafted. *C,* Postsurgical cephalometric radiograph shows good facial balance.

presurgical orthodontics; (2) surgery, including (a) multiple maxillary osteotomies to segmentally advance the maxilla 10 mm at the incisor tip and 5 mm at the level of the maxillary osteotomy, (b) expansion of the maxilla to correct the crossbite in the cuspid area, and (c) bone graft alveolar clefts bilaterally; (3) postsurgical orthodontics; and (4) prosthetic dentistry (Fig. 21–27*B*). The maxilla was approached as previously described and stabilized with bone plates and PBHA grafting. The bilateral alveolar cleft grafting was done with cancellous bone from the iliac crest. Secondarily, an external

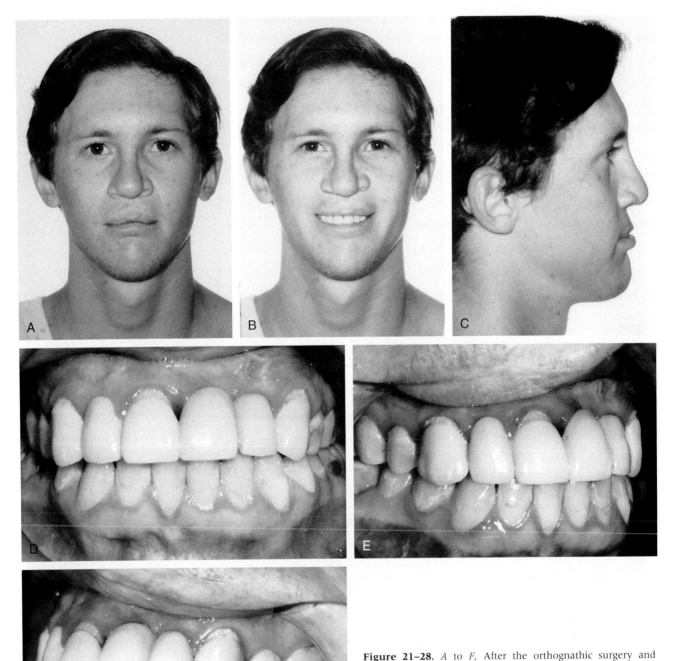

Figure 21–28. *A* to *F*, After the orthognathic surgery and subsequent secondary lip-nose revision and rhinoplasty, an acceptable functional and esthetic result was achieved for this patient.

rhinoplasty with extensive tip work (including recontouring of the lower lateral cartilages, and cartilage graft and lengthening of the columella), was performed to establish more normal nasal morphology. Nasal projection is significantly improved with the columella lengthening procedure and cartilaginous strut graft. The upper lip was revised at the same time as the nasal reconstruction, which included establishing the continuity of the orbicularis oris muscle through the lip revision incisions. Occlusally, space was opened in the maxillary arch for lateral incisor pontics and a class I cuspid-molar relationship was established (Figs. 21–28A–F, 21–27C).

Case 4

A 13-year-old female was born with a bilateral cleft lip and palate, with repair early in infancy. Diagnosis at the age of 13 years was as follows: (1) AP maxillary deficiency, (2) AP mandibular deficiency, (3) AP microgenia, (4) class II occlusion, (5) bilateral oronasal fistulas and alveolar clefts, and (6) missing maxillary lateral incisors (Figs. 21–29A–F, 21–30A). Recommended treatment includes the following:

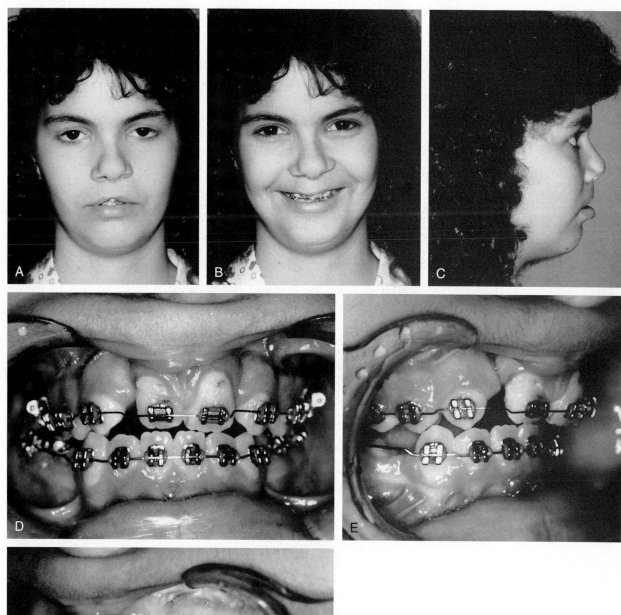

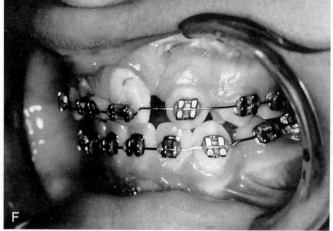

Figure 21–29. *A* to *F*, Case 4: this 15-year-old female presented with a repaired bilateral cleft lip and palate. She was diagnosed as having AP maxillary deficiency and AP mandibular deficiency. She has oronasal fistulas and bilateral alveolar clefts and is missing upper lateral incisors. She has a class II occlusal relationship and palatal inclination of maxillary incisors.

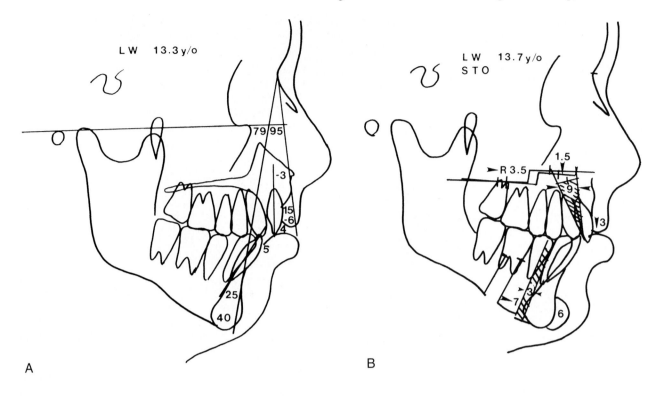

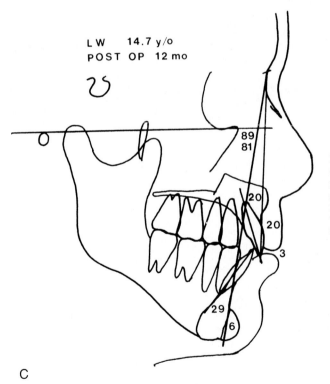

Figure 21–30. *A,* Cephalometrically, the AP maxillary deficiency and AP mandibular deficiency is observed, as well as a palatal inclination of the incisors in the premaxilla. *B,* The surgical treatment objective includes maxillary advancement and reorientation of the premaxilla and mandibular advancement with genioplasty. The secondary stage involved cleft lip reconstruction. *C,* Postsurgical cephalometric changes are noted.

1. Presurgical orthodontics to align and level the maxillary teeth in three segments. The maxillary anterior teeth are to be flared forward. Align and level the mandibular arch.

2. Surgery, including (a) maxillary osteotomies to advance the maxilla 5 mm, (b) mandibular advancement of 8 mm, (c) right mandibular body ostectomy to create lower arch symmetry, and (d) augmentation genioplasty.

3. Postsurgical orthodontics to refine occlusion.

4. Dental reconstruction (Fig. 21–30*B*).

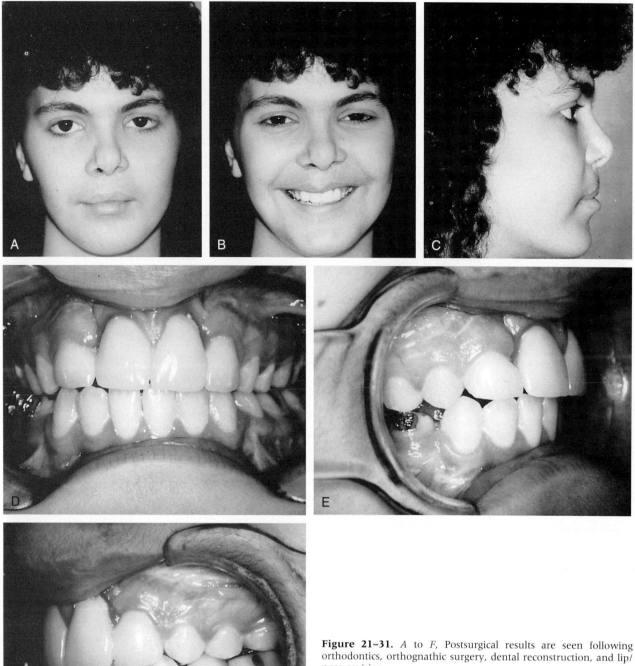

Figure 21–31. *A* to *F*, Postsurgical results are seen following orthodontics, orthognathic surgery, dental reconstruction, and lip/nose revision.

The maxilla was stabilized with bone plates and PBHA and alveolar cleft were grafted with cancellous bone. The mandible was stabilized with bone screws, and an alloplastic chin implant was used to augment the chin. Approximately 8 months later, a lip revision was performed as a secondary procedure. The patient was seen 2 years after treatment with an acceptable functional and esthetic result (Figs. 21–31*A–F*, 21–30*C*).

References

1. Subtelny JD: Width of the nasopharynx and related anatomic structure in normal and unoperated cleft palate children. Am J Orthod 1955; 41:889.
2. Ortiz-Monasterio F, Serrano A, Valderrama M, Cruz R: Cephalometric measurements on adult patients with non-operated cleft palates. Plast Reconstr Surg 1959; 24:53.
3. Ortiz-Monasterio F, Serrano A, Barrera G, et al: A study of untreated adult cleft palate patients. Plast Reconstr Surg 1966; 38:36.
4. Mestre JC, De Jesus J, Subtelny JD: Unoperated oral clefts at maturation. Angle Orthod 1960; 30:78.
5. Atherton JD: Morphology of facial bones in skulls with unoperated unilateral cleft palate. Cleft Palate J 1967; 4:18.
6. Bishara SE, Krause CJ, Olin WH, et al: Facial and dental relationships of individuals with unoperated clefts of the lip and/or palate. Cleft Palate J 1976; 13:238–252.
7. Normando ADC, Silva Filho OG, Capelozza Filho L: Influence of surgery on maxillary growth in cleft lip and/or palate patients. J Craniomaxillofac Surg 1992; 20:111–118.
8. Bardach J, Eishbach KJ: The influence of primary unilateral cleft lip repair on facial growth: Part I. Lip pressure. Cleft Palate J 1977; 14:88.
9. Eisbach KJ, Bardach J, Klausner EC: The influence of primary cleft lip repair on facial growth: Part II. Cleft Palate J 1978, 15:109.
10. Silva Filho OG, Rocha R, Capelozza Filho L: Padrao facial do pacien te portador de fissura pre-forame incisivo unilateral completa. Rev Bras Cirurg 1989; 79:197.
11. Ross BR: Treatment variables affecting facial growth in complete unilateral cleft lip and palate. Part 1: Treatment affecting growth. Cleft Palate J 1987; 24(1):5–23.
12. Rosenstein SW, Monroe CW, Kernahan DA: The case for early bone grafting in cleft lip and cleft palate. Plast Reconstr Surg 1982; 70:297.
13. Semb G: Effect of alveolar bone grafting on maxillary growth in unilateral cleft lip and palate patients. Cleft Palate J 1988; 25(3):288–295.
14. Ross RB: Treatment variables affecting facial growth in complete cleft lip and palate. Part 3: Alveolus repair and bone grafting. Cleft Palate J 1987; 24(1):33–44.
15. Nelson CL: Primary alveolar cleft bone grafting. Oral Maxillofac Surg Clin North Am 1991; 3(3):599–608.
16. Hall DH, Werther JR: Conventional alveolar cleft bone grafting. Oral Maxillofac Surg Clin North Am 1991; 3(3):609–616.
17. Dahl E: Craniofacial morphology in congenital clefts of the lip and palate. Acta Odont Scand 1970; 28[Suppl 57]:1.
18. Ross BR: Treatment variables affecting growth in cleft lip and palate. Part 6: Techniques of palate repair. Cleft Palate J 1987; 24(1):64–70.
19. Ross BR: Facial growth in cleft lip and palate. In McCarthy JG: Plastic Surgery, vol 4. Cleft Lip and Palate and Craniofacial Anomalies, pp 2553–2580. Philadelphia: WB Saunders, 1990.
20. Long RE Jr, McNamara JA: Facial growth following pharyngeal flap surgery: Skeletal assessment on serial lateral cephalometric radiographs. Am J Orthod 1985; 87:187.
21. Wolford LM, Cooper RL, El Deeb M: Orthognathic surgery on the young cleft patient and the effect on growth. Abstract presented at American Cleft Palate Association Annual Meeting, St. Louis, May, 1990.
22. Millard DR Jr: Cleft Craft, vol II, pp 28–31. Boston: Little, Brown, 1977.
23. Epker BN, Wolford LM: Dentofacial Deformities: Surgical-Orthodontic Correction. St. Louis: CV Mosby, 1980.
24. Bennett MA, Wolford LM: The maxillary step osteotomy modification and Steinmann pin stabilization. J Oral Maxillofac Surg 1985; 43:307–311.
25. Holmes RE, Wardrop RW, Wolford LM: Hydroxylapatite as a bone graft substitute in orthognathic surgery. J Oral Maxillofac Surg 1988; 46:661–671.
26. Moenning JE, Wolford LM: Coralline porous hydroxyapatite as a bone graft substitute in orthognathic surgery: 24-month follow-up results. Int J Adult Orthod Orthognath Surg 1989; 4:105–117.
27. Wardrop RW, Wolford LM: Maxillary stability following downgraft and/or advancement procedures with stabilization using rigid fixation and porous block hydroxyapaptite implants. J Oral Maxillofac Surg 1989; 47:336–342.
28. Guymon M, Crosby DR, Wolford LM: The alar base cinch suture to control nasal width in maxillary osteotomies. Int J Adult Orthod Orthognath Surg 1988; 2:89–95.
29. Kawauchi M, Sachdeva R, Bossolla E, et al: Frontal and lateral changes in lip and chin morphology as a result of orthognathic surgery. Abstract presented at the AADR Annual Meeting, Boston, March 1992.
30. Kawauchi M, Sachdeva R, Bossolla E, et al: Nasal dimensional changes in response to maxillary surgery in the lateral and frontal perspective. Abstract presented at the AADR Annual Meeting, Boston, March 1992.
31. Epker BN, Schendel SA, Washburn M: Effects of early surgical superior repositioning of the maxilla on subsequent growth: III. Biomechanical considerations. In McNamara JA: The Effects of Surgical Intervention on Craniofacial Growth.
32. Vig KWL, Turvey TA: Surgical correction of vertical maxillary excess during adolescence. Int J Orthod Orthognath Surg 1989; 4:119–128.
33. Mogavero FJ, Buschang PH, Wolford LM: The effects of orthognathic surgery on growth of the maxilla in patients with vertical maxillary excess. In Bell WM (ed): Modern Practice in Orthognathic and Reconstructive Surgery, pp 1932–1955. Philadelphia: WB Saunders, 1991.
34. Freihofer HP Jr: Results of osteotomies of the facial skeleton in adolescence. J Maxillofac Surg 1977; 5:267.
35. Wolford LM: Effects of orthognathic surgery on nasal form and function in the cleft patient. Cleft Palate Craniofac J 1992; 29(6):546–555.
36. Wolford LM, Bennett MA, Rafferty CG: Modification of the mandibular ramus sagittal split osteotomy. Oral Surg Oral Med Oral Pathol 1987; 64:146–155.

37. Wolford LM, LeBanc JP: Effectiveness of condylectomies in controlling class III disproportionate mandibular growth. Abstract presented at the American Cleft Palate Association Annual Meeting, New York, May 16–19, 1986.
38. Mason R, Turvey TA, Warren DW: Speech considerations with maxillary advancement procedures. J Oral Surg 1980; 38:752–758.
39. Schendel SA, Oeschlaeger M, Wolford LM, Epker BN: Velopharyngeal anatomy and maxillary advancement. J Maxillofac Surg 1979; 7:116–124.

22

Comprehensive Surgical and Orthodontic Management of Hemifacial Microsomia

Karin Vargervik, William Hoffman, and Leonard B. Kaban

GENERAL CONSIDERATIONS

Hemifacial microsomia (HFM) is a variable, progressive, and asymmetric craniofacial anomaly. The term was first used by Gorlin and Pindborg[12] in 1964, although the anomaly was well known long before this date. Some of the other labels that have been suggested include asymmetric first and second branchial arch deformity,[13] oculo-auriculovertebral spectrum,[7] otomandibular dysostosis,[10] oculo-auriculovertebral dysplasia,[11] lateral facial dysplasia,[35] and unilateral craniofacial microsomia.[14] The variety of names reflects an incomplete understanding of etiology, genetics, and pathogenesis, as well as the wide spectrum of clinical deformities that are included in this category by different authors.[7] Mulliken[31] proposed the most likely reason why HFM, more than all the other terms, remains in common usage. He stated that HFM "endures perhaps because of its brevity, clarity, and euphony."

HFM involves the skeletal, soft tissue, and neuromuscular components of the first and second branchial arches, and it is the second most common congenital facial anomaly after cleft lip and palate.[23, 35] The reported incidence of HFM ranges from 1 in 3500 births[37] to 1 in 26,500 live births.[26] The most frequently quoted incidence rate is 1 in 5600 live births,[13] which is reportedly in accordance with the experience of Gorlin and Cohen,[7] although they presented no data.

The wide spectrum of clinical malformations suggests that the etiology of HFM may be variable and heterogenous. Although most cases are isolated and sporadic, multiple occurrences in families have been reported.[8,13] Both discordance[2,46] and concordance[40, 43] have been reported in monozygotic twins. Exposure of the pregnant mother to thalidomide,[13] primidone,[15] and retinoic acid[24] has been associated with congenital first and second branchial arch defects in humans.

The mechanism by which HFM develops in humans is unknown, but Poswillo[38] described an animal phenocopy in mice after administration of triazine to the pregnant mothers. Hemorrhage from the developing stapedial artery produced a hematoma in the area of the first and second branchial arches. The size of the hematoma and resultant tissue destruction determined the morphology and variability of HFM in the experimental model. This sequence may be applicable to the human condition as it explains the spectrum of involvement. In addition, hematoma formation may be the result of a variety of causes such as hypoxia, hypertension, anticoagulants,[38] or anomalous development of the carotid artery system.[45]

Treatment of HFM requires an integrated plan taking into account all aspects of this complex anomaly. In the past, individual specialists who became interested in treating these patients had a tendency to concentrate exclusively on their own area of expertise. Today, the majority of these patients are cared for in centers for craniomaxillofacial anomalies staffed by multidisciplinary professional groups. This chapter presents an integrated approach to analysis and treatment of HFM.

Acknowledgment

We acknowledge Marilyn Hersh and Sherlyn Jimenez, administrative assistants, Department of Oral and Maxillofacial Surgery, for their valuable work on the preparation of this manuscript. This work was supported in part by National Institutes of Health Grant No. DE 04940, Dr. Vargervik, PI, and the UCSF Oral and Maxillofacial Surgery Research Fund.

CLINICAL FINDINGS

Skeletal Defects

Asymmetric mandibular growth is the earliest skeletal manifestation of HFM, and it plays an important role in progressive deformity of the ipsilateral and contralateral facial skeleton. The mandible is short, retrusive, and narrow at birth and may become progressively more asymmetric with time as growth of the contralateral side outpaces that of the affected side. The spectrum of mandibular malformation ranges from a small but normally shaped ramus and condyle to complete absence of these structures. The midface (nose, maxilla, zygomas, and orbits) normally grows downward and forward away from the cranial base. In patients with HFM, temporal bone abnormalities, mandibular hypoplasia, and neuromuscular defects inhibit normal downward growth of the maxilla and midface on the affected side. This prevents progressive lowering of the pyriform aperture and maxillary alveolus from the orbit. The result is a short maxilla with an occlusal plane that is tilted upward on the abnormal side; in some cases the orbit is inferiorly displaced.[23,33,34] The untreated end-stage skeletal malformation of HFM shows considerable variation. The abnormality of the mandible is a short, medially displaced, or absent ramus. If present, the ramus and body are usually flat in contour and the chin point is deviated toward the affected side (Figs. 22–1 and 22–2). There may be a crossbite on the affected side, although the occlusion is usually quite good because the dentoalveolar adaptations tend to keep up with the slowly progressing skeletal asymmetry. In addition to classic HFM, microphthalmic, frontonasal, and Goldenhar types have been reported.[51]

Soft Tissue Defects

The soft tissue defect is analyzed by physical examination; review of frontal, lateral, oblique, and submental photographs; computed tomography (CT) scans, and electromyelogram (EMG) recordings.[51] Components of the soft tissue to consider include bulk of subcutaneous soft tissue; muscles of mastication and facial expression; presence or absence of macrostomia, skin tags, and facial clefts; cranial nerve function (particularly VII nerve); and soft palate function.

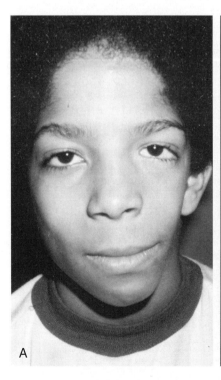

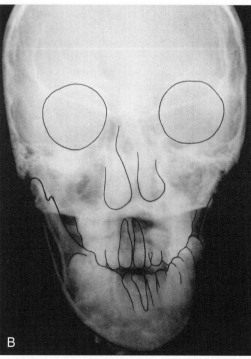

A

B

Figure 22–1. *A,* Classic hemifacial microsomia. Frontal photograph of a teenager with end-stage hemifacial microsomia demonstrating the following features: Deviation of the chin point toward the left, macrostomia on the left, marked flattening of the contour of the left side of the face, low set ear on left and decreased midface height (decreased distance from the infraorbital rim to the alar base). *B,* AP cephalogram demonstrating the short hypoplastic ramus with an absent temporomandibular joint on the left. There is also a decreased distance between the infraorbital rim and the pyriform aperture on the left and marked deviation of the chin point to the left.

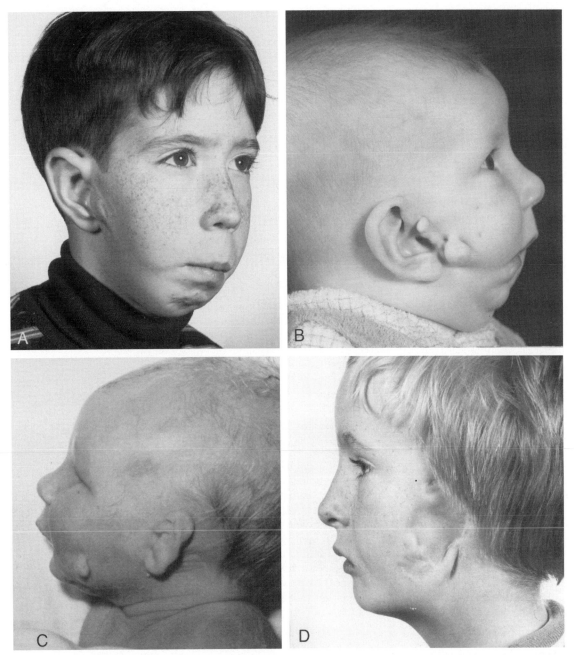

Figure 22–2. Ear abnormalities in hemifacial microsomia. *A*, Grade 1 ear with preauricular scar after excision of skin tags. *B*, Grade 1 ear with somewhat more inferior and anterior displacement and with multiple preauricular skin tags. *C*, Grade 2 ear with absence of the external auditory canal, marked hypoplasia of concha, and large skin tag near mouth. *D*, Grade 3 ear with absent auricle.

The soft tissue abnormalities seen in HFM involve the first and second branchial arch structures—the ear, the facial nerve, and the soft tissues of the face (i.e., subcutaneous fat).

Skin Tags

Skin tags are small vestigial rests of epithelial tissue that usually lie along the cleft between the first and second branchial arches. These are frequently associated with small cartilaginous remnants that may lie in a subcutaneous position, and with sinus tracts that may form inclusion cysts if obstructed. The skin tags and small lesions may be of considerable concern to the parents, especially when they lie in positions on the cheek rather than in the preauricular area.

Macrostomia

Macrostomia results from a failure of fusion of the maxillary and mandibular processes, which are derived from the first and second branchial arches. In most cases this is fairly subtle, although the deformity may be increased by correction of the skeletal abnormalities. Inevitably there is a cleft of the orbicularis oris muscle, and the most critical aspect of surgical correction is the repair of the muscle; Z-plasty of the skin closure is preferred over straight line closure to avoid late contracture of the repair.

Ear Abnormalities

The ear can range from virtually normal to completely absent (see Fig. 22–2) Meurman's classification of ear deformity in HFM is the most widely used.[28]

Grade I: Smaller ear with obvious malformation but all structures present
Grade II ("classic" microtia): Vertically oriented cartilaginous remnant and lobule, complete atresia of the canal
Grade III: Minimal tissue present (e.g., small lobular remnant).

Pruzansky evaluated 101 patients with HFM and found a moderate correlation between the degree of ear deformity and the degree of skeletal deformity.[39] Murray and coworkers[33] did not confirm this association in their review of 62 patients but did find a direct association between the degree of ear deformity and the presence of seventh nerve deficits. Interestingly, it has been estimated that approximately 50% of children with microtia do not have an obvious skeletal anomaly.[3]

Patients who present with grade II or III ear deformity have hearing loss that must be assessed carefully. Audiometry will delineate the nature of the loss, which is usually conductive in nature, although neurosensory loss may be seen as well. High-resolution CT scans of the temporal bone are necessary to define the presence or absence of middle ear structures to determine whether reconstruction of a canal and typanic membrane is feasible. If the contralateral side has normal hearing, this is usually adequate for daily activities, and reconstruction is not performed. With only one ear functioning, the major problem is difficulty in determining the direction of sounds rather than the content.

Reconstruction of the external ear is a high priority for patients and parents alike. Complete microtia may be more obvious than a subtle type I deformity of the mandible in some patients. The decreased anteroposterior distance in the upper face and the absence of an adequate platform (i.e., temporal bone cavity) are two factors that may compromise the best efforts at surgical reconstruction. The quality and location of the soft tissue remnant are also important factors; it may be necessary to reposition or remove the remnant if it is too far anterior and/or inferior (Fig. 22–3).

Soft Tissue Hypoplasia

The temporalis and masseter muscles may be deficient or absent in HFM, and this is frequently related to the degree of bony abnormality: if the temporalis is absent, there is an absent coronoid process, and there is a similar correlation between the masseter muscle and the gonial angle. The surgical correction of the bony abnormality may actually increase the observed degree of soft tissue hypoplasia. As the maxilla and mandible are shifted downward on the affected side and the midline is shifted toward the contralateral side, the soft tissue on the "normal" side is increased whereas the already deficient soft tissue on the "abnormal" side is further stretched and attenuated.

More than 25% of patients have cranial nerve abnormalities, usually consisting of facial nerve palsy and/or deviation of the palate toward the affected side with motion. Palatal deviation may be the result of a combination of structural asymmetry, muscle hypoplasia, and cranial nerve weakness. Presence or absence of seventh nerve palsy correlates with severity of the ear and not the skeletal defect (i.e., those patients with more severe ear abnormality are more likely to have seventh nerve deficit) (Fig. 22–4). The most common facial nerve weakness involves the marginal mandibular

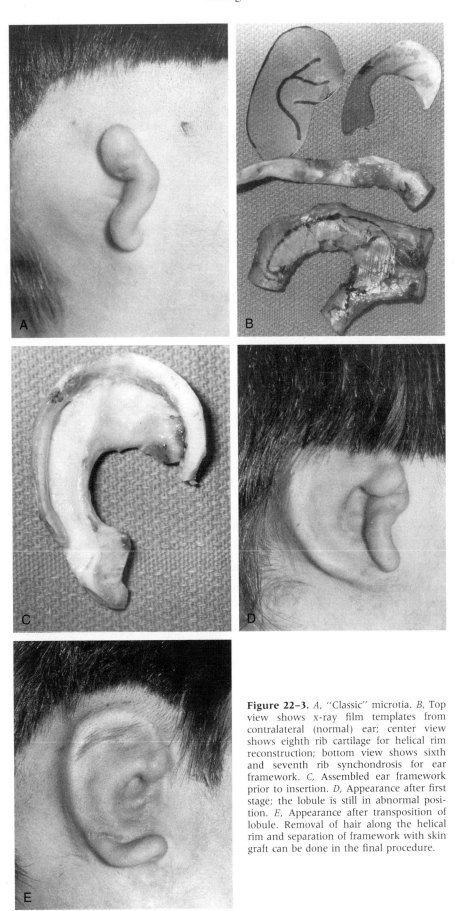

Figure 22–3. *A*, "Classic" microtia. *B*, Top view shows x-ray film templates from contralateral (normal) ear; center view shows eighth rib cartilage for helical rim reconstruction; bottom view shows sixth and seventh rib synchondrosis for ear framework. *C*, Assembled ear framework prior to insertion. *D*, Appearance after first stage; the lobule is still in abnormal position. *E*, Appearance after transposition of lobule. Removal of hair along the helical rim and separation of framework with skin graft can be done in the final procedure.

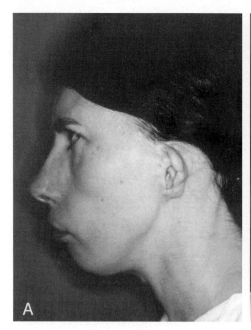
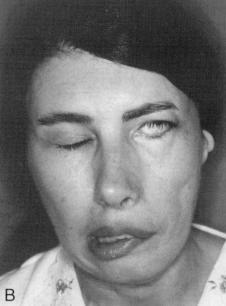

Figure 22–4. Facial nerve abnormalities. *A,* Adult patient with a partially reconstructed left ear. This was originally a grade 3 ear deformity. *B,* The patient has total facial nerve palsy on the left side in the presence of a severe ear defect and only a mild skeletal defect.

branch followed by the branch to the frontalis muscle. Rarely, a patient has total seventh nerve weakness or a sensory deficit in the fifth nerve distribution.[21, 22] Hypoplasia of the lateral pterygoid muscle ranges from mild to complete absence of the muscle and correlates with the severity of the skeletal defect. This muscle hypoplasia, the short ramus, abnormal location of the temporomandibular joint (TMJ), or absence of joint structures results in deviation of the mandible toward the abnormal side on opening.

CLINICAL CLASSIFICATION OF HEMIFACIAL MICROSOMIA

The classification presented (Table 22–1) is based on discrete findings of presence or absence of critical structures rather than on degree of deficiencies in terms of size and shape. It also is well related to treatment. In type I HFM, the existing joint can be maintained; in types II and III HFM, a joint usually has to be created. Type I patients may respond well to functional appliance treatment, whereas patients with types II and III almost always require surgical construction of missing structures and lengthening of the mandibular ramus by an extension bone graft.

Type I

Skeletal

All components are present but hypoplastic to varying degree. The temporomandibular joint is present, but there is reduced cartilage and joint space. Hinge movement is normal, but there is reduced translation during jaw opening. Type I is equivalent to Pruzansky[39] grade I, Harvold and coworkers[18] type I, and Kaban and coworkers[23] type I (Fig. 22–5).

Muscles

All masticatory muscles are present but small with inclusions of fatty tissue, as seen on CT scans.[25, 51] Patterns of muscle use are within normal variation.

Table 22–1. HEMIFACIAL MICROSOMIA TREATMENT PLAN BY AGE AND SKELETAL TYPE

Skeletal Type*	Deciduous Dentition	Mixed Dentition	Permanent Dentition
I—Equivalent to Pruzansky grade I Harvold et al type I Kaban et al type I	Observation Remove ear tags if indicated	Activator appliance in cooperative patient to develop normal closing patterns and prevent progressive asymmetric development. Mandibular advancement and rotation to create open bite when occlusal cant and mandibular asymmetry progress	Orthodontic treatment preparation for surgical correction if not done previously. Maxillary and mandibular osteotomies to correct endstage asymmetry
IIA—Equivalent to Pruzansky grade II Harvold et al type II Kaban et al type IIA	Same as for type I	Same as for type I. Less effect of activator treatment on jaw asymmetry than in type I	Same as for type I
IIB—Equivalent to Pruzansky grade II or III Harvold et al type IV Kaban et al type IIB or III	Same as for type I	Construction of glenoid fossa, condyle, and ramus. Surgically created open bite maintained with appliance to permit vertical midface growth. Assisted by active extrusion of teeth	Same presurgical preparation, total TMJ construction plus maxillary and mandibular osteotomies to correct endstage asymmetry
III—Equivalent to Pruzansky grade III Harvold et al type V Kaban et al type III	Construction of glenoid fossa, condyle and ramus if function such as opening, chewing and speech are severely affected by the condition	Construction of glenoid fossa, condyle, and ramus, if not done previously. Surgically created open bite maintained with appliance to permit vertical midface growth, assisted by active extrusion of teeth	Same as for type IIB

* As described in this chapter.

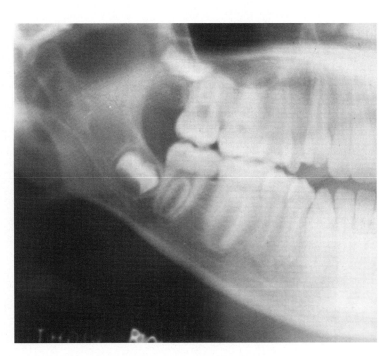

Figure 22–5. Radiographic example of type I mandible. Note the absence of the glenoid fossa and atypical position of mandibular canal and foramina.

Type IIA

Skeletal

An articulation that allows hinge but not translatory movement is present; there is no morphologically normal joint. The condylar process is cone-shaped and positioned anterior and medial of normal position. Coronoid process and gonial angle are well developed. Type IIA is equivalent to Pruzansky grade II, Harvold and coworkers type II, and Kaban and coworkers (Fig. 22–6).

Muscles

All muscles are present but hypoplastic, and because of the anterior and medial position of the condylar process, contraction of the lateral pterygoid muscle does not advance the affected side of the mandible.

Type IIB

Skeletal

No condylar process that articulates with the temporal bone is present, but there is presence of a coronoid process of varying size. In some individuals, a small bony extension is present at the posterior border of the ramus. Type IIB is equivalent to Pruzansky grade II or III, Harvold and coworkers type IV, and Kaban and coworkers type IIB or III (Fig. 22–7).

Muscles

No lateral pterygoid muscle is attached to mandibular structures. There are variable deficiencies of masseter and medial pterygoid muscles. The temporal muscle is small but easily palpated and attached to the coronoid process.

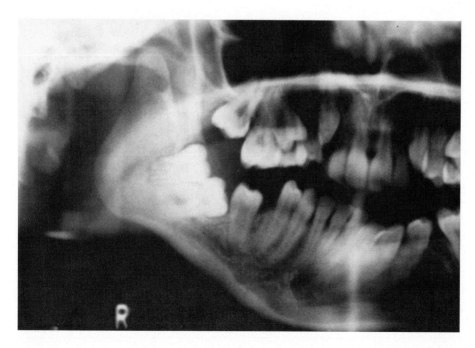

Figure 22–6. Radiographic example of type IIa mandible; cone-shaped anteriorly and medially displaced condylar process, absence of TMJ structures, well-developed gonial area.

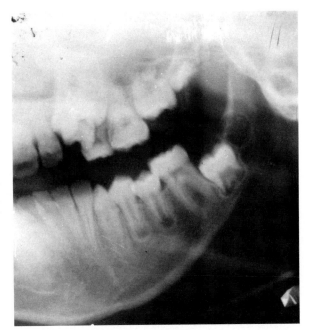

Figure 22–7. Radiographic example of type IIb mandible; absence of TMJ structures, condylar process and gonial area; presence of a short, underdeveloped coronoid process with attached temporalis muscle. There is no evidence of masseter or medial and lateral pterygoid muscles attached to mandible as seen on CT scans.

Type III

Skeletal

No condylar or coronoid process and no gonial angle area are present. Type III is equivalent to Pruzansky grade III, Harvold and coworkers type V, and Kaban and coworkers type III (Fig. 22–8).

Muscles

Masticatory muscles are severely hypoplastic; the lateral pterygoid and temporalis are not attached to mandibular structures.

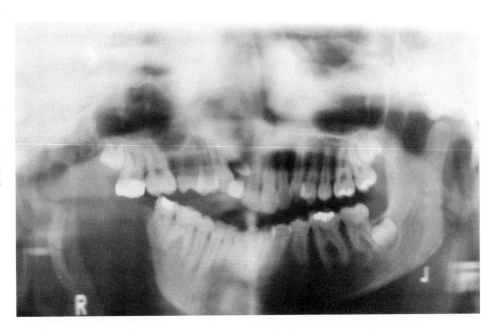

Figure 22–8. Radiographic example of type III mandible; there is absence of TMJ structures and the entire mandibular ramus with all associated muscles.

MANDIBULAR GROWTH IN PATIENTS WITH HEMIFACIAL MICROSOMIA

Type I

In the mildest form of mandibular involvement, the condylar cartilage is minimal and the disc may be missing. This is determined radiographically by a clear cortical outline of the condyle and reduced joint space (see Fig. 22–5). The shape of the condylar head is usually normal but small, and movements are somewhat restricted, with normal rotation but reduced translation. The glenoid fossa is shallow or missing. The sensory-motor feedback mechanisms between the joint and the musculature appear normal, and joint function is adequate and asymptomatic. This side of the mandible grows but less than the normal side, presumably because the contribution to mandibular growth attributed to condylar cartilage proliferation does not occur. All muscles are present but may be significantly smaller than normal. Fatty and glandular tissues may also be reduced in size, contributing to the facial asymmetry.

If the masseter and medial pterygoid muscles are hypoplastic, the gonial area is also reduced and usually is positioned more medial than the other side. This mildest form of mandibular involvement may or may not manifest seventh nerve impairment and may exhibit any of the four phenotypes.[50] The degree of ear involvement is not closely associated with degree of mandibular malformation. In this mandibular type, the external ear may be missing or near normal. It is quite possible to provide a partial substitute for the deficient condylar cartilage proliferation and to achieve additional mandibular length by the use of a functional appliance.[18,27,51,52]

Type IIA

The next degree of mandibular involvement is a missing TMJ but still with presence of a condylar process and lateral pterygoid muscle attached to the cone-shaped condyle (see Fig. 22–6). This process lacks a defined head and neck and is medial and anterior of normal position. It may have an articulation at the anterior slope of the temporal bone. Contraction of the lateral pterygoid muscle does not advance the mandible under these circumstances, and this condition results in severe asymmetry of the mandible and secondary asymmetry of the maxilla and nasal structures. All muscles are present, and patterns of use are relatively normal. The gonial angle is usually well-developed and the coronoid process and temporalis present and well-developed. During jaw opening, the mandibular asymmetry becomes more marked because the affected side does not translate forward. Excessive movement of the contralateral joint with occasional clicking is not infrequent in teenagers and adults in the two above-described types of HFM. In addition, in this type more mandibular length can be achieved by using a functional appliance.[27,52] However, correction of mandibular deficiency cannot be expected by functional appliance treatment alone.

Type IIB

The next degree of severity is represented by missing condylar process and only the coronoid process present (see Fig. 22–7). The lateral pterygoid is absent or at least not attached to the mandible. The joint structures are missing, and the size of the coronoid process is reduced. The masseter and medial pterygoid muscles are involved to varying degrees, from a few strands of muscle bundles to a broader, but thin band as seen on CT scans. The degree of muscle hypoplasia is reflected in the amount of bony deficiency at the attachment sites. The skeletal deformity is usually rather severe because the mechanism advancing the mandible on that side is missing; the gonial area is poorly developed and the muscles and other soft tissues are deficient. Because there is no glenoid fossa, slope, eminence, and lateral pterygoid function, the body of the mandible with the alveolar process and developing dentition is not disoccluded from the maxilla. Consequently, the down and forward development of the maxilla also becomes inhibited. The result is canting of the occlusal plane and impaired mesial migration of the maxillary teeth on the affected side. This is also the case in type IIA and, to some extent, in type I HFM as well.

Although the upper portion of the coronoid process is in normal position relative to the zygomatic arch and temporal fossa, its height is short because its increase in height depends on down and forward growth of the mandible. The temporal muscle and coronoid process do not contribute to mandibular advancement, but rather develop in response to advancement. By substituting an advancement functional appliance for the missing joint structures and lateral pterygoid function, some height increase of the coronoid process can be achieved. Functional appliance treatment effecting a lowering and advancing of the mandible also allows better maxillary development and less dentoalveolar adaptations during the growth period. An actual lengthening of the mandible can only be achieved by surgically constructing a process that can articulate with the temporal bone.

Type III

The most severe mandibular involvement is absence of both the condylar and coronoid processes, resulting in absence of the entire ramus (see Fig. 22–8). In this condition, only rudiments of masseter, medial, and lateral pterygoid and temporal muscles are present. The bony development of the body of the mandible is limited to alveolar bone surrounding the toothbuds as they form; attachments for muscles may develop at the floor of the mouth. When the affected side is not attached by muscles to the temporal region and zygomatic arch, the mandible has an excessive amount of freedom of movement and can easily be manipulated to an advanced and lowered position. Such a position cannot be sustained, however, because the advancing mechanisms are absent. Alveolar development of the maxilla and mandible may be less impaired under these circumstances than it is in less severely affected individuals. Functional appliance treatment does not have a significant effect in this type, because there are no structures that can respond with bone apposition, and little effect can be achieved on the dentition. Early construction of a mandibular ramus with subsequent functional appliance treatment is the approach of choice in this type of HFM.

TREATMENT

Accurate classification of the skeletal and soft tissue defect is critical in developing a treatment plan. The skeletal type predicts the rate of progression of asymmetry and the end-stage distortion of contiguous and contralateral skeletal structures. Table 22–1 provides a summary of the general treatment principles by age and skeletal type.

Treatment of the Growing Child

The overall goal of treatment is improved function and optimal facial symmetry and esthetics when craniofacial growth is completed. Treatment is therefore directed toward (1) increasing the size of the underdeveloped and malformed mandible and associated soft tissues; (2) creating an articulation between mandible and temporal bone when missing; (3) correcting secondary deformities of the maxilla; and (4) establishing a functional occlusion and esthetic appearance of the face and dentition.

The treatment approach of choice for the growing child with HFM is indicated by morphologic and functional findings, age at presentation, psychosocial functioning of the child, and availability for treatment visits.

Treatment must proceed stepwise, conforming to a predictable sequence of biologic development, and is in general characterized by several sequential phases, consisting of presurgical jaw orthopedic treatment when indicated; mandibular surgery including joint reconstruction, if necessary; immediate postsurgical treatment to support graft remodeling; maxillary correction when necessary; final orthodontic treatment; and soft tissue augmentation.[18, 23, 32, 33, 51, 52]

Presurgical Orthopedic Treatment

As mentioned earlier, growth impairment of the mandible may be the result of absent or reduced condylar cartilage proliferation and reduced protrusive action of the condylar process as a result of missing joint proprioception and reduced or missing lateral pterygoid function. According to the condylar growth theory, it can be expected that additional bone apposition on the condylar process will take place if a substitute for the missing advancement mechanism can be provided. The bone apposition thus occurring would be similar to that which takes place on the coronoid process in normal mandibular growth. A functional appliance constructed to hold the affected side of the mandible in a lowered, forward position can therefore be expected to stimulate additional length increase of both the condylar and coronoid processes. This treatment principle is applied routinely on young patients during the presurgical growth management phase. Response to this type of treatment has been found to be beneficial, particularly in type I individuals (Fig. 22–9).

Results of a study of 15 patients with type I HFM showed that during the functional appliance treatment period, the affected side increased more than the contralateral side in four individuals, an amount equal to the contralateral side in another four, and slightly less in the remaining seven subjects. There was no significant group mean difference in growth of the two sides in this sample.[52] A similar response to this type of treatment was reported by Melsen and coworkers.[27]

When treatment response is good, surgical lengthening may be avoided if the canting of the occlusal plane is acceptable. If the occlusal plane is severely affected early, it will be necessary to set the mandible down on the affected side rather early, either after eruption of the first molars or close to the time of eruption of the premolars. The open bite thus created can be closed by active orthodontic extrusion of maxillary teeth. The need for a LeFort I osteotomy is usually avoided (Figs. 22–10, 22–11, 22–12). In type IIA HFM, a similar presurgical treatment phase may be beneficial.[18, 27]

When the condyle is missing, as in type IIB and type III HFM, additional length of the mandible can only be achieved effectively by surgical reconstruction. This should be done early in development, particularly if movements are severely restricted or functions such as chewing and manipulation of food are impaired by the lack of a ramus and severe distortion of the tongue and floor of the mouth to the affected side. The need for a second mandibular lengthening procedure should be anticipated if the costochondral grafting procedures are done early; a considerable amount of additional length is required for symmetry in the adult face.

After operative joint construction and mandibular lengthening and repositioning has been done in the growing child, it is recommended that a functional appliance be used for continued growth management to support the deficient joint structure and asymmetric muscle function.

Orthodontic Treatment

Orthodontic treatment of the growing child should be focused on control of tooth eruption and prevention or correction of dentoalveolar adaptations to the asymmetric position of the maxilla and the mandible. There may be delayed tooth eruption and dental irregularities on the affected side,[8] and crowding of teeth is common. The orthodontist should be actively involved and should coordinate the treatment for children with HFM throughout their growth period.

Surgical Correction of Mandibular Deformity

Operative correction of the skeletal defect is indicated in selected growing children with HFM. If mandibular lengthening and creation of an open bite is done early in the mixed dentition stage, vertical growth potential of the midface can be used to minimize secondary deformity and often prevent the need for a maxillary osteotomy. In type I and IIA HFM, the mandible is elongated and rotated to the proper midline, leaving the TMJ in place (Figs. 22–4, 22–12). A compensatory osteotomy of the normal side is usually not required in the young child. This may be determined preoperatively by model surgery or intraoperatively, depending on the magnitude of the correction and flexibility of the TMJ. No surgery is performed on the maxilla of the young child; an open bite is created on the affected side by the mandibular elongation. This open bite is maintained and regulated by an orthodontic appliance.

Text continued on page 555

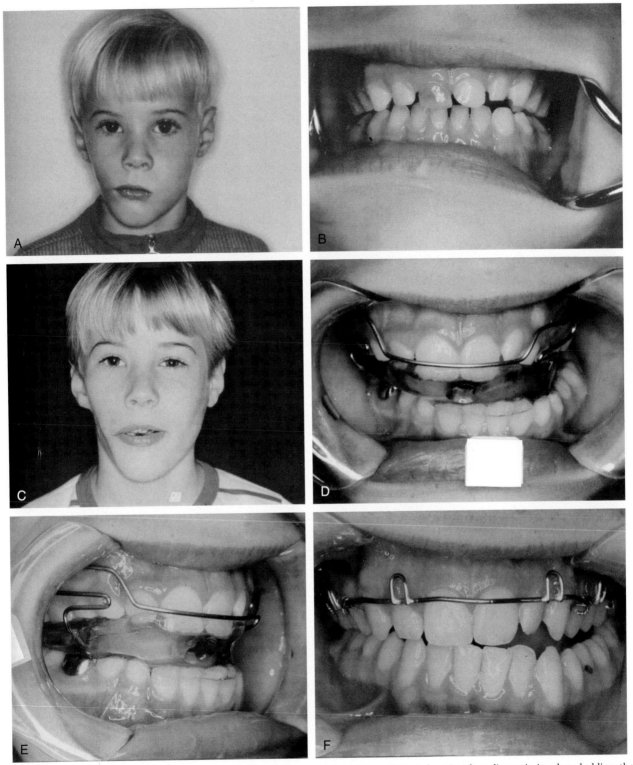

Figure 22–9. *A* and *B*, Six-year old with right hemifacial microsomia. *C, D,* and *E,* A functional appliance is in place holding the affected side down and forward. The acrylic is removed below the maxillary posterior teeth on the affected side, allowing further vertical dentoalveolar development. The appliance serves as a biteblock for the teeth on the contralateral side, inhibiting vertical development. *F,* The maxillary occlusal plane has improved, resulting in an open bite on the contralateral side. The lower dental midline is now further over to the contralateral side, indicating more length increase of the mandible on the affected than on the contralateral side. A surgical arch bar has been placed on the maxillary teeth, and one will also be placed on the mandibular teeth in preparation for the mandibular surgery. Maxillary surgery can be avoided owing to favorable response to functional appliance treatment.

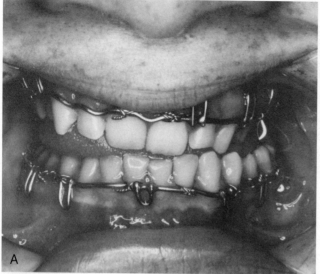

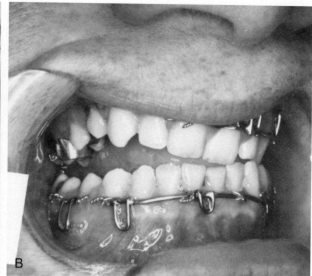

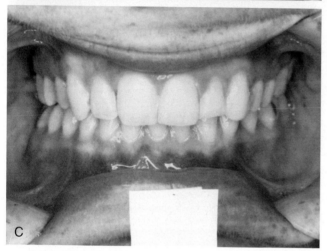

Figure 22–10. Right HFM after ramus-lengthening by an interpositional bone graft. *A,* An open bite has been created by the ramus-lengthening. *B,* The maxillary first molar is being extruded by a spring from a plate. *C,* The maxillary teeth have been brought down to the occlusal level and the left side crossbite has been corrected. When maxillary surgery is not planned, the final orthodontic treatment is done after the corrected mandibular position has been established and the maxillary occlusal plane has been corrected.

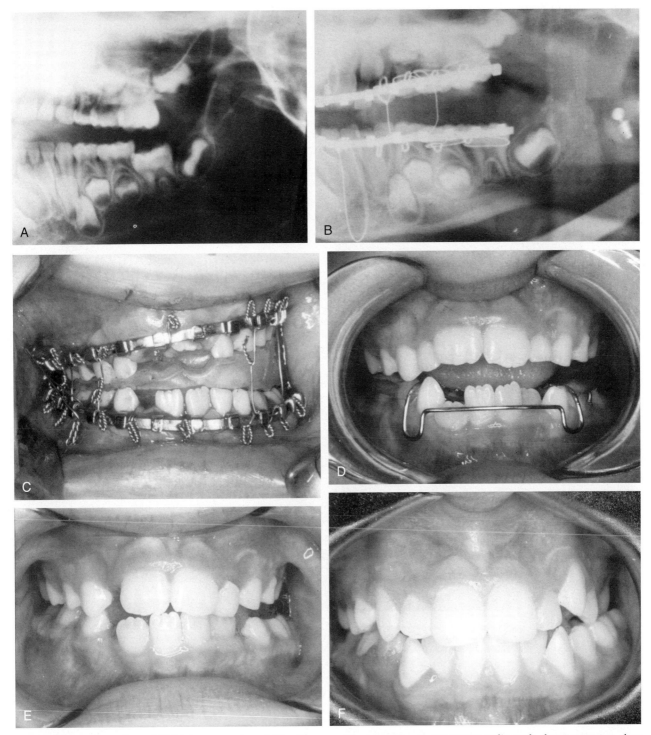

Figure 22–11. Correction of HFM in a growing child with type IIA mandible. *A,* Panoramic radiograph demonstrates a short, abnormally shaped ramus and a very narrow sigmoid notch with slight elongation of the coronoid process. *B,* Immediate postoperative panorex after vertical lengthening of the mandibular ramus. A vertical osteotomy was performed via an extraoral approach. Coronoidectomy was also done at this time. The mandible was lengthened and the proximal portion of the ramus was placed into a notch in the distal fragment. An open bite was created at the time of the surgery. *C,* Immediate postoperative photograph demonstrating the surgically created open bite. Note the diversion of maxillary and mandibular arch bars, which demonstrates the tilting of the maxillary occlusal plane and the postoperative leveling of the mandibular occlusal plane. *D* and *E,* These views demonstrate progressive closure of the open bite over an 18-month period postoperatively. *F,* Intraoral photograph of the same patient 5 years postoperatively demonstrates coincident maxillary and mandibular dental midlines and a level occlusal plane. The patient will have conventional orthodontic treatment for crowding and the slight maxillary width discrepancy.

Illustration continued on following page

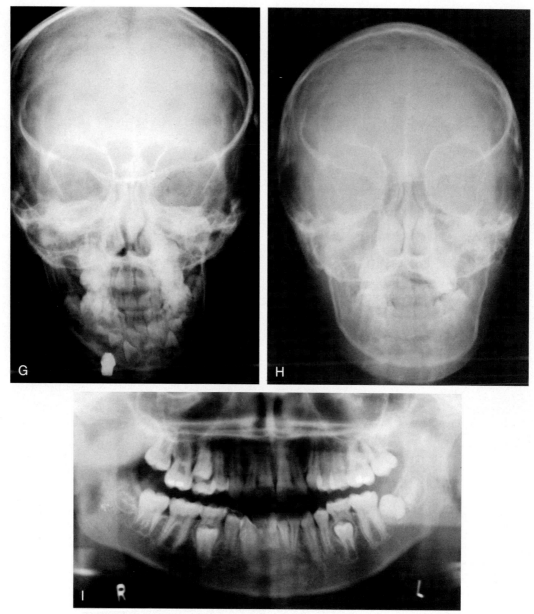

Figure 22–11. *Continued* Preoperative (*G*) and 5-year postoperative (*H*) AP cephalograms and 5-year postoperative panoramic views (*I*) demonstrating mandibular symmetry and remodeling of the angle of the mandible. (Fig. 22–11 is partially reproduced with permission from Kaban LB: Pediatric Oral and Maxillofacial Surgery, pp 284–286. Philadelphia: WB Saunders, 1990.)

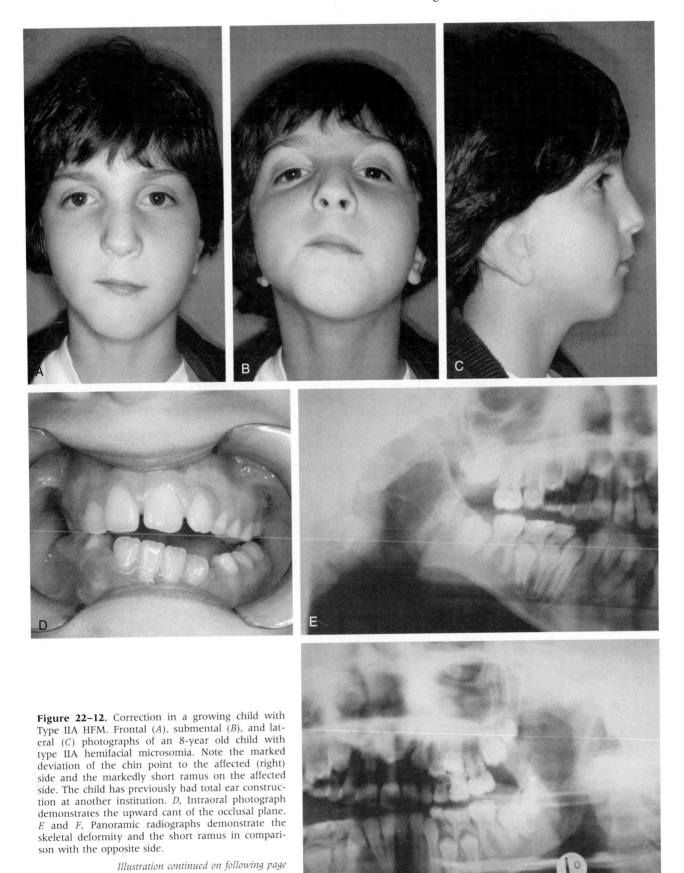

Figure 22–12. Correction in a growing child with Type IIA HFM. Frontal (*A*), submental (*B*), and lateral (*C*) photographs of an 8-year old child with type IIA hemifacial microsomia. Note the marked deviation of the chin point to the affected (right) side and the markedly short ramus on the affected side. The child has previously had total ear construction at another institution. *D*, Intraoral photograph demonstrates the upward cant of the occlusal plane. *E* and *F*, Panoramic radiographs demonstrate the skeletal deformity and the short ramus in comparison with the opposite side.

Illustration continued on following page

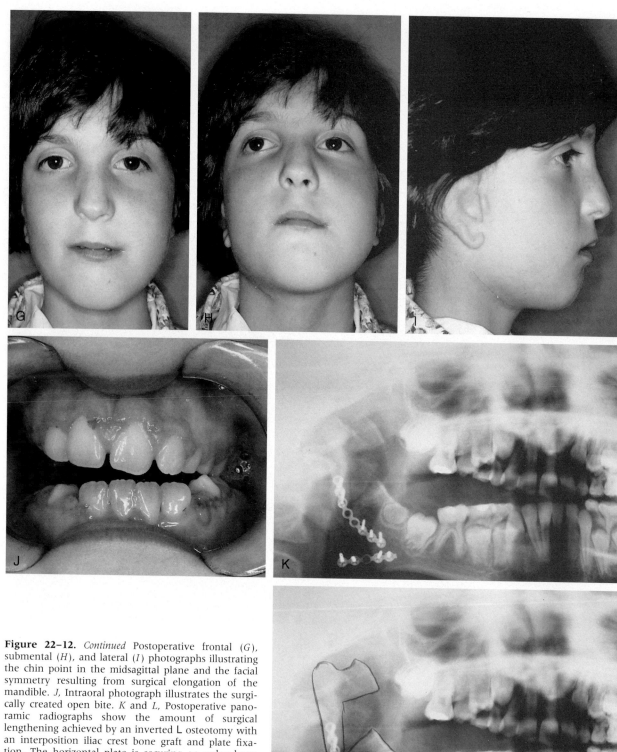

Figure 22–12. *Continued* Postoperative frontal (*G*), submental (*H*), and lateral (*I*) photographs illustrating the chin point in the midsagittal plane and the facial symmetry resulting from surgical elongation of the mandible. *J,* Intraoral photograph illustrates the surgically created open bite. *K* and *L,* Postoperative panoramic radiographs show the amount of surgical lengthening achieved by an inverted L osteotomy with an interposition iliac crest bone graft and plate fixation. The horizontal plate is securing an onlay bone graft to construct the angle.

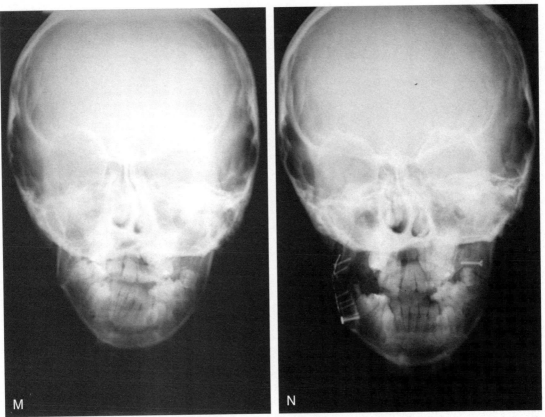

Figure 22–12. *Continued* Preoperative (*M*) and postoperative (*N*) AP cephalograms demonstrating the skeletal symmetry achieved by lengthening of the right ramus of the mandible.

The maxilla grows vertically down into the created space with eruption of the permanent teeth, thus leveling the occlusal plane.[21,22,33] To accelerate this process, active orthodontic extrusion of the maxillary teeth is recommended (Figs. 22–10, 22–12). In type IIB and III HFM, the mandible is elongated and rotated by construction of a mandibular ramus and TMJ with costochondral junction and rib and/or iliac crest bone grafts (Fig. 22–13). The operation and orthodontic procedures are otherwise the same as for patients with types I and IIA HFM.

The results of treatment of HFM in growing children have been reviewed and reported. The Boston Children's Hospital Group[21,22] studied 20 patients who were classified as having type I or IIA (group 1, n = 10) and type IIB or III (group 2, n = 10). They were treated by the protocol described in this chapter, and the mean follow-up was 50.9 months (group 1) and 45 months (group 2). In all cases, the midface grew vertically to close the surgically created open bite, and the occlusal plane was leveled without a maxillary osteotomy. Of the patients with type I or IIA HFM who were observed to completion of growth (9 of 10), none required a maxillary osteotomy or a second operation in the mandible. In patients with type IIB or III HFM who were operated upon during the deciduous dentition period (below age 5), it appears that the affected mandible may require a second elongation procedure in the late mixed dentition period or early teens. Midface osteotomy was not necessary in this series. The patients were reclassified from type IIB or III to type IIA HFM.

The University of California, San Francisco, Group[52] reported continued growth of the lengthened mandibular ramus in the majority of their 10 patients operated on early in their growth period and followed until growth was completed. In three of these subjects, however, growth of the affected side did not keep up with the contralateral side and asymmetry recurred, requiring a second surgical procedure that also involved the maxilla. Otherwise, the maxilla was corrected orthodontically in all these patients.

In summary, the midface hypoplasia that is a progressive secondary deformation due to the restriction of midface growth by the small mandible and underdeveloped musculature can be intercepted or corrected. Elongation of the mandible and creation

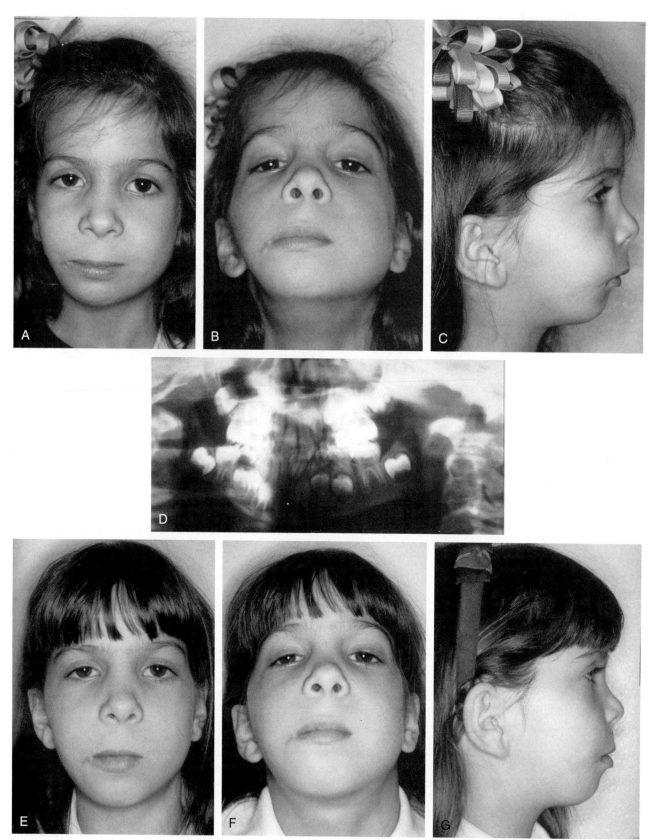

Figure 22–13. Surgical correction of type III HFM in growing child. *A*, Preoperative frontal photograph of a 6-year old child with type III HFM with congenital absence of the ramus of the mandible. *B*, Submental photograph shows the marked deviation of the chin point and the contour deficit of the right face. *C*, Lateral photograph. *D*, Preoperative panoramic radiograph demonstrating the absence of right mandibular ramus. Frontal (*E*), submental (*F*), and lateral (*G*) photographs 1 year postoperatively. Note the marked improvement in the symmetry of the face with the chin point being in the midline and marked improvement of the contour.

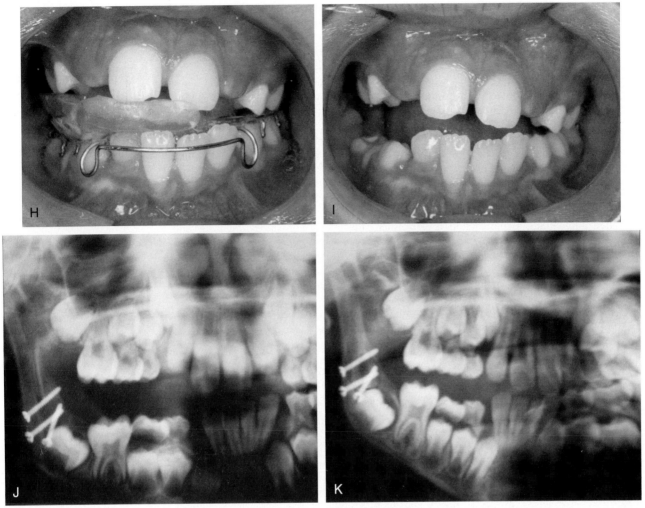

Figure 22–13. *Continued* Intraoral photographs with splint (*H*) and without the splint (*I*) demonstrating the surgically created open bite. Immediate postoperative (*J*) and 1-year postoperative (*K*) panoramic radiographs showing the constructed ramus, the surgically created open bite with progressive closure, and the remodeling of the constructed ramus.

of an open bite on the affected side, in growing children with HFM, decreases and may eliminate the need for bimaxillary surgery in adulthood.[21, 22, 33, 52]

Surgical Correction of Soft Tissue Defects

The correction of the soft tissue abnormalities associated with HFM must be coordinated with the treatment of bony problems. Frequently, small procedures to correct minor but obvious anomalies may alleviate parents' concerns in the first year of life.

Skin Tags

Excision of skin tags can be performed at any age; great care must be exercised in the removal of deep cartilage, because the facial nerve may be quite superficial in small children and can be injured in deep dissection. Sinus tracts can be injected with vital dyes (e.g., methylene blue), and complete removal of stained tissue is critical to avoid subsequent cyst formation.

Ear Abnormalities

The ideal patient for external ear reconstruction has a well-formed lobule in a relatively normal position, although vertically oriented. A large cartilaginous remnant provides a form of autogenous tissue expansion, with thin, pliable skin for coverage of the carved cartilaginous framework. These patients would be classified as having Meurman grade II ear deformities. In these cases, the use of autogenous rib cartilage, as described by Tanzer[48] and later refined by Brent,[3-5] is an ideal method. The optimal age for reconstruction is around 6 years: the ear is approximately 90% of adult size by that age (this age also correlates to the body size) and provides adequate cartilage for reconstruction. This is also a time when body image is becoming important for young children. The precise timing of the surgical intervention must be individualized, taking into account the relative sizes of the ear and the chest cartilage as well as the child's emotional development.

Contralateral rib cartilage is generally used for external ear reconstruction. A Silastic framework has also been used for this purpose, but the lack of resistance to trauma and the incidence of late infection and extrusion makes its use in children questionable. More recently, the use of porous alloplastic material has been advocated, which permits ingrowth of soft tissue; long-term results from the use of this material are not yet available.

When autogenous reconstruction is performed, the synchondrosis of the sixth and seventh ribs is used as a framework, with the cartilage of the eighth rib being attached to provide a helical rim. It is necessary to exaggerate certain features to approximate the appearance of an ear, especially the concha and the antihelical fold. The position of the framework should be as closely symmetric as possible with the contralateral ear, if that is normal.

The vestigial cartilaginous remnant is removed and a thin flap of tissue elevated to cover the carved framework, with adherence maintained by suction drains and dressings for several days. In the absence of adequate skin coverage (grade III deformities or scarring secondary to prior procedures), two alternatives must be considered: tissue expansion or use of temporoparietal fascia as vascularized cover with skin graft closure over the fascia. Later stages are separated by 4 to 6 months, and they consist of derotation of the lobule, separation of the framework from its base with a posterior skin graft, and construction of a tragus. Thus the entire staged reconstruction is completed in 12 to 18 months (see Fig. 22–3).

Patients with true anotia have no lobule and no cartilaginous remnant; these are the most severe deformities and are fortunately quite rare. These patients should be considered for ear prostheses, because reconstruction of the lobule may be quite difficult, especially in light of the associated soft tissue deficit. Glue may separate and cause embarrassment in social situations; reports indicate that the placement of osseointegrated implants in the temporal bone may be useful for supporting prostheses when autogenous reconstruction is not considered for either physical or psychological reasons.[53]

Treatment of the Skeletal Defect in Nongrowing Patients

Orthodontic Management

In the nongrowing patient with HFM, the dento-alveolar adaptations to the asymmetries must be corrected and the arches coordinated before the corrective jaw surgery is done. The principles for this treatment are similar to those that apply to any jaw asymmetries requiring orthognathic surgical correction.

Surgical Correction of Skeletal Defects

Treatment strategy depends on the patient's age and skeletal type. Three-dimension correction of the end-stage deformity of HFM consists of an operation to level the maxilla and pyriform apertures, to make the mandible symmetric, and to place the TMJ in its proper location (coronal plane). Abnormalities in mandibular and maxillary width (transverse plane) are corrected orthodontically or at the time of operation. In the sagittal plane, the maxilla and mandible are mobilized in the direction dictated by the relationship of these structures to the cranial base. Contour defects in the skeleton are corrected with onlay bone grafts; the soft tissue and ear defects are usually corrected after skeletal symmetry has been achieved (Fig. 22–14).

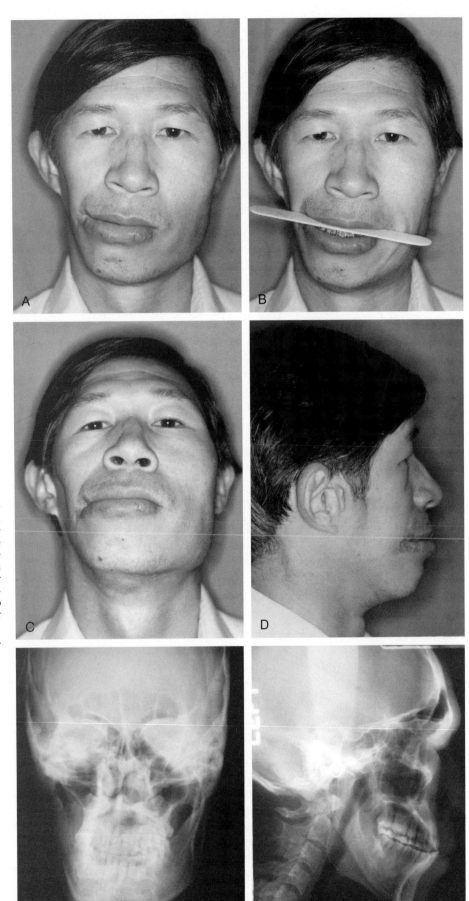

Figure 22–14. Surgical correction of hemifacial microsomia in the adult with end-stage deformity. Frontal (*A* and *B*) and submental (*C*) views of a patient with end-stage type IIA hemifacial microsomia. Note the marked deviation of the chin point to the right, the soft tissue defect, macrostomia, and tilting of occlusal plane. The lateral photograph (*D*) demonstrates the preauricular ear tag, macrostomia and a slightly long and retruded chin. *E,* The AP cephalogram demonstrates marked skeletal asymmetry with an upward cant of the pyriform aperture and occlusal plane on the right side. Maxillary and mandibular dental midlines are also deviated to the right. *F,* The lateral cephalogram demonstrates a double contour at the inferior border indicating the marked discrepancy in ramus height. It also shows bimaxillary dentoalveolar protrusion and a retruded chin.

Illustration continued on following page

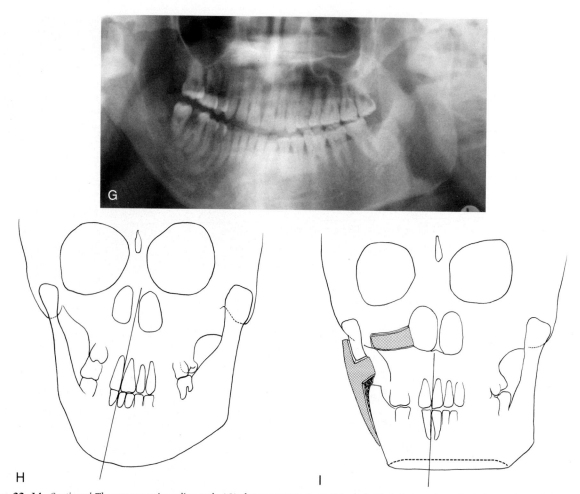

Figure 22–14. *Continued* The panoramic radiograph (*G*) demonstrates type IIA skeletal defect and marked shortening of the ramus on right side. *H,* AP cephalometric tracing demonstrates a plane joining the maxillary and mandibular dental and mandibular skeletal midlines. All lower face midline structures in this patient were deviated to the right of the facial midline. The TMJ was in good position. *I,* The correction included a LeFort 1 osteotomy to correct the maxillary midline and level the occlusal plane. The fulcrum of movement was at the molars on the normal side so that the midface was lengthened maximally on the affected side. Bilateral mandibular osteotomies and an asymmetric advancement genioplasty were planned. Iliac bone grafts were used for the maxillary and mandibular ostectomies and to augment the contour of the right chin and mandible.

In patients with type IIB and type III HFM, a new TMJ and ramus of the mandible are constructed in the correct location. Patients with type III deformity are congenitally missing the ramus and TMJ; the temporal lobe of the brain is visible radiographically where the TMJ would normally be located. In the case of patients with type IIB HFM, the existing ramus is often so hypoplastic and abnormally positioned that it is not useful and must be excised and replaced.[22, 32, 33]

The first step in planning the operation is to determine the proper location for the TMJ. On a coronal or anteroposterior (AP) cephalogram, the true midline (vertical) is drawn from the crista galli through the upper part of the nasal septum. The nasal septum is often in an asymmetric position. The vertical line is then drawn as a perpendicular through crista galli to the line connecting the two zygomaticofrontal sutures (see Fig. 22–1B). The distances from the normal and abnormal TMJs to the midline are measured perpendicular to the true vertical. The vertical distances from the normal and abnormal TMJs to the true horizontal, at the level of the supraorbital rims, are measured. From these measurements it is possible to determine the inferior and medial displacement of the abnormal temporomandibular joint.

At operation, the facial midline is drawn from mid-forehead through the glabella and dorsum of the nose. The distance from the true midline at the glabella to the tragus of the ear is measured on the normal and abnormal sides of the face. The distance from the lateral canthus, on the normal and abnormal sides, to the tragus is

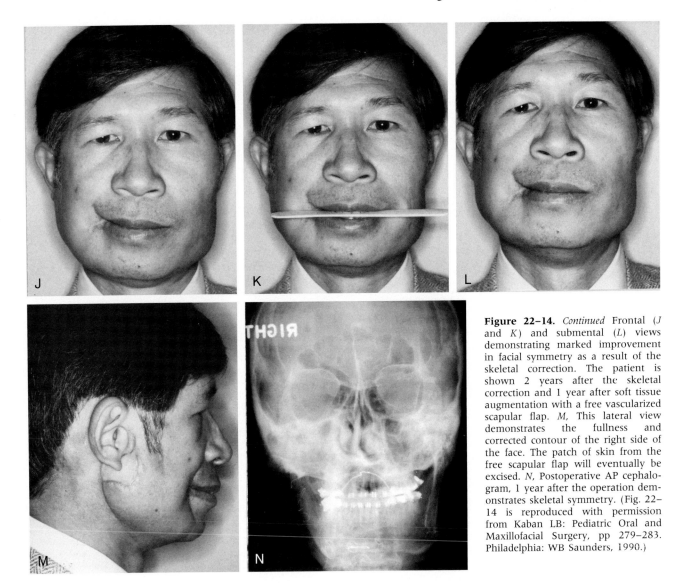

Figure 22–14. *Continued* Frontal (*J* and *K*) and submental (*L*) views demonstrating marked improvement in facial symmetry as a result of the skeletal correction. The patient is shown 2 years after the skeletal correction and 1 year after soft tissue augmentation with a free vascularized scapular flap. *M,* This lateral view demonstrates the fullness and corrected contour of the right side of the face. The patch of skin from the free scapular flap will eventually be excised. *N,* Postoperative AP cephalogram, 1 year after the operation demonstrates skeletal symmetry. (Fig. 22–14 is reproduced with permission from Kaban LB: Pediatric Oral and Maxillofacial Surgery, pp 279–283. Philadelphia: WB Saunders, 1990.)

also documented. The location of the constructed TMJ is determined by these measurements.

The next step in correction of the end-stage adult deformity is to place the maxilla in its correct position by a LeFort I osteotomy (see Fig. 22–14). It is important to choose the correct fulcrum for maxillary repositioning. If there is vertical maxillary excess, the fulcrum of rotation of the maxilla is on the abnormal (short) side, leveling the occlusal plane without midface elongation. If the vertical length of the midface is normal, the fulcrum of rotation is in the midline, and thus midface length does not change. If the midface is short, the fulcrum is on the normal side to provide maximal midface lengthening while leveling the occlusal plane. Once the maxilla is repositioned, bilateral mandibular osteotomies are required to rotate the lower jaw into its correct relation to the maxilla. A new ramus is constructed on the abnormal side, using iliac crest with a costochondral junction for the condylar head. The TMJ is constructed from full thickness rib or iliac crest. It is wired into place lateral to the existing zygomatic arch or to the cranium if no zygomatic arch is present. A glenoid fossa is hollowed out of this graft and lined with perichondrium or temporalis fascia and muscle if present[22, 32, 33] (Fig. 22–15).

Correction of end-stage types I and IIA HFM skeletal defects requires the same planning and operation on the maxilla. The mandible is repositioned with bilateral osteotomies if necessary with or without bone grafts, depending on the anatomy and magnitude of the malformation. The affected TMJ is left intact.

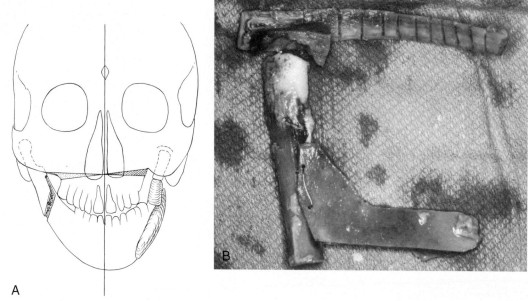

Figure 22–15. *A,* An AP tracing with a proposed operation for correction of another type IIA hemifacial microsomia patient. In this case, the relationship of the maxillary teeth to the upper lip was judged to be satisfactory. Therefore, leveling of the maxillary occlusal plane was achieved by impacting the normal side and lengthening the abnormal side with the fulcrum of rotation in the midline. (This is a more common plan than the maximal lengthening of the midface that was achieved in the patient in Fig. 22–14). A sagittal osteotomy was planned on the normal side because the mandible had to be advanced as well as rotated. Finally, an interpositional and onlay bone graft was planned for the affected mandible to increase its length and contour. *B,* In those patients who require TMJ construction as adults, iliac crest is used for the body, angle, and ramus of the mandible and a costochondral graft is used for the condylar head. The zygomatic arch is constructed with full thickness rib or calvarial bone. The glenoid fossa is constructed medial to the arch and lined with perichondrium or temporalis fascia when present.

Surgical Correction of Soft Tissue Hypoplasia

Correction of soft tissue contour is one of the final steps in surgical reconstruction of HFM, and it must follow skeletal surgery. There is no known alloplastic material that will reliably augment soft tissue contour deformities with long-lasting results. Injection of liquid silicone was tried in the 1970s through a multicenter trial, but early success was followed by late occurrence of severe inflammatory reactions. Minor soft tissue deficits can be corrected with dermal grafts; obtaining such grafts from the buttocks permits an inconspicuous donor scar as well as fairly thick dermis. Although cyst formation has been reported, it is not generally a problem. A study compared dermal grafts to microvascular transfers and revealed that the smaller defects were well corrected by the more minor procedure, whereas the larger defects were better corrected by microvascular tissue transfer.[30]

A variety of donor sites has been proposed for microvascular transfer, the primary distinction being between muscle flaps and de-epithelialized skin and subcutaneous flaps. The recipient vessels, which provide the inflow and outflow in the face, may be anomalous.[20] If muscle is used, either the serratus anterior or the rectus abdominus muscles are those most commonly chosen; the chief problem with muscle transfer is the unpredictable degree of atrophy that occurs after denervation. The use of de-epithelialized flaps is more reliable in this regard and also permits later "fine-tuning" with liposuction if overcorrection has occurred; this is the first choice at most centers (see Fig. 22–14). Omentum was used in early microvascular procedures for contour correction, but this requires a midline abdominal incision and an intra-abdominal procedure, and it also tends to sag with time.

Facial Nerve Palsy

Complete facial palsy in HFM is, fortunately, rare. The chief consideration in infancy is competent eye closure, without which exposure keratitis, corneal ulcerations, and even blindness may occur. An active Bell's phenomenon, involving upward rotation of the globe with eye closure, may be adequate for eye protection; otherwise, patching and lubricants may be required. In older patients, placement of a gold weight in the upper lid to aid in closure has proven to be a useful adjunctive procedure. Lateral tarsorrhaphy has largely been supplanted by procedures that shorten and support the lower eyelid.[44] Correction of paralysis around the mouth is more difficult. An asymmetric smile is of great concern to patients and their families, and the thinning of the soft tissue seen with facial palsy serves only to exaggerate the deformity that is already present. In children with complete paralysis, the best reconstructive approach is a two-stage reconstruction with cross-facial nerve grafting from the contralateral side as the first stage, followed after several months' interval by microneurovascular transfer of muscle. The serratus anterior, the pectoralis minor, and the gracilis muscle have all been used successfully for this purpose. The best results of these transfers are in children, in whom transfers can provide mimetic movement of the commissure and upper lip. Transfer of muscles of mastication (e.g., the temporalis or masseter muscles) provides support for the facial features but does not offer the same degree of coordinated movement, particularly while eating or talking. Static slings should be used only when the patient is a poor candidate for alternative procedures.[19]

SUMMARY

The etiology, pathogenesis, clinical characteristics, diagnosis, and orthodontic and surgical management of HFM have been discussed. We have emphasized the important concept of progression of the deformity with time and growth. The purpose of treatment in the growing child is to enhance growth potential in the mandible, decrease or prevent secondary deformity in contiguous and contralateral facial skeletal structures, and improve body image development by early intervention. In the adult with end-stage malformation, accurate three-dimension analysis and planning, taking into account both the skeletal and soft tissue defects, is critical for the achievement of a satisfactory esthetic and a stable functional result.

The esthetic and functional end result of treatment in HFM is difficult to accurately quantitate because it involves many features, some of which are difficult to assess and some of which are not necessarily associated with the original anomaly. The final form of the new structures depends upon the musculature, other soft tissues, and orofacial functions and can only be predicted in association with assessment of function and neuromuscular characteristics.

References

1. Bennun RD, Mulliken JB, Kaban LB, Murray JE: Microtia: A microform of hemifacial microsomia. Plast Reconstr Surg 1985; 76:859–863.
2. Boles DJ, Bodurtha J, Nance WE: Goldenhar complex in discordant monozygotic twins: A case report and review of the literature. Am J Med Genet 1987, 28:103.
3. Brent B: Auricular repair with autogenous rib cartilage grafts: Two decades of experience with 600 cases. *Plast Reconstr Surg* 1992; 90:355.
4. Brent B: The correction of microtia with autogenous cartilage grafts. 1. The classic deformity. Plast Reconstr Surg 1980; 66:1.
5. Brent B, Byrd HS: Secondary ear reconstruction with cartilage grafts covered by axial, random and free flaps of temporoparietal fascia. Plast Reconstr Surg 1983; 72:141.
6. Chierici G, Miller AJ: Experimental study of muscle reattachment following surgical detachment. J Oral Maxillofac Surg 1984; 42:485.
7. Cohen MM, Rollnick BR, Kaye CI: Oculoauriculovertebral spectrum: An updated critique. Cleft Palate J 1989; 26:276.
8. Cohen MM: Variability versus "incidental findings" in the first and second branchial arch syndrome: Unilateral variants with anophthalmia. Birth Defects 1971; 7:103.
9. Farias M, Vargervik K: Dental development in hemifacial microsomia. I. Eruption and agenesis. Pediatr Dent J 1988; 10:140–143.
10. Francois J, Haustrate L: Anomalies colobomateuses du globe oculaire et syndrome du premier arc. Ann Ocul 1954; 187:340.
11. Gorlin RJ, Jue KL, Jacobson NP, Goldschmidt E: Oculoauriculovertebral dysplasia. J Pediatr 1963; 63:991.
12. Gorlin RJ, Pindborg J: Syndromes of the Head and Neck (1st ed), pp 261–265, 419–425. New York: McGraw-Hill 1964.
13. Grabb WC: The first and second branchial arch syndrome. Plast Reconstr Surg 1965; 36:485.
14. Grayson BH, Boral S, Eisig S, et al: Unilateral craniofacial microsomia. I. Mandibular analysis. Am J Orthodont 1983; 84:225.
15. Gustavson EE, Chen, H: Goldenhar syndrome, anterior encephalocele and aqueductal stenosis following fetal primidone exposure. Teratology 1985, 32:13.

16. Harvold EP: Centric relation. Dent Clin North Am 1975; 19:473.
17. Harvold EP: New treatment principles for mandibular malformations. *In* Transactions of the Third International Orthodontic Congress, 1975, p 148.
18. Harvold EP, Vargervik K, Chierici G (eds): Treatment of Hemifacial Microsomia. New York: Alan R. Liss, 1983.
19. Hoffman WY: Reanimation of the paralyzed face. Otolaryngol Clin North Am 1992; 25:649.
20. Huntsman WT, Lineaweaver W, Ousterhout DK, et al: Recipient vessels for microvascular transplants in patients with hemifacial microsomia. J Craniofacial Surg 1992; 3:187.
21. Kaban LB, Moses ML, Mulliken JB: Correction of hemifacial microsomia in the growing child. Cleft Palate J 1986; 23[Suppl 1]: 50–52.
22. Kaban LB, Moses ML, Mulliken JB: Surgical correction of hemifacial microsomia in the growing child. Plast Reconstr Surg 1988; 82:9–19.
23. Kaban LB, Mulliken JB, Murray JE: Three-dimensional approach to analysis and treatment of hemifacial microsomia. Cleft Palate J 1981; 18:90–99.
24. Lammer EJ, Chen DT, Hoar RM, et al: Retinoic acid embryopathy. N Engl J Med 1985; 313:837.
25. Marsh JL, Baca D, Vannier MW: Facial musculoskeletal asymmetry in hemifacial microsomia. Cleft Palate J 1989; 26:292–302.
26. Melnick M: The etiology of external ear malformations and its relation to abnormalities of the middle ear, inner ear and other organ systems. Birth Defects 1980; 16:303.
27. Melsen B, Bjerregaard J, Bundgaard M: The effect of treatment with functional appliances on a pathologic growth pattern of the condyle. Am J Orthod 1986; 90:503–512.
28. Meurman Y: Congenital microtia and meatal atresia. Arch Otolaryngol 1957; 66:443.
29. Miehlke A, Partsch CJ: Ohrmissbildung, facialis-und abducenslahmung als syndrom der thalidomidschadigung. Arch Ohrenheilkd 1963; 181:154.
30. Mordick TG, Larossa D, Whitaker L: Soft-tissue reconstruction of the face: A comparison of dermal-fat grafting and vascularized tissue transfer. Ann Plast Surg 1992; 29:390.
31. Mulliken JB: Preface. Cleft Palate J 1989; 26:275.
32. Mulliken JB, Kaban LB: Analysis and treatment of hemifacial microsomia. Clin Plast Surg 1987; 14(1):91–100.
33. Murray JE, Kaban LB, Mulliken JB: Analysis and treatment of hemifacial microsomia. Plast Reconstr Surg 1984; 74:186–199.
34. Murray JE, Kaban LB, Mulliken JB, Evans CA: Analysis and treatment of hemifacial microsomia. *In* Caronni EP (ed): Craniofacial Surgery, pp 377–390. Boston: Little, Brown, 1985.
35. Murray JE, Kaban LB, Mulliken JB: Analysis and treatment of hemifacial microsomia. Plast Reconstr Surg 1984; 74:186.
36. Petrovic A, Stutzman J, Oudet C: Control processes in postnatal growth of condylar cartilage of the mandible. *In* McNamara JA Jr (ed): Monograph No. 4, Craniofacial Growth Series, p 100. Ann Arbor: University of Michigan, 1975.
37. Poswillo D: Otomandibular deformity: Pathogenesis as a guide to reconstruction. J Maxillofac Surg 1974; 2:64.
38. Poswillo D: The pathogenesis of 1st and 2nd branchial arch syndrome. Oral Surg 1973; 35:302.
39. Pruzansky S: Not all dwarfed mandibles are alike. Birth Defects 1969; 1:120.
40. Rollnick BR: Oculovertebral anomaly: Variability and causal heterogeneity. Am J Med Genet 1988; [Suppl 4]:41.
41. Ross RB: Lateral facial dysplasia (first and second branchial arch syndrome, hemifacial microsomia). Birth Defects 1975; 11:51.
42. Rune B, Selvik G, Sarnas K, et al: Growth in hemifacial microsomia studied with the aid of roentgen stereophotogrammetry and metallic implants. Cleft Palate J 1981; 17:128.
43. Ryan CA, Finer NN, Ives E: Discordance of signs in monozygotic twins concordant for the Goldenhar anomaly. Am J Med Genet 1988; 29:755.
44. Seiff SR, Chang J: Management of ophthalmic complications of facial nerve palsy. Otolaryngol Clin North Am 1992; 25:669.
45. Soltan HC, Homes LB: Familial occurrence of malformations possibly attributable to vascular abnormalities. J Pediatr 1986; 109:112–114.
46. Stoll C, Roth MP, Dott B, Bigel T: Discordance for skeletal and cardiac defect in monozygotic twins. Acta Genet Med Gemellol 1984; 33:501.
47. Storey A: Temporomandibular joint receptors. *In* Anderson OJ, Matthews B (eds): Mastication, p 50. Bristol: John Wright and Sons, 1976.
48. Tanzer RC: The total reconstruction of the auricle. The evolution of a plan of treatment. Plast Reconstr Surg 1971; 47:523.
49. Tanzer RC: Total reconstruction of the external ear. Plast Reconstr Surg 1959; 23:1.
50. Tenconi R, Hall BD: Hemifacial microsomia: Phenotypic classification, clinical implications, and genetic aspects. *In* Harvold EP, Vargervik K, Chierici G (eds): Treatment of Hemifacial Microsomia, p 40. New York: Alan Liss, 1983.
51. Vargervik K, Miller AJ: Neuromuscular patterns in hemifacial microsomia. Am J Orthod 1984; 86:33–42.
52. Vargervik K, Ousterhout D: Factors affecting long-term results in hemifacial microsomia. Cleft Palate J 1986; 23[Suppl]:53–68.
53. Wilkes GH, Woolfaardt JF: Osseointegrated alloplastic vs. autogenous ear reconstruction: Criteria for treatment selection. Presented at the 71st Annual Meeting of the American Association of Plastic Surgeons, Vancouver BC, Canada, May 20, 1992.

23 | Management of Mandibulofacial Dysostosis*

Paul Tessier and J.-F. Tulasne

ANATOMY

According to Tessier's classification,[1] mandibulofacial dysostosis (MFD) is a compound assemblage of number 6, number 7, and number 8 clefts (Fig. 23–1).

- Number 6 is a *maxillozygomatic* cleft with coloboma of the lower eyelid between the middle and lateral thirds. The cleft is between the maxilla and the zygomatic bone, opening the infraorbital fissure. It is marked on the cheek by a vertical sclerodermic furrow that results from hypoplasia of the subcutaneous tissue and the superficial cheek muscles.
- Number 7 is a *temporozygomatic* cleft, usually with absence of the zygomatic arch and concomitant deformities of the mandibular ramus. Soft tissue abnormalities include malformations of the ear and hypoplasia or absence of the temporal muscle.
- Number 8 is a *frontozygomatic* cleft, with hypoplasia or absence of the frontal process of the zygoma. Because of the lack of malar bone, the lateral orbital rim is formed by the greater wing of the sphenoid.

Combination of the three clefts results in a complex malformation characterized by lack of development of the zygoma, maxilla, and mandible, with associated soft tissue anomalies. MFD, or Treacher Collins syndrome, is always bilateral. Bone and soft tissue anomalies result in impairment of several important functions:

Hearing loss resulting from microtia and middle ear anomalies
Visual disturbance arising from mechanical upper eyelid ptosis or from lower lid coloboma
Breathing difficulties secondary to obstruction of the nasopharynx and hypopharynx
Speech problems as the result of hearing loss and pharyngeal obstruction
Labial incompetence because of the macrostomia, weakness of the levators of the upper lip, and retrogenia pulling away the lower lip

SURGICAL TREATMENT

The surgical treatment of MFD has been well codified by Tessier and Tulasne in several publications.[2–6] This treatment is one of the most difficult and disappointing endeavors in craniofacial surgery. The indications for surgery, timing, and strategy are not yet clearly defined. The central concept is to build a bone structure where there is none, when the orbital complex is absent.

Objectives

The *functional* objectives of treatment of MFD are as follows:

1. To improve hearing function
2. To restore normal nasal and oral breathing
3. To normalize the dental occlusion

---

* Portions of this chapter were previously published in Bell WH (ed): Modern Practice in Orthognathic and Reconstructive Surgery, vol 2, pp 1600–1623. Philadelphia: WB Saunders, 1992.

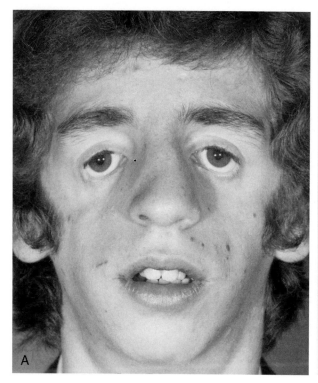

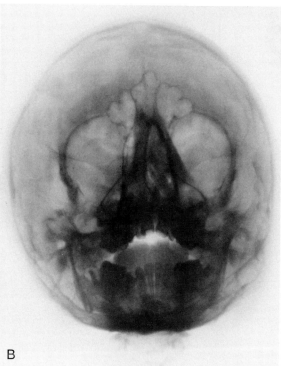

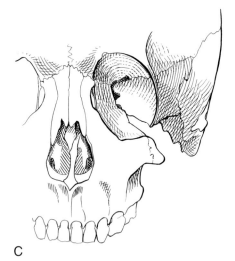

Figure 23–1. Clefts No. 6, No. 7, and No. 8, bilateral: Treacher Collins-Franceschetti syndrome. Frontal view *(A)* and radiographic view *(B)* show complete absence of the malar bone, which appears to be the conjunction of three clefts: maxillozygomatic (between the maxilla and zygomatic bone with eyelid coloboma); temporozygomatic (between the temporal and zygomatic bone with dystopia of the pre-auricular hair line and malformation of the ramus); and frontozygomatic (between the frontal and zygomatic bones with lateral canthal dystopia because of the lack of attachment of the canthus). *C,* Diagram shows typical orbital deformities of MFD, related to the absence of zygomatic bone; prolapsed supra-orbital ridge, lateral wall formed by the greater wing of the sphenoid, infraorbital fissure anteriorly opened.

The *morphologic* objectives are the following:

1. To give projection to the mandible and chin
2. To restore the orbital contours, the malar eminences, and a normal level of the lateral canthi
3. To construct the auricles

Procedures

The procedures used to treat MFD include both displacement of facial segments and bone construction, together with the correction of ear malformations.

Hearing aids are preferred to surgical procedures on the middle ear, which are often unsuccessful and involve the risk of possible damage to the facial nerve.[7]

Auricular construction is done according to Brent's method. It is generally performed in three or four stages, depending on the severity of the malformation. It includes implantation of a costal cartilage framework with later lobule transposition, tragus construction, and conchal excavation.

Endosseous implants placed in the mastoid bone with construction of a prosthetic ear is another treatment alternative. The advantages of this approach include minimal surgical treatment and preservation of the donor sites for use with other reconstructive procedures. The disadvantage of the technique is that it requires maintenance of the implant and the prosthesis. Interested readers are referred to Chapter 23.

Lengthening of the ramus and angle by a V-shaped osteotomy and bone graft advances the mandible and thus expands the floor of the mouth and the pharyngeal space. It also corrects the class II malocclusion and anterior open bite and gives more normal projection to the lower face.

The Obwegeser sagittal split procedure can be applied in some cases. Generally, however, the ramus is so short and narrow that the V-shaped osteotomy with a bone graft inside the gap is preferred. With this procedure, there is no practical limit to lengthening the ramus, and advancement of up to 20 to 25 mm is possible in the mandibular body. In children, the mandible is fixed to the maxilla with a splint in an anterior crossbite position and posterior open bite (Fig. 23–2). Skeletal fixation of the mandible is provided by Kuffner suspension made between two screws in the glabella and the inframandibular rim.

Lowering of the posterior part of the maxilla to open the choanae is achieved by a LeFort I maxillotomy or a LeFort II to III type of midfacial rotation. The latter

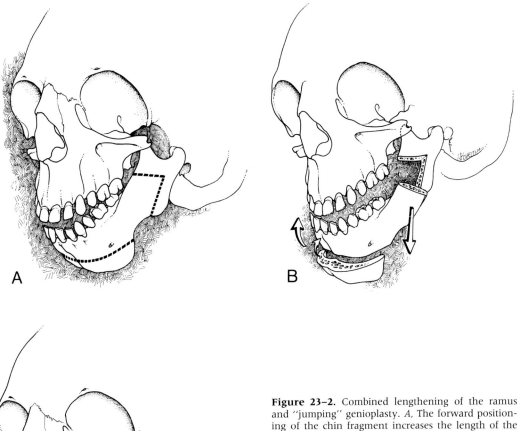

Figure 23–2. Combined lengthening of the ramus and "jumping" genioplasty. *A,* The forward positioning of the chin fragment increases the length of the mandibular body. The osteotomy of the ramus is performed through a combined oral and extraoral route. *B,* A posterior open bite is created. *C,* The bone gap is filled with cranial or tibial grafts. (From Tessier P, Tulasne JF: Surgical correction of Treacher Collins Syndrome. *In* Bell WH (ed): Modern Practice in Orthognathic and Reconstructive Surgery, vol 2, pp 1600–1623. Philadelphia: WB Saunders, 1992.)

procedure is indicated particularly in young children to preserve the dental buds, which could be damaged by an osteotomy at the LeFort I level.

After the osteotomy at the LeFort II or III level (depending on the degree of aplasia of the zygomas), the midfacial segment is rotated around a transverse axis using the frontonasal angle as a fulcrum. A bur is used to remove bone from the frontal region and to allow deeper impaction at the frontonasal angle. The rotation has the following effects: (1) shortening of the anterior face; (2) forward movement of the anterior teeth; (3) downward movement of the posterior maxilla, which also enlarges the nasopharynx; and (4) downward displacement of the zygomatic remnant, which slightly enlarges the vertical diameter of the orbit. As a result, the maxilla approaches the horizontal plane and has a more pronounced projection.

Stability is provided by bone grafts taken from the calvarium in the parietal region. Depending on the patient's age, the graft can be either half thickness taken at intervals or full thickness harvested as a single fragment that is cut in several bands and split.

The frontonasal angle is stabilized with two interosseous wires. The key point for sagittal stability is the bone graft interposed between the temporal bone and the maxilla (Fig. 23–3A).

The parietal area gives the correct curvature to the temporomaxillary bone graft. The posterior end of this graft is fixed to the cranium through a hole that enters the middle cranial fossa anteriorly or above the mastoid process. The anterior end is fixed under the malar stump against the maxilla.

The orbital complex is also constructed with calvarial bone grafts to the lateral orbital wall, the inferior lateral angle, the floor, and the inferior orbital rim.

Cancellous grafts from the tibia can also be used to fill in the dead space between the major grafts (Fig. 23–3B).

Genioplasty with elongation of the suprahyoid tissues lengthens the body of the mandible and achieves a better contour to the chin and the whole lower face. If

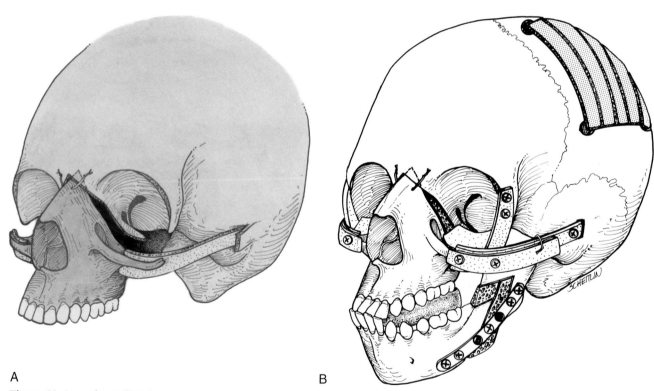

A   B

Figure 23–3. *A*, The midfacial segment is stabilized by two central wires and by lateral bone grafts. The latter abut against the maxilla behind the malar stump. They are pegged either into a groove above the mastoid or in a hole in the median cranial fossa. *B*, Lengthening of the ramus and mandibular body by a V-shaped osteotomy and eventually by a bone graft between the fragments. The mandible is advanced on a splint in an anterior crossbite position and a posterior open bite. Construction of the orbital region and zygoma is completed with calvarial grafts. Tibial or iliac cancellous grafts fill up the dead spaces between the main supporting grafts. The calvarial donor site is covered by the other part of the split strips of the parietal bone. (From Tessier P, Tulasne JF: Surgical correction of Treacher Collins Syndrome. *In* Bell WH (ed): Modern Practice in Orthognathic and Reconstructive Surgery, vol 2, pp 1600–1623. Philadelphia: WB Saunders, 1992.)

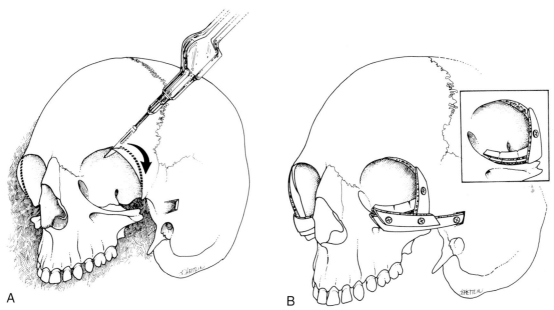

Figure 23–4. Bone grafting required for bilateral construction of the malar bone, zygomatic arch and orbital contours. *A,* Resection of the prolapsed supraorbital ridge. *B,* Cranial or iliac grafts of the orbital floor and the inferior orbital wall. Cranial grafts of the zygomatic arch and the inferior and lateral orbital rims. *Inset* shows detail of grafting on left orbit. (From Tessier P, Tulasne JF: Surgical correction of Treacher Collins Syndrome. *In* Bell WH (ed): Modern Practice in Orthognathic and Reconstructive Surgery, vol 2, pp 1600–1623. Philadelphia: WB Saunders, 1992.)

necessary, another advancement genioplasty can be made after 2 years by means of a transplanted inframandibular segment.

The orbital complex and zygomatic arch are constructed and reshaped in two or three stages with bone grafts from the calvarium, ilium, tibia, or ribs (Fig. 23–4).

Construction of the orbit requires more than the addition of bone grafts where bone is missing. Prior to bone grafting, the prolapsed supralateral orbital angle is recontoured by deepening the curvature. Then the bone graft used to build up the lateral rim is placed in the temporal fossa. It is pegged into a groove on the temporal crest and into another groove made in the long graft, which constitutes the zygoma and inferior rim and extends to the temporal bone.

In the planning of orbital reconstruction, it must never be forgotten that the malar bone is often totally absent, the zygomatic arch is always totally missing, the infraorbital rim and maxillary orbital floor are highly hypoplastic, and the condition is bilateral. Consequently, orbital reconstruction requires considerable amounts of bone graft material. Moreover, all patients with the complete form of the syndrome have short stature, that is, they are hypotrophic children. Therefore, neither the ilium nor the thorax can provide a sufficient amount of bone for such an extensive bilateral construction.

The eyelid coloboma is corrected by dissection of the edges of the cleft and careful approximation of the conjunctiva, orbicularis oculi muscle, and skin (Tessier's procedure). Chondromucosal grafts from the upper lateral cartilage and/or nasal septum are useful in cases of severe hypoplasia of the lower eyelid (Fig. 23–5).

Correction of the coloboma gives a more normal contour to the margin of the lower eyelid. The construction of the inferior rim by bone grafting provides better support to the orbital septum and consequently the lower eyelid. However, all bone grafts to the zygoma and inferior rim make the vertical shortness of the skin more obvious, because the eyelid skin is not supported by a strong orbicularis muscle. In addition, all reoperations through the infraorbital route result in more dense scar tissue, which increases retraction of the eyelid without true ectropion. The final correction consists of resection of the scar, vertical stretching of the edges of the excision, and placement of a large regional full-thickness skin graft.

A *lateral canthopexy* must be done each time the orbital complex is reconstructed or reinforced. However, even after construction of the lateral orbital rim and advancement of the temporal fascia, the lateral canthus tends to return to a lax state despite fixation to the bone and the temporal aponeurosis. The absence or weakness of the orbital

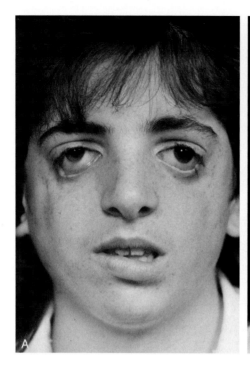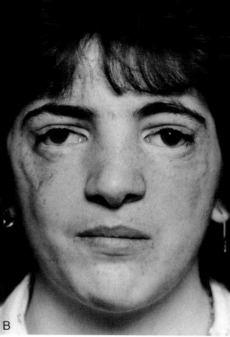

Figure 23–5. Treacher Collins syndrome. *A,* Severe hypoplasia of the lower eyelids. *B,* After reconstruction of the lower eyelids with chondromucosal grafts from the nasal septum and a cutaneous flap from the upper eyelid. The patient also had lateral canthopexy, bone grafting of the orbits, mandibular lengthening, and genioplasty. She still needs additional bone grafts on the zygomas. (Patient operated on by Dr. Tulasne.) (From Tessier P, Tulasne JF: Surgical correction of Treacher Collins Syndrome. *In* Bell WH (ed): Modern Practice in Orthognathic and Reconstructive Surgery, vol 2, pp 1600–1623. Philadelphia: WB Saunders, 1992.)

septum, which is part of the superficial musculoaponeurosis system, may explain the recurrent looseness of the lateral canthus.

Orthodontic treatment is always necessary to align the teeth both preoperatively and after surgical correction.

TIMING

Principles of treatment timing are as follows:

1. Hearing aids should be used as early as possible.
2. Eyelid colobomas can be corrected in the first few years of life.
3. Orbital and zygomatic reconstruction can begin between 6 and 10 years of age.
4. Ear construction can begin after 8 years of age, when substantial rib cartilage is available.
5. Surgery of the jaws should be performed between the ages of 6 and 10 years only when the child has major breathing problems.

The deficiency in oral and nasal breathing causes not only acute and chronic respiratory insufficiency but also the poor development of these children. Early operation is not necessary for correction of facial dysmorphism or dental malocclusion but is performed exclusively for addressing the choanal atresia and hypopharyngeal obstruction.

RESULTS

As previously stated, the treatment of MFD is one of the most disappointing endeavors in craniofacial surgery (Fig. 23–6). Immediate results often are promising, but relapse or deterioration, at least partial, seems inevitable. One reason for this is that resorption of bone grafts in MFD is more severe than in other malformations. In the malar region, this phenomenon may be explained by the absence of periosteum where bone is lacking, coverage of the graft by skin only, precarious contact of the grafts with the temporal bone and the maxilla, and/or minimal stressing of the grafts by muscular function. Although the condition can be much improved after several operations, the patient still looks like someone with MFD, even if cranial grafts seem to be resorbed to a lesser extent than rib or iliac grafts (Fig. 23–7).

Text continued on page 575

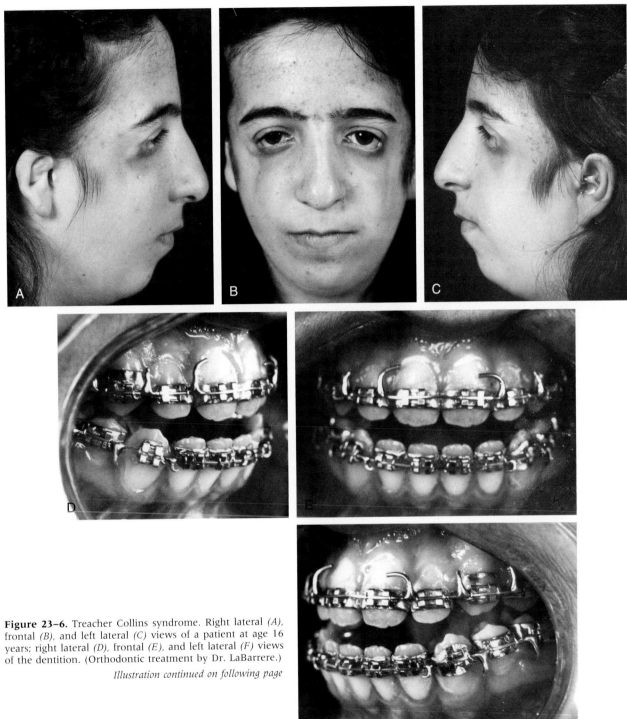

Figure 23–6. Treacher Collins syndrome. Right lateral *(A),* frontal *(B),* and left lateral *(C)* views of a patient at age 16 years; right lateral *(D),* frontal *(E),* and left lateral *(F)* views of the dentition. (Orthodontic treatment by Dr. LaBarrere.)

Illustration continued on following page

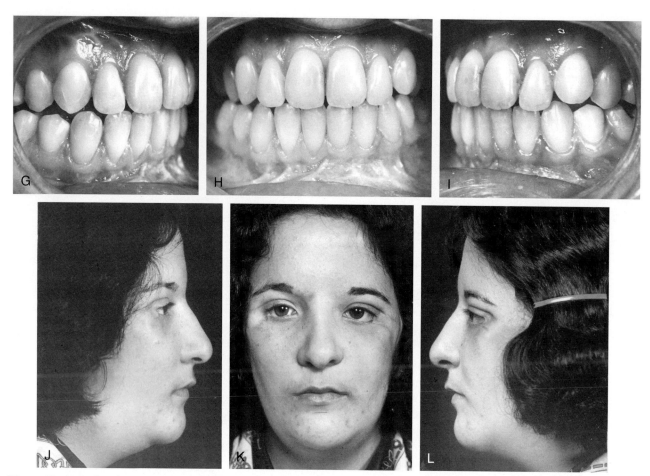

Figure 23–6. *Continued.* At age 20 years, right lateral *(G)*, frontal *(H)*, and left lateral *(I)* views of the dentition and right lateral *(J)*, frontal *(K)*, and left lateral *(L)* views of the patient, after a two-stage radical procedure (with genioplasty) and two additional operations on the orbits and eyelids.

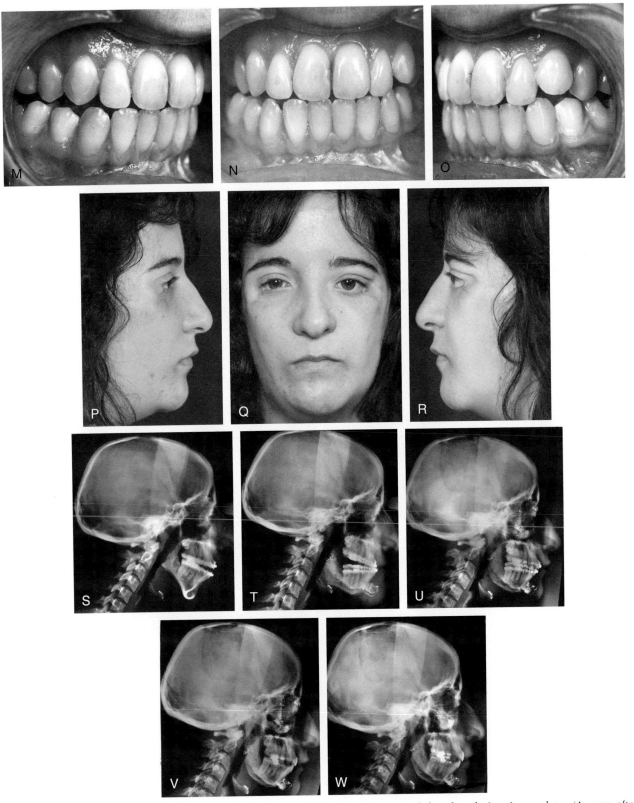

Figure 23–6. *Continued.* Right lateral *(M)*, frontal *(N)*, and left lateral *(O)* views of dental occlusion 1 year later (4 years after mandibular lengthening and 3 years after rotation of the midfacial segment); right lateral *(P)*, frontal *(Q)*, and left lateral *(R)* views of the patient. Cephalometric radiographs before *(S)* and 3 months after *(T)* the first operation, showing lengthening of the ramus with tibial graft and genioplasty. Cephalometric radiographs 6 months *(U)*, 18 months *(V)*, and 4 years *(W)* after rotation of the midfacial segment. (Patient was operated on by Dr. Tulasne.) (From Tessier P, Tulasne JF: Surgical correction of Treacher Collins syndrome. *In* Bell WH (ed): Modern Practice in Orthognathic and Reconstructive Surgery, vol 2, pp 1600–1623. Philadelphia: WB Saunders, 1992.)

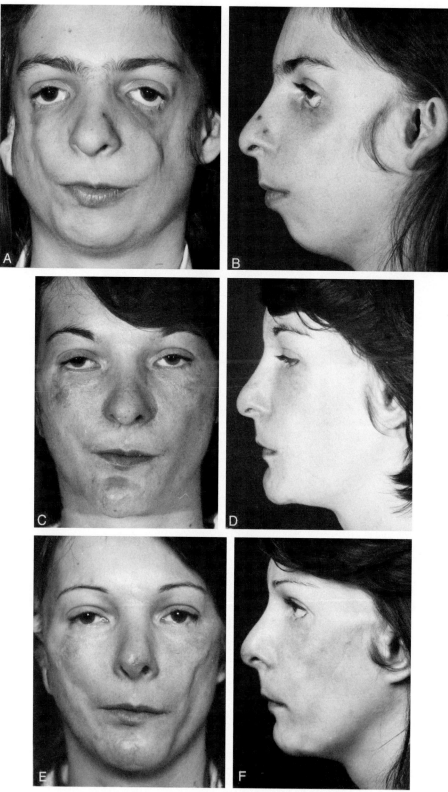

Figure 23–7. Before (*A* and *B*) and 4 years later (*C* and *D*) construction of the orbital contours, posterior displacement of the preauricular hair, and flap advancement genioplasty. *E* and *F*, After 9 years, partial deterioration in the zygomatic regions and cheeks is seen. (Patient was operated on by Dr. Tessier.) (From Tessier P, Tulasne JF: Surgical correction of Treacher Collins Syndrome. *In* Bell WH (ed): Modern Practice in Orthognathic and Reconstructive Surgery, vol 2, pp 1600–1623. Philadelphia: WB Saunders, 1992.)

The position of the midfacial segment is rather stable in both adults and children. There is a strong tendency to relapse after lengthening the mandible in children. This suggests that postponement of mandibular operations until the patient is 12 to 15 years old may be prudent except in the case of major breathing problems.

References

1. Tessier P: Anatomical classification of facial, craniofacial and laterofacial clefts. J Maxillofac Surg 1976; 4:69.
2. Tessier P, Rougier J, Hervouet F, et al: Plastic Surgery of the Orbit and Eyelids. New York: Masson Publishing, 1981, pp 164, 170.
3. Tulasne JF, Tessier P: The logical treatment of Treacher Collins syndrome. Presented at the European Meeting of Plastic and Reconstructive Surgery, Stockholm, 1985.
4. Tulasne JF, Tessier P: Results of the Tessier integral procedure for correction of Treacher Collins syndrome. Cleft Palate J [Suppl 23] 1986.
5. Tessier P, Tulasne JF: Treacher Collins syndrome (Berry, Pires de Lima, Treacher Collins, Franceschetti syndrome): Combined rotation of the midfacial segment and mandibular lengthening. *In* Marchac D (ed): Craniofacial Surgery. Proceedings of the First International Congress of the International Society of Cranio-Maxillo-Facial Surgery. Berlin: Springer-Verlag, 1987, p 369.
6. Tessier P, Tulasne JF: Surgical correction of Treacher Collins syndrome. *In* Bell WH (ed): Modern Practice in Orthognathic and Reconstructive Surgery, vol 2. Philadelphia: WB Saunders, 1992, pp 1600–1623.
7. Brent B: Auricular repair with autogenous rib cartilage grafts: Two decades of experience with 600 cases. Plast Reconstr Surg 1992; 90:355–373.

Distraction Osteogenesis: Indications, Clinical Application, and Preliminary Case Reports

H. Wolfgang Losken, Katherine W. L. Vig, and Fernando Molina

INTRODUCTION

Lengthening of long bones, particularly those of the lower limb, has preoccupied orthopedic surgeons for more than a century. In 1890, Hopkins and Penrose[1] reported a method of extending long bones by a transverse osteotomy that was stabilized by ivory pegs in the medullary cavity. This method was criticized by Magnuson[2] in 1908, who observed "this blocked the ends of the medullary cavity and left no periosteum over the space between the fragments, making it impossible for new bone to be formed in the interspace."

The interest in developing a technique to increase the length of long bones was a direct consequence of the prevalence of poliomyelitis in childhood. Fractures involving the epiphysis in children were another common cause of failure of the long bones to reach their full growth potential. Unfortunately, before the advent of antibiotics in the 1940s, the risk of infection following such procedures made bone lengthening a high-risk venture for patients.

In reviewing mandibular distraction and its application from a century of literature on lengthening long bones, especially the legs, current concepts relate to the Ilizarov era.[3] Deformities of the arms and legs have concerned "Orthopedia" since 1741, when Nicholas Andry[4] recorded a cure that parents could effect on their children by rubbing the affected arm or leg of the child with "a bit of Scarlet cloth." This was supposed to gently cause friction "to bring back the Animal spirits" as reported by Moseley. The introduction into North America and the adoption of the technique by orthopedic surgeons may largely be ascribed to the new understanding and rationale of the biology of lengthening bones. The importance of the intramedullary circulation and preservation of the soft tissues resulted in the introduction of the corticotomy to replace the previous osteotomy procedure. One of the first successful bone lengthening procedures was reported by Codvilla[5] in 1905 after he lengthened a femur to correct limb length discrepancy. Several years elapsed before the procedure was reported again in 1927, when Abbott[6] successfully lengthened a tibia and fibula in the lower leg. The procedure was fraught with problems of infection and malunion and, because of complications, was abandoned until Gavriel A. Ilizarov, a Russian physician, introduced a technically innovative method of bone distraction in the long bones.[7] He described distraction osteogenesis in the femur, tibia, radius, ulna, humerus, iliac crest, and also the bones of the hands.[8,9]

Our current concepts have evolved from distraction appliances with external frames or devices from which alignment of the parts could be maintained as they were slowly moved apart. Complications in the late 1930s included the risk of infection and other complications, about which Compere[10] warned that "some patients were more crippled after the procedure than before." By the 1970s, the Wagner technique[11,12] was introduced into North America, and such advances prepared the scene for the corticotomy of the Ilizarov era. Although this technique was not universally accepted, the delay following the operative procedure *before* starting distraction allowed osteogenesis to begin, and the success rate improved.[13] In addition, stabilization of the fragments after distraction allowed consolidation of the newly formed bone and support while it regained adequate strength. The application of this technique to mandibular distraction obeys many of the same rules, except that the mandible is not a weightbearing bone

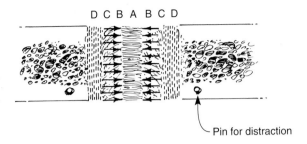

Figure 24–1. Histological appearance of osteogenesis following bone distraction at the corticotomy site in a canine model. *A,* Fibrous tissue; *B,* advancing bone formation; *C,* bone remodeling; *D,* mature bone. (Based on Karp NS, McCarthy JG, Schreiber JS, et al: Membranous bone lengthening: A serial histological study. Ann Plast Surg 1992; 29:2–7.)

and it has multidirectional forces from a variety of muscular attachments, including the pterygomasseteric sling, the suprahyoid musculature, the tongue muscles, and others. Experimental and clinical studies in gradually lengthening the mandible by distraction[14] has provided the biologic basis to rationalize the procedure in the human mandible. The neurosensory deficits in the inferior alveolar nerve, following gradual distraction, have not been fully elucidated in the human. However, Block and co-workers[15] reported on changes in the inferior alveolar nerve following mandibular lengthening in a canine model. Because many of the patients who have had distraction osteogenesis are infants or young children, it has not been possible to use nerve evoked potentials for evaluating the outcome of the treatment with a validated and reliable measure.

Bone lengthening or distraction osteogenesis using circumferential corticotomy and gradual distraction had been developed in the lengthening of long bones, but only recently has it been attempted in the craniofacial region for the correction of unilateral or bilateral mandibular deficiency. Although initially the technique was developed to lengthen the long bones, it was not until the 1970s that the technique of performing a corticotomy with minimal disruption of the periosteum and endosteum was applied to the mandible using an extraoral bone lengthening device in a canine model.[16, 17] Mandibular lengthening by distraction has been evaluated in dogs and sheep. The optimal amount of distraction was considered to be 1 mm per day for 14 days in a canine mandible with an external device. Michieli and Miotti[17] used an orthodontic appliance on the teeth of dogs to examine the histologic changes of collagen fibers with distraction of the bone. More recently, Karp and McCarthy[18] reported membranous bone lengthening with external devices and evaluated the histologic response. This serial histologic study in the canine mandible reveals the mechanism of bone formation during the distraction process to be similar to that in long bones. The gap between the distracted bone edges is filled with fibrous tissue, which becomes oriented in the direction of distraction (Fig. 24–1). Early bone formation advances along the fibrous tissue from the bone ends, with collagen fibers parallel to the tension vectors. Slender trabeculae of bone extend from the bone ends and calcify (Fig. 24–2). At completion of distraction, osteoclastic resorption of bone is noted, and the trabeculae become thicker to form early cortical bone. The vascular spaces increase and bone

Figure 24–2. Schematic view of bone remodeling following osteogenesis in the mandible.

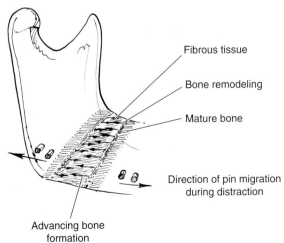

Fibrous tissue

Bone remodeling

Mature bone

Direction of pin migration during distraction

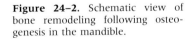

Advancing bone formation

remodeling occurs with increased osteoblastic bone formation and osteoclastic resorption and remodeling. Apparently, bone regains 90% of its original structure within 8 months of distraction, and long-term studies are indicated in the growing individual to ascertain whether the increased bone length is maintained over time and continues to respond to systemic somatic growth stimulation. Intraoral mandibular distraction was attempted by Staffenberg, and also by Wood and coworkers.[19] Extrapolating from contemporary orthodontic treatment involving rapid maxillary expansion, the distraction of the midpalatal suture is not directly applicable, because this involves a reactive sutural response. However, in surgically assisted rapid maxillary expansion, a similar rationale applies to the maxilla in correcting transverse discrepancies.

The purpose of this chapter is to review the application of gradual distraction osteogenesis in the human mandible in those craniofacial anomalies that result in bilateral or unilateral mandibular deficiency.

BIOLOGIC RATIONALE FOR BONE DISTRACTION

In 1992, distraction of the human mandible was reported by McCarthy, Schreiber and coworkers,[20] using a skin incision and external bone distractors. Two pins were inserted into each bony segment. An alternative method by Molina and Ortiz Monasterio[21] involved approaching the mandible through a vestibular incision and performing a corticotomy of the gonial angle, using a single pin fixation to each segment of the mandible in front and behind the corticotomy. They also reported a double bone corticotomy of the mandible involving the ascending ramus and the mandibular body with a pin in each of the three segments to differentially distract the vertical and horizontal rami (Fig. 24–3).

The rationale for distraction osteogenesis relies on the premise that the regeneration of bone between the distracted ends will result in a lengthening of bones that will remain stable. This is predicated on the biologic response of bony healing. Because much of our understanding of bone remodeling has been derived from skeletal fractures, it is incumbent on those clinicians using the techniques to evaluate new procedures with reliable and valid outcome measures to ascertain the utility and efficacy of bone distraction in comparison with alternative methods of treatment.

Ilizarov proposed the tension-stress model as an explanation, in which ''the gradual traction on living tissue creates stress that can stimulate and maintain the regeneration and active growth of certain tissue structures, through metabolic stimulation.''

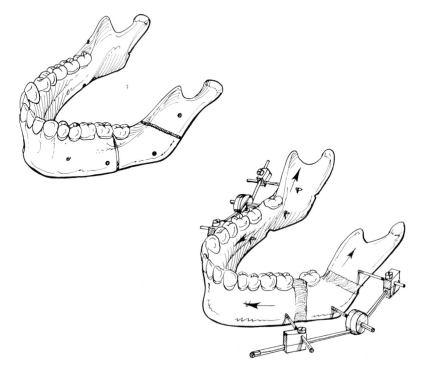

Figure 24–3. Bidirectional distraction to effect an elongation of both the vertical ramus and the horizontal body of the mandible.

INDICATIONS FOR MANDIBULAR DISTRACTION IN HUMANS

Severe mandibular deficiency in infants and children may be unilateral or bilateral. Birth defects with craniofacial manifestations may fall into the classification of malformations, deformations, or disruptions, depending on their etiology.[22, 23] The prognosis for future growth and development is considered to be related closely to the etiology. For instance, the small mandible associated with the Robin sequence has a different prognosis for "catch up" growth than that of a child with Treacher Collins syndrome. Likewise, hemifacial microsomia/craniofacial microsomia differs from a fractured mandibular condyle due to birth injury or an acquired injury for future facial asymmetry with continued growth in the child. In determining the appropriate treatment plan, it is important that the initial defect be accurately diagnosed and managed. Traditionally, costochondral grafts have been recommended in the early management of unilateral or bilateral mandibular deficiency when the condyle is absent or severely hypoplastic. The size and shape of the mandible during the growth period of the child can be unpredictable, with either overgrowth or undergrowth. In most birth defects involving mandibular deficiency, there is also the consequence of respiratory and feeding difficulties in the neonatal period. These vital functions take precedence over the developing malocclusion, and the role of the orthodontist is adjunctive to surgical intervention. However, in the 6- to 8-year-old child, an orthodontic evaluation is appropriate, not only in assessing future growth and development but also in managing the cant of the occlusal plane, which may develop as a consequence of the unilateral skeletal and soft tissue deficiencies in hemifacial microsomia. Differential modification of the dentoalveolar process may be accomplished by controlling eruption of the permanent successors in the mixed dentition. A hybrid functional type of appliance[24] may be indicated, but expectations of promoting or accelerating growth on the affected side are usually unrealistic in effecting a marked skeletal change that would avoid surgical intervention to correct the facial asymmetry.

MANDIBULAR DISTRACTION OSTEOGENESIS

Procedures to correct mandibular skeletal deficiency in the infant or young child to promote improvement in airway function and feeding capability have had unpredictable results. The advent of distraction osteogenesis to lengthen the mandible provides the clinician with an effective means of increasing mandibular length by promoting an increase in the amount of new bone at the corticotomy site in the mandible. This method of slowly distracting the bone ends at 1 mm per day allows stretching and adaptation of the musculotendinous attachments to the mandible, with the assumption that serial sarcomere additions may allow neuromuscular adaptation to gradual alteration in mandibular morphology. Previous unrealistic claims that have been made for functional appliances have now been realized in this innovative method of lengthening the mandible.

DUAL PIN: PITTSBURGH EXPERIENCE

(Case Report 1)

Distraction osteogenesis is performed (HWL) using an external bone lengthening device (Fig. 24–4A,B) (Howmedica Corporation, Rutherford, NJ). Initially the procedure was performed under general anaesthetic with orotracheal intubation, and a modified Risdon incision was made over the lower border of the mandible. The dissection is performed carefully to avoid the mandibular nerve; the mandible is exposed extraperiosteally and the site of the corticotomy established. The corticotomy is typically made behind the terminal molar tooth (Fig. 24–5) and radiographs confirm the exact location of the corticotomy site and placement of the pins. In the young child with unerupted teeth, it is important not to damage the tooth germs or dental lamina. The corticotomy may be made along the horizontal ramus, at the angle of the mandible, or on the ascending ramus. If the deficiency is mainly in the vertical ramus, the corticotomy should be on the vertical ramus, but if the deficiency includes the

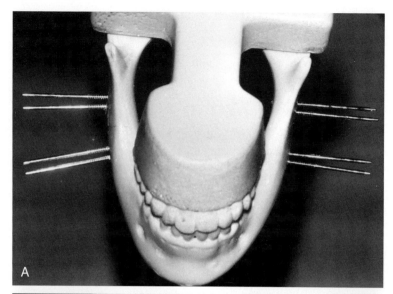

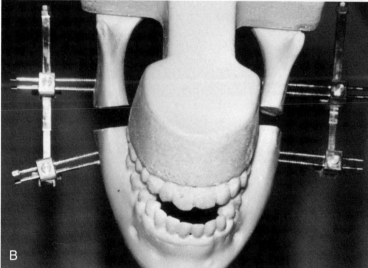

Figure 24–4. *A,* Model illustrating direction of dual pin approach with placement of the pins on either side of the corticotomy site. *B,* Model illustrating the effect of opening the attached distraction device. Note angulation of pins and the effect on the occlusal relationship.

Figure 24–5. Dual pin technique with position of corticotomy distal to terminal molar.

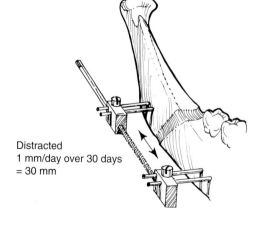

Distracted
1 mm/day over 30 days
= 30 mm

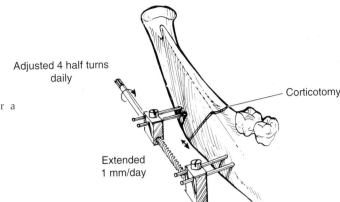

Figure 24–6. Following activation of distraction device over a month period at a rate of 1 mm per day.

vertical and horizontal ramus equally, the bone is divided at the angle. If the deficiency is predominantly of the horizontal body of the mandible, the corticotomy is made on the body of the mandible. The pins are inserted on each side of the corticotomy site (Fig. 24–6). The pin sites are marked off on the mandible so that the pin placement is at the preplanned angle to the lower border of the mandible, taking care to avoid the inferior alveolar nerve.

Dual Pin Procedure

Planning

The object of treatment is to correct the mandibular deficiency. The deformity may be more correctly altered by assessing the extent of deficiency in three dimensions compared with normative gender- and age-related standards. If the pin placement can be mathematically determined in the vertical and horizontal direction, an approximate model for planning direction and position may be estimated. However, because syndromic patients may have intrinsic potential deficiencies for growth and development, a mathematical model may only approximate the biologic response. In a mandible that is bilaterally deficient (10 mm each side) in the vertical and horizontal ramus, with a gonial angle of 140 degrees, the pin placement angle is adjusted accordingly from the lower border of the mandible (Fig. 24–7A,B).

To decide the exact placement of the pins in relation to the lower border of the mandible, the following formula has been devised:[25]

$$\text{Pin placement angle} = 180 - \text{gonial angle} \times \frac{\text{vertical deficiency}}{\text{total deficiency}}$$

$$\text{In the above example:} \quad 180 - 140 \times \frac{10}{20} = 40 \times \frac{1}{2} = 20°$$

With the use of the formula, placement of the pins can be planned accurately, but the resultant distraction is predicated on the biologic response. This method was used in Case 1 (HWL).

Surgical Technique

The holes for the pins are drilled at 90 degrees to the mandible and parallel to each. A 1.5-mm drill is used at a low speed to avoid heating the bone. Single or bicortical drill holes are made and the four half-pins are inserted (Fig. 24–8). The pins must be long enough to ensure that the distractor device is not impinging on the skin and does not irritate the ear. Typically, 50-mm pins are used, and when inserting the pins, the depth of the mandible is measured on the pin to ensure that the pins are inserted bicortically. If the pin is inserted too deeply and withdrawn, it will lose stability. In young children under the age of 2 years (Case Report 1) the bone of the mandible is soft, whereas in older children the bone is more solid, and the fixation of the pins to the bone is improved.

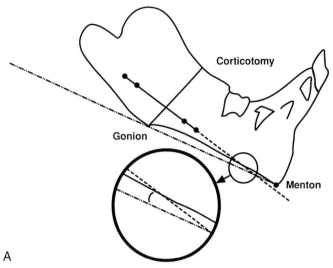

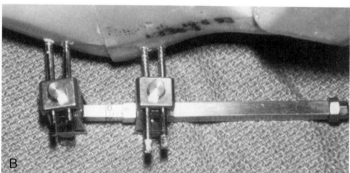

Figure 24–7. *A,* Positioning of dual pins in a straight line to allow distraction. Note angle to lower border of the mandible. *B,* Close-up view of distraction device with calibration in millimeters.

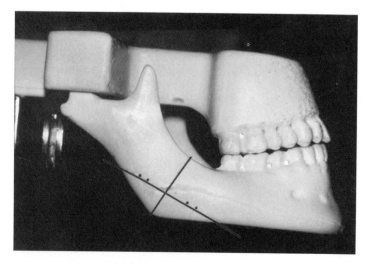

Figure 24–8. Position of the pin in a straight line perpendicular to the corticotomy line.

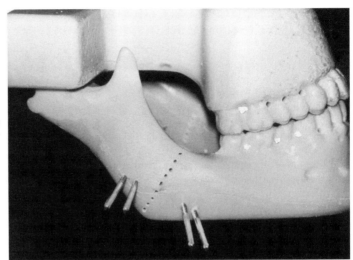

Figure 24–9. Pins inserted into a model of the mandible with corticotomy cut prepared to avoid damage to the inferior alveolar nerve.

If the angle of the mandible is more obtuse than normal, this may be altered by placing the proximal pin inferior to the distraction line. The distal end of the mandible will rotate up and reduce the gonial angle. Mandibular distraction may result in an open bite, because of increase in the gonial angle, and thus manipulation of the pin positions may avoid an open bite developing after distraction.

The corticotomy is performed by making multiple drill holes through the periosteum (Fig. 24–9) and through the outer cortex over the center of the mandible to avoid damage to the inferior alveolar nerve. In the upper and lower third of the mandible, the drill holes are made bicortically. Care is taken to keep the periosteum intact between the drill holes. The corticotomy is completed on the anterior surface of the mandible with a 2-mm osteotome, leaving as much periosteum intact as possible. The posterior surface of the mandible is divided with a 2-mm osteotome, making the bone cut a corticotomy and not an osteotomy. At the completion of the corticotomy, mobility at the corticotomy site is expected and denotes that the cortex has been adequately divided.

An alternative method is through an intraoral incision with nasotracheal intubation. A lateral vestibular incision is made and the bone is exposed on the anterior surface, between the periosteum and the temporalis muscle. Percutaneous incisions are made at the site of the pin protrusion. Undue tension on the skin resulting in scarring from the tension of the pins during distraction can be reduced by constricting the skin between the proximal and distal pins. The corticotomy is completed along the outer cortex with a 2-mm osteotome, taking care to leave as much periosteum intact as is possible and not to damage the inferior alveolar nerve, with the marrow cavity maintained intact. The inner cortex is then divided, leaving as much of the periosteum undisturbed as possible. After the pins are placed, an 8-mm osteotome is used to complete the corticotomy, with a slight twist of the bone ends. The neck incision is closed with 4–0 chromic deep sutures and 6–0 nylon interrupted skin sutures. Meticulous skin closure around the pins is essential. The intraoral incision is repaired with 4–0 chromic sutures. Following closure of the extra oral or intraoral surgical sites, the pins are inserted into the lengthening device with the distraction device angulated distally. The distraction distance is set to 0 and the screw bolts are all tightened. The distraction apparatus is placed clear of the skin and ear, and care is taken to have the fixation on the pins proximal to the flat distal end of the pins. The pins are dressed with Xeroform dressing. Postoperatively, care is taken to protect the distraction device from trauma. Ear protectors are placed over the distraction apparatus and are protected with sponge. The protectors may be left in position all the time or only at night when the child sleeps. The patient is kept in the hospital 1 to 2 days until oral fluids are tolerated. Anteroposterior and lateral skull radiographs are taken at this stage.

SINGLE-PIN, DOUBLE CORTICOTOMY: MEXICO EXPERIENCE (CASE REPORTS 2 AND 3)

Surgical Technique

This alternative method (FM) involves a 3-cm incision on the oral mucosa along the mandibular vestibule. The periosteum is elevated, exposing the gonial angle. With the side-cutting burr, an external corticotomy is performed on the lateral aspect of the mandible of patients with hemifacial microsomia. The corticotomy must be extended inferiorly around the inferior edge of the mandible and superiorly to the alveolar ridge. The lingual cortex and the inner periosteum remain untouched. An external bone lengthening device is used (Wells Johnson Company, Tucson, AZ). With a hand driver, two stainless steel screws are introduced percutaneously through the whole thickness of the mandible, separated by 5 mm from the corticotomy. The cheek skin is pinched between the thumb and the index finger before introducing the second screw to allow for stretching and to minimize the scar. The site of the screw insertions is determined preoperatively according to the growth prediction, the location of the tooth buds, and the direction of the desired mandibular distraction. By using the panorex view, damage can be avoided to the inferior alveolar nerve and tooth germs. The caudal pin always must be placed inferior to the nerve canal. The mucosa is closed with absorbable sutures and the distraction device is applied.

Patients are discharged from the hospital on the same day with instructions for a soft diet and antibiotics during the ensuing 5 days. Soap and water are used to clean the skin around the pins every day.

The elongation starts at the fifth postoperative day at a rate of 1 mm per day. This is done by the patient and causes minimal discomfort. Usually, the elongation is completed in 3 to 4 weeks. The screws are left in place for 6 to 8 weeks more, until radiologic evidence of new cortical bone formation is found at the elongated segment. Then the screws are removed.

Patients with micrognathia and Treacher Collins syndrome present with bilateral deformities and a different bone hypoplasia because the mandibular body and the ascending ramus are affected, requiring bidirectional distraction. In this group of patients, two corticotomies must be performed, one vertical on the mandibular body and the other roughly horizontal on the ascending ramus. Three screws are used: a central one at the mandibular angle, the second into the body in front of the vertical corticotomy, and the third in the ascending ramus. A bidirectional device (Wells Johnson Company, Tucson, AZ) is used to allow independent and more precise elongation of each segment using the central screw as the fixed pivot for both of them.

Measurements of the distance between the screws and soft tissue structures (external canthus–buccal commissure and inferior orbital rim–buccal commissure) are recorded weekly. Dental casts and radiographs are taken at the end of the distraction period to assess osteogenesis and occlusal changes.

The total distraction is planned depending on the grade of bone hypoplasia of the mandible. Patients with hemifacial microsomia have been classified into one of three degrees. In grade I, the hypoplasia affects the gonial angle. In grade IIA, the hypoplasia affects the angle and the initial portion of the ascending ramus. In grade IIB, the angle and the entire ramus are affected, with presence of a rudimentary condyle. Grade III shows a complete absence of the ramus and condyle.

Careful planning of the corticotomy depending on the degree of bony hypoplasia allows mandibular elongation that follows the direction of the normal growth of the mandible. We produce different resistance to the distraction forces at the external and internal cortices of the mandible by performing only an external corticotomy. This point is important to produce elongation and simultaneously bone remodeling in a tridimensional direction, closely resembling the normal curve of the mandibular growth. When the distraction procedure starts, the bone elongation occurs mainly in the external cortex and cancellous bone, positioning the pins in a triangular pattern. At the end of the second week, the distraction forces produce fracture of the lingual cortex. The distraction procedure continues until the projected elongation of the hypoplastic mandible is achieved.

Criteria to end the distraction period depend on facial and occlusal outcomes:

1. To obtain optimal aesthetic results with restored facial symmetry. This includes descent of the buccal commissure to the level of the contralateral side and positioning of the chin horizontally and at the midline.

2. To obtain a final stable dental occlusion. In grade I hypoplasia dental occlusion remains stable, without posterior open bite. No functional orthodontics appliances are used. In grade IIA, a posterior open bite of 3 mm is produced. Bite blocks are used to maintain the elongation and to stabilize the occlusion. Patients with grade IIB present a stable but inadequate occlusion with marked lateral deviation of the midline teeth to the affected side. The distraction may reproduce this malocclusion on the opposite side as a result of overcorrection.

In all of these patients, bite blocks and dynamic orthodontic appliances (Bionator) are used at an early stage. Use of the posterior bite blocks is gradually reduced to allow vertical maxillary growth.

Management of the Mandibular Distractor

After the surgical intervention to place the pins and perform the corticotomy, the *latency period* is the time between insertion of the distractor and occurrence of activation. Ilizarov suggested that 5 to 7 days elapse before distraction forces are activated. The pin sites and skin suture line are cleaned three times a day with saline and Xeroform dressings are applied.

The *distraction period* covers the time during which activation occurs at 0.5 mm twice a day or 0.25 mm four times a day. One complete turn of the distractor in an anticlockwise direction results in 0.5 mm of movement. The parents or caregivers are advised to keep a record of the measurement on the distractor at the end of each day. The total distraction distance is planned depending on the deficiency of the mandible. If the deficiency is only in the vertical or horizontal ramus, the distraction is the same as the deficiency. If the gonial angle is near 180 degrees, the total distraction distance is the sum of the vertical and horizontal deficiency. For all other situations, the total distraction distance is not the sum of the vertical and horizontal deficiencies. The more acute the gonial angle is, the lower the distraction distance will be. Those mandibles in which there is an intrinsic growth deficiency or dysmorphology may be overcorrected within the limits of the appliance. The extent of distraction depends on the age and size of the mandible; the greatest distraction distance reported in the mandible is 38 mm by McCarthy.[20] Documentation at the end of active movement include antero-posterior and lateral skull radiographs, intraoral photographs, and study models to record the occlusal change.

The *fixation period* occurs after completion of the distraction and is retained for 9 weeks. It is suggested that the fixation period be at least twice as long as the distraction period to allow healing and consolidation of the bone at the corticotomy site.

Distractors are carefully and slowly removed in the outpatient clinic without anesthesia being necessary and with minimal discomfort. Lateral and anteroposterior skull radiographs are taken again at 6-month intervals, and dental impressions are taken at the time of the appliance placement and at the end of distraction. The effect of distraction is reflected in the occlusal relationship, which is a useful outcome measure at the end of active treatment.

Preliminary case reports to illustrate the method of mandibular osteosynthesis include cases of bilateral mandibular deficiency in an infant with Nager syndrome (Case Report 1) and a child with Treacher Collins syndrome (Case Report 2). The management of unilateral mandibular deficiency is illustrated in Case Report 3 in a child with hemifacial (craniofacial) microsomia.

CASE REPORT 1 (HWL)

A 2-year-old boy with Nager syndrome presented with severe micrognathia (bilateral deficiency) (Fig. 24–10A,B). A tracheostomy had been performed for airway management, and mandibular size and position was evaluated on three-dimension

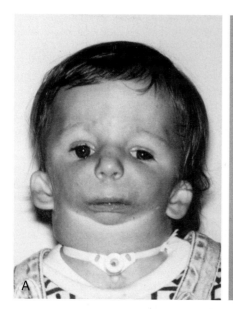
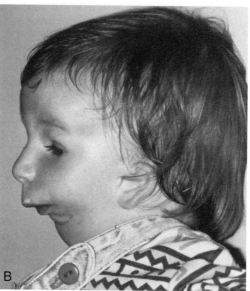

Figure 24–10. *A,* Case Report 1: Full face view to illustrate severe mandibular deficiency, apparent "low set ears" and tracheotomy. Patient diagnosed with Nagers syndrome. *B,* Profile view to illustrate mandibular deficiency, retrogenia, and obliteration of the chin/neck angle. (From Losken HW, Patterson GT, et al: Planning mandibular distraction: Preliminary report. Cleft Palate-Craniofac J 1995; 32:71–76.)

computed tomography (3D CT) scans. Measurements were taken from the computer image of the mandible and the cephalometric landmark condylion was taken as the most posterior superior point of the condyle of the mandible. The zygomatic arch was removed on the image to identify the head of the mandible (Fig. 24–11*A,B*). The pogonion landmark was the most anterior point of the mandibular symphysis and, despite the dysmorphology of the mandible, "gonion" at the angle of the mandible was identified. A tracing of the mandible "gonion" at the angle of the mandible was identified. A tracing of the lateral skull radiograph was made and radiographs of the posterior border of the vertical ramus and the inferior mandibular border were made to identify anatomic gonion and the gonial angle. The vertical ramus was measured from the condylion to the anatomic gonion, although standardization of these measurements on serial radiographs tends to be inaccurate.

The distance from condylion to gonion was measured as 27 mm, which is several standard deviations below the 41 mm mean for a 2-year-old boy from published longitudinal normative data in the Bolton/Brush Archive.[26] The gonion to pogonion distance was 35 mm (mean 52 mm) and the gonial angle was 158 degrees (mean 134 degrees).

The mandible was exposed through a Risdon incision, and a corticotomy was

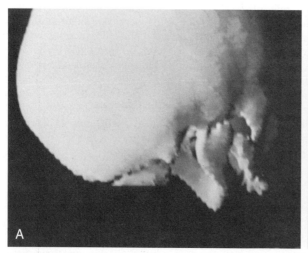
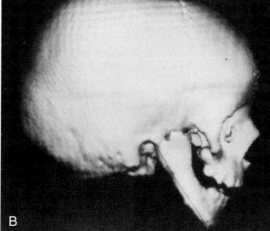

Figure 24–11. *A,* Three-dimensional CT scan to illustrate dysmorphology of the mandible with hypoplastic condyle. *B,* Lateral view of three-dimensional CT scan with the zygomatic arch removed for illustrative purposes to show absence of the gonial angle of the mandible. (From Losken HW, Patterson GT, et al: Planning mandibular distraction: Preliminary report. Cleft Palate-Craniofac J 1995; 32:71–76.)

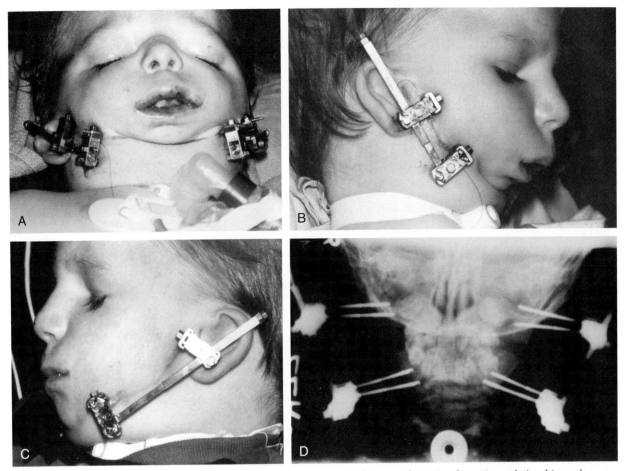

Figure 24–12. *A*, Postoperative view of the placement of the dual pins with distractor device in place. Note relationship to the external ear. *B*, Profile view of pins in place with the distractor activated. *C*, Profile view showing full activation of the distractor device equal to 30 mm. *D*, Posteroanterior cephalogram following distraction to illustrate fixation period until osteogenesis and bone consolidation occur before removal of the pins.

performed. After a 7-day latency period, the mandible was distracted at 1 mm a day for 31 days (Fig. 24–12*A,B,C,D*). A fixation period of 9 weeks was maintained before the pins were removed in the outpatient clinic, and a repeat 3D CT scan was taken (Fig. 24–13). Follow-up photographs 1 year later show improvement of the facial scars and the patient feeding orally instead of using the gastric tube (Fig. 24–14).

Figure 24–13. Profile view illustrating an increase in mandibular length following mandibular distraction. Note scars from pins on the cheek and the chin/neck angle, which is restored. (From Losken HW, Patterson GT, et al: Planning mandibular distraction: Preliminary report. Cleft Palate-Craniofac J 1995; 32:71–76.)

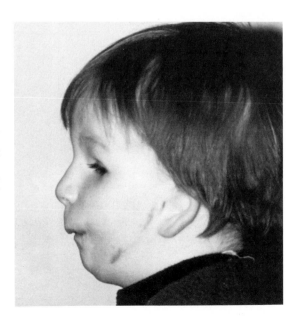

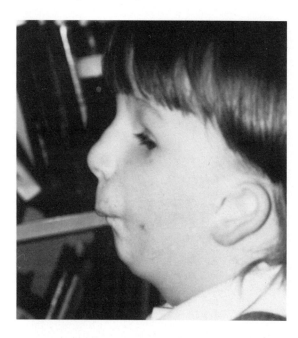

Figure 24–14. Profile view 1 year later. Note fading of scars on the cheek.

CASE REPORT 2 (FM)

A 3-year-old female patient had severe Treacher Collins syndrome (Fig. 24–15A,B) in whom we initially performed a bilateral and bidirectional mandibular distraction, which elongated the dimensions of the ascending ramus and the mandibular body simultaneously (Fig. 24–16A,B). In a period of 3 weeks, a bone elongation of 8 mm was achieved on the ascending ramus and 11 mm on the mandibular body bilaterally and symmetrically. The bidirectional distraction overcame the problems associated with the control of both the vertical and sagittal dimensions, correcting the anterior open bite characteristic of this syndrome by elongation of the ascending ramus. The distraction device was maintained during the next 8 weeks to obtain bone consolidation. In the frontal view (Fig. 24–17), we observed an increased dimension of the lower third of the face produced by the anterior rotation of the mandible as a result of the distraction procedure. In the lateral view (Fig. 24–18) the dimensions of the

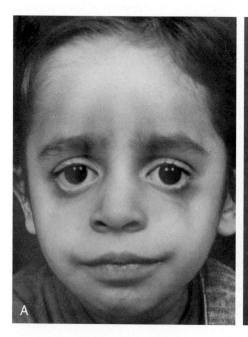
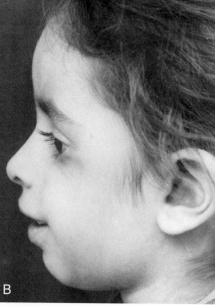

Figure 24–15. *A,* Full face view of a child with Treacher Collins syndrome. *B,* Profile view of the same child with Treacher Collins syndrome.

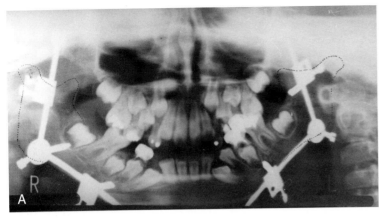

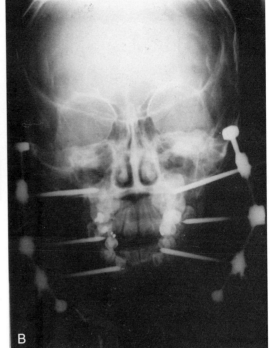

Figure 24–16. *A,* Panorex radiograph showing placement of single pins bilaterally. *B,* Posteroanterior radiograph of the child in case report 2 with single pins in bidirectional distraction for vertical and horizontal lengthening of the mandible.

mandibular body and the ascending ramus are significantly increased postoperatively, and the change in position of the gonial angle is evident. The soft tissue distribution is greatly improved, the neck has a defined angle, and the menton has become more prominent. The pre- and postoperative occlusion (Fig. 24–19*A,B*) indicate some increase in the anterior open bite. A myofunctional appliance was fitted after the distraction device was removed.

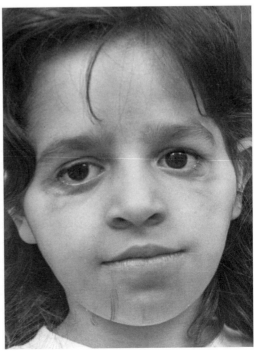

Figure 24–17. Full face view illustrating changes from increase in mandibular lengthening.

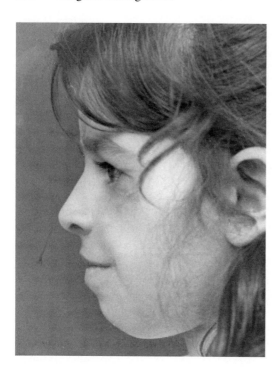

Figure 24–18. Profile view postoperatively. Note changes in facial appearance following mandibular lengthening procedure.

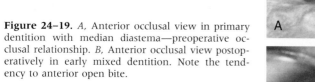

Figure 24–19. A, Anterior occlusal view in primary dentition with median diastema—preoperative occlusal relationship. B, Anterior occlusal view postoperatively in early mixed dentition. Note the tendency to anterior open bite.

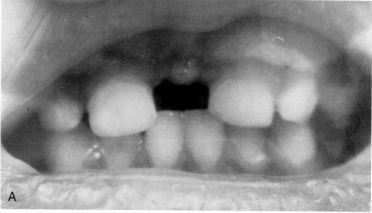

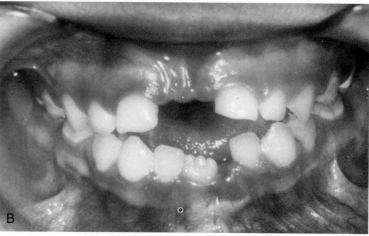

CASE REPORT 3 (FM)

A 6-year-old patient with left hemifacial microsomia (grade II) (Fig. 24–20A) presented with mandibular hypoplasia of both the gonial angle and the ascending ramus with a hypoplastic condyle (Fig. 24–21A,B,C). Through a vestibular incision, an oblique corticotomy was performed, and two pins were inserted in an almost vertical position (Fig. 24–22). During the next 4 weeks, mandibular elongation of 22 mm was obtained (Fig. 24–23A,B,C). There was remodeling of the bone at the gonial angle. The clinical result comparing the pre- and postoperative frontal view is illustrated (see Fig. 24–20B). Improved facial appearance includes the descending buccal commissure with a marked increase in the distance between the lateral canthus and buccal commissure. In addition, the distance between the tragus and the commissure is increased, resulting in a considerable improvement in the facial symmetry (see Fig. 24–20B).

DISCUSSION

These case reports illustrate distraction techniques with single and dual pins. The second case, with the typical dysmorphic antegonial notch at the mandibular angle characteristic of Treacher Collins syndrome, was lengthened both in the vertical and sagittal dimensions by two corticotomies (see Fig. 24–3). The introduction of bidirectional distractor devices overcomes the problems associated with control of both the vertical and horizontal dimensions. If the process of distraction results in an obtuse gonial angle and increased vertical lower facial height, this may be reflected in a dental open bite malocclusion.

In developing process and outcome measures to establish the efficacy and effectiveness of alternative treatments, a prerequisite is to evaluate risks-cost-benefit ratios. In symmetric or asymmetric lengthening of the mandible, especially as a direct consequence of syndromic malformations characterized by mandibular deficiency, costochondral grafts have been an effective method of lengthening the mandible. When performed in the young child, continued increase in the size of the affected side of the mandible occurs in response to systemic growth hormone and circulating growth factors. However, problems have been experienced with overgrowth, undergrowth, and unpredictable amount of growth of costochondral grafts. In comparing mandibular distraction against this "yardstick," there is little long-term evidence to show that after the initial lengthening procedure the increase in mandibular size and change in shape and position are maintained over time. Until long-term data are available, the efficacy of distraction osteogenesis can only be evaluated in the context of the initial

Figure 24–20. A, Case report 3 of a child with hemifacial microsomia affecting the left side with microcrotia of the left ear—preoperative appearance. B, Full face postoperative appearance following mandibular distraction. Note changes in facial appearance including the cant of the oral commissure and the chin in midsagittal facial plane.

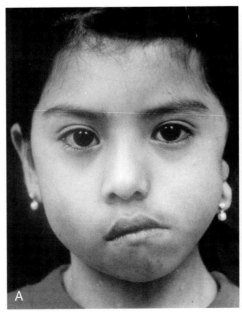
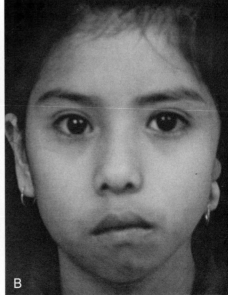

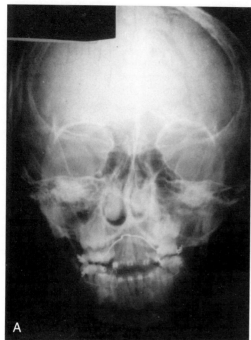

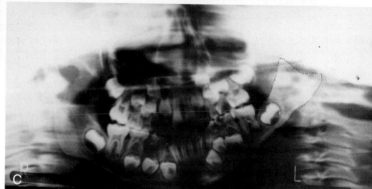

Figure 24–21. *A,* Preoperative posteroanterior radiograph of a patient with hemifacial microsomia. *B,* Preoperative lateral skull radiograph of a patient. *C,* Panoramic radiograph of a patient with hemifacial microsomia.

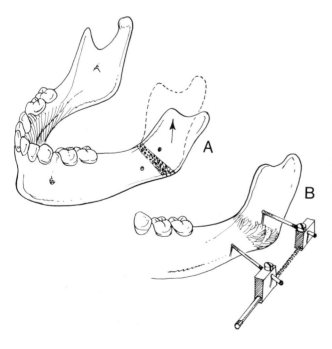

Figure 24–22. Illustration of single pin placement in the patient in case report 3 with angulation of distraction to increase vertical height and length of the mandibular ramus.

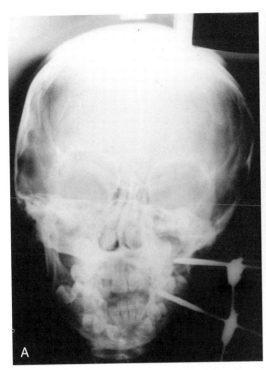

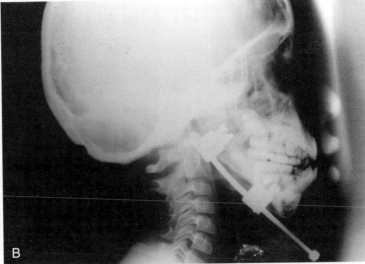

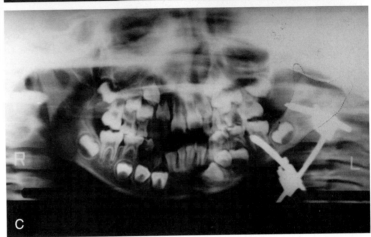

Figure 24–23. *A,* Postoperative posteroanterior radiograph following mandibular distraction on left side only. *B,* Lateral skull radiograph showing the mandibular distraction device. Note that extension is anterior instead of posterior against the external ear. *C,* Panorex radiograph postoperatively to illustrate lengthening of the left ramus of the mandible.

change and anecdotal case reports, which has significant implications as an alternative procedure to orthognathic surgery.

Sagittal split mandibular osteotomy is limited in the young child by the dimensions of the mandibular ramus and the extent to which the mandible may be advanced. Although distraction devices may allow greater lengthening of the mandible and may contribute to a reduction in airway obstruction,[27] the effect on the condylar head and its close association with the external auditory canal may also have long-term implications.[28] The morphology and functional aspects of the temporomandibular joint and the glenoid fossa may also result in adaptive changes of size and shape from the forces of mandibular distraction, especially in the infant and young child.[29,30] In the child represented in case report 3 with hemifacial microsomia, the example shows that the more affected the condyle, coronoid, and ramal height, the greater the vertical distance before the cranial base is contacted with distraction of the proximal segment. The addition of serial sarcomeres to increase musculotendinous length may also be assumed to occur if muscle lengthening is an adaptive component to the ultimate stability of the long-term result.

The importance of recognizing and selecting cases appropriate for mandibular distraction osteogenesis includes considering severe syndromic patients. Selection criteria should consider those patients with mandibular deficiency that compromises respiratory and feeding functions. Because slow distraction of the mandible following corticotomy results in adaptation of the soft tissues and an increase in mandibular mass and length by the osteogenesis process, elongation of the mandible over a period of 4 to 6 weeks may result in an increase in size and change in position and shape, which would not be possible with conventional orthognathic surgery with the sagittal split osteotomy procedure. Those severe unilateral cases of hemifacial microsomia with an absent or severely hypoplastic condyle, rudimentary coronoid, and no zygomatic arch have responded satisfactorily to distraction devices, which simultaneously affect both the skeletal and soft tissues by gradually increasing and stretching the musculoskeletal complex, which in the young child rapidly responds and adapts. However, how this will be maintained during the child's subsequent growth and development remains to be seen as these preliminary results are followed over time.

Complications that may occur include migration of the pins through the mandible. Not only may this overestimate the distraction distance achieved, but also they may loosen and move out of the cortical bone. In addition, the extraoral distraction device is vulnerable in the young child who may be learning to walk and may have traumatic incidents with furniture and other impediments.

Mandibular distraction osteogenesis has definite benefits. With further refinements such as an intraoral device to prevent facial scarring, which is a consequence of the extraoral technique, further benefits may be achieved. The biology of distraction osteogenesis[31,32] and its application to mandibular deficiency has far-reaching benefits and consequences for the practicing clinician, whether this be the surgeon, the orthodontist, or the craniofacial biologist.

References

1. Hopkins WB, Penrose CB: On the organization and absorption of sterilized dead bone dowels. JAMA 1890; 14:505–508.
2. Magnuson PB: Lengthening shortened bones of the leg by operation. University of Pennsylvania Med Bull 1908; 21:103–110.
3. Moseley CF: Leg lengthening: The historical perspective. Orthop Clin North Am 1991; 22:555–561.
4. Andry N: Orthopedia or The Art of Correcting and Preventing Deformities in Children. London: A Millar, 1741.
5. Codvilla A: On the means of lengthening, in the lower limbs, the muscles and tissues which are shortened through deformity. Am J Orthop Surg 1905; 2:353.
6. Abbott LC: The operative lengthening of the tibia and fibula. J Bone Joint Surg 1927; 9:128.
7. Ilizarov GA: The principles of the Ilizarov method. Bull Hosp Joint Dis Orthop Inst 1988; 48:1.
8. Ilizarov GA: The tension-stress effect on the genesis and growth of tissues; part 1: The influence of stability of fixation and soft tissue preservation. Clin Orthop 1989; 238:249–281.
9. Ilizarov GA: The tension-stress effect on the genesis and growth of tissues; part 2: The influence of stability of fixation and soft tissue preservation. Clin Orthop 1989; 239:263–285.
10. Compere E: Indications for and against the leg lengthening operation. J Bone Joint Surg 1936; 18:692–705.
11. Wagner H: Surgical lengthening or shortening of femur and tibia: Technique and indications. Prog Orthop Surg 1977; 1:71–94.
12. Wagner H: Surgical lengthening of the femur. Report of 58 Cases. Am Chir 1980; 34:263–275.
13. Paley D: Current techniques of limb lengthening. J Pediat Orthop 1988; 8:73–92.
14. McCarthy JG, Karp N, et al: Lengthening of the mandible by gradual distraction: Experimental and clinical studies. Craniofac Surg 1992; 4:85–88.
15. Block MS, Daire J, Stover J, et al: Changes in the inferior alveolar nerve following mandibular lengthening in the dog using distraction osteogenesis. J Oral Maxillofac Surg 1993; 51:652–660.
16. Snyder CC, Levine GA, et al: Mandibular lengthening by gradual distraction. Plast Reconstr Surg 1973; 51:506–508.
17. Michieli S, Miotti B: Surgical-orthodontic mandibular body lengthening by gradual distraction. Minerva Stomatol 1976; 25:77–78.
18. Karp NS, McCarthy JG, Schreiber JS, et al: Membranous bone lengthening: A serial histological study. Annals of Plast. Surg. 1992; 29:2–7.
19. Staffenberg DA, Wood RJ, McCarthy JG: Mandibular lengthening in the canine using an intraoral device. Proceedings of the Fifth International Craniofacial Congress 1993; 5:77.
20. McCarthy JG, Schreiber J, et al: Lengthening the human mandible by gradual distraction. Plast Reconstr Surg 1992; 89:1–8.
21. Molina F, Ortiz Monasterio F: Extended indications for mandibular distraction: Unilateral, bilateral and bidirectional. Proceedings of the Fifth International Craniofacial Congress 1993; 5:79.
22. Cohen MM Jr: The Child With Multiple Birth Defects. New York: Raven Press, 1982.
23. Vig KWL: Orthodontic perspectives in craniofacial dysmorphology. In Vig KWL, Burdi AR (eds): Craniofacial Morphogenesis and Dysmorphogenesis. Monograph 21, CHGD. Ann Arbor: University of Michigan, 1988.
24. Vig PS, Vig KWL: Hybrid appliances: A component approach to dentofacial orthopedics. Am J Orthodont Dentofac Orthop 1986; 90(4):273–285.
25. Losken HW, Patterson GT, et al: Planning mandibular distraction: Preliminary report. Cleft Palate-Craniofac J 1995; 32:71–76.
26. Broadbent BH, Golden HH: Bolton Standards of Dentofacial Developmental Growth. St. Louis: CV Mosby, 1975.
27. Moore HH, Guzman-Stein G, Proudman TW, et al: Mandibular lengthening by distraction for airway obstruction in Treacher-Collins Syndrome. J Craniofac Surg 1994; 5:22–25.
28. McCormick S, Grayson B, et al: The effect of mandibular lengthening on the condylar head and neck. Abstract of the International Craniofacial Surgery Society Meeting. 1993, p 164.

29. Molina F: Mandibular distraction in hemifacial microsomia, technique and results in 56 patients. Abstract of the Craniofacial Society of Great Britain, Cambridge, 1994.
30. Vig KWL, Losken HW, Patterson G: Mandibular manipulations of unknown efficacy and utility. Abstract of the Craniofacial Society of Great Britain, Cambridge, 1994.
31. Aronson J: The biology of distraction osteogenesis. *In* Chapman MC (ed): Operative Orthopaedics. Philadelphia: JB Lippincott, 1993.
32. Constantino PD, Friedman CS, et al: Experimental mandibular regrowth by distraction osteogenesis. Arch Otolaryngol Head Neck Surg 1993; 119:511–516.

Nonsyndromic Craniosynostosis

25

Timothy A. Turvey and Steven K. Gudeman

Craniosynostosis (premature fusion of cranial sutures) is a complex condition that occurs as an isolated event or in association with other malformations. One or more cranial vault sutures may be involved, and Cohen identified at least 64 syndromes in which craniosynostosis is a feature.[1] The cranial vault normally enlarges rapidly during fetal development and continues at a rapid rate of growth postnatally. Diagnosis is made generally during the first year of life and is based on head shape.

Craniosynostosis exists in primary and secondary forms, and there are important therapeutic implications for this distinction. Patients with primary craniosynostosis possess a brain of normal growth potential, and premature suture closure precludes appropriate skull expansion. Therefore, patients with primary craniosynostosis are generally surgical candidates. Secondary craniosynostosis occurs when the brain lacks growth potential or in the presence of other medical conditions, such as blood dyscrasias (e.g., thalassemia) that result in suture immobility but not necessarily bony fusion. Infants with secondary craniosynostosis may lack the normal stimulus for cranial development (neural tissues), which results in severe neurologic impairment, or they may have serious medical problems that have caused the condition. They are not good surgical candidates because the underlying conditions do not support favorable head and/or brain growth.

Craniosynostosis is an expression of pathology, but it may not be the disease itself. Sometimes the prematurely fused suture is the only malformation. In other instances, craniosynostosis is found to coexist with other congenital findings and is part of an identifiable syndrome. In the syndromic forms of craniofacial dysostosis (e.g., Apert, Crouzon, and Pfeiffer syndromes), craniosynostosis is a component and the cranial base is thought to be a region of primary pathology; this also affects midface growth.[2, 3]

The focus of this chapter is on nonsyndromic craniosynostosis. Chapter 26 deals with the management of the craniofacial dysostosis syndromes. The etiopathogenetic diversity of craniosynostosis is significant and is responsible for varying treatment outcomes.

BIOLOGY AND PHYSIOLOGY OF CRANIAL SUTURES

Cranial sutures represent a form of bone articulation in which the margins of the cranial vault bones are suspended by a thin layer of fibrous tissues. The cranial vault is composed of six major sutral areas and multiple minor sutures (Fig. 25–1). The bones of the cranial vault originate as ossification centers within the fibrous tissue desmocranium that surrounds the fetal brain. The edges of the bone plates are not enveloped by this tissue. As the bones enlarge, they split the fibrous tissue layers into an outer periosteal surface and an inner layer (the dura mater).[4] Experimental data indicates that the dura possesses significant osteogenic potential. In fact, the entire calvaria can be removed during infancy, as is done in the treatment of some forms of severe craniosynostosis, and it regenerates along with the cranial sutures. However, if the dura is resected with the calvaria, bone and suture regeneration are limited.[5]

Cranial vault sutures have several functions. During postnatal development, cranial vault sutures facilitate head expansion to accommodate brain growth.[6] Only small amounts of pressure (5 mm Hg) from the growing brain are required to stimulate bone deposition at the margins of the cranial bone.[7, 8] Another function of cranial vault sutures is to permit head deformation during vaginal delivery. As the fetus squeezes through the narrow pelvic canal, deformation must occur to permit passage. Under normal circumstances, cranial vault shape is restored within weeks after birth.

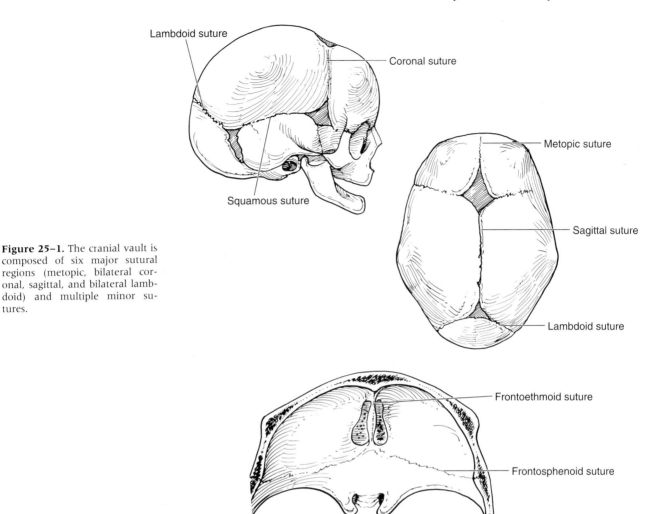

Figure 25–1. The cranial vault is composed of six major sutural regions (metopic, bilateral coronal, sagittal, and bilateral lambdoid) and multiple minor sutures.

Under normal conditions, growth of the calvaria is a reflection of the growth and shape of the brain (Fig. 25–2). Most calvarial sutures are normally inactive by 8 years of age. Closure of cranial vault sutures occurs earlier than the membranous facial bone sutures, which may remain patent until adulthood. At birth, the cranial vault sutures should be widely open and then close during development in a consistent pattern. Synchondroses at the skull base exist between the cartilaginous bones and remain active growth centers until adulthood.

Figure 25–2. This anencephalic human specimen demonstrates lack of forehead and cranial vault development. Without adequate brain growth, the cranium fails to develop normally. Notice the lack of midfacial development, which may also be related.

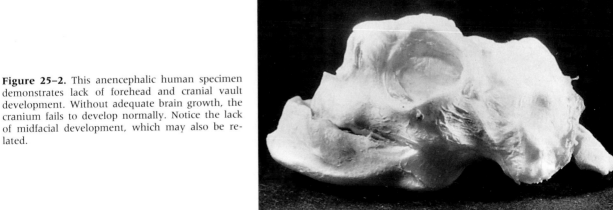

Cranial sutures are not primary growth centers; expansion of the underlying brain results in tension on the suspensory tissue with apposition of bone along the edges of the sutures. As the brain grows, cranial sutures widen at areas of least resistance, resulting in bone apposition perpendicular to the suture (Virchow's law).[9] Cranial growth also occurs by a process of gradual resorption along the inner surface of the cranial bones (endocranial) with deposition on the outer surface (exocranial). This type of brain growth is common at areas of calvarial curvature, such as the forehead and occipitoparietal areas.[10] Clinically, this may be of importance when nonresorbable fixation devices (interosseous wires or bone plates and screws) are used during cranial vault reconstruction performed early in infancy. When these regions are reexamined at surgery several years later, the nonresorbable devices may be covered entirely with bone, and in some instances are found in contact with the dura.

ETIOLOGY OF CRANIOSYNOSTOSIS

There are multiple etiologies for craniosynostosis, including genetic factors, mechanical factors, metabolic disturbances, bone and dural pathologies, and teratogens. Abnormalities of the cranial base that result in abnormal tensions on dural attachments were cited by Moss and Greenberg as possible causes of premature fusion.[11] Park and Powers suggested that intrauterine injury to the blastomal suture anlage prevents differentiation into normal sutures.[12] Metabolic disturbances (such as hyperthyroidism), nutritional deficiencies (such as rickets), and hematologic disorders (such as sickle cell anemia) have also been associated with this disturbance of development.[13] Higgenbottom and associates linked intrauterine constraint to craniosynostosis.[14] Because there is etiologic heterogeneity with craniosynostosis, pathogenetic diversity is typical and dependent on the etiology. Consequently, response to treatment is also diverse and dependent on the exact cause of the condition, its pathogenesis, the treatment, and the timing of treatment.

CONSEQUENCES OF CRANIOSYNOSTOSIS

Single-suture craniosynostosis is primarily a problem of skull shape. This should not be viewed casually, since the face can also be affected and the abnormality may lead to psychosocial difficulties.[15-17] In the presence of craniosynostosis, the cranial vault does not grow perpendicular to the fused suture, and so growth is expressed in a parallel direction with compensations occurring at other areas of least resistance. Even with single-suture craniosynostosis, the entire calvaria, portions of the cranial base, and sometimes the face become secondarily affected[18,19] (Figs. 25–3 to 25–5).

The age at which the synostosis occurs and the extent of suture involvement determines the severity of distortion. With unilateral coronal synostosis, the affected side of the forehead flattens, whereas the opposite side overgrows. The contralateral lambdoid region also overgrows, whereas the ipsilateral region flattens (see Fig. 25–3). Orbital dystopia (in which the orbit on the affected side does not descend enough, whereas the orbit on the contralateral side compensates by moving inferiorly), nasal bridge asymmetry, hypoplasia of the zygoma on the affected side, and mandibular asymmetry caused by inferior overgrowth of the temporal fossa and displacement of the glenoid fossa on the affected side are other secondary distortions that can occur.

Multiple-suture craniosynostosis is more commonly associated with functional disorders (i.e., increased intracranial pressure, visual deficits, developmental delay). The greater the extent of suture fusion and the number of sutures involved, the greater the likelihood of functional disorders. The worrisome data published by Renier and co-workers indicate that single-suture fusion may be associated with increased intracranial pressure (>15 mm Hg), as it was in 14% of their patients. These authors also reported that 47% of their patients with multiple-suture fusion had increased intracranial pressure.[20-22]

For normal cranial vault development, brain expansion must occur to displace the bony plates. The classical signs of acute increased intracranial pressure (papilledema,

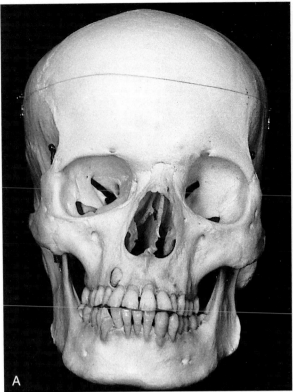

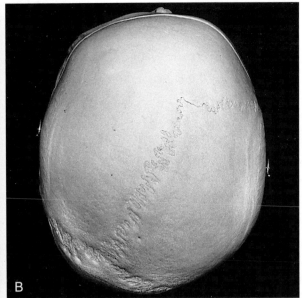

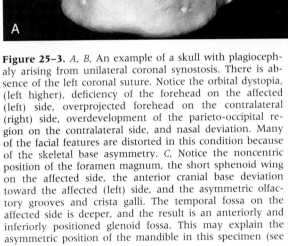

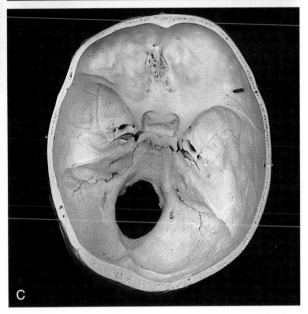

Figure 25–3. *A, B,* An example of a skull with plagiocephaly arising from unilateral coronal synostosis. There is absence of the left coronal suture. Notice the orbital dystopia, (left higher), deficiency of the forehead on the affected (left) side, overprojected forehead on the contralateral (right) side, overdevelopment of the parieto-occipital region on the contralateral side, and nasal deviation. Many of the facial features are distorted in this condition because of the skeletal base asymmetry. *C,* Notice the noncentric position of the foramen magnum, the short sphenoid wing on the affected side, the anterior cranial base deviation toward the affected (left) side, and the asymmetric olfactory grooves and crista galli. The temporal fossa on the affected side is deeper, and the result is an anteriorly and inferiorly positioned glenoid fossa. This may explain the asymmetric position of the mandible in this specimen (see Fig. 25–12*A*).

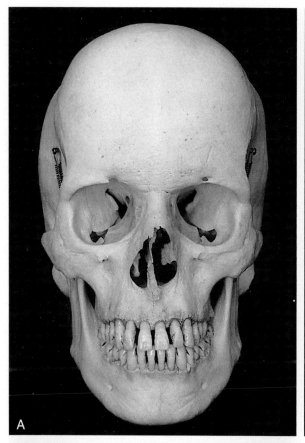

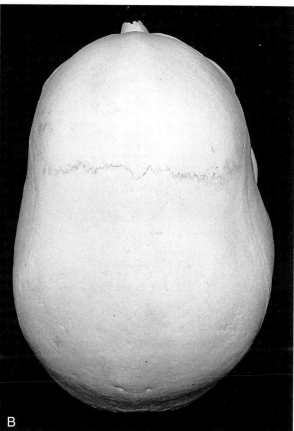

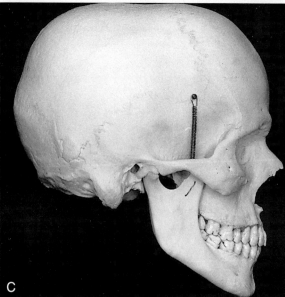

Figure 25–4. *A, B, C,* An example of scaphocephaly secondary to sagittal synostosis. The head is very long, the sagittal suture is absent, and the bitemporal width is narrow. The facial features (from nasion inferiorly) are not grossly abnormal in this condition, as is reflected in proportional facial skeletal development and class I jaw relationships.

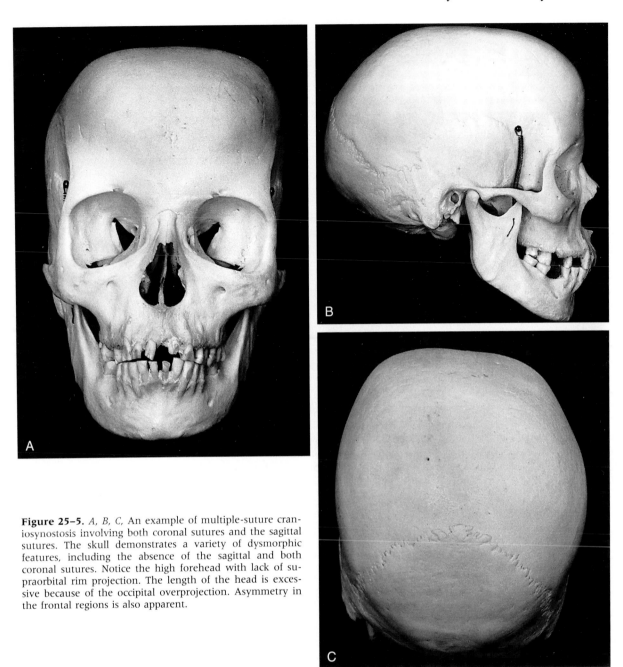

Figure 25–5. *A, B, C,* An example of multiple-suture craniosynostosis involving both coronal sutures and the sagittal sutures. The skull demonstrates a variety of dysmorphic features, including the absence of the sagittal and both coronal sutures. Notice the high forehead with lack of supraorbital rim projection. The length of the head is excessive because of the occipital overprojection. Asymmetry in the frontal regions is also apparent.

vomiting, headache, and so forth) are rarely seen even in the presence of multiple-suture craniosynostosis. The long-term consequences of significantly increased intracranial pressure include optic atrophy, blindness, and cerebral atrophy with reduced cerebral function. The onset of these consequences in the presence of craniosynostosis may be gradual, difficult to detect, and irreversible. The young age of the patient population may contribute to difficulty in detecting the signs and symptoms of increased intracranial pressure, because infants and young children do not communicate effectively. Funduscopic and neurologic examinations of infants and small children require the special services of a pediatric ophthalmologist and a pediatric neurosurgeon.

Developmental delay is occasionally associated with craniosynostosis. Renier and coworkers found a significant relationship between increased intracranial pressure and mental function; higher intracranial pressure was associated with lower mental levels in their patients with craniosynostosis.[20–22] Cohen and Kreiborg suggested that abnormal cerebral development, not necessarily increased intracranial pressure, in patients with Apert syndrome may be the cause of the delay.[23]

The psychosocial consequences of head and facial deformation can be considerable, but individual response varies and is not predictable.[15–17, 24, 25] Mildly dysmorphic craniofacial features can result in profound psychosocial adjustment disorders, whereas severe deformities from craniosynostosis may have minimal effect on psychosocial adjustment. It is postulated that early surgery may prevent adverse psychosocial problems by improving the appearance of the patient, but there are minimal data to support this contention. A prospective, randomized study requires long-term observations of an affected untreated population and a population that has undergone surgical reconstruction. Ethical issues are major considerations that make conducting such a study difficult.

Hydrocephalus appears to be a finding that may occur independently of this condition, not a consequence of craniosynostosis. It is seen in approximately 10% of patients with multiple cranial sutures involved.[26–28] The diagnosis of hydrocephalus, especially in patients with craniofacial dysostosis syndromes, can be confused with ventriculomegaly, which can also be seen with some forms of brachycephaly and Apert syndrome.[23] Only by careful neurologic evaluation and sequential radiographic examination can the diagnosis be made and plans for treatment developed. (See the section on management of hydrocephalus and craniosynostosis in Chapter 26.)

DIAGNOSIS

The diagnosis of craniosynostosis is made primarily from clinical examination and is confirmed with radiographs. Abnormal head shape is key and should alert the examiner to the possibility of this condition. However, abnormal head shape can also result from other causes, from which craniosynostosis must be distinguished. Palpation of the head to detect movement between the bones of the cranial vault is a helpful maneuver, especially in infants and young children. In infants, immobility between the cranial vault bones or early closure of fontanelles suggests premature suture fusion. Ridging (elevation) along the suture is another classical diagnostic feature that is detected by palpation and inspection. It has been suggested that ridging is likely to occur only in synostosed midline sutures because the bone plates are abutted, not obliquely associated.[6] The findings of other malformations in a child with suspected craniosynostosis should raise the index of suspicion for the presence of a syndrome, because craniosynostosis is commonly associated with other congenital anomalies. A change over time in the child's cephalic index (the ratio of head length to head width) is another feature that may alert the examiner to the possibility of craniosynostosis.

When craniosynostosis occurs, distinct patterns of abnormal head shape result. Head shape is determined by which sutures are prematurely fused, the order in which they synostose, the extent of synostosis, and the timing of synostosis. The earlier the synostosis occurs, the more dramatic the skull deformation. The asymmetric head shape resulting from unilateral coronal synostosis is referred to as *plagiocephaly*. Lambdoid synostosis, congenital muscular torticollis, and infant positioning may also result in plagiocephaly. *Scaphocephaly* is the term for a long, narrow head and is

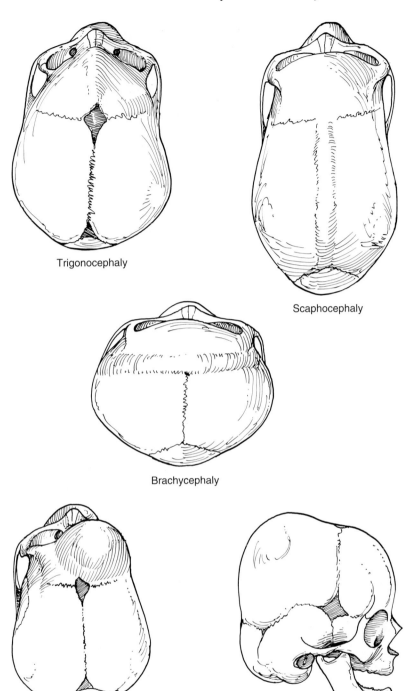

Figure 25–6. A variety of dysmorphic skulls resulting from craniosynostosis. The extent of cranial dysmorphology varies and is dependent on the sutures involved, the extent of sutural synostosis, the cause of the condition, the age at which the premature fusion occurs, and the order in which the fusion occurred. A compounding influence on head shape is the effect of head position and posture.

associated with sagittal synostosis. *Brachycephaly* is the term for a wide, short head commonly associated with bilateral coronal synostosis. *Trigonocephaly* is characteristic of premature fusion of the metopic suture that results in a triangular forehead and orbits. *Oxycephaly, acrocephaly,* and *turricephaly* are terms descriptive of high heads (Fig. 25–6). It is emphasized that these terms describe head shapes and are not related to the etiology. The head shapes are findings that may be consistent with one or more diagnoses.

Plain anteroposterior and lateral skull radiographs remain helpful in determining the presence of craniosynostosis. Complete or incomplete hyperostosis of the suture con-

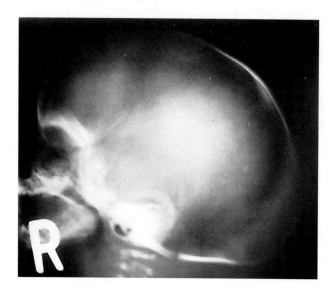

Figure 25–7. Lateral skull radiograph demonstrating hyperostosis of the sagittal suture.

firms the diagnosis (Fig. 25–7). Cranial base distortion, such as that seen when the coronal suture is synostosed and results in the harlequin eye deformity, is also a characteristic and confirmatory radiographic finding (Fig. 25–8). Digital markings (the so-called beaten copper appearance) along the inner table of the cranial vault represent indentations of the convolutions of the brain and are suggestive of increased intracranial pressure, sometimes seen with craniosynostosis (Fig. 25–9A,B). Scintigraphy is a method of determining metabolic activity at cranial sutures and may be helpful in establishing the diagnosis of craniosynostosis (Fig. 25–10). Computed tomography is now the standard method of confirming the diagnosis and is also a screening tool for other pathologic findings (Fig. 25–11).

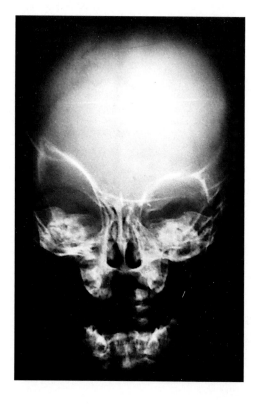

Figure 25–8. Harlequin eye is demonstrated on this posteroanterior skull radiograph, suggesting unilateral coronal synostosis. The shortened anterior cranial base and flattened supraorbital rim contribute to this distortion.

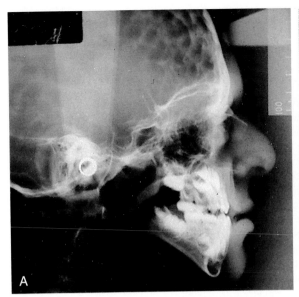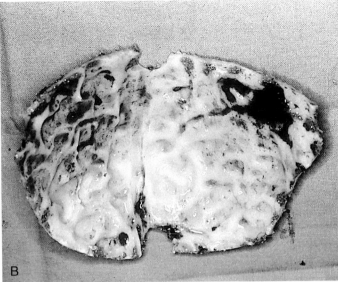

Figure 25–9. *A,* The "beaten copper" appearance demonstrated by the forehead region on this cephalogram represents indentations of the convolutions of the brain on the inner table of the cranial vault. This radiographic finding suggests increased intracranial pressure. *B,* This forehead bone plate demonstrates the irregular inner cortex of the patient whose radiograph appears in part *A.*

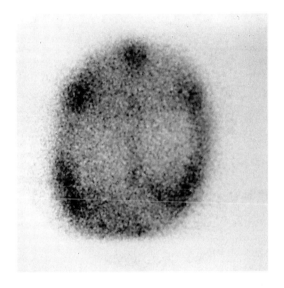

Figure 25–10. This scintigraphic study demonstrates asymmetric uptake of the marker at the lambdoid suture region. The increased metabolic activity observed on the left suggests premature synostosis. Proponents of scintigraphy believe that the metabolic activity at the suture is a more accurate indicator of premature synostosis than is the anatomy of the suture, which is revealed by plain radiography or computed tomography.

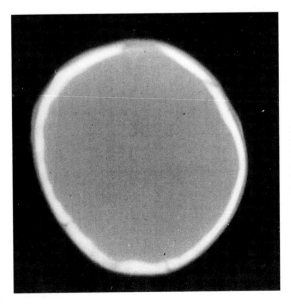

Figure 25–11. Computed tomography is now the standard method of confirming the diagnosis of craniosynostosis and is used to screen for other pathology. This scan indicates premature fusion of the left coronal suture.

SURGICAL CONSIDERATIONS

Timing of Surgery

The optimal timing of surgery for managing the craniosynostosis deformities remains controversial. Some authors believe that surgery performed early (within 6 months) is advisable because it takes advantage of the rapid brain growth that occurs within the first year.[29,30] Normally, the frontal lobes quadruple in weight during the first year, and early surgery may allow this propulsive brain expansion to support the advanced forehead and supraorbital rims. In addition, early surgery may positively affect facial growth. Best results with this approach occur when the brain is normal and has normal growth. Other authors believe that delaying surgery until the 9th to 12th month is advisable, because the bones are better developed then and there is less reliance on growth of the operated bones and brain to maintain the initial surgical results.[31] Allowing the child to age also enables other medical problems to be identified, and this may alter the decision-making process. Nevertheless, some authors believe that single-suture craniosynostosis is of minimal cosmetic and/or functional concern and therefore should not be treated unless the deformity is moderate to severe.

All of these approaches have merit, and there is ample empiric evidence that each approach has merit. A singular approach is not effective for each of the various types of craniosynostosis. A greater understanding of these conditions, identification of the exact etiology, and improved diagnostic skills will enhance the criteria for the selection of patients for surgery and long-term results.

In the absence of clear outcome studies, the preferred timing of surgery for improvement of nonsyndromic craniosynostosis must be made on an individual basis. If the brain and neurologic development are normal (no overt pathology) and the head shape remains abnormal for several months postnatally without appreciable change in configuration, early surgery or continued observation may be indicated, depending on other circumstances. Delaying surgery may allow the condition to improve, but it may also allow greater compensatory changes to occur over time that may make correction more extensive and difficult.

The need for and optimal timing of skull reshaping becomes easier to ascertain when the etiology is understood. For instance, if intrauterine constraint is responsible for the abnormal head shape without craniosynostosis, observation of the condition is wisest, because postnatal growth and remodeling generally compensate sufficiently as the infant grows. If craniosynostosis is diagnosed, a separate set of criteria for surgery is utilized. If microcephaly is the cause of the craniosynostosis, surgical intervention may not be indicated because greater intracranial volume is not required for brain growth. Surgery is indicated (1) when primary craniosynostosis is diagnosed, the head shape is noticeably distorted, and the brain is normal or (2) when secondary craniosynostosis is present, the head is noticeably distorted, and the underlying medical condition has been corrected. In the presence of brain abnormalities and/or other uncorrected medical conditions, the benefits of surgery must be determined in relation to the prognosis.

The surgery carried out to release prematurely fused sutures and to reshape the skull positively affects cranial vault shape. Any adverse effects that the surgery itself may have on further growth of the operated bones are difficult to determine. The development of such effects may be dependent on the details of the surgery performed, the method of stabilization, scarring, and so forth.

Adverse postsurgical growth may also be consistent with the original condition and may have little to do with the surgery.[32] Growth of the head in untreated craniosynostosis conditions and in postsurgical conditions requires further investigation.

Historical Perspective

Craniectomy for relief of imbecility secondary to microcephaly was first attempted by the French and American pioneers Lannelongue and Lane in the late 19th century.[33,34] Because of their poor results, the surgeons and the neurosurgical procedures were denounced, and more than 20 years elapsed before surgery for craniosynostosis reappeared in the literature. Strip craniectomy and/or decompression and morcellation have been employed for improvement of craniosynostosis for many years.[35–39] During this era, concepts such as wrapping the bone margins with alloplasts and treating the dura with caustic agents to prevent reossification were introduced.[40–42]

Extensive cranial vault resection was also attempted for improvement in cases of severe craniosynostosis.[43,44] Bertelsen, Seeger and Gabrielson, and Burdi and colleagues made critical observations about the extension of coronal synostosis into the cranial base and are credited for citing the "coronal ring" in these conditions.[45–47] As a result of their observation, it is currently appreciated that the anterior cranial base (frontosphenoidal and frontoethmoidal sutures), as well as the coronal sutures, must also be released to improve coronal synostosis.[48] Rougerie and associates applied the original principles of craniofacial surgery as described by Tessier to infants affected with craniosynostosis.[49,50] In 1976, Hoffman and Mohr published and popularized the technique of lateral canthal advancement for patients with coronal synostosis who required forehead reconstruction.[51] This is the basic technique that most craniofacial surgeons employ today, with modification, for improvement of these conditions. McCarthy, Jane, Marchac, Whitaker, Munro, Posnick, Persing, Van der Meuhlen, Ortiz-Monasterio, and many other authors are also credited for their contributions to the current concepts of surgical correction of craniosynostosis.[48,52–59] In the future, surgical techniques will be refined, these conditions will be better understood, and therapeutic algorithms will improve.

Necessity and Extent of Surgery

The forehead and orbits are esthetic units that cannot easily be disguised. The nonfacial regions of the head are less noticeable because they are covered with hair and the hair camouflages irregular head form well. Surgery to release isolated suture fusion, not involving the forehead and orbital region, is much more elective, especially if there is no functional impairment.

Some authors have questioned the value of early correction of nonsyndromic craniosynostosis in the absence of signs and symptoms of increased intracranial pressure.

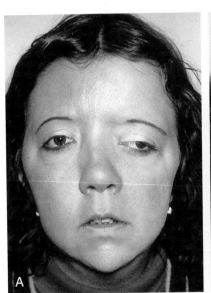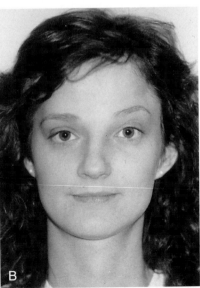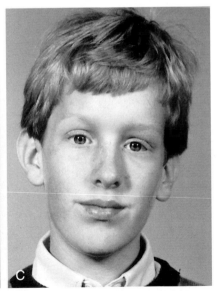

Figure 25–12. All patients shown had unilateral coronal synostosis. *A,* This patient has untreated right unilateral coronal synostosis. She demonstrates all the craniofacial compensations discussed in the section "Consequences of Craniosynostosis," including orbital dystopia (elevation of right globe, inferior position of left globe). *B,* This patient had undergone left unilateral coronal craniectomy at age 4 months. Note the residual forehead deficiency and the elevated eyebrow position on the affected side. *C,* This patient had undergone right unilateral coronal craniectomy and fronto-orbital remodeling at age 3 months (see Case 1). Minimal asymmetry persists, and this treatment has produced the most predictable long-term result for this condition.

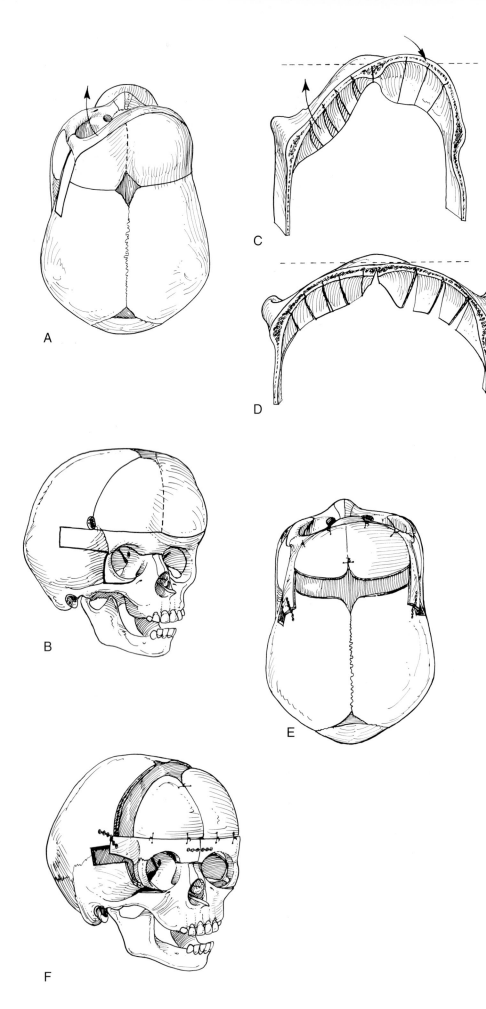

Figure 25–13. This modified osteotomy by Persing extends to include the lateral and inferior orbital rim. This method was suggested in order to minimize irregularity of the orbital rim after advancement. *A,* Original condition with bilateral expression. *B,* A bifrontal craniotomy is performed, and the entire fronto-orbital unit is removed. Notice the extension of the osteotomy to include the entire lateral orbital rim and a portion of the inferior orbital rim. *C,* With the fronto-orbital unit removed, bilateral contouring can be achieved by removing wedges from the left orbital roof to facilitate bending and scoring the right orbital roof to facilitate straightening. *D,* Symmetric contour is achieved by bending the unit's left side and straightening the right. *E* and *F,* Stabilization is achieved with either wires or microplates and microscrews.

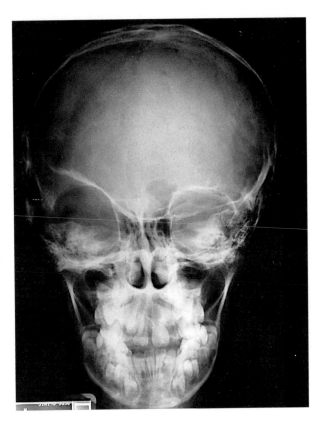

Figure 25–14. This skull radiograph of an unoperated 7-year-old demonstrates the "harlequin eye" deformity on the right, which is consistent with plagiocephaly secondary to right coronal synostosis. Note the lack of frontal sinus development on the right but presence of sinus on the left. This suggests that the lack of development of the sinus may be associated with the pathology and not a consequence of surgery.

Head molding with helmets and no surgical intervention has been suggested by some authors.[60,61] Others believe that simple surgical release of the suture allows the head to expand more normally and that remodeling is not necessary. The authors' experience suggests that if the fronto-orbital esthetic units are affected by craniosynostosis, self-correction without surgical intervention does not occur. Simple craniectomy alone is inadequate for restoring normal forehead and orbital esthetics. Craniectomy combined with fronto-orbital remodeling is the most predictable way of improving the condition. Fronto-orbital remodeling includes osteotomies of the orbital roof (cranial base) and orbital rim as well as forehead reconstruction (Figs. 25–12, 25–13).

When fronto-orbital remodeling is undertaken, the level of the osteotomy through the orbit is determined by the level of deficiency. As originally described by Hoffman and Mohr, the lateral canthal advancement is conducted just at or slightly inferior to the frontozygomatic suture.[51] Some authors have observed irregular contour of the lateral orbital rim after this procedure. Modifications for including the entire lateral orbital rim and a portion of the inferior orbital rim in the osteotomy design have been described.[57] Advocates for these modifications contend that a smoother orbital rim contour is achievable and maintainable (see Fig. 25–13).

Some authors advocate the avoidance of unilateral fronto-orbital remodeling during infancy and early childhood because in plagiocephaly associated with unilateral coronal synostosis, there is no "normal" side.[62] The contentions are that (1) bilateral remodeling produces the best result because both sides require alteration for optimal improvement and (2) it is easiest to achieve this by removing the entire supraorbital rim and forehead, reshaping these units, and replacing them in the desired position. An additional concern is the symmetric development of the frontal sinuses and maintenance of forehead symmetry after surgery. Some authors believe that unilateral fronto-orbital remodeling results in adverse effects on frontal sinus development unilaterally and that this causes forehead asymmetry to recur as the frontal sinus develops.[62] This observation must be critically considered because asymmetric frontal sinus development is also observed in nonsurgically treated patients with unilateral coronal synostosis and plagiocephaly and it may therefore be a feature of the deformity and not an effect of surgery (Fig. 25–14).

Other authors believe that unilateral fronto-orbital remodeling performed during infancy on the affected side alone is adequate for improving the condition.[63,64] This technique relies on normal brain and head development to self-correct many of the compensatory head shape changes. It is also dependent on the surgery's being conducted within the first year to take advantage of brain growth and development. Still other authors have suggested that delaying treatment until later in life will produce the best results, because the reconstruction can be done more precisely and the result is not as dependent on brain growth. If this approach is undertaken, more extensive surgery is necessary.[65,66]

Stabilization of the Osteotomy, Bone Grafting, and Prevention of Reossification

When prematurely fused sutures are released and fronto-orbital reconstruction is performed during infancy, stabilization of the repositioned forehead segment is critical, as it is when surgery is performed at any age. Tongue and groove osteotomies and/or bone grafts strategically placed along the anterior cranial base or in the temporoparietal regions and stabilized with wires are usually sufficient to support the position of the reconstructed supraorbital region (Figs. 25–15, 25–16). Another possibility is the use of microplates and microscrews to add support and rigidity to the reconstruction (Fig. 25–17A). With all of these choices, dilemmas exist.

Bone grafts and/or osteotomy extensions that bridge the region of prematurely fused sutures may promote early reossification. Therefore, the wisdom of using bone grafts and/or tongue-in-groove extensions that cross the prematurely fused region must be questioned. Although their use is to retain the reconstructed position of the forehead, they may also promote refusion at the region of the synostosed suture and therefore may be detrimental to head growth over the long term.

Another area of controversy with cranial remodeling procedures during infancy and childhood is the use of nonresorbable bone plates, screws, and wires. Although the nonresorbable microplates offer more stability and rigidity to the reconstructed bone segments, some investigators have observed varying degrees of restriction of head growth after placement.[67,68] Some of these observations have been made from animal models that demonstrated a variety of growth responses, including restriction. The applicability of these studies to the human condition is questionable, but the concept merits further investigation.[32]

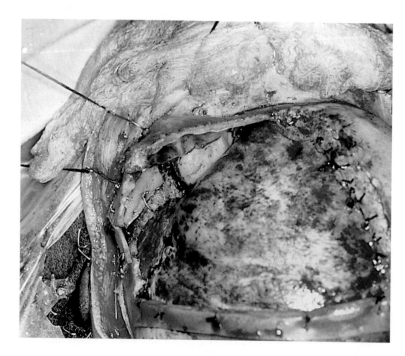

Figure 25–15. Bone grafts can be placed along the anterior cranial base (self-retained) and temporoparietal regions (secured with wire fixation) to support the repositioned supraorbital rim.

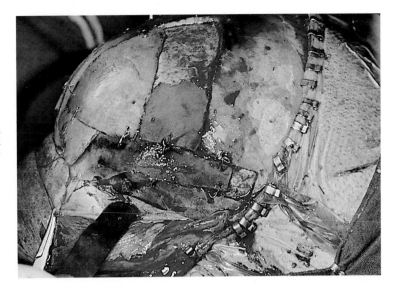

Figure 25–16. Tongue-in-groove osteotomy design extends into the temporoparietal region to control the position of the supraorbital rim after advancement.

The use of interosseous screws, plates, and/or wire during infant cranial remodeling procedures has raised concerns about the migration of the fixation devices: namely, that the hardware will eventually contact the dura and irritate the brain. Although there is evidence that hardware used during infant remodeling procedures does eventually contact and even perforate the dura, there is no conclusive evidence that this results in any adverse neurologic effects (see Fig. 25–17B). Migration in the true sense of the word does not occur. What occurs is a combination of endocranial bone resorption and exocranial bone deposition, especially in areas that lack the potential for sutural growth.[10] Some authors have suggested that if bone plates are used during infant cranial remodeling procedures, consideration should be given to removing them within 9 months of their placement to avoid long-term complications.[69]

Another area of surgical controversy is the efficacy of attempting to prevent reossification at the suture area. A consideration is the use of alloplastic material to wrap

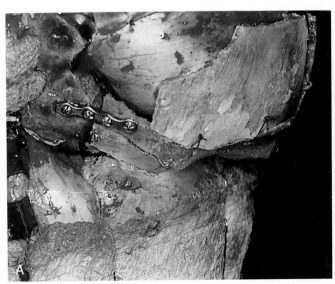

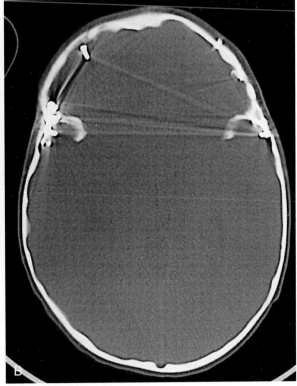

Figure 25–17. *A,* Metallic bone plates may also be used to stabilize the repositioned forehead units of a 3-month-old. *B,* Six years after placement of the bone plates used in the patient described in part *A,* the plates and screws are seen contacting and perforating the dura mater.

the bone margins. Some authors have suggested that the introduction of an alloplast into the surgical field increases the likelihood of infection.[70] The authors have observed infection with the use of an alloplastic wrap, as well as reossification over the alloplastic covering previously placed at suture regions. Most authors have abandoned applying caustic agents such as Zenker's solution to the dura to prevent reossification because of the accompanying damage to the dura and lack of adequate results.[71] Some authors advocate splitting the dura and covering the bone margins with the outer layer in an attempt to prevent ossification. Long-term effectiveness of this maneuver is unknown.

The method of stabilizing osteotomies, the efficacy of placing bone grafts into surgically created defects in regions of craniosynostosis, and attempts to prevent reossification require further investigation.

A serious consideration with the performance of this surgery during infancy and early childhood is the need to transfuse blood products. The risks of homologous blood transfusion must be addressed with family members and must also be factored into the risk/benefit ratio when surgery for improvement of isolated craniosynostosis is considered. Autologous or donor-directed blood programs and the use of laboratory-produced erythropoietin are alternatives to be considered when blood replacement is necessary.

CASE REPORTS

Since the introduction of surgical techniques to address craniosynostosis by craniectomy and reshaping by osteotomies of the fronto-orbital units and bone grafting, many modifications and surgical innovations have been developed. The patients described in this section represent follow-up observations of procedures and techniques used more than 15 years earlier. The techniques used were prototypes, but the basic principles of releasing sutures and reconstruction of the fronto-orbital region by osteotomies and reshaping are similar to those followed today. Results with these approaches for isolated craniosynostosis have been good in general. Until improved results with other more involved, time-consuming, and expensive techniques are demonstrated, simplicity should govern the choice of surgical procedures.

What appears critical with this approach is freeing the fused suture and achieving symmetric fronto-orbital units. In general, the best and most predictable results with nonsyndromic craniosynostosis are seen with isolated sagittal synostosis and unilateral coronal synostosis. Metopic synostosis and bilateral coronal synostosis respond favorably to these procedures, but programmed cerebral and cranial development appear to have a greater influence on results, and some patients benefit from revisions later in life. Patients in whom multiple sutures are involved respond with less predictability to these procedures, probably because the initial pathology is more complex and adversely affects their growth pattern. Patients with craniofacial dysostosis respond the least favorably to the procedures, and all eventually require additional surgery.

Case 1 (Figs. 25–18 to 25–23)

Right coronal synostosis was diagnosed in a 3-month-old who presented with a flattened forehead, orbital dystopia, nasal asymmetry, and hypoplasia of the right zygoma. There were no abnormal ophthalmologic findings or signs of increased intracranial pressure, but the right coronal suture was ridged. Plain skull radiographs revealed a harlequin eye deformity and hyperostosis of the right coronal suture.

According to the parents, the deformities were present at birth, but the parents were assured of the transient nature by the pediatrician, who believed that the deformities had resulted from intrauterine molding. Despite continued reassurances by the pediatrician of the self-correcting nature of this problem, the actual worsening of the situation alarmed the parents, and they sought another opinion.

The child underwent surgery soon after the initial evaluation. The decision to operate was based on the diagnosis of craniosynostosis and the progressive nature of the problem. A unilateral release of the coronal suture to the level of the temporal fossa was carried out. With the frontal bone plate removed, the anterior cranial base and supraorbital rim were separated on the right from the midline to the craniectomy

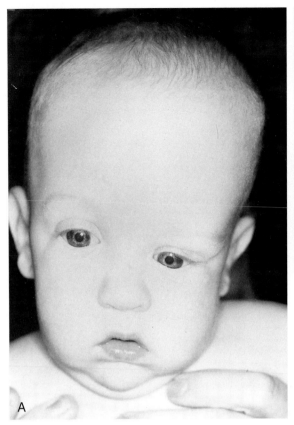

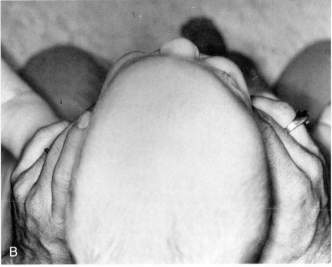

Figure 25–18. *A, B,* A 3-month-old boy with right coronal synostosis. Notice the abnormal forehead contour (projection on the nonaffected side and flattening on the affected side), uneven eyebrow position, orbital dystopia, and nasal bridge deviation.

Figure 25–19. Illustration of the surgery. Unilaterally, the coronal suture was released and the supraorbital rim was advanced, contoured, wired into position, and further stabilized with bone grafts in the temporal region and in the anterior cranial base. The osteotomy extended to the frontozygomatic suture only, and did not include the lateral orbital rim or infraorbital rim.

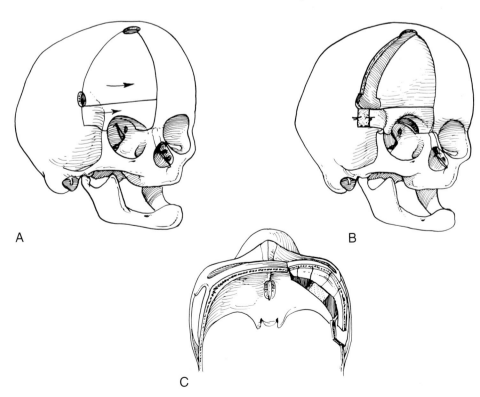

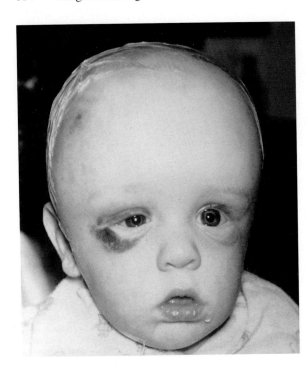

Figure 25–20. Result 1 week after surgery.

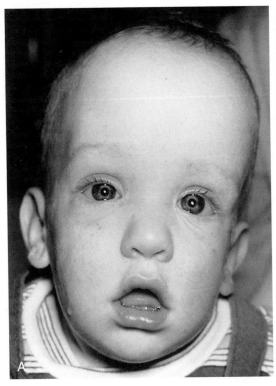

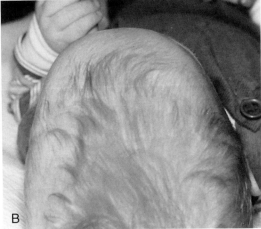

Figure 25–21. *A, B,* Result 6 months after surgery (9 months of age). Notice the improved forehead contour and facial symmetry. The orbital dystopia and nasal bridge deviation have self-corrected with continued growth. Had surgery not been undertaken early, the autocorrection may not have been possible.

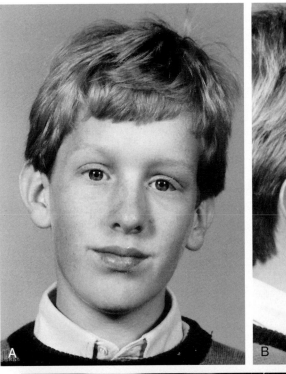

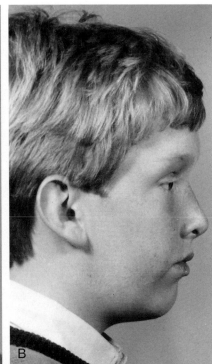

Figure 25–22. *A, B, C,* At 13 years, the patient's forehead, orbital, and facial development have remained satisfactory. There is some depression (banding) of the forehead above the supraorbital rim on the affected side. The patient had no concerns about this and does not desire revision. The lateral orbital rim has a smooth and symmetric contour even though the lateral and infraorbital rims were not included in the osteotomy.

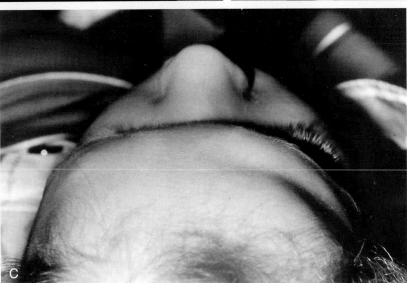

site. A greenstick fracture at the midforehead region allowed the segment to be hinged forward. Score osteotomies were placed on the internal surface of the supraorbital ridge, and contouring forceps were used to achieve the appropriate bend to the repositioned segment. Wire fixation and bone grafts at the temporal region and anterior cranial base were used to stabilize the position of the advanced orbit. The remaining forehead bone segments were trimmed and rotated to achieve the desired contour. They were secured to the supraorbital rim with wire fixation anteriorly and were supported by the brain posteriorly. A large defect remained at the area of the coronal suture.

This case illustrates a very satisfactory long-term result achieved by utilizing a unilateral operation and the principles of releasing the suture and performing simultaneous fronto-orbital remodeling.

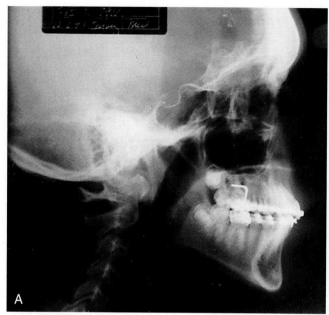

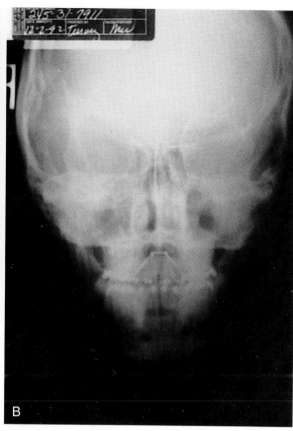

Figure 25–23. *A, B,* Lateral and posteroanterior cephalograms demonstrate favorable facial growth and symmetric class I occlusion. The frontal sinus on the left has begun developing, but there is none on the right. Although some surgeons implicate surgery as the cause of the sinus agenesis, it may also be a component of the original condition (see Fig. 25–14).

Case 2 (Figs. 25–24 to 25–27)

A 7-month-old with an asymmetric and flattened occiput was referred for evaluation and treatment. According to the parents, abnormal head shape was noted at birth, and this progressively worsened. The forehead and orbital regions were normal. The occiput was asymmetric with flattening on the right and bossing on the left. The right lambdoid suture was elevated and was immobile. Plain radiographs confirmed hyperostosis of the right lambdoid suture.

There were no abnormal neurologic or ophthalmologic findings, and surgical treatment was very optional. The parents opted for surgical reconstruction because of the abnormal head shape and its potential adverse effect on social acceptance.

Surgery was performed with the patient in the prone position. The occipitoparietal regions were exposed with a coronal incision, and two plates of bone from the right and left were removed. The left bone plate was convex and was placed on the right. The left side remained open.

Postsurgical recovery was uneventful.

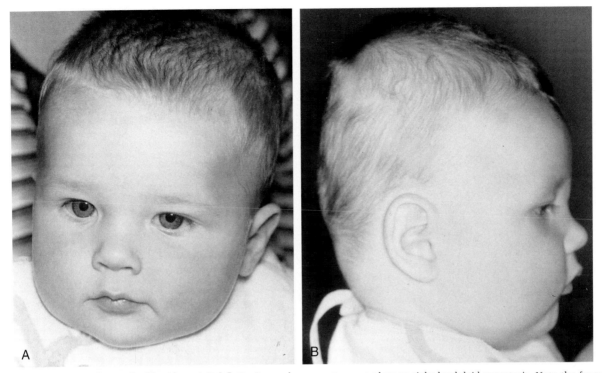

Figure 25–24. *A, B,* A 7-month-old with occipital flattening and asymmetry secondary to right lambdoid synostosis. Note the favorable forehead and orbital development.

Figure 25–25. Lateral skull radiograph demonstrates the abnormal head shape and hyperostosis of the lambdoid suture.

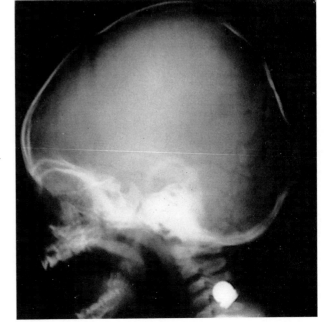

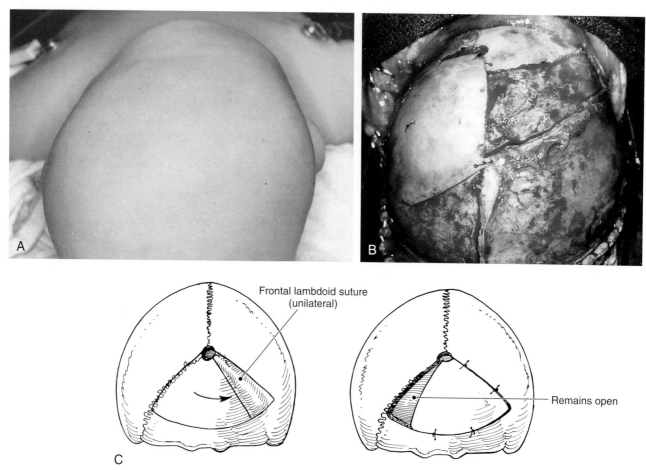

Figure 25–26. *A, B,* The surgery was performed with the patient in the prone position. The lambdoid suture was widely excised on the right. The left occipitoparietal convexity was removed and transferred to the right and wired in place. *C,* Illustration of the surgery for lambdoid synostosis.

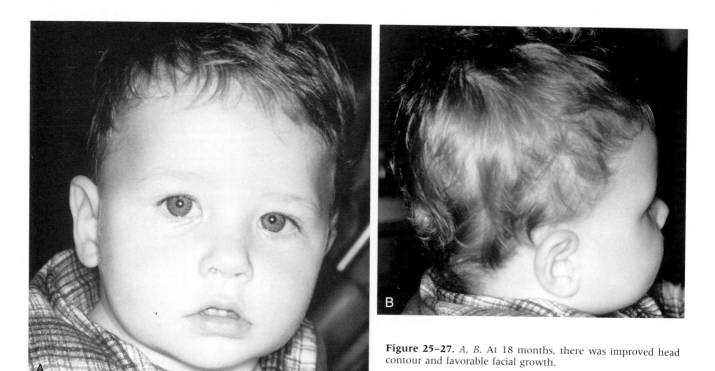

Figure 25–27. *A, B,* At 18 months, there was improved head contour and favorable facial growth.

Case 3 (Figs. 25–28 to 25–32)

A 9-month-old with trigonocephaly secondary to metopic synostosis was seen incidentally after a fall in which he sustained a linear skull fracture. The parents were aware of the abnormal head shape but had been advised by the pediatrician that it would improve with time. A triangular forehead with prominent metopic ridging and bitemporal narrowing were the obvious findings. There were no abnormal neurologic or ophthalmologic findings, other than hypotelorism and epicanthal folds. Surgery was elected.

Bilateral frontal bone plates were removed, preserving the ridged metopic suture. The anterior cranial base was dissected, as were the orbital roofs. Bilateral supraorbital rim advancements were performed with a greenstick fracture in the glabellar region, which served as a hinge. Long tongue-in-groove osteotomies into the temporal region, controlled the position of the segments, and score osteotomies on the internal surface of the segments facilitated the desired contour. The frontal plates were carved and rotated to the desired forehead contour and were wired to the repositioned supraorbital rims and midline strut.

At the age of 13 years, lateral forehead and orbital rim deficiencies were obvious, and there was some return of the original triangular forehead shape. Although the patient was advised that the situation could be improved again, he was not concerned enough to pursue further treatment.

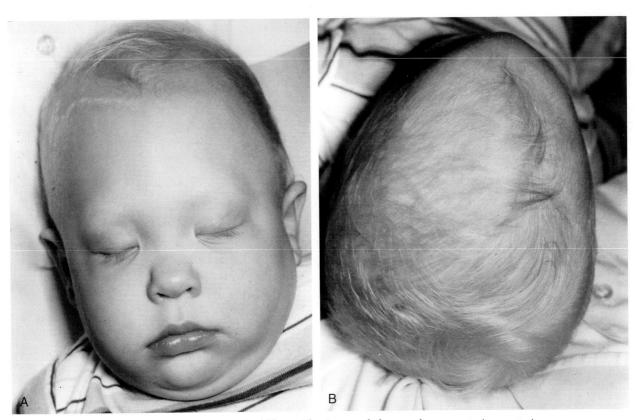

Figure 25–28. *A, B,* A 9-month-old boy with trigonocephaly secondary to metopic synostosis.

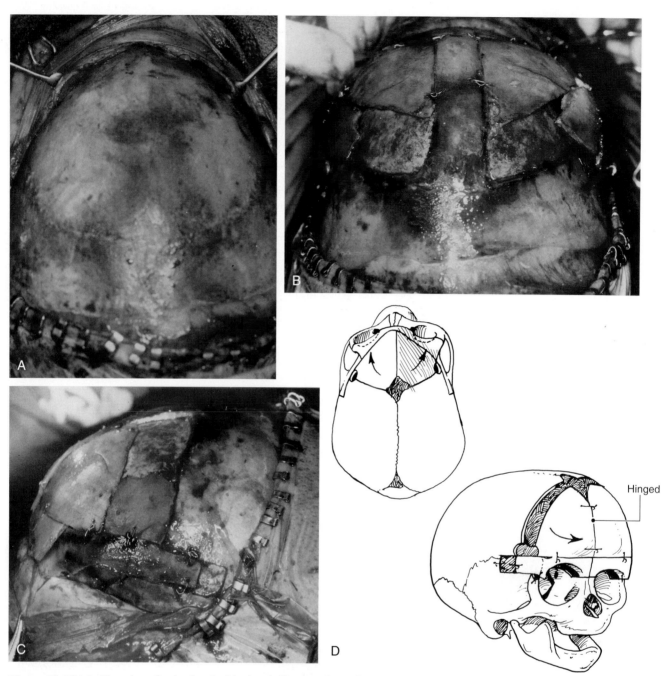

Figure 25–29. *A,* The triangular forehead with the skull exposed. *B,* The surgery involved bilateral fronto-orbital expansion. The glabellar region was the point of fracture to advance and laterally expand the supraorbital rims. *C,* The tongue-in-groove extensions and bilateral scoring of the internal surface of the supraorbital rims enabled reshaping as well as repositioning of the forehead. *D,* Illustration of the surgery.

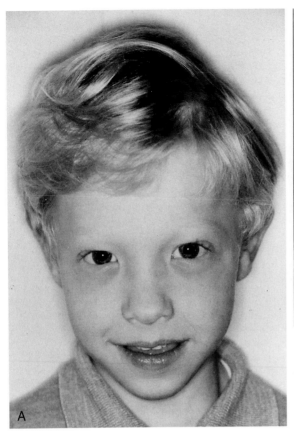

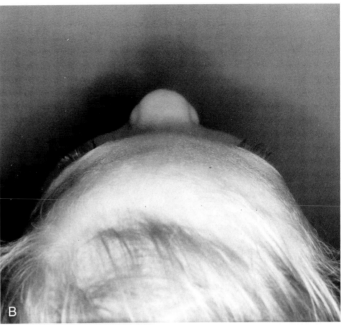

Figure 25–30. *A, B,* Two years after surgery, a satisfactory change was appreciated.

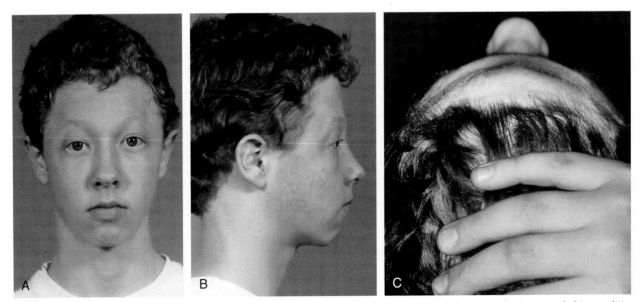

Figure 25–31. *A, B, C,* Twelve years after surgery (age 13), there was return of some of the original stigmata of this condition. Deficiency of projection of the lateral aspects of the forehead and supraorbital rims as well as the lateral orbital rim are noticeable.

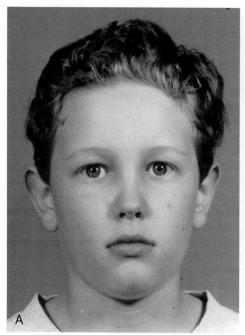 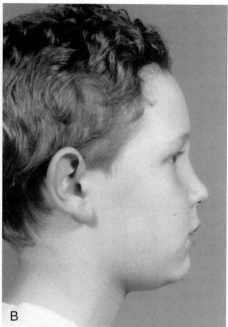

Figure 25–32. *A, B,* This is the 11-year-old brother of the patient shown in Figures 25–24 to 25–31. At 1 year of age, he underwent sagittal craniectomy for relief of sagittal synostosis. Head and forehead development as well as orbital development have been favorable. In a comparison of the forehead shapes of the brothers, the one with metopic synostosis (see Fig. 25–31) has had much less anterior and lateral development of the lower forehead and supraorbital regions. In addition, he lacks the normal forehead curvature. The different growth responses after surgery are reflective of the different conditions and the programmed cerebral and cranial development. These two cases also highlight the possibility of a hereditary aspect of craniosynostosis.

Case 4 (Figs. 25–33 to 25–35)

A 9-month-old was referred for evaluation of abnormal head shape. There was ridging and immobility of the sagittal and coronal sutures. The posterior fontanelle was open, but the anterior fontanelle was closed and immobile. Plain radiographs indicated hyperostosis of the sagittal suture and fusion of the coronal sutures bilaterally. Neurologic testing failed to demonstrate any abnormalities, and there were no signs of increased intracranial pressure.

A wide sagittal craniectomy was carried out from the lambdoid region anteriorly to the coronal suture. Bilateral coronal craniectomies to the temporal fossa region were performed next. Removal of a large frontal bone plate allowed access to the anterior cranial base. The supraorbital rims were then advanced and held in place with wire fixation. The osteotomy was designed with tongue-in-groove extensions into the temporal region, and so bone grafts were not used to stabilize this segment. Back cuts were then placed in the lambdoid and coronal areas on each side to allow for temporal and parietal widening, which occurred within minutes. The frontal bone plate was halved, and the forehead contour was reconstructed by reversing and inverting the two plates. These were attached to the supraorbital rim and stabilized with wire fixation. Several bone strips were wired into the widened sagittal craniectomy site, but large bone defects remained at both the coronal and sagittal suture sites.

At age 13, normal head and facial configurations had been maintained. This case demonstrates favorable head and facial development after sutural release, forehead and orbital reshaping, and remodeling for multiple synostosed sutures.

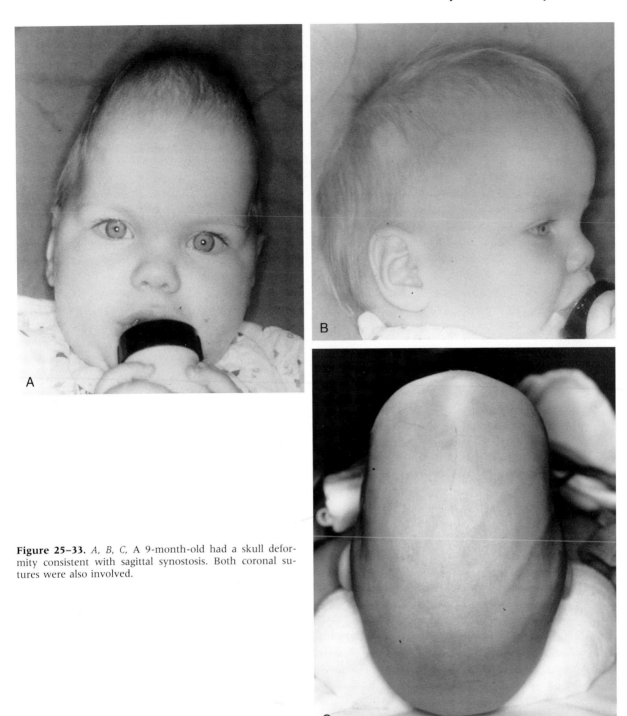

Figure 25–33. *A, B, C,* A 9-month-old had a skull deformity consistent with sagittal synostosis. Both coronal sutures were also involved.

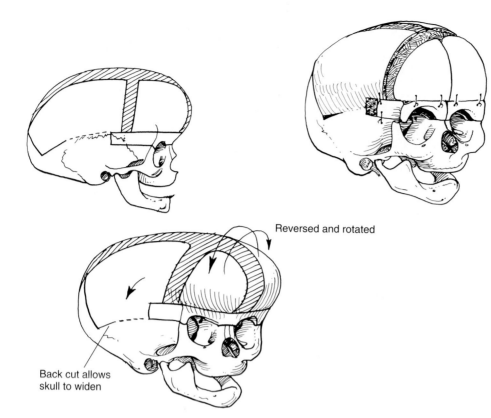

Reversed and rotated

Back cut allows
skull to widen

Figure 25–34. The surgery involved a wide sagittal craniectomy with relief cuts in the temporal and parietal regions to permit lateral skull expansion. Bilateral coronal craniectomies and supraorbital rim advancements were simultaneously performed and stabilized with wire fixation. The forehead was reconstructed by reversing the two frontal bone plates and securing them with wire fixation.

Figure 25–35. *A, B,* Twelve years after surgery, at age 13, there was favorable head and facial development.

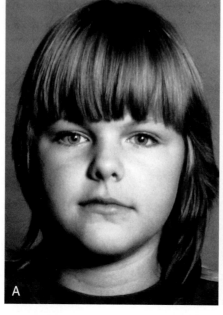

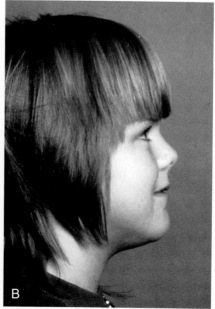

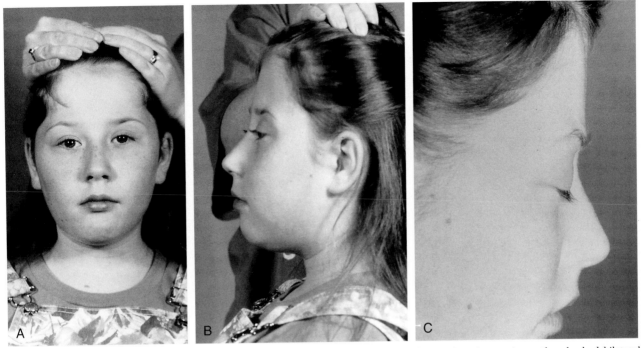

Figure 25–36. *A, B, C,* An 11-year-old with oxycephaly and lack of supraorbital rim projection. At age 6 months, she had bilateral coronal craniectomy and fronto-orbital advancement performed elsewhere. Her osteotomies were stabilized with wire fixation. Note the temporal banding.

Case 5 (Figs. 25–36 to 25–40)

An 11-year-old girl was referred because of her concern about fronto-orbital appearance and ''a long forehead.'' In addition, she complained of frequent frontal headaches. The patient had undergone bilateral coronal craniectomy and fronto-orbital advancement at approximately 6 months of age elsewhere.

Her examination revealed deficient supraorbital projection and a high, straight forehead with temporal banding bilaterally (oxycephaly). The same growth pattern after

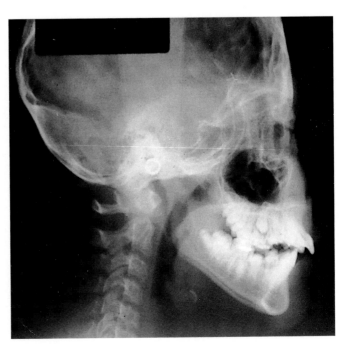

Figure 25–37. The lateral cephalogram demonstrates the distorted anterior cranial base and the vertical projection without curvature of the forehead.

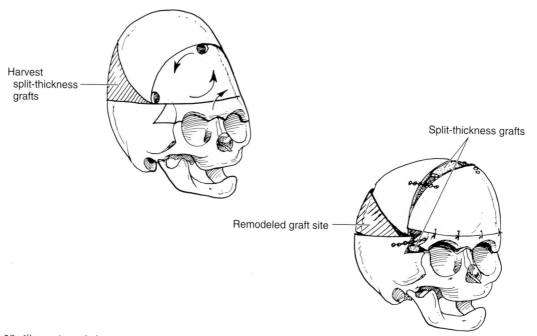

Harvest
split-thickness
grafts

Split-thickness grafts

Remodeled graft site

Figure 25–38. Illustration of the surgery, which consisted of advancement of the supraorbital rim and forehead reconstruction, as originally described by Marchac.

surgery has been observed in some of the authors' patients with bilateral coronal synostosis who underwent similar surgery within the first year as well. Her neurologic examination and computed tomographic scans failed to reveal any abnormalities other than the abnormal head shape. Funduscopic examination was also normal. The headaches were believed to be nonspecific and incidental to the condition.

At surgery, a frontal bone plate was removed, and the supraorbital rim and lower forehead were advanced approximately 15 mm. They were stabilized with microplates and microscrews. The frontal bone was sectioned and reversed to achieve appropriate forehead contour. The segments were stabilized with microplates and microscrews. Split-thickness bone grafts were harvested from the parietal region, and the anterior defects were grafted.

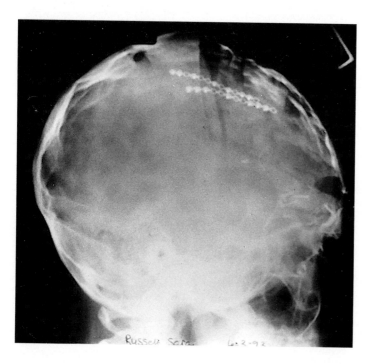

Figure 25–39. Postoperative skull radiograph demonstrating the improved head configuration and stabilization of the segments with microplates and microscrews.

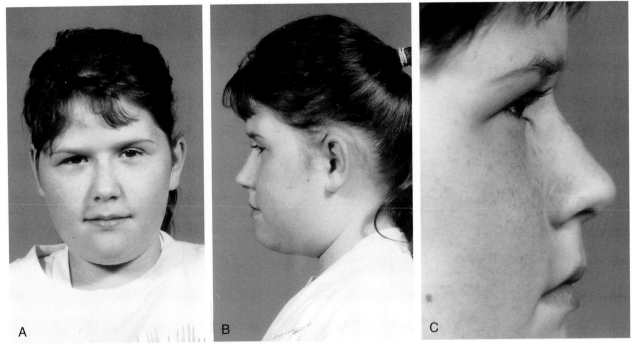

Figure 25–40. *A, B, C,* One-year postoperative photograph demonstrating improved forehead contour, elimination of the temporal banding, and adequate projection of the eyebrows. Upper eyelid edema continued to resolve.

After surgery, the patient's headaches resolved, and she recovered quickly. One year later, she and her family were happy with the esthetic result.

In contrast to surgery for craniosynostosis undertaken during infancy, it must be conducted more precisely when performed at this age. The result is more dependent on the surgeon's diagnostic and reconstructive skills and less dependent on brain growth for support.

Acknowledgments

The primary author acknowledges the following neurosurgeons who invited his participation in the care of these patients: Dr. Steven K. Gudeman, Professor and Chief, Division of Neurosurgery, University of North Carolina School of Medicine, Chapel Hill; Dr. Steven K. Powers, Professor and Chairman, Department of Neurosurgery, Pennsylvania State Medical School, Hershey; and Dr. Ronald Woosley, Tulsa, Oklahoma.

References

1. Cohen MM Jr: Syndromes with craniosynostosis. *In* Cohen MM Jr (ed): Craniosynostosis: Diagnosis, Evaluation, and Management, pp 413–590. New York: Raven Press, 1986.
2. Moss ML: The pathogenesis of premature cranial synostosis in man. Acta Anat (Basal) 1959; 37:351–370.
3. Stewart RE, Dixon G, Cohen A: The pathogenesis of premature craniosynostosis in acrocephalosyndactyly (Apert's syndrome): A reconsideration. Plast Reconstr Surg 1977; 59:699–703.
4. Kokich VG: The biology of sutures. *In* Cohen MM Jr (ed): Craniosynostosis: Diagnosis, Evaluation, and Management, pp 81–105. New York: Raven Press, 1986.
5. Mossaz CF, Kokich VG: Redevelopment of the calvaria following partial craniectomy in growing rabbits: The effect of altering dural continuity. Acta Anat (Basal) 1981; 109:321–331.
6. Cohen MM Jr: Sutural biology and the correlates of craniosynostosis. Am J Med Genet 1993; 47:581–616.
7. Renier D: Intracranial pressure in craniosynostosis: Pre- and postoperative recordings. Correlation with functional results. *In* Persing JA, Jane JA, Edgerton MT (eds): Scientific Foundations and Surgical Treatment of Craniosynostosis, p 263. Baltimore: Williams & Wilkins, 1989.
8. Gault DT, Renier D, Marchac D, Jones BM: Intracranial pressure and intracranial volume in children with craniosynostosis. Plast Reconstr Surg 1992; 90:377–381.
9. Virchow R: Uber den cretinismus, nametlich in Franken, under uber pathologische: Schadelformen. Verk Phys Med Gessellsch Wurzburg 1851; 2:230–271.
10. Enlow DH: Normal craniofacial growth. *In* Cohen MM Jr (ed): Craniosynostosis: Diagnosis, Evaluation, and Management, pp 131–156. New York: Raven Press, 1986.

11. Moss ML, Greenberg SV: Postnatal growth of the human skull base. Angle Orthod 1955; 25:77–84.
12. Park EA, Powers GF: Acrocephaly and scaphocephaly with symmetrically disturbed malformations of the extremities. Am J Dis Child 1920; 20:235–315.
13. Cohen MM Jr: Etiology of craniosynostosis. In Cohen MM Jr (ed): Craniosynostosis: Diagnosis, Evaluation, and Management, pp 131–156. New York: Raven Press, 1986.
14. Higgenbottom MC, Jones KL, James HE: Intrauterine constraint and craniosynostosis. Neurosurgery 1980; 6:39–49.
15. MacGregor FC: Transformation and identity—The face and plastic surgery. New York Times, Quadrangle section, 1974.
16. MacGregor FC: Facial disfigurement: Problems and management of social interaction and implications for mental health. Aesthetic Plast Surg 1990; 14:249.
17. Bull R, Ramsey VL: The social psychology of facial appearance. New York: Springer-Verlag, 1988.
18. Babler WJ, Persing JA, Winn HR, Rodeheaver GT: Compensatory growth following premature closure of the coronal suture in rabbits. J Neurosurg 1982; 57:533–542.
19. Babler WJ: Relationship of altered cranial suture growth to the cranial base and midface. In Persing JA, Edgerton MT, Jane JA (eds): Scientific Foundations and Surgical Treatment of Craniosynostosis, pp 87–95. Baltimore: Williams & Wilkins, 1989.
20. Renier D, Sainte-Rose C, Marchac D, Hirsch JF: Intracranial pressure in craniostenosis. J Neurosurg 1982; 57:370–377.
21. Renier D: Intracranial pressure in craniosynostosis: Pre- and postoperative recordings: Correlation with functional results. In Persing JA, Edgerton MT, Jane JA (eds): Scientific Foundations and Surgical Treatment of Craniosynostosis, pp 263–269. Baltimore: Williams & Wilkins, 1989.
22. Gault DT, Renier D, Marchac D, Jones BM: Intracranial pressure and intracranial volume in children with craniosynostosis. Plast Reconstr Surg 1992; 90:377–381.
23. Cohen MM Jr, Kreiborg S: The central nervous system in the Apert syndrome. Am J Med Genet 1990; 35:36–45.
24. LeFebvre A, Munro I: The role of psychiatry in a craniofacial team. Plast Reconstr Surg 1978; 61:564–569.
25. Pertschuk MS, Whitaker LA: Psychosocial outcome of craniofacial surgery in children. Plast Reconstr Surg 1988; 82:741.
26. Hogan GR, Bauman ML: Hydrocephalus in Apert's syndrome. J Pediatr 1971; 79:782.
27. Golabi M, Edwards MSB, Ousterhout DK: Craniosynostosis and hydrocephalus. Neurosurgery 1987; 21:63.
28. Fishman MA, Hogan GR, Dodge PR: The concurrence of hydrocephalus and craniosynostosis. J Neurosurg 1971; 36:621–629.
29. Marchac D: Discussion of Whitaker FA, Bartlett SP, Schut L, Bruce D: Craniosynostosis: An analysis of the timing, treatment and complications in 164 consecutive patients. Plast Reconstr Surg 1987; 20:207–212.
30. Shillito J: A plea for early operation for craniosynostosis. Surg Neurol 1992; 37:182–188.
31. Posnick JC: Craniosynostosis: Diagnosis and treatment in infancy and early childhood. In Bell WH (ed): Modern Practice in Orthognathic and Reconstructive Surgery, vol 3, p 1845. Philadelphia: WB Saunders, 1992.
32. Posnick J: Discussion of Yaremchuk MJ, Fiala TG, Barker F, Ragland R: The effects of rigid fixation on craniofacial growth of rhesus monkeys. Plast Reconstr Surg 1994; 93:11–15.
33. Lannelongue M: De la craniectomie dans la microcephalic. Compte-Rondu Academie des Sciences 1890; 110:1382.
34. Lane LC: Pioneer craniectomy for relief of mental imbecility due to premature sutural closure and microcephalus. JAMA 1892; 18:49.
35. Faber HK: The importance of early diagnosis in oxycephaly and allied cranial deformities with reference to the prevention of blindness and other sequelae. Calif West Med 1924; 22:542–545.
36. Faber HK, Towne EB: Early craniectomy as a preventive measure in oxycephaly and allied conditions, with special reference to the prevention of blindness. Am J Med Sci 1927; 173:701–711.
37. Mehner A: Beitrage zu den augenverandewingen bie der schadel-deformitat des saq. Turnschadelsmit besonderer beruchsichtegung des rontgenbildes. Klin Monatsbl Augenheilmd 1921; 61:204.
38. King J: Oxycephaly. Ann Surg 1942; 115:488–506.
39. Anderson FM, Johnson FC: Craniosynostosis: A modification and surgical treatment. Surgery 1956; 40:961–970.
40. Simmons DR, Peyton WT: Premature closure of cranial sutures. J Pediatr 1947; 31:528–546.
41. Ingraham FD, Alexander E, Matson DD: Clinical studies in craniosynostosis: Analysis of fifty cases and description of a method of surgical treatment. Surgery 1948; 24:518–541.
42. Ingraham FD, Matson DD: Neurosurgery of Infancy and Childhood. Springfield, MA: Charles C Thomas, 1954.
43. Powiertowski H, Matlosz Z: The treatment of craniosynostosis by a method of extensive resection of the vault of the skull. In Proceedings of the Third International Congress on Neurosurgery, Surgical Excerpts Medical International Congress Series 110, p 834, 1965.
44. Hanson JW, Sayers MP, Known LM, et al: Subtotal neonatal calveriectomy for severe craniosynostosis. J Pediatr 1977; 91:251–260.
45. Bertelsen TI: The premature synostosis of the cranial sutures. Acta Ophthalmol Suppl 1958; 51:24–174.
46. Seeger JF, Gabrielson TO: Premature closure of the frontosphenoidal suture. Radiology 1971; 101:631–635.
47. Burdi AR, Kusnetz AB, Venes JL, Gebarski SS: The natural history and pathogenesis of the cranial coronal ring articulations: Implications in understanding the pathogenesis of the Crouzon craniostenotic defects. Cleft Palate J 1986; 23:28–39.
48. McCarthy JG, Coccaro PJ, Epstein F, Converse JM: Early skeletal relapse in the infant with craniofacial dysostosis. The role of the sphenozygomatic suture. Plast Reconstr Surg 1978; 62:335.

49. Rougerie J, Derome P, Anques L: Craniosténoses et dysmorphosies cranio-faciales. Principes d'une nouvelle technique de traitement et ses résultats. Neurochirurgie 1972; 18:429–440.

50. Tessier P: The definitive plastic surgical treatment of the severe facial deformities of craniofacial dysostosies. Crouzon and Apert's diseases. Plast Reconstr Surg 1971; 48:419.

51. Hoffman HJ, Mohr G: Lateral canthal advancement of the superorbital margin. J Neurosurg 1976; 45:376–381.

52. Jane JA, Persing JA: Neurosurgical treatment of craniosynostosis. In Cohen MM Jr (ed): Craniosynostosis: Diagnosis, Evaluation, and Management, pp 249–320. New York: Raven Press, 1986.

53. Marchac D, Renier D: Craniofacial Surgery for Craniosynostosis. Boston: Little, Brown, 1982.

54. Whitaker LA, Schut L, Kerr LP: Early surgery for isolated craniofacial dysostosis. Plast Reconstr Surg 1977; 60:575.

55. Munro IR, Sabatier RE: An analysis of 12 years of craniofacial surgery in Toronto. Plast Reconstr Surg 1985; 76:29.

56. Posnick JC: Craniofacial dysostosis: Staging of reconstruction and management of the midface deformity. Neurosurg Clin North Am 1991; 2(3):638–702.

57. Persing JA, Jane JA, Edgerton MT: Surgical treatment of craniosynostosis. In Persing JA, Edgerton MT, Jane JA (eds): Scientific Foundations and Surgical Treatment of Craniosynostosis, pp 117–238. Baltimore: Williams & Wilkins, 1989.

58. Van der Meuhlen JCH: Medial fasciotomy. Br J Plast Surg 1979; 32:339.

59. Ortiz-Monasterio F, Fuente del Carupo A, Carillo A: Advancement of the orbits and the midface in one piece, combined with frontal positioning for the correction of Crouzon's deformities. Plast Reconstr Surg 1978; 61:507.

60. Clarren SK, Smith DW, Hanson JW: Helmet treatment for plagiocephaly and congenital muscular torticollis. J Pediatr 1979; 94:43–46.

61. Clarren SK: Plagiocephaly and torticollis: Etiology, natural history and helmet treatment. J Pediatr 1981; 98:92–95.

62. McCarthy JG, Karp NS, LaTrenta GS, Thorpe CH: The effect of early fronto-orbital advancement on frontal sinus development and forehead aesthetics. Plast Reconstr Surg 1990; 86:1078–1084.

63. Bartlett SP, Whitaker LA, Marchac D: The operative treatment of isolated craniofacial dysostosis (plagiocephaly): A comparison of the unilateral and bilateral techniques. Plast Reconstr Surg 1990; 85:677–683.

64. Whitaker LA, Bartlett SP, Schut L, Bruce D: Craniosynostosis: An analysis of the timing, treatment, and complications in 166 consecutive patients. Plast Reconstr Surg 1987; 80:195–212.

65. Raulo Y: Radical surgery of plagiocephaly. In Caronni E (ed): Craniofacial Surgery, pp 275–279. Boston: Little, Brown, 1985.

66. Tulasne JF, Tessier P: Analysis and late treatment of plagiocephaly. Scand J Plast Reconstr Surg 1981; 15:257.

67. Manson PN: Commentary on the long-term effects of rigid fixation on the growing craniomaxillofacial skeleton. J Craniofac Surg 1991; 2:69.

68. Yaremchuk MJ, Fiala TG, Barker F, Ragland R: The effects of rigid fixation on craniofacial growth of rhesus monkeys. Plast Reconstr Surg 1994; 93:1–10.

69. Muhling J: Treatment of craniofacial synostosis in early infancy: Educational summaries and outlines. J Oral Maxillofac Surg 1993; 51(Suppl 3):146.

70. McComb JG, Raffel C: Craniosynostosis. In Apuzzo LJ (ed): Brain Surgery: Complication Avoidance and Management, p 1458. New York: Churchill Livingstone, 1993.

71. Martin AE, Brown WE, Huntington HW, Epstein F: Effect of the dura application of Zenker's solution on the feline brain. Neurosurgery 1982; 6:45–48.

Craniofacial Dysostosis Syndromes: A Staged Reconstructive Approach

26

Jeffrey C. Posnick

Premature fusion of the cranial vault sutures has been recognized since the time of the ancient Greeks. Galen introduced the term *oxycephaly* to describe the condition. In the 19th century, Virchow coined the term *craniosynostosis* and formulated the classic theory known as Virchow's law: that premature fushion (synostosis) of a cranial vault suture inhibits normal skull growth perpendicular to the fused suture and that compensatory growth occurs at the open sutures and that the general direction of growth after synostosis is parallel to the fused suture.[1]

The term *craniofacial dysostosis* is generally used to describe familial forms of synostosis involving not only the cranial vault but various cranial base and midface sutures as well. Familial types of craniofacial dysostosis were described by Apert in 1906,[2] Crouzon in 1912,[3] Pfeiffer in 1964,[4] Saethre and Chotzen in 1931,[5] and Carpenter in 1901. *Kleeblattschädel anomaly* refers to the overall shape of the skull and face (cloverleaf) that results when specific cranial vault and cranial base sutures fuse prematurely.[6]

The incidence of craniosynostosis is about 0.4:1000 in the general population.[5] Most cases of simple craniosynostosis are sporadic. However, if both a parent and a child are affected, the risk for each subsequent child approaches 50%. Syndromal craniosynostosis is usually genetic. The mode of transmission may be either autosomal dominant, as in Crouzon syndrome, or autosomal recessive, as in Apert syndrome.

The treatment for these conditions has been surgical, but the indications, timing, type, and effectiveness of reconstruction have not been well evaluated. This chapter describes a philosophy and a rationale for treatment intervention.

CROUZON SYNDROME

The incidence of Crouzon syndrome is 1:25,000 in the general population. The inheritance pattern is autosomal dominant, and the trait is noted for its variable expression.[7-25]

Crouzon described an affected family pedigree in 1912.[3] He listed four major characteristics of the disease: exorbitism, retromaxillism, inframaxillism, and paradoxic retrogenia. Premature fusion of sutures may occur at the level of the cranial vault; bilateral coronal premature fusion is the most common and results in a brachycephalic appearance. Other forms of premature suture synostosis (i.e., sagittal, lambdoid, or metopic) may also occur in Crouzon syndrome. In addition to cranial vault synostosis, there is a poorly defined effect on the anterior cranial base and facial sutures that results in a variable degree of symmetric hypoplasia or dysplasia of the orbits, zygomas, and maxilla.[3, 8, 13–16, 19–23, 25–33] The mandible has normal growth but may become secondarily deformed with an obtuse ramus/inferior border angle and a vertically long chin.[34] In general, the soft tissue envelope is normal except for a variable degree of upper eyelid ptosis and inferiorly positioned lateral canthi. In patients with classical findings, the cranial vault is either brachycephalic or oxycephalic, the orbits are shallow with proptotic eyes, and the midface is flat with an Angle class III malocclusion. Nasal airflow is diminished with partial obstruction, and a mouth-breathing pattern is common.[16]

APERT SYNDROME

Most cases of Apert syndrome have occurred sporadically.[4,5,35] Pedigrees of dominant transmission with complete penetrance have been documented. However, sufficient numbers of adults with Apert syndrome have not been observed in order to ascertain a genetic pattern.[35] This syndrome has been observed in white, black, and Asian populations, and advanced paternal age is thought to be a factor in producing new gene mutations. The incidence is thought to be 1 : 100,000 in the general population.[5] Results of postmortem studies suggest that skeletal deficiencies in the Apert face result from reduced growth of the cranial base, which leads to premature fusion of the midline sutures from the occiput to the anterior nasal septum.[23,31,33,36–38] Results of some studies suggest that synostosis of the sphenoid bone to the adjacent vomer may be a factor.[30]

Apert first described the syndrome as a combination of multiple physical findings, including severe cranial vault deformities, syndactylism, mental retardation, and blindness.[2] It is now known that the craniofacial skeletal abnormality of Apert syndrome is complex and includes fusion of the coronal sutures and abnormal formation or fusion of the anterior cranial base and midface sutures. In addition, the syndrome is characterised by four-limb symmetric complex syndactylies of the hands and feet. Fusion or malformation of other joints, including the elbows and shoulders, often occurs. Although the syndrome has features in the general craniofacial skeletal dysmorphology that are similar to those of Crouzon syndrome, expressivity of the trait in Apert syndrome is more severe and with less variation in expression.[35,38] Shallowness and hypertelorism of the orbits and proptotis of the eyes (exophthalmus) are more severe. Midface hypoplasia is more marked both vertically and horizontally with a greater upper face transverse width than seen in Crouzon syndrome. The soft tissue drape also varies from that seen in Crouzon syndrome, with a greater downward slant to the lateral canthi and a distinctive, S-shaped ptosis of the upper eyelids. Hydrocephalus necessitating ventriculoperitoneal shunting is also a more common finding in Apert syndrome.[39–42] Apert syndrome is frequently associated with a degree of developmental delay. Cohen clarified some of these issues by documenting central nervous system variations in Apert syndrome patients.[43–46] A conductive hearing loss may be present and is characterized by a 30%–40% incidence of congenital fixation of the middle ear structures and a high incidence of poorly treated otitis media.[6]

PFEIFFER SYNDROME

In 1964, Pfeiffer described a syndrome consisting of craniosynostosis, broad thumbs, broad great toes, and, occasionally, partial soft tissue syndactyly of the hand.[6] An autosomal dominant inheritance pattern has been recognized. Penetrance is complete, whereas expressivity is variable. Sporadic cases have been reported. Bilateral coronal suture synostosis with midface deficiency, exorbitism, and exophthalmus are frequent findings. This disorder should be distinguished from Apert syndrome, Crouzon syndrome, Saethre-Chotzen syndrome, Carpenter syndrome, and simple craniosynostosis.

CARPENTER SYNDROME

Carpenter syndrome is characterized by craniosynostosis often associated with preaxial polysyndactyly of the feet, short fingers with clinodactyly and variable soft tissue syndactyly, sometimes postaxial polydactyly, and other anomalies such as congenital heart defects, short stature, obesity, and mental deficiency.[6] It was first described by Carpenter in 1901 and was later recognized as an autosomal recessive syndrome.

SAETHRE-CHOTZEN SYNDROME

Saethre-Chotzen syndrome is characterized by great variation in the pattern of malformations, including craniosynostosis, low-set frontal hairline, facial asymmetry, ptosis of the upper eyelids, brachydactyly, partial cutaneous syndactyly, and other skeletal anomalies.[6] An autosomal dominant inheritance pattern with a high degree of penetrance and variable expressivity is seen.

KLEEBLATTSCHÄDEL ANOMALY

Kleeblattschädel (cloverleaf) skull anomaly is a trilobular shape of the skull secondary to craniosynostosis.[6] The cloverleaf skull anomaly is known to be both etiologically and pathogenetically heterogenous. The cloverleaf skull malformation is nonspecific: It may be observed as an isolated anomaly or together with other anomalies, making up various syndromes (i.e., Apert, Crouzon, Carpenter, Pfeiffer, and Saethre-Chotzen syndromes). The severity varies, and different sutures may be involved, including the coronal, lambdoidal, and metopic sutures, with bulging of the cerebrum through an open sagittal suture or through open squamosal sutures. Synostosis of the sagittal and squamosal sutures with cerebral bulging through a widely patent anterior fontanelle may also be observed. As a result of the cranial base synostosis, the ears are displaced downward. Midface hypoplasia is a common finding.

FUNCTIONAL CONSIDERATIONS

Brain Growth

Brain volume in normal children almost triples during the first year (Table 26–1). By age 2 years, the cranial capacity is four times that at birth. If this rapid brain growth is to proceed unhindered, the open cranial vault and base sutures must spread during phases of rapid growth, resulting in marginal ossification.

In craniosynostosis, premature suture fusion is combined with continuing brain growth. The upper orbital and cranial vault shape is determined by Virchow's law.[1] Depending on the number and location of prematurely fused sutures and the timing of closure, the growth of the brain may be restricted. If surgical intervention, with suture release and reshaping to restore a more normal intracranial volume and configuration, does not reverse the process, diminished central nervous system function is often the end result.[46]

Intracranial Pressure

Elevated intracranial pressure is the most important functional problem that is associated with premature suture fusion. Its late and devastating effect can be identified on plain radiographs from the fingerprinting or beaten-copper appearance along the inner table of the cranial vault and base. Early signs of pressure apparent from a

Table 26–1. CRANIAL AND BRAIN GROWTH DURING THE FIRST 20 YEARS OF LIFE*

Age	Volume of Brain (cm³)	Cranial Capacity (cm³)
Newborn	330	350
3 months	550	600
6 months	575	775
9 months	675	925
1 year	750	1000
2 years	900	1100
3 years	960	1225
4 years	1000	1300
6 years	1060	1350
9 years	1100	1400
12 years	1150	1450
20 years	1200	1500

* From Blinkov SM, Glezer II: The Human Brain in Figures and Tables. A Quantitative Handbook (Haigh B, Trans). Leningrad: Meditsina Press, 1964. Copyright © 1968 by Plenum Press and Basic Books, Inc. Reprinted by permission of Basic Books, New York.

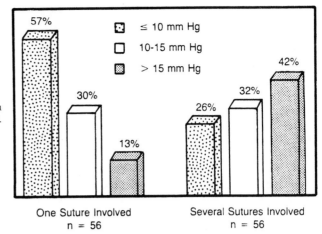

Figure 26–1. Craniosynostosis and intracranial pressure. (From Marchac D, Renier D: Craniofacial Surgery for Craniosynostosis. Boston: Little, Brown, 1982.)

computed tomographic (CT) scan include the loss of cisternae, but this is considered a soft finding. If intracranial hypertension goes untreated, it affects brain function. Fundoscopic examination of the eyes may reveal papilledema and, later, optic atrophy.

Intracranial hypertension can be documented invasively by means of a craniotomy used to place an epidural pressure sensor or by lumbar puncture monitoring. Increased intracranial pressure is most likely to affect patients with great disparity between brain growth and intracranial capacity and may occur in as many as 42% of untreated children in whom more than one suture is affected[47,48] (Fig. 26–1). Standard CT scans can be used to indirectly measure intracranial volume, but reliable mean and standard deviation values of age-matched cohorts are not available.[49,50] It is not yet possible to make objective judgments on the basis of CT scans alone as to who requires craniotomy for decompression. A specific head shape in conjunction with radiographic findings of synostosis is not definitive for increased intracranial pressure.

Vision

Craniosynostosis may lead to increased intracranial pressure. If this pressure is left untreated, papilledema and eventual optic atrophy develop, resulting in partial or complete blindness.

If the orbits are shallow (exorbitism) and the eyes proptotic (exophthalmus), as occurs in the craniofacial dysostosis syndromes, the cornea may be exposed and abrasions or ulcerations may occur. An eyeball extending outside of a shallow orbit is also at risk for trauma. If the orbits are extremely shallow, herniation of the globe itself may occur, necessitating emergency reduction followed by tarsorrhaphies or urgent orbital decompression.

Some forms of craniofacial dysostosis result in marked degrees of orbital hypertelorism, which may compromise visual acuity and restrict binocular vision. Divergent or convergent nonparalytic strabismus or exotrophia occurs frequently and should be looked for. This may be the result of congenital anomalies of the extraocular muscles themselves. Paralytic or nonparalytic unilateral or bilateral upper eyelid ptosis also occurs with greater frequency than would be expected by chance alone.

Hydrocephalus

Hydrocephalus affects as many as 10% of patients with a craniofacial dysostosis syndrome.[39–42] Although the etiology is not always clear, hydrocephalus may be secondary to a generalized cranial base stenosis with constriction of all cranial base foramina. It may be identified with the help of a CT scan or a magnetic resonance image (MRI) to document progressively enlarging ventricles. Confusion may arise in interpreting the ventricular findings as seen on a CT scan when the skull and cranial base are brachycephalic, because the ventricles will take on an abnormal shape. This finding by itself is not consistent with hydrocephalus; serial imaging and clinical correlation are required. A high index of suspicion should be maintained, with early diagnosis and prompt ventriculoperitoneal shunting when indicated. A great deal of clinical judgment is often required in order to make this assessment.

Breathing

All newborns are obligate nasal breathers. A percentage of infants born with a craniofacial dysostosis syndrome, including severe hypoplasia of the midface, have diminished nasal and nasopharyngeal spaces with increased nasal airway resistance.[16] An affected child is forced to breath through the mouth, and the mouth may simultaneously be filled with a normal-sized tongue confined within an abnormally small oropharyngeal space. A long and floppy soft palate may further complicate the situation. Sleep apnea of either central or peripheral origin may also be present. An affected infant expends greater energy respiring, which may result in a catabolic state (negative nitrogen balance) unless supportive treatment (i.e., tracheostomy and gastrostomy) is undertaken. If a peripheral origin is documented in the sleep laboratory, the tracheostomy may be indicated. Central apnea may result from poorly treated intracranial hypertension as well as from other causes. The condition may be improved by reducing elevated intracranial pressure through cranio-orbital decompression.

Nutrition

Newborns with limited nasal airflow experience difficulty with oral feeding. To ingest food through the mouth requires both sucking from a nipple to achieve negative pressure and an intact swallowing mechanism. Affected infants are unable to accomplish this complicated task while breathing through the mouth at the same time. Nutritional imbalance and failure to thrive results if the infants are untreated. The treatment is either nasogastric feeding or a temporary feeding gastrostomy. Evaluation by a skilled therapist can help distinguish minor feeding difficulties from those that necessitate more aggressive treatment.

Dentition and Occlusion

The incidence of dental and oral anomalies is higher among children with craniofacial dysostosis syndromes than among normal children. In Apert syndrome in particular, the palate is high and constricted in width. The incidence of isolated cleft palate in patients with Apert syndrome approaches 30%. Clefting of the secondary palate may be submucous, incomplete, or complete. Confusion has arisen over whether the malformations and absence of teeth that are often characteristic of these conditions are a result of congenital or iatrogenic factors (injury to dental follicles with early midface surgery). The midface hypoplasia seen in craniofacial dysostosis results in limited maxillary alveolar bone to house a full complement of teeth. There is severe crowding, and extractions are often required to alleviate it. An Angle class III skeletal pattern combined with an anterior open bite is typical.

Extremity Anomalies

Apert syndrome results in joint fusion and bony and soft tissue syndactylism of the digits of all four limbs.[6] Partial or complete fusion of the shoulder, elbow, or other joints is common. Broad thumbs, broad great toes, and partial soft tissue syndactyly of the hands may be seen in Pfeiffer syndrome, but these are variable features. Preaxial polysyndactyly of the feet may be seen in Carpenter syndrome.

Hearing

Hearing deficits are more common among patients with the craniofacial dysostosis syndromes than among the general population.[6] In Crouzon syndrome, conductive hearing deficit is common and atresia of the external auditory canals may also occur. Otitis media is common in Apert syndrome, although the exact incidence is unknown. Middle ear disease may be related to the presence of a cleft palate that results in eustachian tube dysfunction. Congenital fixation of the stapedial footplate is also believed to be a frequent finding. The possibility of significant hearing loss is paramount in importance and should not be overlooked because of preoccupation with other more easily appreciated craniofacial findings.

ESTHETIC ASSESSMENT

Examination of the entire craniofacial region should be meticulous and systematic. The skeleton and soft tissues are assessed in a standard way to identify all normal and abnormal anatomy. Specific features tend to occur in particular malformations, but each patient is unique. A quantitative analysis of measurements taken from CT scans,[20, 25, 51–56] surface anthropometry,[57–62] cephalometry,[34, 63] and dental models are valuable parts of the craniofacial assessment. The achievement of symmetry, proportionality, and balance and the reconstruction of specific esthetic units is critical to forming a normal face in a child born with one of the craniofacial dysostosis syndromes.

Fronto-Forehead Esthetic Unit

The fronto-forehead region is dysmorphic in an infant with craniofacial dysostosis. The establishment of the position of the forehead is crucial for overall facial balance. The forehead is divided into two separate components: the supraorbital ridge and the superior forehead. The supraorbital ridge includes the glabella region and supraorbital rim, extending lateral and inferiorly down the frontozygomatic sutures and posteriorly along the temporoparietal bones. The morphology and position of the supraorbital ridge component is key to upper face esthetics. In the normal forehead at the level of the frontonasal suture, an angle ranging from 90 to 110 degrees is formed by the supraorbital ridge and the nasal bones when viewed in profile. In addition, the eyebrows, overlying the supraorbital ridges, should be anterior to the cornea. When the supraorbital ridge is viewed from above, the rim should gently arc posteriorly to achieve a 90° angle at the temporal fossa with a center point of the arc at the level of each frontozygomatic suture. The superior forehead component (about 1.0–1.5 cm up from the supraorbital rim) has a gentle posterior curve of about 60° leveling out at the coronal suture region, when seen in profile.

Posterior Cranial Vault Esthetic Unit

Esthetics, form, and normal intracranial volume of the posterior cranial vault are closely linked. Posterior cranial vault flattening may result from a unilateral or bilateral lambdoidal synostosis, from previous craniectomy with reossification in a dysplastic flat shape, or from postural molding caused by frequent lying in the supine position early in infancy. A short anteroposterior cephalic length may be misinterpreted as a forehead problem when the occipitoparietal portion of the skull is at least partially to blame. Therefore, careful serial examination of the posterior cranial vault is necessary.

Orbitonasozygomatic Esthetic Unit

In the craniofacial dysostosis syndromes, the orbitonasozygomatic region is often dysmorphic and consistent with a short and wide anterior cranial base, as is seen with bilateral coronal suture synostosis extending into the base. For example, in Apert syndrome, the nasal bones, orbits, and zygomas are transversely wide and horizontally short (retruded), resulting in shallow hyperteloric orbits and bulging eyes.[25,56]

Maxillary-Midface Esthetic Unit

In the craniofacial dysostosis patient with midface deficiency, the upper anterior face is vertically short from the nasion to the maxillary central incisors, and there is a lack of horizontal projection of the midface. These findings may be confirmed through cephalometric analysis, which indicates an s-n-a angle that is below the mean value and a short upper anterior facial height. The width of the maxilla at the dentoalveolar region is generally constricted, with a high, arched palate. In order to normalize the maxillary-midface region, three-dimensional multidirectional expansion is generally required. The maxillary lip-to-tooth relationship and occlusion should be normalized.

QUANTITATIVE ASSESSMENT

The purpose of quantitative assessment by CT scan analysis, anthropometric measurements, cephalometric analysis, or dental model analysis is to help predict growth patterns, confirm or refute clinical impressions, aid in treatment planning, and provide a framework for objective assessment of immediate and long-term results.

These methods of assessment show the measurement, based on specific anatomic landmarks, of linear distances, angles, and proportions are are useful in evaluation of patients.

CT Scan Analysis

Accurate standardized points of reference have been defined in the cranio-orbito-zygomatic region on the basis of axial CT.[51,52] The normal range of specific measurement values and growth patterns for the cranial vault and the orbital and upper midface (zygomatic) regions have been tabulated. Knowledge of the differential facial bone growth patterns and normal measurement values can be used to improve diagnostic accuracy, assist in the staging of reconstruction, and offer the option of making intraoperative measurements that correlate and relate to the preoperative CT scan measurements.[20,25,53-56] The information may guide the reconstruction and allow for accurate postoperative reassessment.

Anthropometric Surface Measurements

Cross-sectional studies of the patterns of postnatal facial growth based on anthropometric surface measurements have been carried out in growing Caucasian children.[57] This previously published material has proved useful in the quantitative evaluation and the understanding of deviant postnatal development in the head and face of patients with specific craniofacial syndromes such as craniofacial dysostosis.[58-62] This is particularly useful for evaluating basic distance, angles, and proportions of the head, face, orbits, nose, lips, and ears.

Cephalometric Radiography

Cephalometric radiography, first introduced by Broadbent in 1931, has traditionally been used to study the morphology and patterns of growth in the maxillofacial skeleton and to develop standards for it. The substantial normative data that has been collected allow clinicans to monitor an individual patient's development. The interpretation of cephalometric films remains useful in the analysis of facial heights and of maxillary, mandibular, and chin positions and their relationships to each other, to the cranial base, and to the incisors. Cephalometry provides a view through the midsagittal plane if the face being analyzed is relatively symmetric. The number of anatomic landmarks that can be identified accurately in the cranio-orbitozygomatic region by cephalometry is limited because the overlap of structures makes locating these landmarks difficult.

Dental Model Analysis

The analysis of accurately articulated dental models is useful in the diagnostic assessment and the orthodontic and surgical planning for a child or adolescent with craniofacial dysostosis. The extrapolation of the data to the upper face deformity is limited because deficiencies between these esthetic units are frequently nonuniform.

SURGICAL APPROACH

Historical Perspective: The Pioneers

The first recorded surgical approach to craniosynostosis was performed by Lannelongue in 1890[64] and Lane in 1892,[65] who completed strip craniectomies. Their aim was to control the problem of brain compression (intracranial hypertension) within a small cranial vault.

The classical neurosurgical techniques developed over the ensuing decades were geared toward resecting the synostotic sutures in the hope that the "released" skull would reshape itself and continue to grow in a normal and symmetric manner.[17] The strip craniectomy was supposed to allow for a creation of a new suture line at the site of the previous synostosis. With the realization that this goal was rarely achieved, attempts were made to fragment the cranial vault surgically with pieces of flat bone used as free grafts to reshape the cranial vault. These techniques occasionally resulted in cerebral decompression, but they rarely produced an adequate shape. In addition, uncontrolled postoperative skull molding generally resulted in significant distortion. Furthermore, reossification after craniectomy was unpredictable; often there was rapid reossification, and at other times, significant cranial vault defects remained.

The thousands of combined soft tissue and hard tissue facial injuries that resulted from the trench warfare of World War I required urgent and secondary reconstructions. Two doctors in particular, Kazanjian[66] and Gillies,[67] were notable for their work in the treatment of craniomaxillofacial war injuries during this period. During and after World War I and again during World War II, these men laid the foundation for what is now known as craniomaxillofacial surgery. Their successful repair of war injuries brought hope to people with congenital facial anomalies.

Between the wars and after World War II, Gillies applied the knowledge that he had gained from treating wartime facial injuries to the previously untreated congenital facial deformities of the increasing numbers of patients seeking his help. In 1950, he reported an encouraging experience involving total midface (LeFort III) advancement for a patient with Crouzon syndrome.[68] His early enthusiasm later turned to discouragement when the patient's facial skeleton relapsed to its preoperative status.

In 1967, Tessier described a new approach to the management of Crouzon and Apert syndromes.[24] His landmark presentation and publications were the beginning of modern craniofacial surgery.[69-75] To overcome Gillies' earlier problems, Tessier developed a new basic surgical approach that included new locations for the LeFort III osteotomy, a combined intracranial-extracranial approach, the use of a coronal (skin) incision, and an autogenous bone graft. He also applied an external fixation device to help maintain bony stability until healing had occurred. The next year, Murray and Swanson from Boston Children's Hospital published their experience with Tessier's LeFort III midface advancement for Crouzon syndrome.[76]

Rougerie and associates applied this concept of simultaneous suture release and cranial vault reshaping to infants in 1972.[77] In 1976, Hoffman and Mohr advanced the concept of suture release and a degree of cranial vault and orbital reshaping for unilateral coronal synostosis in infancy.[78] They coined the term *lateral canthal advancement* to describe the procedure. In 1977, Whitaker and colleagues proposed a more formal cranial vault and orbital reshaping procedure for unilateral coronal synostosis.[79] In 1979, Marchac and Renier published their experience with the "floating forehead" technique for simultaneous suture release and cranial vault and orbital reshaping to manage bilateral coronal synostosis in infancy.[80] They hoped that the growing brain would further push the orbits and midface forward and allow for correction over time. Unfortunately, this does not occur predictably.[81]

During the same time period in which Tessier was introducing craniofacial surgery, Luhr, a young maxillofacial surgeon, learned of the benefit of internal fixation (bone plates and screws) for healing fractures of the extremities. In 1968, he proposed that miniature bone plates and screws could be constructed and used to provide stability and compression for mandibular fracture healing.[82] Despite his initial enthusiasm, these concepts of internal plate and screw fixation for the craniofacial skeleton were not put into practice.

Bone Grafting and Fixation Techniques

The widespread use of the autogenous cranial bone grafting has virtually eliminated rib and hip grafts when bone replacement or augmentation is required in cranio-orbitozygomatic procedures. This represents another of Tessier's contributions to craniofacial surgery.[71] Tessier's rationale for using autogenous cranial grafts included its easy access within the operative field, avoiding the need for a second surgical site, and a clinical impression that the grafts healed well with less need for secondary revision. A review of the experimental studies in which cranial bone grafts were used also clarifies the shift from hip and rib to cranial bone as a preferred donor site when grafting material was required.[83-94]

Peer showed that human membranous autogenous bone grafts placed in a subcutaneous pocket reabsorbed less over time than did endochondral grafts.[83] Zins and Whitaker,[84] working with both New Zealand rabbits and rhesus monkeys, placed membranous and endochondral autogenous onlay bone grafts in a subperiosteal pocket but without any form of fixation. They demonstrated less resorption of the membranous than of the endochrondral bone grafts. Kusiak and coworkers also demonstrated that membranous onlay grafts revascularized earlier and resorbed less over time.[85]

Phillips and Rahn studied onlay autogenous bone grafts in mature sheep from a slightly different perspective.[86] They examined the differences between membranous and endochondral onlay autogenous bone grafts and considered fixation techniques an additional variable. They concluded that the stable fixation of grafts (lag screw technique) result in less graft resorption. The nonfixed membranous graft resorbed less than did the nonfixed endochondral graft, but the difference in graft resorption patterns was much less when a stable form of fixation (lag screw technique) was used.

In summary, these experimental studies indicate that onlay bone graft resorption is less when grafts are stably fixed (plate and screw fixation), that membranous onlay bone grafts are likely to resorb less than endochondral grafts, and that bone graft resorption patterns may vary with the region grafted.[87,88] This experimental work, coupled with clinical studies, has resulted in the universal use of autogenous cranial bone grafts when either onlay or interpositional grafts are required in the cranial vault, orbits, and zygomas.[71,89-91] The use of internal mini- and microplate and screw fixation is also a preferred form of fixation when stability and complex three-dimensional reconstruction of multiple segments of bone are required.[91-94]

Incisions

For exposure of the craniofacial skeleton above the LeFort I level, the most frequently used approach is the coronal (skin) incision. This versatile incision allows for camouflaged access to the anterior and posterior portions of the cranial vault, the orbits, the nasal dorsum, the zygomas, the upper maxilla, the ptygeroid fossa, and the temporomandibular joints. For added cosmetic advantage, placement of the coronal incision posterior on the scalp and with postauricular rather than preauricular extension is useful.[95] When exposure at the maxillary LeFort I level is required, a circumvestibular maxillary (intraoral) incision is needed. Unless there are complications that necessitate unusual exposure, no other incisions are required for managing the patient with craniofacial dysostosis. The coronal (skin) incision may be reopened as many times as necessary to complete the patient's staged reconstruction.

Airway

Rarely is it necessary to perform a tracheostomy for perioperative airway management during the reconstruction for craniofacial dysostosis. In cranial vault and upper orbital procedures, orotracheal intubation is preferred. When total midface osteotomies (LeFort III, monobloc, and facial bipartition) are carried out, nasotracheal intubation can be used. If the nasotracheal route is used, the surgeon must exercise care not to sever the endotracheal tube during the septal osteotomy or, in small children, not to dislodge the tube from the larynx during maxillary disimpaction. The orotracheal route is not preferred because occlusal contact is required in order to obtain correct occlusion and jaw relationships. When the orotracheal route must be used, a modified occlusal splint may be used in conjunction to avoid tracheostomy when a total midface osteotomy is required.[96] The author often prefers another option: to begin the operation with an orotracheal tube and then, after completion of the midface osteotomy and disimpaction, convert to the nasotracheal route.

Management of Hydrocephalus

In a patient with craniofacial dysostosis, the decision for ventriculoperitoneal shunting for the management of hydrocephalus is a neursurgical one. The presence of an adequately functioning ventriculoperitoneal shunt, located in the posterior third of the cranial vault and passing through the subcutaneous tissues of the posterior portion of the neck, should not interfere with the decision-making process for or against craniotomy/decompression and reshaping. Shunt infection may result in these circumstances, but it is infrequent.

The infant or young child with craniofacial dysostosis who requires suture release, decompression, and reshaping and who is also believed to require ventriculoperitoneal shunting poses a difficult problem. Lack of precision in the technology of ventriculoperitoneal shunting may result in overshunting with the collapse of the ventricles and shrinkage of the intracranial contents. If an unstable shunt is placed just before cranial vault decompression and reshaping, any unsupported bone segments could collapse as the intracranial contents shrink. The avoidance of this scenario is preferred to the secondary management of the complication. When there are marginal indications for ventriculoperitoneal shunting, it is best to proceed with craniotomy, decompression, and reshaping first, followed by postoperative reassessment and shunting 3 to 6 months later if indications remain. The use of more stable forms of fixation (microplates and screws), rather than the "floating forehead" concept of Marchac, has also limited the importance of precise ventricular drainage as an issue when timing of reconstruction is being considered.

The Effect of Early Surgery on Growth

When considering the timing, extent, and preferred staging of reconstruction of a craniofacial malformation, a risk/benefit analysis is essential. For example, Renier and

Marchac showed that of children with isolated forms of craniosynostosis (i.e., lambdoid, sagittal, metopic, or coronal), only 14% present with significantly increased intracranial pressure (>15 mm Hg). The corollary is that 86% are not known to have pressure elevations necessitating decompression.[47,48] Furthermore, there is little documentation that the initial presenting morphologic deformity in isolated forms of craniosynostosis, if left untreated, worsens over time. By operating early (before 1 year of age), there may not be functional problems that necessitate resolution. Further distortions with ongoing growth may occur. Yaremchuk[97] and others[98,99] have shown that the surgical intervention itself may result in growth distortion, or unpredictable further growth within the operated bones. Our current strategies including the preferred timing of reconstruction may have to be rethought to achieve ideal long-term, three-dimensional morphologic results. The initial satisfactory cranio-orbital results achieved on the operating table in an infant are not always maintained, as growth distortions may occur over time.

In patients with craniofacial dysostosis syndromes, more than one cranial vault suture is generally closed prematurely, and a much higher percentage of children are at risk for significantly increased intracranial pressure. For this reason, craniotomy, decompression, and reconstruction are carried out at an early age (before 1 year) in most cases, even thought repeat procedures are likely to be required in order to maintain intracranial volume and to improve the morphology later.

Intracranial Approach to the Midface (see Fig. 26–2)

The presumed presence within the anterior cranial vault of an extradural (retrofrontal) dead space that communicates with the nasal cavity after an intracranial LeFort III, monobloc, or facial bipartition osteotomy with advancement is considered a major factor in postoperative morbidity.[100] This concern has heavily influenced the thinking of craniofacial surgeons and limited their perceived options for the reconstruction of the midface deformity in patients with craniofacial dysostosis syndromes.[101]

It is generally accepted as fact that the infants's brain is able to expand and fill the surgically created extradural dead space after an advancement procedure of the cranial vault, whereas such expansion is assumed not to occur in older children and young adults. The veracity of these assumptions has not been proved.[101]

As part of a total midface osteotomy with advancement, carried out through an intracranial approach (LeFort III, monobloc, or facial bipartition), nasocranial communication occurs in *all* patients. Application of sound surgical principles and then allowing this communication to seal itself by the process of nasal mucosa re-epithelialization enables this surgery to be performed successfully. The constricted brain rapidly expands to fill the extradural dead space created by the expanded anterior cranial fossa volume. The surgical principles include maintenance of separate oral and cranial surgical fields; prevention of bubbling of mucus and air into the intracranial cavity during ventilation; avoidance of operating through multiple surgical sites (i.e., tracheostomy and rib or hip graft donor sites); use of stable forms of fixation for all osteotomies and placed bone grafts (mini- and microplates and screws); the use of perioperative intravenous antibiotics for 10 days after surgery; elective maintenance of endotracheal intubation for 3 to 5 days after operation to prevent an air or fluid gradient from occurring across the upper nasal cavity and the anterior cranial vault; and prevention of suctioning through or blowing of the nose for 6 weeks after the operation.

CURRENT SURGICAL APPROACH: STAGING OF RECONSTRUCTION (see Figs. 26–1 to 26–11)

Primary Cranio-Orbital Decompression-Reshaping in Infancy

Once a craniofacial dysostosis syndrome is recognized, the child should undergo an assessment by the full craniofacial team. The planning of the timing and type of surgical intervention must account for the functions, future growth, and development of the craniofacial skeleton as well as the achievement of a satisfactory body image and self-esteem.

The term *brachycephaly* is derived from the Greek word for "short head." It results from bilateral, premature coronal suture fusion that extends into the cranial base. This is the most common cranial vault suture synostosis pattern associated with Apert, Crouzon, and Pfeiffer syndromes. In infancy and early childhood, it is not always possible to distinguish simple brachycephaly from Crouzon syndrome unless either midface hypoplasia is evident or a family pedigree with an autosomal dominant inheritance pattern is known. The midface deficiency associated with Crouzon syndrome is variable and, when present, is not always obvious until later in childhood.

In bilateral coronal synostosis, the supraorbital ridge is recessed and the overlying eyebrows sit posterior to the corneas of the eyes. The anterior cranial base is short in the anteroposterior dimension and wide transversely. The overlying cranial vault is high in the superoinferior dimension, with anterior bulging of the upper forehead that results from compensatory growth through the open metopic and sagittal sutures. The orbits are often shallow (exorbitism) and the eyes proptotic (exophthalmos) and abnormally widely separated (orbital hypertelorism). The sphenoid wings are elevated bilaterally, producing a harlequin appearance as seen on the anteroposterior plane radiographs or the CT scan.

In the craniofacial dysostosis syndromes, in addition to premature fusion of multiple cranial vault sutures, there is a poorly defined effect on the anterior cranial base and facial sutures that results in a variable degree of symmetric hypoplasia of the orbits, zygomas, and maxilla.

Initial treatment requires suture release and simultaneous cranial vault and upper orbital osteotomies with reshaping and advancement in infancy.[17,67,78,80,81,102–104] The preferred age at surgery is 10 to 12 months unless signs of increased intracranial pressure are present.[56,105] If they are present, decompression and reshaping are carried out earlier. The reshaping of the upper three fourths of the orbits and supraorbital ridge component is geared to decreasing bitemporal and anterior cranial base width (slightly) with simultaneous horizontal advancement to increase the anteroposterior dimension. The depth of the upper orbits is increased, resulting in some improvement of the exophthalmos. Once this is accomplished, the overlying forehead is reconstructed. The overall improved shape also provides a needed increase in intracranial volume within the anterior cranial vault. A degree of overcorrection is preferred to undercorrection at the level of the supraorbital ridge.

Repeat Craniotomy and Decompression-Reshaping in Young Children

Once the initial suture release, decompression, and reshaping are conducted during infancy, the young children are observed at intervals by the pediatric craniofacial surgeon, pediatric neurosurgeon, pediatric neuro-ophthalmologist, and neuroradiologist with interval CT scanning. If signs of increased intracranial pressure develop, urgent decompression with further reshaping to expand the intracranial volume is performed. When increased intracranial pressure is suspected, the location of cranial vault constriction influences the region of the skull earmarked for decompression and reshaping. Head shape and CT scan findings are helpful in determining the location requiring decompression.

If the problem is judged to be anterior, further anterior cranial vault and upper orbital osteotomies with reshaping and advancement are carried out. The technique is similar to that described earlier. Decompression and expansion of the posterior cranial vault may also be required; if so, they are completed with the patient in the prone position. The second craniotomy for decompression and reshaping is often complicated by brittle bone, previous fixation devices in the operative field (i.e., Silastic sheeting with metal clips, stainless steel wires, microplates, and screws), and compression (herniation) of the convoluted dura into the inner table of the skull, which results in more frequent dural tears during the dissection. An increased amount of blood loss is likely when the scalp flaps are elevated and at the time of craniotomy.

Management of the Total Midface Deformity in Childhood

The type of osteotomy selected to manage the total midface deficiency should depend on the presenting deformity rather than on a fixed universal approach to the management of the midface. In 1971, Tessier described a single-stage intracranial frontofacial advancement in which the orbitofrontal bandeau was advanced as a separate element but in conjunction with the LeFort III complex below and frontal bone above.[75] Seven years later, Ortiz-Monasterio and associates developed the monobloc osteotomy to advance the orbits and midface as one unit. The procedure was combined with frontal bone repositioning to correct the Crouzon deformity.[106, 107] In 1979, van der Meulen described the ''medial faciotomy'' for the correction of midline facial clefting.[108] By splitting the monobloc osteotomy vertically in the midline, he moved the two halves of the face together to correct orbital hypertelorism. To correct midface dysplasia and the associated orbital hypertelorism in patients with Apert syndrome, Tessier refined the vertical splitting and reshaping of the monobloc segment, thus improving the midface deformity in three dimensions through a procedure now known as facial bipartition.

The decision to complete a monobloc, facial bipartition, or LeFort III osteotomy to manage the horizontal, transverse, and vertical midface deficiency should depend on the patient's skeletal morphology.[19] If the supraorbital ridge with its overlying eyebrows sits in good position when viewed from the sagittal plane with adequate depth to the orbits, if there is a normal arc of rotation to the midface and forehead, and if the root of the nose is not wide with resulting orbital hypertelorism, then there is no need to reconstruct this region further. In such cases, the total midface deficiency may be effectively managed by a LeFort III osteotomy. If the supraorbital ridge and the anterior cranial base are both deficient in the sagittal plane along with the zygomas, nose, lower orbits, and maxilla, a monobloc osteotomy with differential (orbital and occlusal) anterior repositioning is indicated. Because the deficiencies noted at the orbit and at the occlusal plane are rarely uniform, segmentation of the structures at the LeFort I level enables more precise reconstruction. If orbital hypertelorism and midface flattening with loss of the normal facial curvature is obvious, the monobloc is split vertically in the midline (facial bipartition), a wedge of interorbital (nasal and ethmoidal) bone is removed, and the orbits are repositioned medially while the maxillary arch is widened. In Apert syndrome, facial bipartition osteotomy enables more complete correction of the abnormal craniofacial skeleton. A more normal arc of rotation to the midface complex is achieved with the midline split, which reduces the stigmata of the preoperative Apert ''flat face'' appearance. The medial and lateral orbital rims are shifted to the midline while the maxillary arch width is spread. Bipartition of the monobloc complex is less commonly required for the Crouzon and Pfeiffer midface deformity.

A common error may occur if the surgeon attempts to simultaneously adjust the orbits and idealize the occlusion by using the LeFort III, monobloc, or facial bipartition procedure without completing a separate LeFort I osteotomy. Rarely is it possible to normalize the orbits and occlusion without additional horizontal segmentalization of the total midface complex. If LeFort I segmentalization is not carried out and the surgeon attempts to achieve a positive overjet and overbite at the incisors, enophthalmos (sunken eyes) may occur. The degree depends on the degree of nonuniform skeletal deficiencies.

Problems unique to the LeFort III osteotomy when the indications are less than ideal include unesthetic step-offs in the lateral orbital rims that occurs when a moderate to extensive advancement is carried out. These step-offs are difficult, if not impossible, to modify later. With the LeFort III osteotomy, the ideal orbital depth is more difficult to judge, and either residual proptosis or enophthalmos is more likely to occur.[19] Simultaneous correction of orbital hypertelorism cannot be effectively managed with the LeFort III procedure. Excessive lengthening of the nose, accompanied by flattening of the nasofrontal angle, may also occur when the LeFort III osteotomy, rather than the monobloc or facial bipartition procedure, is selected.

Total midface deficiency is managed as early as age 5 to 7 years.[19] By this age, the cranial vault and orbits have attained approximately 85% to 90% of their adult size.[52] When the procedure is carried out after this age, the reconstructive result in the cranio-orbital region is permanent once healing has occurred. If surgery is performed at this age, additional orthognathic surgery will be necessary later in life to achieve ideal occlusion. Psychosocial considerations weigh heavily in selecting the time frame for the total midface advancement: surgery at 5 to 7 years of age allows the child to enter the first grade with an improved chance for satisfactory self-esteem.

In fact, some surgeons have advocated that the total midface osteotomy be carried out in infancy or very early in childhood (before the age of 2 years). Their hope is that early surgery would improve nasal breathing to avoid tracheostomy, improve long-term function (i.e., brain and eye development), and achieve midface projection in the operating room that would continue with ongoing growth. Unfortunately, these hoped-for benefits have not been documented. Furthermore, the early midface osteotomies (before 2 years of age) carried out have been accompanied by a high complication rate.[16]

Management of the Orthognathic Deformity in Adolescence

The mandible, which has normal growth in the craniofacial dysostosis syndromes, continues to develop throughout childhood and adolescence. The maxilla does not have this same growth potential, and as a result, a class III malocclusion with anterior open bite often results.[34] A LeFort I osteotomy (horizontal advancement, transverse widening, and vertical lengthening) is required in combination with a genioplasty (vertical reduction and horizontal advancement) to further correct the lower face deformity during the teen years. Bilateral sagittal split osteotomies of the mandible may also be required for management of minor discrepancies. The orthognathic surgery is carried out in conjunction with orthodontic intervention planned for completion at skeletal maturity (approximately age 14 to 16 years in females and 16 to 18 years in males). Stabilization is achieved both with miniplates and screws and with autogenous bone grafts.

CONCLUSION

Staged surgery performed at intervals to coincide with facial growth and viscera (brain, eyes, teeth, paranasal, and sinus) function is the current approach to the correction of the skeletal deformities seen in the craniofacial dysostosis syndromes. The recognition of this need for a staged approach serves to clarify the reconstructive goals of treatment. This allows the surgeon to take advantage of known differences in craniofacial growth patterns between normal and affected children and between the different bones within the craniofacial skeleton. By continuing to define the rationale for the timing of surgical intervention and then evaluating both function and morphologic results in an objective way, craniofacial teams will make further advances for patients affected by these disorders.

CASE REPORTS

Case 1 (Fig. 26–2)

A 12-year-old girl born with Pfeiffer syndrome underwent a facial bipartition osteotomy combined with cranial vault reshaping. The cranial vault length (85% of normal), medial orbital wall length (68% of normal), zygomatic arch length (83% of normal), and extent of globe protrusion (140% of normal) all indicated horizontal deficiency of the upper and middle face. In addition, the anterior interorbital distance (136% of normal), mid-interorbital distance (129% of normal), lateral orbital distance (121% of normal), and intertemporal distance (132% of normal) all indicated a degree of upper face hypertelorism. As a result of the facial bipartition osteotomy, improved horizontal facial depth was achieved and maintained. The upper face hypertelorism was improved but fell short of age-matched normal values.

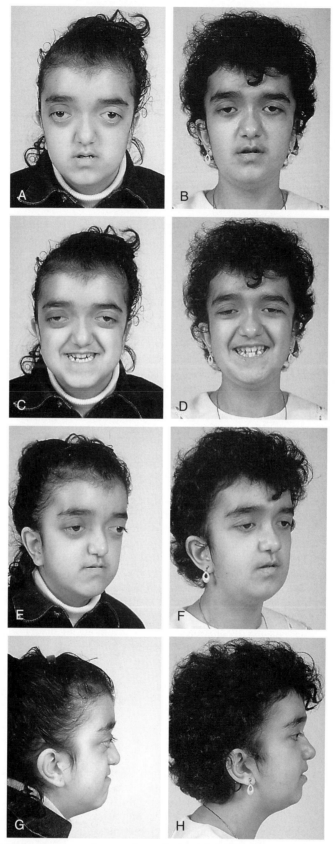

Figure 26–2. Twelve-year-old girl with Pfeiffer syndrome, who underwent facial bipartition. *A*, Preoperative frontal view in repose. *B*, Postoperative frontal view in repose. *C*, Preoperative frontal view with smile. *D*, Postoperative view with smile. *E*, Preoperative oblique view. *F*, Postoperative oblique view. *G*, Preoperative profile view. *H*, Postoperative profile view.

A step-by-step description of the monobloc and facial bipartition osteotomies is helpful for understanding the safe execution of the procedures. The detailed operative technique is illustrated as follows.

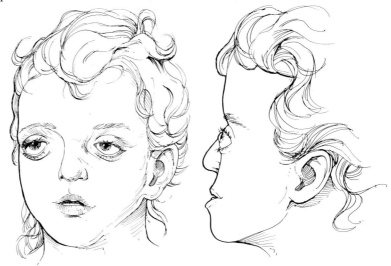

Illustrations of patient before
facial bipartition

1. Illustration of preoperative oblique and profile facial views.

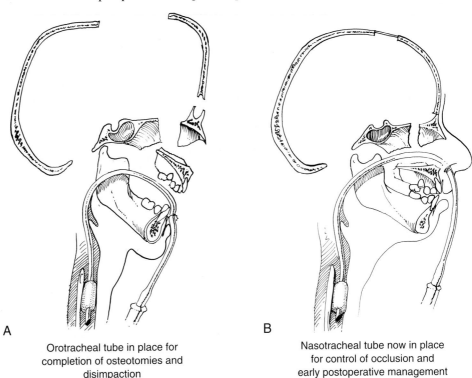

A

Orotracheal tube in place for
completion of osteotomies and
disimpaction

B

Nasotracheal tube now in place
for control of occlusion and
early postoperative management

2. Illustration of airway management in a patient undergoing total midface osteotomy.
   A. An orotracheal tube is secured adjacent to the incisal edge of the mandibular central incisors with a circummandibular wire.
   B. After the midface osteotomy and disimpaction are completed, a nasotracheal tube is placed and the orotracheal tube is removed. Through this controlled approach, endotracheal tube injury or dislodgment is prevented, direct occlusal contact between the maxillary and mandibular teeth can be achieved, and a nasotracheal tube is in place at the end of the surgical procedure to allow for increased patient comfort and nasal mucosal stenting during the initial postoperative phase.

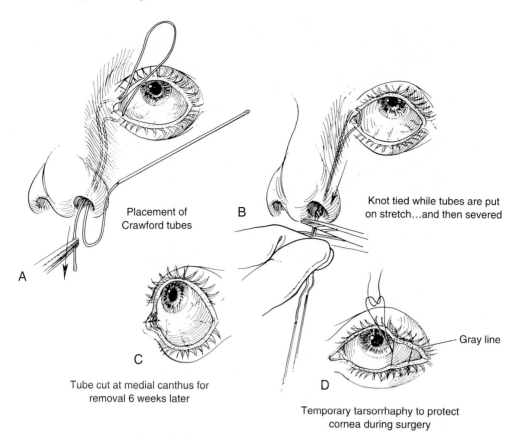

Placement of
Crawford tubes

Knot tied while tubes are put
on stretch...and then severed

Tube cut at medial canthus for
removal 6 weeks later

Gray line

Temporary tarsorrhaphy to protect
cornea during surgery

3. A,B,C. The insertion of Crawford nasolacrimal tubes: the puncta are dilated; a probe in inserted through each puncta to confirm entrance into the nose; the Crawford tube is inserted through each puncta and pulled through the nose; within the nose, the Silastic sheeting is stripped; and the tubing is tied in the nose, and the excess is cut (in the nose) with a scissors.

   D. Temporary tarsorrhaphies are placed with 6–0 nylon suture from gray line to gray line just lateral to the pupil of each eye.

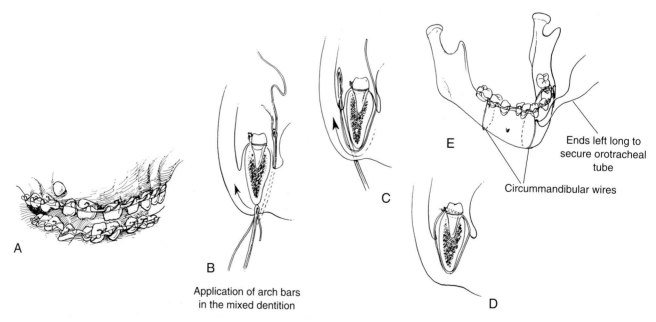

Ends left long to
secure orotracheal
tube

Circummandibular wires

Application of arch bars
in the mixed dentition

4. Application of surgical arch bars: a throat pack is placed; the mouth is cleaned; Erich arch bars are applied to the maxillary and mandibular teeth; circummandibular wires are placed to further stabilize the mandibular arch bar; and the orotracheal tube is secured to the symphyseal region with a circummandibular wire.

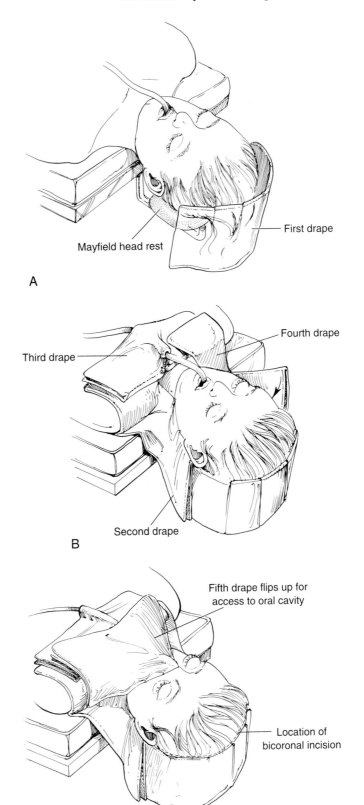

5. Patient preparation and drape: Exposure of the neck, face, and anterior scalp is essential.
   A. The patient's head is placed in a Mayfield head rest in the neutral neck position.
   B. Sterile towels are stapled in place for adequate exposure.
   C. Separation of the mouth-nose portion from the eyes-forehead portion by an additional sterile drape is useful.

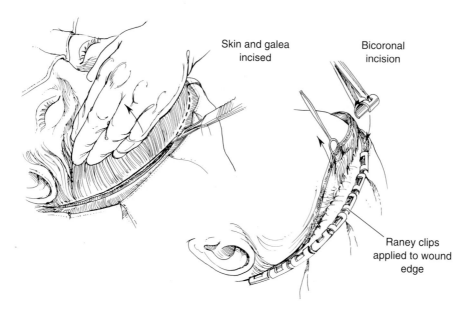

Skin and galea incised

Bicoronal incision

Raney clips applied to wound edge

6. Completion of the coronal incision: The incision is located postauricular and posterior in the scalp. Raney clips are applied for hemostasis.

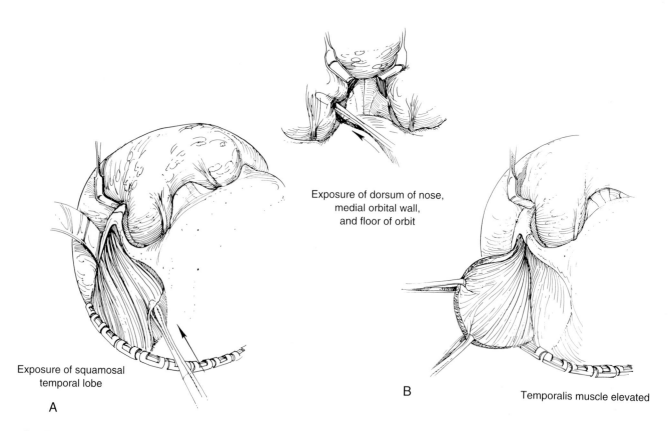

Exposure of dorsum of nose, medial orbital wall, and floor of orbit

Exposure of squamosal temporal lobe

A

B

Temporalis muscle elevated

7. The anterior scalp flap is elevated by remaining superficial to the superficial layer of the deep temporal fascia; subperiosteal over the midforehead region; subperiosteal down the lateral orbital rims; subperiosteal with exposure of the anterior maxilla; subperiosteal for exposure of the zygomatic arches; (A) subperiosteal exposure over the dorsum of the nose; and (B) with elevation of the temporalis muscle(s) off the squamosal bones.

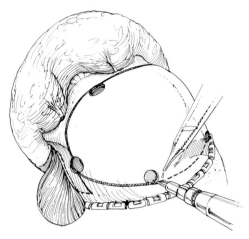

Bifrontal craniotomy completed

8. Bifrontal craniotomy: The craniotomy lines are drawn with a sterile pencil; bur holes are completed with a perforator; the craniotomies are completed with a craniotome; the frontal bones are separated from the underlying dura and then removed; and the frontal and temporal lobes of the brain are retracted and protected with Cottonoid strips.

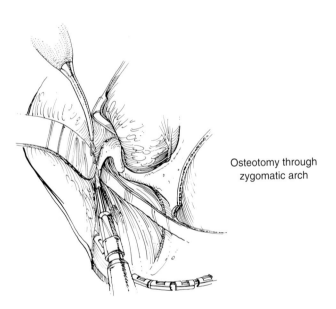

Osteotomy through zygomatic arch

9. Zygomatic arch osteotomies: Retractors are placed, and an osteotomy is completed through the midzygomatic arch on each side with a sagittal saw.

The orbital osteotomies are completed:

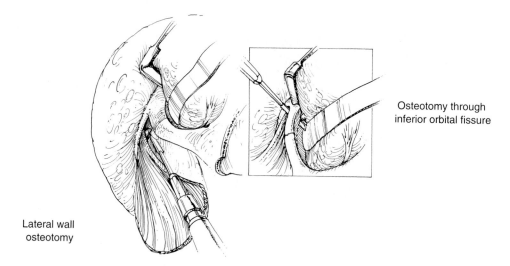

Osteotomy through
inferior orbital fissure

Lateral wall
osteotomy

10. With the use of a sagittal saw, the lateral orbital wall osteotomy is initiated through the inferior orbital fissure and then extended superiorly.

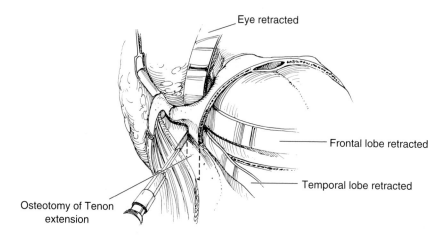

Eye retracted

Frontal lobe retracted

Temporal lobe retracted

Osteotomy of Tenon
extension

11. With continued use of the sagittal saw the lateral Tenon extension of the osteotomy is carried out.

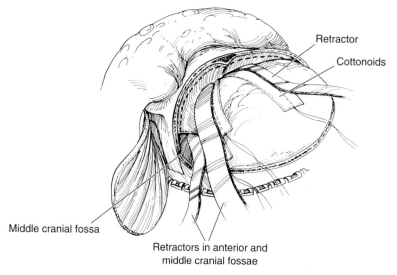

Retractor

Cottonoids

Middle cranial fossa

Retractors in anterior and
middle cranial fossae

12. The orbital roof osteotomy is completed with the sagittal saw through the anterior skull base.

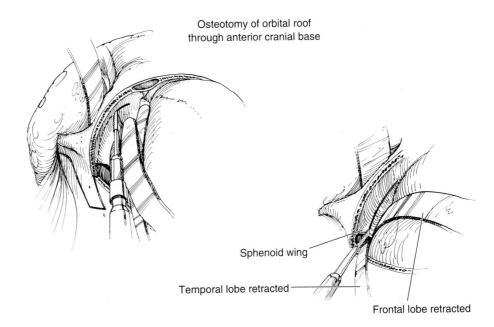

13. The orbital roof osteotomy continues laterally through the sphenoid wing.

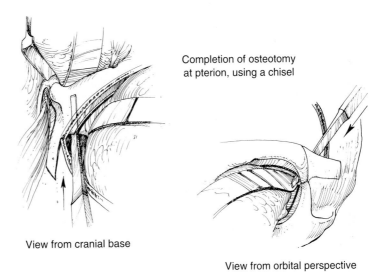

14. A thin chisel placed through the anterior skull base is used to confirm the sphenoid wing cuts.

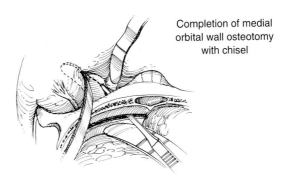

15. With the use of a thin chisel, the medial orbital wall osteotomy is completed posterior to the medial canthus and nasolacrimal apparatus and inferiorly into the inferior orbital fissure.

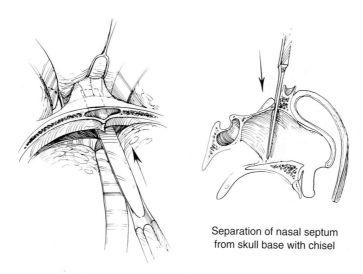

Separation of nasal septum
from skull base with chisel

16. Separation of the bony nasal septum from the anterior cranial base: A straight (15-mm) chisel placed through the cranial base just anterior to the crista galli is used to further separate the midface from the base of the skull.

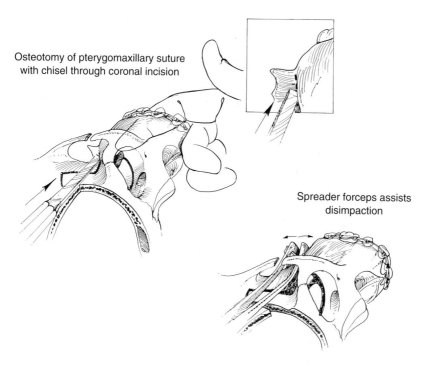

Osteotomy of pterygomaxillary suture
with chisel through coronal incision

Spreader forceps assists
disimpaction

17. Separation of the pterygomaxillary (P-M) sutures is completed: A long chisel is placed through the coronal incision and infratemporal fossa to the P-M suture; one hand (double-gloved) is placed in the patient's mouth, and the other hand is used to place the chisel through the coronal incision into the infratemporal fossa; a mallet is then used to separate the P-M suture with the chisel; the success of the separation is confirmed with the P-M spreader forceps.

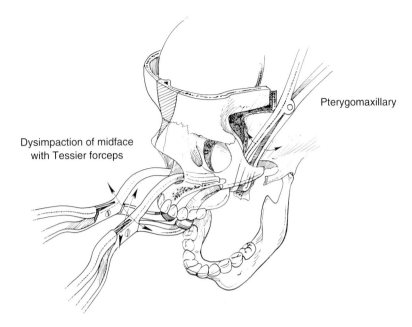

Pterygomaxillary

Dysimpaction of midface
with Tessier forceps

18. The midface is dysimpacted: With the use of nasomaxillary forceps placed in the nose and the mouth and P-M spreader forceps placed through the coronal incision, the midface is dysimpacted.

Note: At this stage, the endotracheal airway exchange is completed. Additional sterile drapes are placed over the scalp and face-neck regions; the throat pack is removed; the surgeon places the nasotracheal tube through the nose and into the oral pharynx; and the anesthesiologist removes the orotracheal tube and completes the insertion of the nasotracheal tube through the larynx.

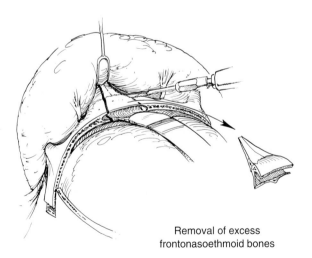

Removal of excess
frontonasoethmoid bones

19. For facial bipartition, a midnasal ostectomy is completed: Working through the coronal incision, the surgeon marks out the proposed midnasal ostectomy with caliper and pencil and then completes it with a sagittal saw with removal of portions of cartilaginous nasal septum.

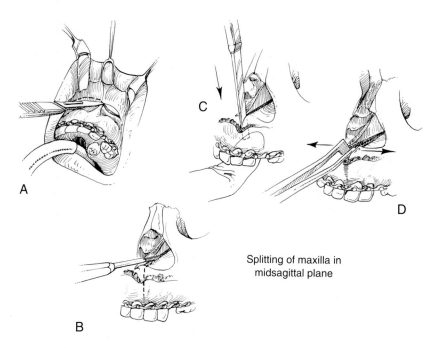

Splitting of maxilla in
midsagittal plane

20. For facial bipartition, sagittal splitting of the maxilla is completed: An anterior
    maxillary vestibular incision is made; subperiosteal exposure of the anterior nasal
    spine and nasal floor is completed; with a sagittal saw, a midline osteotomy is
    completed between the central incisors and down the palate; the final separation is
    completed with a thin, straight chisel; further release and separation at the osteot-
    omy site is completed with a P-M spreader forceps; and the oral wound is closed.

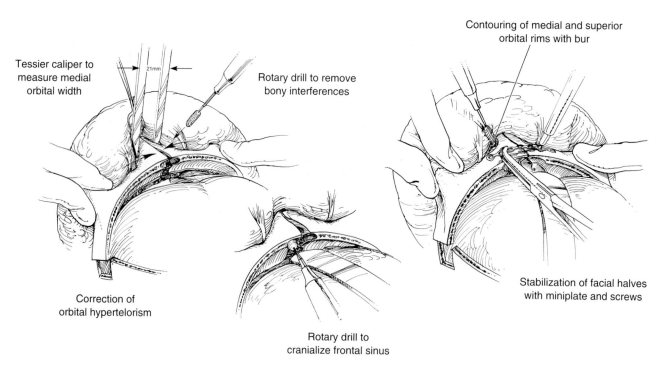

Tessier caliper to
measure medial
orbital width

Rotary drill to remove
bony interferences

Contouring of medial and superior
orbital rims with bur

Correction of
orbital hypertelorism

Rotary drill to
cranialize frontal sinus

Stabilization of facial halves
with miniplate and screws

21–22. For facial bipartition: Stabilization of the upper orbits and nasal bones is
       completed; repositioning of the facial halves medially with adjustment of the
       midface arc of rotation is completed (this will require refinement with a rotary
       drill); and the upper orbits and nasal bones are fixed with mini- and microplates
       and screws. A rotary drill is used to cranialize the frontal sinus.

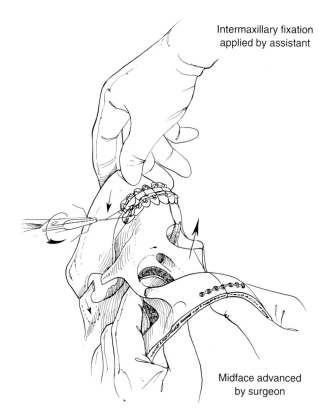

Intermaxillary fixation
applied by assistant

Midface advanced
by surgeon

23. Establishing midface advancement at the maxillary teeth: Working through the coronal incision, one surgeon advances the midface, and two assistants wire the jaws together through the mouth.

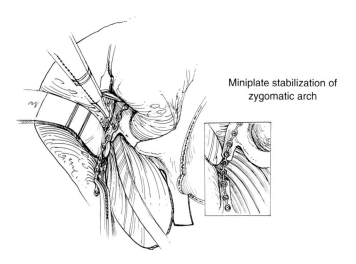

Miniplate stabilization of
zygomatic arch

24. The midface advancement is established at the zygomatic arches: The desired amount of advancement at each zygomatic arch is measured with a caliper, and a miniplate is conformed to extend from the anterior maxilla across the arch to the posterior zygoma on each side.

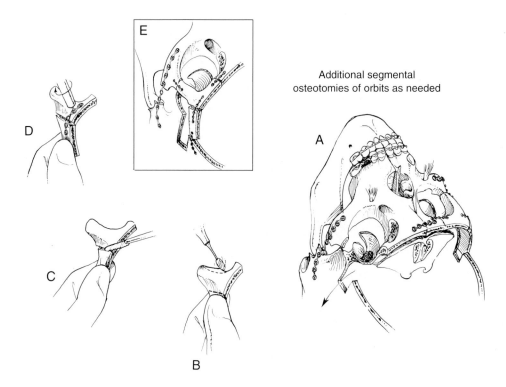

Additional segmental
osteotomies of orbits as needed

25. Additional segmental osteotomies of orbits: Occasionally, the lateral superior orbits have further dysplasia and require segmental osteotomies with reshaping or reconstruction. The locations for the segmental orbital osteotomies are marked out and completed with a reciprocating saw, and the lateral orbital rim–superior orbital rim segments are reshaped with a rotary drill, reinserted, and fixed with mini- and microplates and screws.

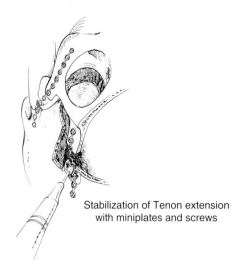

Stabilization of Tenon extension
with miniplates and screws

26. Stabilizing midface advancement at upper orbital (Tenon) extension: The desired advancement is measured with a caliper; a miniplate is adapted to bridge across gap; and screws are used for stabilization.

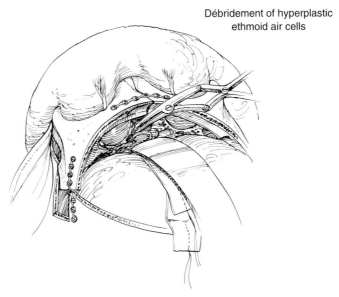

Débridement of hyperplastic
ethmoid air cells

Opening between nasal cavity and
anterior cranial fossa is evident

27. Débridement of hyperplastic ethmoid air cells: Double-action rongeurs, with visualization through anterior cranial base, are used for débridement of ethmoid air
cells for correction of midorbital hypertelorism.

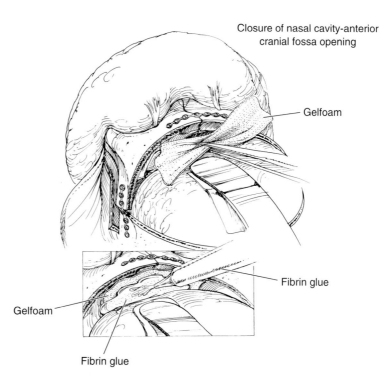

Closure of nasal cavity-anterior
cranial fossa opening

Gelfoam

Fibrin glue

Gelfoam

Fibrin glue

28. Separating opening from anterior cranial fossa into nasal cavity: The surgeon
irrigates and suctions the intranasal cavity through anterior cranial base exposure,
applies a sheet of Gelfoam to separate the opening between the two cavities, and
applies Tissel (fibrin glue) over the Gelfoam to seal the separation.

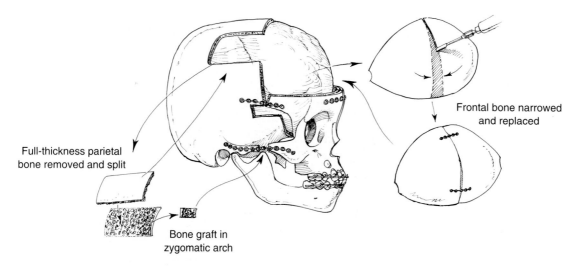

Full-thickness parietal
bone removed and split

Frontal bone narrowed
and replaced

Bone graft in
zygomatic arch

29. Reshaping, advancing, and fixing forehead bones: The desired shape of the forehead is achieved as needed, with the use of a reciprocating saw and a rotary drill; split- or full-thickness cranial bone graft is harvested; the forehead segments are fixed to the upper orbital rims with micro- and miniplates and screws; and the split-thickness cranial bone graft is placed in the midzygomatic arch segmental defects.

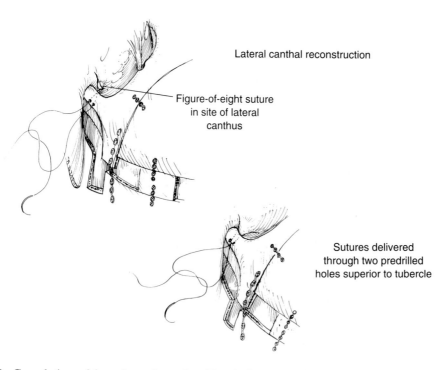

Lateral canthal reconstruction

Figure-of-eight suture
in site of lateral
canthus

Sutures delivered
through two predrilled
holes superior to tubercle

30. Completion of lateral canthopexies: Two holes are drilled at each (new) frontozygomatic suture region; the lateral canthi are identified with a skin hook through the coronal incisions; a figure-of-eight wire suture is placed through the lateral canthi (through coronal incision); and each lateral canthus is fixed through drill holes.

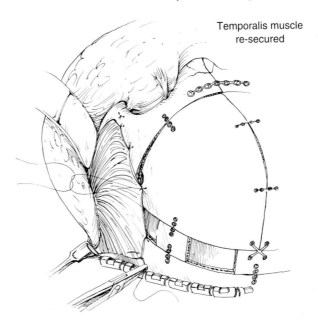

31. Securing the temporalis muscles: The temporalis muscles are repositioned anteriorly; the muscle flaps are secured to the lateral orbital rims and temporal bones.

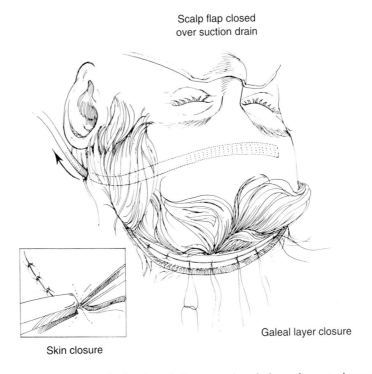

32. Closing the scalp wound: Suction drains are placed through posterior scalp flap (one on each side) with one drain tip anterior and the other posterior; the galea closure is completed with interrupted sutures; and skin layer closure is completed with staples.

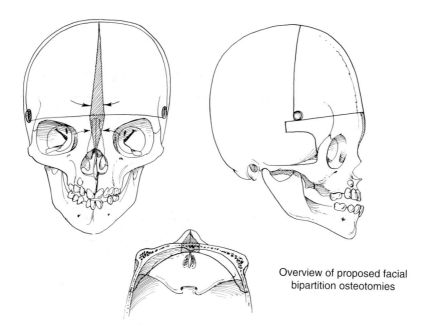

Overview of proposed facial
bipartition osteotomies

33. Overview of skeletal morphology prior to osteotomies. Location of proposed osteotomies indicated.

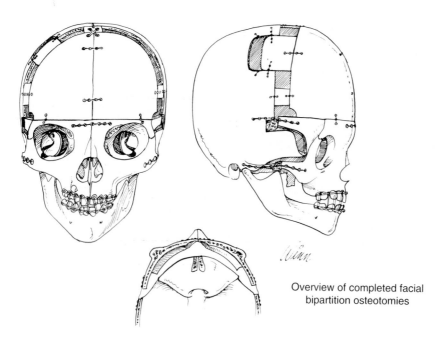

Overview of completed facial
bipartition osteotomies

34. Overview of skeletal morphology after facial bipartition osteotomies with repositioning and stabilization.

Overview of completed
facial bipartition osteotomies

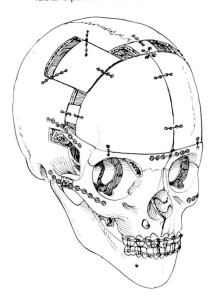

35. Oblique view of skeletal morphology after completion of osteotomies with placement of mini- and microplate and screw fixation and cranial bone grafts.

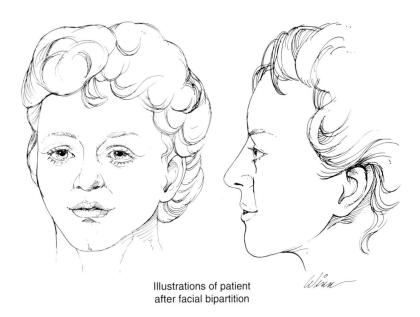

Illustrations of patient
after facial bipartition

36. Postoperative oblique and lateral views after facial bipartition osteotomies with anterior cranial vault reshaping.

Case 2 (Fig. 26–3)

Diagnosis: Crouzon syndrome (bilateral coronal synostosis)
Procedures: 1. Anterior cranial vault and three-quarter orbital osteotomies with reshaping and advancement.
            2. Posterior cranial vault reshaping.

A patient who had abnormal craniofacial morphology at birth also had a family history positive for Crouzon syndrome: the father had a degree of midface hypoplasia, shallow orbits, and bulging eyes; one sibling had a congenital midline dermoid cyst over the sagittal suture; another sibling had bicoronal suture synostosis and midface hypoplasia. Examination of the patient revealed symmetric bony recession at the level of the supraorbital ridges with resulting shallow orbits and bulging eyes. The forehead was wide, and there was compensatory bulging superiorly. Bony ridges were palpable over the coronal suture regions. Midface hypoplasia was minimal.

CT scans of the craniofacial skeleton were obtained in both axial and coronal planes. The anterior cranial base was short and wide as a result of bilateral coronal synostosis, which was indicative of brachycephaly. The orbits were shallow with globes protruded and without evidence of orbital hypertelorism. Review of the midface suggested the presence of mild hypoplasia.

The patient underwent anterior cranial vault and three-quarter orbital osteotomies with reshaping and advancement through an intracranial approach. The postoperative recovery was rapid and without complications.

Three years later, the occipitoparietal region demonstrated severe flattening. The posterior cranial vault was reshaped through an intracranial approach. This not only improved the shape of the back of the head but also provided increased intracranial volume for brain expansion. Further staged reconstruction may necessitate orbital and midface osteotomies, but midface deficiency is not a prominent part of the deformity.

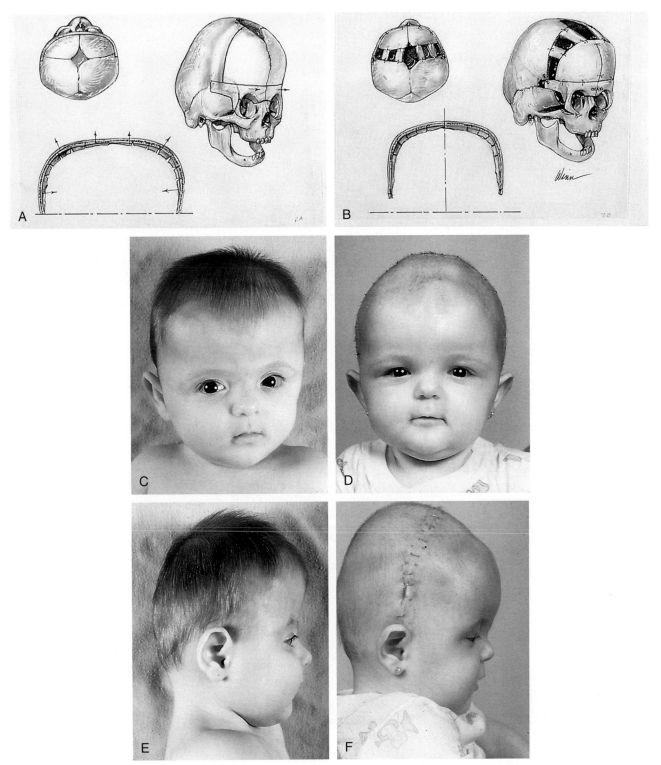

Figure 26–3. A 10-month-old girl with unrepaired bilateral coronal synostosis as part of Crouzon syndrome. *A,* Craniofacial morphology resulting from bicoronal synostosis; proposed osteotomies outlined. *B,* Craniofacial morphology after cranial vault and three-quarter orbital osteotomies with reshaping, advancement, and fixation. *C,* Preoperative frontal view. *D,* Frontal view 10 days after reconstruction. *E,* Preoperative profile view. *F,* Profile view 10 days after reconstruction.

Illustration continued on following page

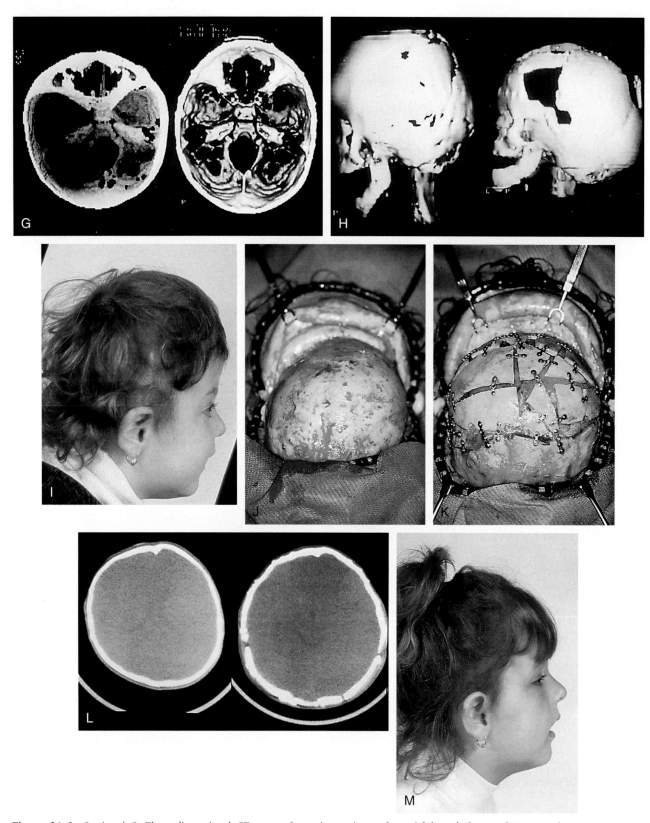

Figure 26–3. *Continued G,* Three-dimensional CT scan reformations; views of cranial base before and 1 year after reconstruction demonstrate improvement in brachycephalic shape. *H,* Three-dimensional CT scan reformations before and immediately after reconstruction, demonstrating upper orbital and forehead advancement. *I,* Lateral view at 3 years of age with flattening of the posterior cranial vault. *J,* Intraoperative view of posterior cranial vault prior to reshaping. *K,* After posterior cranial vault reshaping and stabilization with miniplates and screws. *L,* CT scan view before posterior vault reshaping (left) and early after reshaping (right). *M,* Lateral facial view 1 year after posterior cranial vault reshaping. (Parts *C* to *F* from Posnick JC: Craniofacial dysostosis: Management of the midface deformity. *In* Bell WH [ed]: Modern Practice in Orthognathic and Reconstructive Surgery, vol 3, p 1873. Philadelphia: WB Saunders, 1992.)

Case 3 (Fig. 26–4)

Diagnosis: Apert syndrome (bilateral coronal synostosis)
Procedure: Anterior cranial vault and three-quarter osteotomies with reshaping and advancement

Abnormal craniofacial morphology and four-limb complex syndactylies were noted in a female newborn. The obstetrician and pediatrician obtained a craniofacial consultation for her evaluation and treatment.

Examination revealed ridging over both coronal sutures, a short and wide anterior cranial base, shallow orbits, bulging eyes, and orbital hypertelorism in combination with midface hypoplasia. There was a large soft spot over the region where the metopic and anterior sagittal sutures are normally expected.

CT scans of the craniofacial skeleton were obtained in both axial and coronal planes. The anterior cranial base was short in the anteroposterior dimension and extremely wide transversely. Ridging evident over the left and right coronal sutures confirmed synostosis, and a bony defect was noted over the metopic and sagittal suture regions. The ventricles were of normal size, and the midface was hypoplastic. The patient appeared to have premature closure of the left and right coronal sutures with additional orbital and midface findings that were consistent with Apert syndrome.

Anterior cranial vault and three-quarter orbital osteotomies with reshaping and advancement were carried out through an intracranial approach. Postoperative recovery was uneventful. The need for further staged reconstruction of the cranial vault and total midface is anticipated.

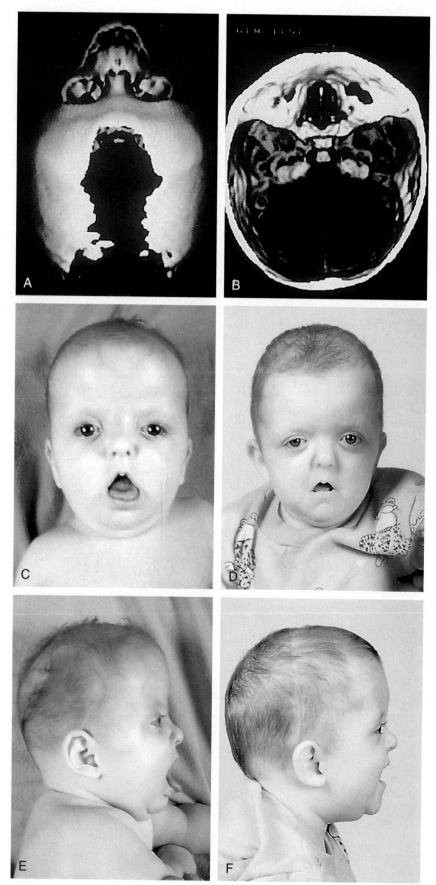

Figure 26–4. A 10-month-old with unrepaired bicoronal synostosis as part of Apert syndrome. *A,B* Three-dimensional CT scan reformations; bird's-eye view (*A*) and cranial base view (*B*) before surgery. *C,* Preoperative frontal view. *D,* Frontal view soon after cranio-orbital reconstruction. *E,* Preoperative profile view. *F,* Profile view early after reconstruction.

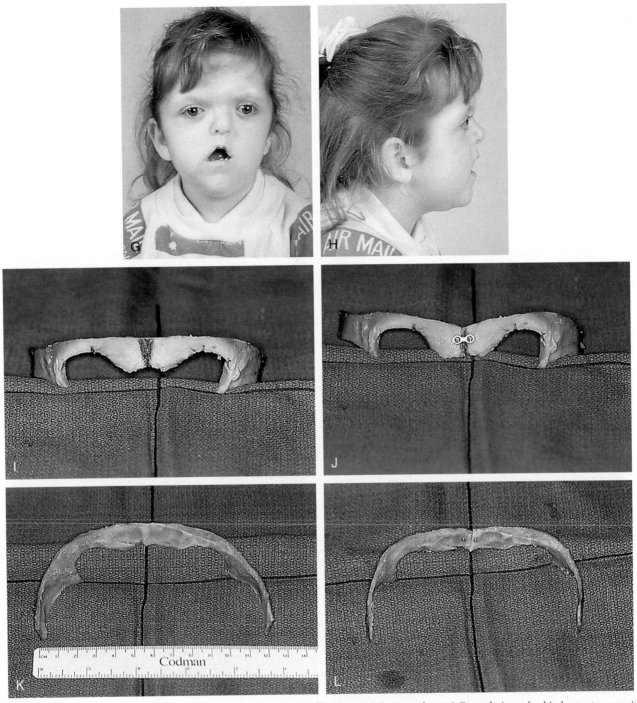

Figure 26–4. *Continued G,* Frontal view at 2.5 years of age. *H,* Profile view at 2.5 years of age. *I,* Frontal view of orbital osteotomy unit before reshaping. *J,* Same view after reshaping; stabilization with titanium miniplates and screws. *K,* Bird's-eye view of orbital osteotomy unit before reshaping. *L,* Same view after reshaping. (Parts *C* to *L* from Posnick JC: Craniofacial dysostosis: Management of the midface deformity. *In* Bell WH [ed]: Modern Practice in Orthognathic and Reconstructive Surgery, vol 3, pp 1876–1877. Philadelphia: WB Saunders, 1992.)

Case 4 (Fig. 26–5)

Diagnosis: Crouzon syndrome (bilateral coronal synostosis)
Previous Surgeries: 1. Bilateral "lateral canthal advancements"
2. Ventriculoperitoneal shunt placement
Procedure: Repeat cranial vault and three-quarter orbital osteotomies with reshaping and advancement

Shortly after birth, an infant was noted to have palpable ridges over both coronal suture regions. Plane skull radiographs documented bicoronal synostosis. She initially underwent bilateral "lateral canthal advancements" as described by Hoffman in 1976.[78] At 18 months of age, the child was found to have an extremely short anteroposterior dimension to the cranial vault with shallow orbits and bulging eyes. The bitemporal width was enlarged.

A ventriculoperitoneal shunt had been positioned in the left ventricle for management of hydrocephalus. The anterior cranial base was short and extremely wide. The cephalic height was increased, resulting in an tower shape to the cranial vault.

Overall, the patient appeared to have oxycephaly resulting from refusion of both coronal sutures with an overall diminished anteroposterior skull dimension and increased bitemporal width.

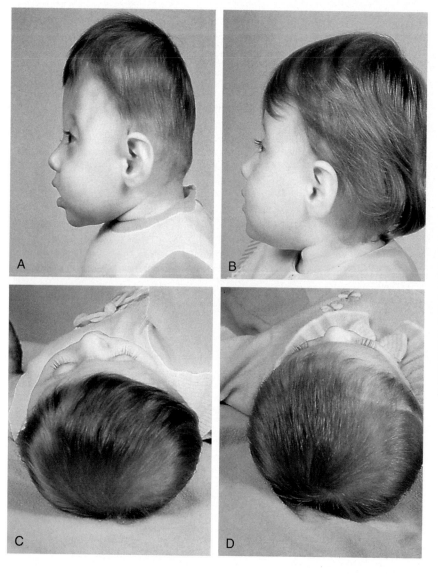

Figure 26–5. A 2.5-year-old female with Crouzon syndrome. She had previously undergone bilateral "lateral canthal advancement" for coronal suture release and reshaping. *A*, Preoperative profile view before repeat craniotomy, upper orbital osteotomies, and cranial vault reshaping. *B*, Profile view after repeat cranio-orbital reconstruction. *C*, Preoperative bird's-eye view before repeat craniotomy. *D*, Bird's-eye view after repeat cranio-orbital reconstruction. (From Posnick JC: Craniofacial dysostosis: Management of the midface deformity. *In* Bell WH [ed]: Modern Practice in Orthognathic and Reconstructive Surgery, vol 3, p 1882. Philadelphia: WB Saunders, 1992.)

Repeat craniotomy was carried out, with total cranial vault and three-quarter orbital osteotomies and reshaping to narrow the bitemporal width, lengthen the cranial vault dimension, and increase the orbital depth through an intracranial approach. The postoperative recovery and follow-up was uneventful. Additional staged reconstruction is required in order to gain adequate projection to the midface.

Case 5 (Fig. 26–6)

Diagnosis: Crouzon syndrome (bilateral coronal synostosis)
Previous Surgeries: 1. Bilateral ''lateral canthal advancements''
       2. Ventriculoperitoneal shunt placement
Procedure: Anterior cranial vault and monobloc osteotomies with reshaping and advancement

An 8-year-old boy who was born with Crouzon syndrome underwent bilateral ''lateral canthal advancements'' at 6 months of age. The family history was positive: the father had severe oxycephaly, proptosis, and midface deficiency. Later the boy required placement of a ventriculoperitoneal shunt for management of hydrocephalus. He was unavailable for follow-up observation for a number of years; when he returned, he had a history of recent onset of severe headaches and bed-wetting, he was 1 year behind in school, and he had been subjected to teasing by his peers because of his bulging eyes and flat face.

Physical examination revealed a flat and wide forehead. The supraorbital ridges as well as the infraorbital rims were recessed, resulting in shallow orbits and bulging eyes (proptosis). The total midface was flat with an Angle class III malocclusion. His teeth were noticeably crowded on the maxillary arch and moderately crowded on the mandibular arch. Psychological testing showed a degree of developmental delay. His self-esteem scores were very low, and he was noted to have a generally inhibited nature with a tendency to cling to his mother. Fundoscopic examination revealed mild optic atrophy, strabismus, and amblyopia.

CT scans were obtained in both axial and coronal planes. The ventricles were mildly enlarged, and a ventriculoperitoneal shunt was in place. A fingerprinting appearance was seen along the inner table of the skull and the anterior cranial base, resulting from long-standing increased intracranial pressure. The orbits were shallow and the zygomas retruded. Cephalometric analysis showed an S-N-A angle greater than two standard deviations below the norm, confirming maxillary retrognathism. The S-N-B angle was within the normal range.

Anterior cranial vault and monobloc osteotomies with reshaping and advancement were carried out through an intracranial approach. The airway was managed with endotracheal intubation. Bone grafts were from the cranium, and stabilization of the osteotomies and grafts was with titanium miniplates and screws.

The patient's recovery was uneventful, and he resumed all age-appropriate activities. A LeFort I osteotomy and a genioplasty in combination with orthodontic treatment will be required at the time of skeletal maturation as part of the staged reconstruction.

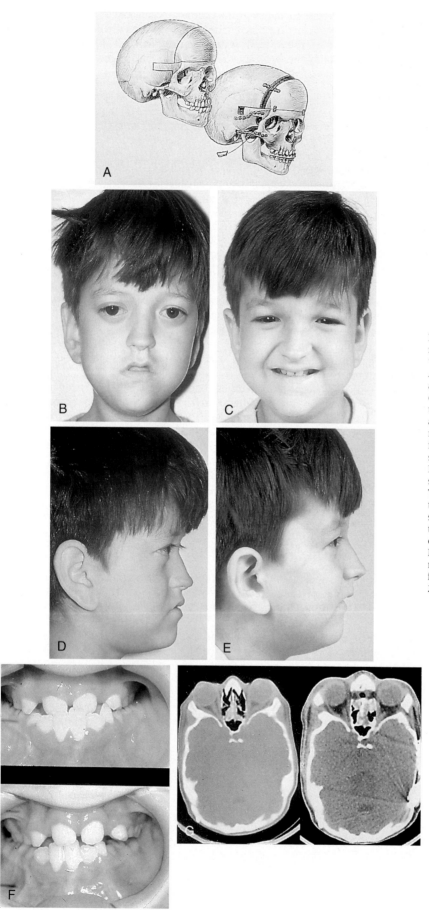

Figure 26–6. An 8-year-old boy with Crouzon syndrome who had undergone bilateral "lateral canthal advancements" in infancy. *A,* Craniofacial morphology before and after anterior cranial vault and monobloc osteotomies with advancement. Osteotomy locations are indicated. Stabilization was achieved with cranial bone grafts and titanium miniplates and screws. *B,* Preoperative frontal view. *C,* Frontal view after reconstruction. *D,* Preoperative profile view. *E,* Profile view after reconstruction. *F,* Occlusion before and after reconstruction. *G,* Two-dimensional axial CT scans; views through the orbits before and after reconstruction indicate resulting increased intraorbital depth and achievement of decreased proptosis. (From Posnick JC, Nakano P: Craniofacial dysostosis: Staging of reconstruction and management of the midface deformity. Neurosurg Clin North Am 2[3]:683–702, 1991.)

Case 6 (Fig. 26–7)

Diagnosis: Crouzon syndrome (bilateral coronal synostosis)
Previous Surgery: Ventriculoperitoneal shunt placement
Procedure: Total cranial vault and monobloc osteotomies with reshaping and advancement (late primary reconstruction)

A 12-year-old boy from Nicaragua presented with unrepaired Crouzon syndrome. He had previously undergone placement of two ventriculoperitoneal shunts. He required eyeglasses for strabismus and astigmatism. He was severely ostracized in his rural village because of his facial appearance.

Physical examination revealed an oxycephalic skull. The anterior cranial base was short and wide (brachycephaly). The forehead sloped posteriorly, reaching a point at the junction of the metopic and sagittal suture regions. The orbits were shallow and the eyes proptotic. The total midface was deficient in the horizontal plane. There was mild Angle class III malocclusion with dental compensation built into the bite. The mandible was somewhat retrognathic, which masked the midface deficiency, and the chin was vertically long and retrognathic. Fundoscopic examination revealed mild optic atrophy and corneal abrasions from keratitis that resulted from chronic exposure. Psychological testing suggested an average intelligence level.

CT scan examination confirmed the oxycephalic appearance of the cranial vault and a fingerprinting appearance along the inner table of the skull and the cranial base. The ventricles were of normal size. The orbits were shallow, and the midface was deficient.

The patient's findings were consistent with Crouzon syndrome, with bicoronal synostosis and horizontal midface deficiency that was greater at the supraorbital and infraorbital ridges than at the occlusal level.

Total cranial vault and monobloc osteotomies with reshaping and advancement were carried out through an intracranial approach. Stabilization was with autogenous cranial bone graft, while fixation was with miniplates and screws. The airway was managed through endotracheal intubation.

The patient was discharged from hospital on the 10th postoperative day. After an additional 6-week stay in the author's community, he returned to his home town in Nicaragua. He continues to do well 8 years later.

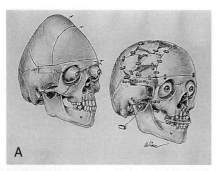

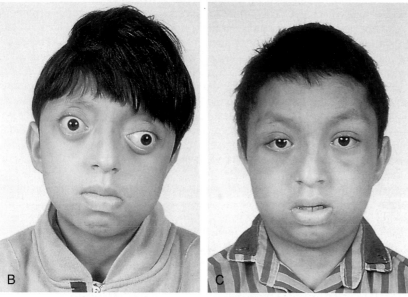

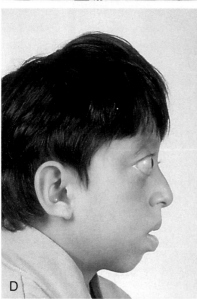

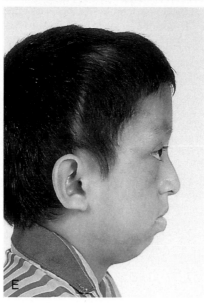

Figure 26–7. A 12-year-old boy with unrepaired Crouzon syndrome who had undergone total cranial vault and monobloc osteotomies with reshaping and advancement. *A*, Illustrations of the patient's craniofacial morphology before surgery: osteotomy locations are indicated, and a second illustration after osteotomies were completed with reshaping and advancement. *B*, Preoperative frontal view. *C*, Postoperative frontal view. *D*, Preoperative lateral view. *E*, Postoperative lateral view.

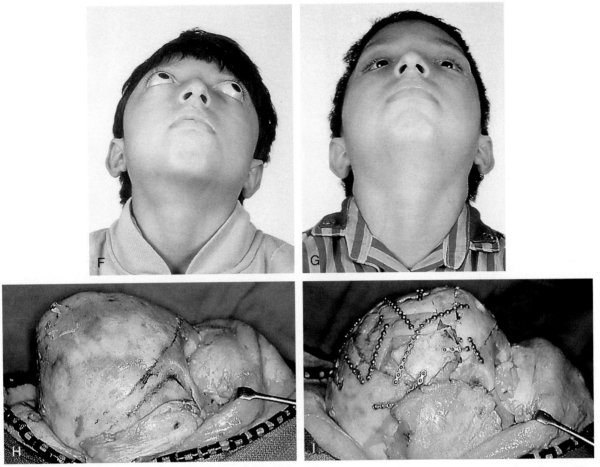

Figure 26–7. *Continued F,* Preoperative worm's-eye view. *G,* Postoperative worm's-eye view. *H,* Intraoperative lateral view of cranial vault and orbits through coronal incision before osteotomies. *I,* Same view after osteotomies, reshaping, cranial bone grafting, and titanium bone plate and screw fixation. (From Posnick JC, Nakano P: Craniofacial dysostosis: Staging of reconstruction and management of the midface deformity. Neurosurg Clin North Am 2[3]:689–692, 1991.)

Case 7 (Fig. 26–8)

Diagnosis: Apert syndrome (bilateral coronal synostosis)
Previous Surgeries: 1. Suture release and forehead reshaping at 6 months
                       2. Staged syndactyly reconstruction
Procedure: Total cranial vault and facial bipartition osteotomies with reshaping and advancement

A 5-year-old girl born with Apert syndrome had undergone suture release and forehead reshaping at 6 months of age. She was in the process of staged reconstruction of her four-limb syndactyly. She had strabismus and amblyopia, for which she wore eyeglasses and was undergoing eye patching.

She presented with a retruded and wide anterior cranial base (residual brachycephaly). The forehead was flat at the supraorbital ridge level with bitemporal constrictions and bulged superiorly. The orbits were shallow with bulging eyes and orbital hypertelorism. The midface was flat and lacked a normal convexity when viewed from above. The total midface was deficient, with a marked anterior open bite and full Angle class III malocclusion. Nasal airflow was poor, and the patient habitually breathed through her mouth.

Craniofacial CT scans were obtained in both axial and coronal planes. The ventricles were of normal size and shape. There was evidence of a fingerprinting appearance along the inner table of the cranial vault and anterior cranial base. The CT scans confirmed that the anterior cranial base was short, with bitemporal constrictions and a

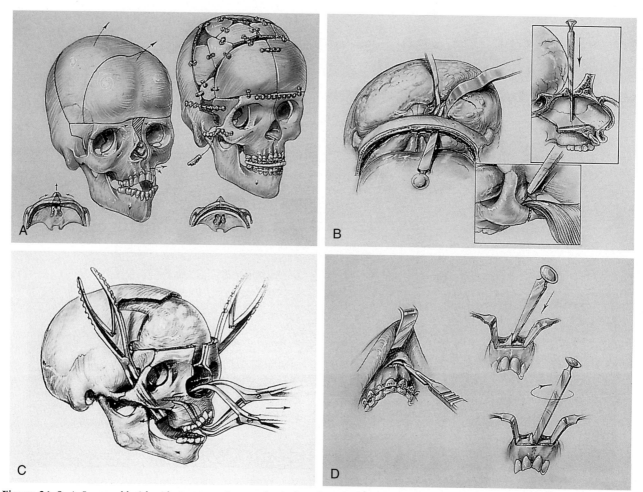

Figure 26–8. A 5-year-old girl with Apert syndrome who had undergone suture release and forehead reshaping at 6 months of age. She presented for cranial vault and facial bipartition osteotomies with reshaping and anterior repositioning. *A,* Illustration of preoperative craniofacial morphology with planned and completed osteotomies and reshaping; stabilization was achieved with cranial bone grafts and miniplate fixation. *B,* Osteotomies requiring completion with a chisel; osteotomy of the medial orbital wall is completed posterior to the medial canthi and nasolacrimal apparatus, with the chisel placement through the anterior cranial base; osteotomy through the anterior cranial base down through the bony septum of the nose; osteotomy through the coronal incision and infratemporal fossa to the pterygomaxillary suture, which is then separated. *C,* Completed facial bipartition osteotomies; Tessier disimpaction forceps placed through the nose and mouth, and pterygomaxillary spreader forceps placed through coronal incision and infratemporal fossa to the pterygomaxillary suture regions for disimpaction of the midface. *D,* Illustration of intraoral buccal vestibular incision, dissection down to anterior nasal spine region, and osteotomy down midline of hard palate as part of facial bipartition osteotomy.

recessed supraorbital ridge. The superior forehead bulged anteriorly. The orbits were shallow, and moderate orbital hypertelorism was present.

The patient appeared to have Apert syndrome with residual cranial vault dysplasia, proptosis, orbital hypertelorism, and total midface deficiency.

Total cranial vault and facial bipartition osteotomies with reshaping and advancement were carried out through an intracranial approach. The airway was managed by endotracheal intubation. The osteotomies were stabilized with autogenous cranial graft and miniplates and screws.

She was discharged from hospital and returned to her home town. At 3 years after surgery, she maintained good function and facial esthetics. A LeFort I osteotomy and genioplasty will be required in combination with orthodontic treatment when the skeleton reaches maturity.

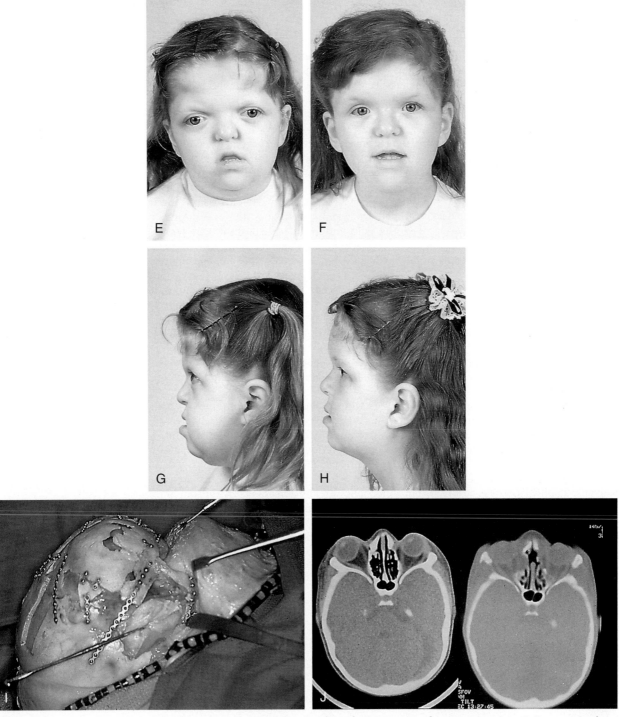

Figure 26–8. *Continued E,* Preoperative frontal view. *F,* Postoperative frontal view 2 years after reconstruction. *G,* Preoperative lateral view. *H,* Postoperative lateral view 2 years after reconstruction. *I,* Intraoperative lateral view of cranial vault, orbits, and zygomatic arch through the coronal incision after osteotomies; stabilization was achieved with cranial bone grafts and miniplate fixation. *J,* Pre- and postoperative axial sliced CT scans through the midorbits, demonstrating improvement in orbital hypertelorism and orbital depth with diminished proptosis (right). (From Posnick JC, Nakano P: Craniofacial dysostosis: Staging of reconstruction and management of the midface deformity. Neurosurg Clin North Am 2[3]:693–695, 1991.)

Case 8 (Fig. 26–9)

Diagnosis: Pfeiffer syndrome (bilateral coronal synostosis)
Previous Surgeries: 1. Bilateral "lateral canthal advancements"
                      2. Ventriculoperitoneal shunt placement
Procedure: Total cranial vault and monobloc osteotomies with reshaping and advancement

A 7-year-old boy born with Pfeiffer syndrome underwent bilateral "lateral canthal advancements" through an intracranial approach at approximately 3 months of age. Later, he required placement of a ventriculoperitoneal shunt for management of hydrocephalus. He was referred to the author because of poor nasal airflow, obstructive sleep apnea, developmental delay, corneal exposure, and herniation of his globe, which had necessitated emergency reduction in the past.

Physical examination revealed multiple cranial vault defects, a decreased head circumference, and bulging eyes. The total midface was hypoplastic with severe Angle class III malocclusion and anterior open bite deformity. The nasal airflow was poor, and a sleep study revealed obstructive sleep apnea. Papilledema with mild optic atrophy was combined with severe strabismus, amblyopia, corneal exposure, and upper eyelid ptosis.

CT scans were obtained in both axial and coronal planes. The ventricles were mildly enlarged, and a ventriculoperitoneal shunt was in place. Multiple cranial vault bony defects were present, and a fingerprinting appearance was observed along the inner table of the skull and the anterior cranial base, caused by long-standing increased intracranial pressure. The orbits were extremely shallow with globe proptosis. There was severe hypoplasia of the midface, which was also documented through cephalometric analysis. The mandible showed a normal anteroposterior growth pattern, as documented by the s-n-b angle.

Total cranial vault and monobloc osteotomies with reshaping and advancement were carried out through an intracranial approach. Autogenous cranial bone grafts were placed at cranial vault defects and osteotomy sites. Stabilization was with multiple titanium miniplates and screws. The airway was managed with endotracheal intubation.

At 1 year after operation, a sleep study revealed resolution of the previous significant oxygen desaturation. Corneal exposure and globe herniation were no longer problems. Papilledema was resolved, but mild optic atrophy remained. Occlusion and chewing were improved, but an Angle class III malocclusion remained. A LeFort I osteotomy and genioplasty in combination with orthodontic treatment will be required when the skeleton matures. Extraocular eye muscle procedures have been carried out to improve the strabismus.

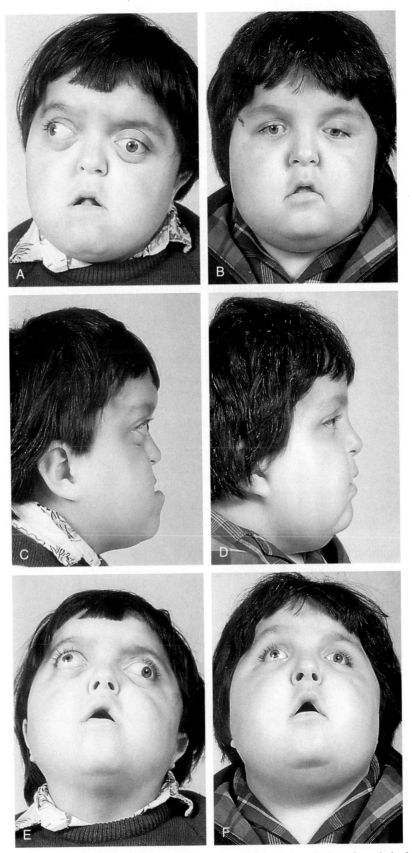

Figure 26–9. A 7-year-old boy born with Pfeiffer syndrome who had undergone bilateral "lateral canthal advancements" through an intracranial approach at 8 months of age and later required placement of a ventriculoperitoneal shunt. He presented for total cranial vault and monobloc osteotomies with reshaping and advancement. *A*, Preoperative front view. *B*, Postoperative frontal view 1 year after reconstruction. *C*, Preoperative lateral view. *D*, Postoperative lateral view 1 year after reconstruction. *E*, Preoperative worm's-eye view. *F*, Postoperative worm's-eye view. (From Posnick JC, Nakano P: Craniofacial dysostosis: Staging of reconstruction and management of the midface deformity. Neurosurg Clin North Am 2[3]:683–702, 1991.)

Case 9 (Fig. 26–10)

Diagnosis: Apert syndrome (bilateral coronal synostosis)
Previous Surgeries: 1. Strip craniectomies of coronal sutures
2. Anterior cranial vault and upper orbital osteotomies with advancement
3. Attempted cranioplasty and LeFort III osteotomy
4. Ventriculoperitoneal shunt placement on three occasions
Procedure: 1. Total cranial vault and facial bipartition osteotomies with reshaping and advancement
2. Repair of encephalocele and frontal and orbital defects

An 8-year-old girl born with Apert syndrome underwent strip craniectomy of stenotic coronal sutures in infancy while living in the Middle East. When signs of increased intracranial pressure appeared, upper orbital and cranial vault osteotomies were performed. Her surgery was complicated by infection and loss of bone in the right fronto-orbital region. A cranioplasty was later attempted, but another infection occurred. Herniation of the brain through the resulting defect in the orbital roof and medial orbital wall resulted in further orbital dystopia and proptosis. She was taken to another country, where a LeFort III osteotomy was attempted. Ventriculoperitoneal shunting was carried out on three occasions.

She was sent to the author as a cheerful, good-natured child whose intelligence was just below normal. Strabismus, amblyopia, and astigmatism with mild optic atrophy were present. She had four-limb complex syndactylies that had not been previously reconstructed. Previous infections and fistula tracts had resulted in multiple well-healed scars over her forehead. A large encephalocele was evident through the bony defect in the right medial supraorbital ridge, orbital roof, and upper aspect of the medial orbital wall. The orbits were shallow, the eyes were bulging, and orbital hypertelorism was present. An Angle class III malocclusion with an anterior open bite was also present. Nasal airflow was poor, and the patient habitually breathed through her mouth. Her forehead was flat and wide, indicative of unresolved brachycephaly.

Total cranial vault and facial bipartition osteotomies with reshaping and advancement were carried out through an intracranial approach. The traumatic encephalocele was repaired while the cranial base and orbital defects were reconstructed with autogenous cranial grafts. Fixation was with multiple titanium miniplates and screws.

The postoperative course was uneventful. The vertical component of the right orbital dystopia was improved but not corrected. Three months postoperatively, the staged four-limbed syndactyly release and reconstruction began. A LeFort I osteotomy and genioplasty in combination with orthodontic treatment will be required when the skeleton reaches maturity.

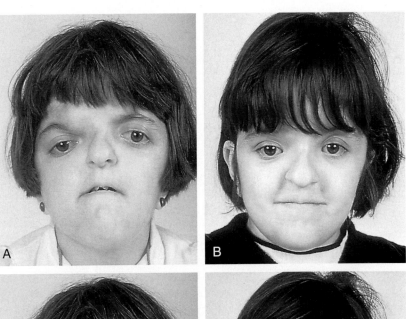

Figure 26–10. An 8-year-old girl with Apert syndrome who had undergone multiple intracranial surgical procedures in the past, including an attempted LeFort III osteotomy. She was referred for management of her residual problems and underwent repair of the fronto-orbital encephalocele and reconstruction of orbital wall defects, combined with total cranial vault and facial bipartition osteotomies, reshaping, and advancement. *A,* Preoperative frontal view. *B,* Frontal view 1 year after reconstruction. *C,* Preoperative front view with smile. *D,* Frontal view with smile 1 year after reconstruction. *E,* Preoperative oblique view. *F,* Oblique view 1 year after reconstruction.

Illustration continued on following page

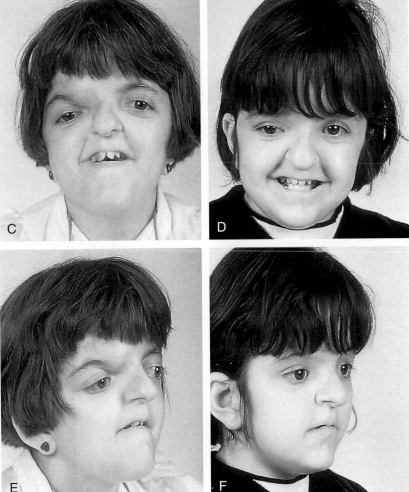

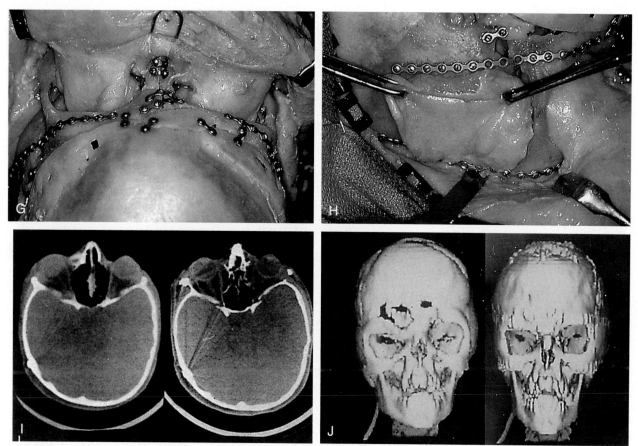

Figure 26–10. *Continued G,* Intraoperative close-up view of anterior cranial vault and orbits after reconstruction; stabilization was achieved with cranial bone grafts and miniplate fixation. *H,* Intraoperative close-up lateral view of craniofacial region with miniplate fixation across the zygomatic arch–anterior maxilla and supraorbital ridge–temporal bone regions demonstrated. *I,* Axial sliced CT scans through the midorbits before and after reconstruction, confirming diminished orbital proptosis and improvement of midorbital hypertelorism. *J,* Three-dimensional CT scan reformations of craniofacial skeleton; frontal views before and after reconstruction. (From Posnick JC: Craniosynostosis: Surgical management in infancy. *In* Bell WH [ed]: Modern Practice in Orthognathic and Reconstructive Surgery, vol 3, pp 1922–1923. Philadelphia: WB Saunders, 1992.)

Case 10 (Fig. 26–11)

Diagnosis: Crouzon syndrome (bilateral coronal synostosis)
Previous Surgery: None
Procedure: Anterior cranial vault and monobloc osteotomies with reshaping and advancement

A 6-year-old girl was born with Crouzon syndrome. Her mother had bicoronal synostosis, proptosis, and midface deficiency. The child had constant headaches and difficulty with her vision when her mother brought her for medical examination.

Physical examination revealed a flat, wide forehead with recessed supraorbital ridges, shallow orbits, and bulging eyes. The total midface was flat with an Angle class III malocclusion. There was evidence of poor nasal airflow and a mouth-breathing habit. Fundoscopic examination revealed papilledema with mild optic atrophy, strabismus, and amblyopia.

CT scans were obtained in both the axial and coronal planes. The ventricles were mildly enlarged. A fingerprinting appearance was obvious along the inner table of the skull and the anterior cranial base, resulting from long-standing increased intracranial pressure. The orbits were shallow with proptosis. The midface deficiency was also confirmed through cephalometric analysis, which revealed an S-N-A angle greater than two standard deviations below the norm. The S-N-B angle was within normal limits.

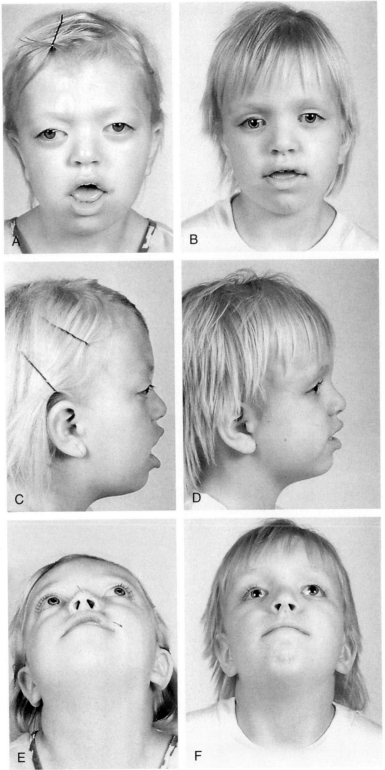

Figure 26–11. A 6-year-old girl with Crouzon syndrome who had undergone anterior cranial vault and monobloc osteotomies with reshaping and advancement. *A,* Preoperative frontal view. *B,* Frontal view 1 year after reconstruction. *C,* Preoperative lateral view. *D,* Lateral view 1 year after reconstruction. *E,* Preoperative worm's-eye view. *F,* Worms's-eye view 1 year after reconstruction.

Illustration continued on following page

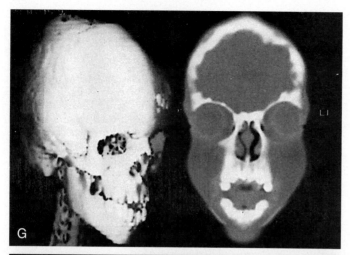

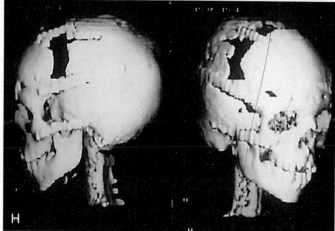

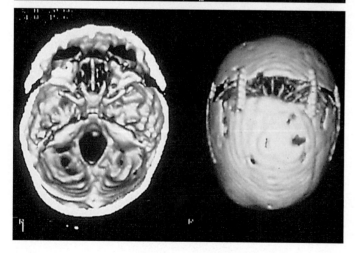

Figure 26–11. *Continued G,* Two- and three-dimensional CT scan reformation before operation. *H,* Three-dimensional CT scan reformation after early reconstruction. *I,* Additional three-dimensional CT scan reformations after early reconstruction, including cranial base view demonstrating increase in anteroposterior length. (From Posnick JC, Nakano P: Craniofacial dysostosis: Staging of reconstruction and management of the midface deformity. Neurosurg Clin North Am 2[3]:683–702, 1991.)

Anterior cranial vault and monobloc osteotomies with reshaping and advancement were carried out through an intracranial approach. Stabilization was with cranial grafts, miniplates, and screws. The airway was managed with endotracheal intubation.

Recovery was uneventful. Orthognathic surgery combined with orthodontic treatment will be required later in adolescence as part of the staged reconstruction.

References

1. Virchow R: Uber den Cretinismus, nametlich in Franken und uber pathologische Schadelforamen. Ver Phys Med Cesselsch Wurzburg 1881; 2:230.
2. Apert E: De l'acrocephalosyndactylie. Bulletins et Memoires Societé Medicale des Hopitaux de Paris 1906; 23:1310.
3. Crouzon O: Dysostose cranio-faciale hereditaire. Bulletins et Memoires Societé Medicale des Hopitaux de Paris 1912; 33:545.
4. Cohen MM Jr: An etiologic and nosologic overview of craniosynostosis syndromes. Birth Defects 1975; 11:137.
5. Cohen MM Jr: Craniosynostosis: Diagnosis, Evaluation and Management. New York: Raven Press, 1986.
6. Gorlin RJ, Cohen MM Jr, Levin LS: Syndromes of the Head and Neck, 3rd ed, Chap. 14. New York: Oxford University Press, 1990.
7. Cohen MM Jr: Syndromes with craniosynostosis. In Cohen MM Jr (ed): Craniosynostosis: Diagnosis, Evaluation and Management, pp 447–461. New York: Raven Press, 1986.
8. David DJ, Sheen R: Surgical correction of Crouzon syndrome. Plast Reconstr Surg 1990; 85:344.
9. Friede H, Lilja J, Lauritzen C, et al: Skull morphology after early craniotomy in patients with premature synostosis of the coronal suture. Cleft Palate J 1986; 23(Suppl 1):1.
10. Hogeman KE, Willmar K: On LeFort III osteotomy for Crouzon's disease in children: Report of a four year follow-up in one patient. Scand J Plast Reconstr Surg 1974; 8:169.
11. Kolar JC, Munro IR, Farkas LG: Patterns of dysmorphology in Crouzon syndrome: An anthropometric study. Cleft Palate J 1988; 25:235.
12. Kreiborg S, Aduss H: Pre- and postsurgical facial growth in patients with Crouzon's and Apert's syndromes. Cleft Palate J 1986; 23(Suppl):78.
13. Kreiborg S, Bjork A: Description of a dry skull with Crouzon syndrome. Scand J Plast Reconstr Surg 1982; 16:245.
14. Kreiborg S: Crouzon syndrome. A clinical and roentgencephalometric study. Scand J Plast Reconstr Surg 1981; 18(Suppl):1.
15. Kreiborg S: Craniofacial growth in plagiocephaly and Crouzon syndrome. Scand J Plast Reconstr Surg 1981; 15:187.
16. Lauritzen C, Lilja J, Jarlstedt J: Airway obstruction and sleep apnea in children with craniofacial anomalies. Plast Reconstr Surg 1986; 77:1.
17. McCarthy JG, Epstein FJ, Wood-Smith D: Craniosynostosis. In McCarthy JG (ed): Plastic Surgery, vol 4, pp 3013–3053. Philadelphia: WB Saunders, 1990.
18. Obwegeser HL: Surgical correction of small or retrodisplaced maxillae: The "dish-face" deformity. Plast Reconstr Surg 1969; 43:351.
19. Posnick JC: Craniofacial dysostosis: Staging of reconstruction and management of the midface deformity. Neurosurg Clin North Am 1991; 2(3):638–702.
20. Posnick JC, Lin KY, Jhawar BJ, et al: Crouzon syndrome: Quantitative assessment of presenting deformity and surgical results based on CT scans. Plast Reconstr Surg 1993; 92:1027.
21. Posnick JC: Craniofacial dysostosis: Management of the midface deformity. In Bell WH (ed): Modern Practice in Orthognathic and Reconstructive Surgery, vol 3, pp 1839–1887. Philadelphia: WB Saunders, 1992.
22. Rune B, Selvik G, Kreiborg S, et al: Motion of bones and volume changes in the neurocranium after craniectomy in Crouzon's disease. A roentgen stereometric study. J Neurosurg 1979; 50:494.
23. Richtsmeier JT, Grausz HM, Morris GR, et al: Growth of the cranial base in craniosynostosis. Cleft Palate-Craniofac J 1991; 28:55.
24. Tessier P: Osteotomies totales de la face. Syndrome de Crouzon, syndrome d'Apert: Oxycephalies, scaphocephalies, turricephalies. Ann Chir Plast 1967; 12:273.
25. Carr M, Posnick J, Armstrong D, et al: Cranio-orbito-zygomatic measurements from standard CT scans in unoperated Crouzon and Apert infants: Comparison with normal controls. Cleft Palate-Craniofac J 1992; 29:129.
26. Bjork A: Cranial base development. Am J Orthod 1955; 41:198.
27. Enlow DH, Azuma M: Functional growth boundaries in the human and mammalian face. Birth Defects 1975; 11:217.
28. Enlow DH, McNamara JA Jr: The neurocranial basis for facial form and pattern. Angle Orthod 1973; 43:256.
29. Moss ML: The pathogensis of premature cranial synostosis in man. Acta Anat 1959; 37:351.
30. Norgaard JO, Kvinnsland S: Influence of submucous septal resection on facial growth in the rat. Plast Reconstr Surg 1979; 64:84.
31. Seeger JF, Gabrielsen TO: Premature closure of the frontosphenoidal suture in synostosis of the coronal suture. Radiology 1971; 101:631.
32. Sarnet BG: Differential craniofacial skeletal changes after postnatal experimental surgery in young and adult animals. Ann Plast Surg 1978; 1:131.
33. Stewart RE, Dixon G, Cohen A: The pathogenesis of premature craniosynostosis in acrocephalosyndactyly (Apert syndrome): A reconsideration. Plast Reconstr Surg 1977; 59:699.

34. Bu BH, Kaban LB, Vargervik K: Effect of LeFort III osteotomy on mandibular growth in patients with Crouzon and Apert syndrome. J Oral Maxillofac Surg 1989; 47:666.
35. Cohen MM Jr: Craniostenoses and syndromes with craniosynostosis. Incidence, genetics, penetrance, variability and new syndrome updating. Birth Defects 1979; 15:13–63.
36. Kreiborg S, Cohen MM Jr: The infant Apert skull. Neurosurg Clin North Am 1991; 2(3):551–554.
37. Ousterhout DK, Melsen B: Cranial base deformity in Apert's syndrome. Plast Reconstr Surg 1982; 69:254.
38. Cohen MM Jr, Gorlin RJ, Berkman MD, et al: Facial variability in the Apert type acrocephalosyndactyly. Birth Defects 1971; 7:143–146.
39. Golabi M, Edwards MSB, Ousterhout DK: Craniosynostosis and hydrocephalus. Neurosurgery 1987; 21:63.
40. Hogan GR, Bauman ML: Hydrocephalus in Apert's syndrome. J Pediatr 1971; 79:782.
41. Murovic JA, Posnick JC, Drake JM, et al: Hydrocephalus in Apert syndrome: A retrospective review. Pediatr Neurosurg 1993; 19:151–155.
42. Fishman MA, Hogan GR, Dodge PR: The concurrence of hydrocephalus and craniosynostosis. J Neurosurg 1971; 34:621.
43. Cohen MM Jr: Perspectives on craniosynostosis. West J Med 1980; 132:508.
44. Cohen MM Jr: Agenesis of the corpus collosum and limbic malformations revisited [Letter]. Arch Neurol 1989; 46:1270.
45. Cohen MM Jr, Kreiborg S: The central nervous system in the Apert syndrome. Am J Med Genet 1990: 35:36.
46. Cohen MM Jr, Kreiborg S: Agenesis of the corpus callosum. Its associated anomalies and syndromes, with special reference to the Apert syndrome. Neurosurg Clin North Am 1991; 2:565.
47. Renier D, Sainte-Rose C, Marchac D, et al: Intracranial pressure in craniosynostosis. J Neurosurg 1982; 57:370.
48. Renier D: Intracranial pressure in craniosynostosis: Pre- and postoperative recordings—Correlation with functional results. In Persing JA, Edgerton MT, Jane JA (eds): Scientific Foundations and Surgical Treatment of Craniosynostosis, pp 263–269. Baltimore: Williams & Wilkins, 1989.
49. Posnick JC, Bite U, Nakano P, et al: Indirect intracranial volume measurements using CT scans: Clinical applications for craniosynostosis. Plast Reconstr Surg 1992; 89:1.
50. Gault DT, Renier D, Marchac D, et al: Intracranial volume in children with craniosynostosis. J Craniofac Surg 1990; 1:1.
51. Waitzman AA, Posnick JC, Armstrong D, et al: Craniofacial skeletal measurements based on computed tomography: Part 1. Accuracy and reproducibility. Cleft Palate-Craniofac J 1992; 29:112.
52. Waitzman AA, Posnick JC, Armstrong D, et al: Craniofacial skeletal measurements based on computed tomography: Part 2. Normal values and growth trends. Cleft Palate-Craniofac J 1992; 29:118.
53. Posnick JC, Goldstein JA, Waitzman A: Surgical correction of the Treacher-Collins malar deficiency with quantitative CT scan analysis of long-term results. Plast Reconstr Surg 1993; 92:12.
54. Posnick JC, Lin KY, Chen P, et al: Sagittal synostosis: Quantitative assessment of presenting deformity and surgical results based on CT scans. Plast Reconstr Surg 1993; 92:1027.
55. Posnick JC, Lin KY, Chen P, et al: Metopic synostosis: Quantitative assessment of presenting deformity and surgical results based on CT scans. Plast Reconstr Surg 1994; 93:16.
56. Posnick JC, Lin KY, Jhawar BJ, et al: Apert syndrome: Quantitative assessment of presenting deformity and surgical results after first-stage reconstruction by CT scan. Plast Reconstr Surg 1994; 93:489.
57. Farkas LG, Posnick JC: Growth and development of regional units in the head and face based on anthropometric measurements. Cleft Palate-Craniofac J 1992; 29:301.
58. Farkas LG, Posnick JC, Hreczko T: Growth patterns of the face: A morphometric study. Cleft Palate-Craniofac J 1992; 29:308.
59. Farkas LG, Posnick JC, Hreczko T: Anthropometric growth study of the head. Cleft Palate-Craniofac J 1992; 29:303.
60. Farkas LG, Posnick JC, Hreczko T: Anthropometric growth study of the ear. Cleft Palate-Craniofac J 1992; 29:324.
61. Farkas LG, Posnick JC, Hreczko T, et al: Growth patterns of the nasolabial region: A morphometric study. Cleft Palate-Craniofac J 1992; 29:318.
62. Farkas LG, Posnick JC, Hreczko T, et al: Growth patterns of the orbital region: A morphometric study. Cleft Palate-Craniofac J 1992; 29:315.
63. Kaban LB, Conover M, Mulliken J: Midface position after LeFort III advancement: A long-term follow-up study. Cleft Palate J 1986; 23(Suppl 1):75.
64. Lannelongue M: De la craniectomie dans la microcephalie. Compte-Rendu Academie des Sciences 1890; 110:1382.
65. Lane LC: Pioneer craniectomy for relief of mental imbecility due to premature sutural closure and microcephalus. JAMA 1892; 18:49.
66. Converse JM, Kazanjian VH: Surgical Treatment of Facial Injuries, 2nd ed. Baltimore: Williams & Wilkins, 1982.
67. Gillies H, Millard DR Jr: The Principles and Art of Plastic Surgery. Boston: Little, Brown, 1957.
68. Gillies H, Harrison SH: Operative correction by osteotomy of recessed malar maxillary compound in case of oxycephaly. Br J Plast Surg 1950; 3:123–127.
69. Tessier P: Dysostoses cranio-faciales (syndromes de Crouzon et d'Apert). Osteotomies totales de la face. In Transactions of the Fourth International Congress of Plastic and Reconstructive Surgery, Amsterdam, p 774, 1969.
70. Tessier P: Relationship of craniostenoses to craniofacial dysostosis and to faciostenoses: a study with therapeutic implications. Plast Reconstr Surg 1971; 48:224.
71. Tessier P: Autogenous bone grafts taken from the calvarium [sic] or facial and cranial applications. Clin Plast Surg 1982; 9:531.

72. Tessier P: Total osteotomy of the middle third of the face for faciostenosis or for sequelae of the LeFort III fractures. Plast Reconstr Surg 1971; 48:533.

73. Tessier P: Recent improvement in the treatment of facial and cranial deformities in Crouzon's disease and Apert's syndrome. *In* Symposium of Plastic Surgery of the Orbital Region, p 271. St. Louis: CV Mosby, 1976.

74. Tessier P: Apert's syndrome: Acrocephalosyndactyly type I. *In* Caronni EP (ed): Craniofacial Surgery, p 280. Boston: Little, Brown, 1985.

75. Tessier P: The definitive plastic surgical treatment of the severe facial deformities of craniofacial dysostosis: Crouzon and Apert's diseases. Plast Reconstr Surg 1971; 48:419.

76. Murray JE, Swanson LT: Mid-face osteotomy and advancement for craniosynostosis. Plast Reconstr Surg 1968; 41:299.

77. Rougerie J, Derome P. Anquez L: Craniostenosis et dysmorphies cranio-faciales. Principes d'une nouvelle technique de traitement et ses resultats. Neurochirurgie 1972; 18:429.

78. Hoffman HJ, Mohr G: Lateral canthal advancement of the supraorbital margin: A new corrective technique in the treatment of coronal synostosis. J Neurosurg 1976; 45:376.

79. Whitaker LA, Schut L, Kerr LP: Early surgery for isolated craniofacial dysostosis. Plast Reconstr Surg 1977; 60:575.

80. Marchac D, Renier D: "Le front flottant." Traitement precoce des facio-craniostenoses. Ann Chir Plast 1979; 24:121–126.

81. Marchac D, Renier D, Jones BM: Experience with the "floating forehead." Br J Plast Surg 1988; 41:1–15.

82. Luhr HG: Zur stabilen Osteosynthese bei Unterkieferfrakturen. Deutsch Zahnaerztl Z 1968; 23:754.

83. Peer LA: Transplantation of Tissues. Baltimore: Williams & Wilkins, 1955.

84. Zins JE, Whitaker LA: Membranous versus endochondral bone: Implications for craniofacial reconstruction. Plast Reconstr Surg 1983; 72:778.

85. Kusiak JF, Zin JE, Whitaker LA: The early revascularization of membranous bone. Plast Reconstr Surg 1985; 76:510.

86. Phillips JH, Rahn BA: Fixation effects on membranous and endochondral onlay bone graft resorption. Plast Reconstr Surg 1988; 82:872.

87. Zins JE, Kusiak JF, Whitaker LA, et al: The influence of the recipient site on bone grafts to the face. Plast Reconstr Surg 1984; 73:371.

88. Perren SM: Physical and biological aspects of fracture healing with special reference to internal fixation. Clin Orthop 1979; 138:175.

89. Jackson IT, Adham M, Bite U, et al: Update on cranial bone grafts in craniofacial surgery. Ann Plast Surg 1987; 18:37.

90. Jackson IT, Hide TAH, Barker DT: Transposition cranioplasty to restore forehead contour in craniofacial deformities. Br J Plast Surg 1978; 31:127.

91. Posnick JC, Goldstein JA, Armstrong D, et al: Reconstruction of skull defects in children and adolescents using fixed cranial bone grafts: Long term results. Neurosurg 1993: 32:785.

92. Posnick JC: The role of plate and screw fixation in the treatment of craniofacial malformations. *In* Gruss JS, Manson PM, Yaremchuk MJ (eds): Rigid Fixation of the Craniomaxillofacial Skeleton, pp 512–526. Stoneham, MA: Butterworth, 1992.

93. Posnick JC: The role of plate and screw fixation in the management of pediatric head and neck tumors. *In* Gruss JS, Manson PM, Yaremchuk MJ (eds): Rigid Fixation of the Craniomaxillofacial Skeleton, pp 556–670. Stoneham, MA: Butterworth, 1992.

94. Posnick JC: The role of plate and screw fixation in the treatment of pediatric facial fractures. *In* Gruss JS, Manson PM, Yaremchuk MJ (eds): Rigid Fixation of the Craniomaxillofacial Skeleton, pp 396–419. Stoneham, MA: Butterworth, 1992.

95. Posnick JC, Goldstein JA, Clokie C: Advantages of the postauricular coronal incision. Ann Plast Surg 1992; 29:114–116.

96. Posnick JC, Nakano P. Taylor M: A modified occlusal splint to avoid tracheostomy for total midface osteotomies. Ann Plast Surg 1992; 29:223–230.

97. Yaremchuk MJ, Fiala TGS, Barker F, et al: The effects of rigid fixation on craniofacial growth of rhesus monkeys. Plast Reconstr Surg 1994; 93:1.

98. Posnick JC: Discussion of "The effects of rigid fixation on the craniofacial growth in rhesus monkeys." Plast Reconstr Surg 1994; 93:11.

99. Manson P: Commentary on the long-term effects of rigid fixation on the growing craniomaxillofacial skeleton. J Craniofac Surg 1991; 2:69.

100. Israele V, Siegel JD: Infectious complications of craniofacial surgery in children. Rev Infect Dis 1989; 11:9.

101. Posnick JC, Al-Qattan MM, Armstrong D: Monobloc and facial bipartition osteotomies for reconstruction of craniofacial malformations: A study of extradural dead space. Plast Reconstr Surg, in press.

102. Epstein F, McCarthy J: Neonatal craniofacial surgery. J Plast Reconstr Surg 1981; 15:217.

103. McCarthy JG, Cutting CB: The timing of surgical intervention in craniofacial anomalies. Clin Plast Surg 1990; 17(1):161.

104. McCarthy JG, Epstein F, Sadove M, et al: Early surgery for craniofacial synostosis an 8 year experience. Plast Reconstr Surg 1984; 73:521.

105. Posnick JC: Craniosynostosis: Surgical management in infancy. *In* Bell WH (ed): Modern Practice in Orthognathic and Reconstructive Surgery, vol 3, pp 1889–1931. Philadelphia: WB Saunders, 1992.

106. Ortiz-Monasterio F, Fuente del Campo A, Carillo A: Advancement of the orbits and the midface in one piece, combined with frontal repositioning for the correction of Crouzon's deformities. Plast Reconstr Surg 1978; 61:507.

107. Ortiz-Monasterio F, Fuente del Campo A: Refinements on the bloc orbitofacial advancement. *In* Caronni EP (ed): Craniofacial Surgery, pp 263–264. Boston: Little, Brown, 1985.

108. van der Meulen JCH: Medical faciotomy. Br J Plast Surg 1979; 32:339.

Surgical Treatment of Hypertelorism

27

Herman F. Sailer and Klaus W. Grätz

DEFINITION

Orbital hypertelorism, or hypertelorbitism, is an increased distance between both orbits. The distance between the medial and lateral orbital walls is also increased. The normal interorbital distance (IOD) of an adult individual is approximately 25 mm. Tessier classified three types of hypertelorism in adults: In type I, the IOD is between 30 and 34 mm; in type II, between 35 and 39 mm; and in type III, wider than 39 mm.[1] In infants and children, the IOD is much smaller and age dependent. An IOD of 25 mm in a 1-year-old child is considered hyperteloric and must be closely observed, and the etiology must be investigated. The IOD (Fig. 27–1) may be measured with a caliper, the arms of which are pressed upon the medial orbital rims. Accurate measurements can be made by posteroanterior cephalometric radiograph and by computed tomography (Fig. 27–2). The intercanthal soft tissue distance (ICD) is measured with a ruler. In an adult, the normal ICD is approximately 30 mm; in a 3-year-old child, approximately 26 mm.[2,3] There is no direct correlation between the IOD and the ICD. Often both distances necessitate independent corrections. Hypertelorism is practically always combined with a malformation of the nose, ranging from wide nasal bones over a bifid nose to complete or partial nasal duplication and also hypoplasia or aplasia of parts of the nasal hard and soft tissue structures.

FORMS OF HYPERTELORISM

Hypertelorism is either symmetric or asymmetric (Fig. 27–3). In addition, the orbits can have an "antimongoloid" position, or they can have a normal shape and volume but can also be shallow, as in Crouzon and Apert syndromes (Fig. 27–4). The four orbital rims can be situated symmetrically in the three planes, or they may be individually malpositioned. These rims must be correctly positioned during the operation. There are also unilateral forms of hypertelorism (Fig. 27–5; see also Fig. 27–11A) as well as cases of hypertelorism with eyeless orbits (Fig. 27–6).

ETIOLOGY

Hypertelorism is not a pathologic entity. It is usually a symptom and can be caused by hyperpneumatization of the ethmoids, craniostenosis of the anterior skull base, persistence of the metopic suture, syndromes such as Crouzon or Apert, medial facial clefts, or meningoencephaloceles (Fig. 27–7; see also Fig. 27–24). Many patients with cleft lip and palate present with mild hypertelorism (Fig. 27–8). Tumors situated between the orbits (osseous keloids, fibrous dysplasia, neurofibromastosis), mucoceles of the frontal and ethmoidal sinuses, and massive facial trauma may induce hypertelorism (Fig. 27–9): only the medial orbital walls show an increased distance from each other, but not the lateral walls. A condition like this is defined as pseudohypertelorism, and correction is often possible by subcranial procedures (to be described).

Text continued on page 691

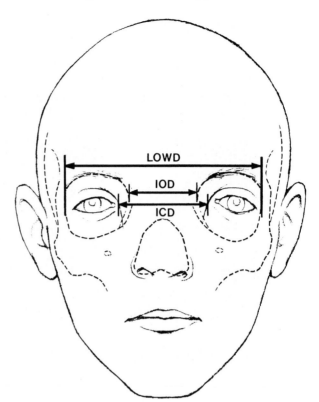

Figure 27–1. The interorbital distance (IOD) is difficult to determine because of the overlying soft tissues; the intercanthal distance (ICD), which is very important for esthetic reasons, is easily measured by a ruler. In true hypertelorism, the distance of the lateral orbital walls (LOWD) is also increased, in contrast to cases of pseudohypertelorism.

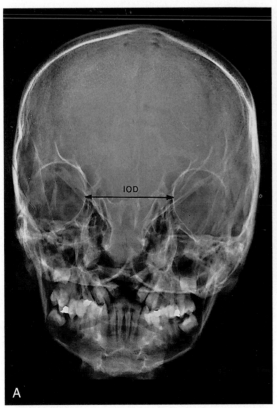

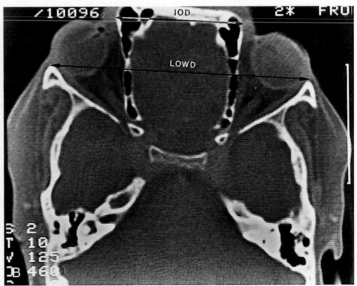

Figure 27–2. Accurate measurement for interorbital distance (IOD) can be made by posteroanterior cephalometry *(A)* and by computed tomography *(B)*.

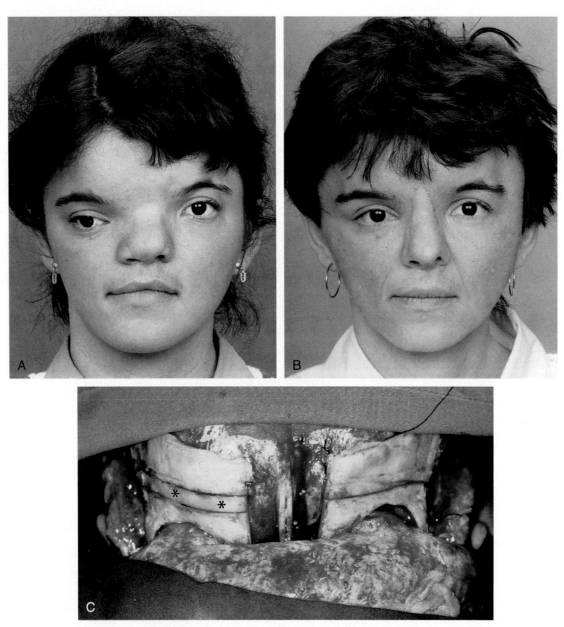

Figure 27–3. Case of asymmetric hypertelorism before *(A)* and after *(B)* correction. The intraoperative picture *(C)* shows the condition after interorbital osteotomy and before removal of the supraorbital horizontal bone band *(asterisk)* to elevate the right orbit.

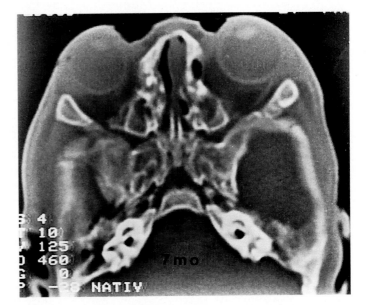

Figure 27–4. Extremely shallow orbits in a case of Crouzon syndrome with medium degree of hypertelorism.

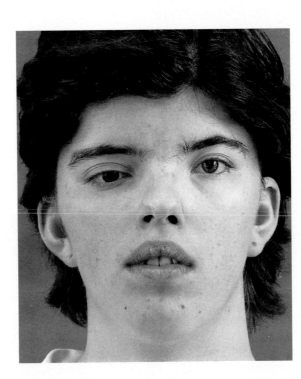

Figure 27–5. Unilateral form of hypertelorism (see also Fig. 27–11*A*) in a case of plagiocephaly.

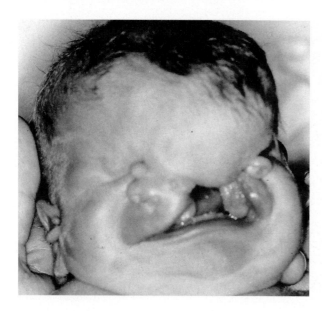

Figure 27–6. Monstrous malformation, including extremely hyperteloric, eyeless orbits, several kinds of facial clefts, and interorbital encephalocele.

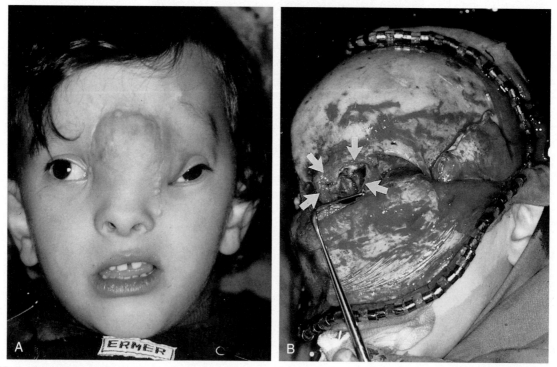

Figure 27–7. *A*, Meningoencephalocele causing hypertelorism; *B*, the intraoperative picture shows the perforation of the encephalocele (already resected) into the left orbit *(arrows)*.

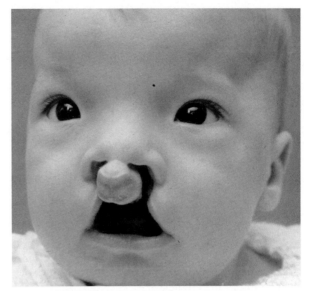

Figure 27–8. Bilateral cleft lip, cleft palate, and orbital hypertelorism.

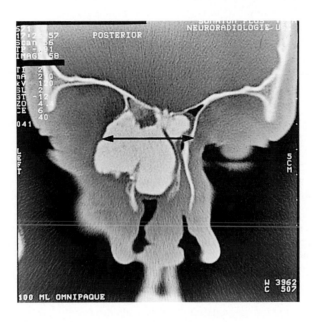

Figure 27–9. Interorbital tumor-like lesion (osseous keloid) causing widening of the interorbital distance (IOD) but not of the lateral walls.

TIME OF SURGERY

The development of the deciduous and permanent dentition is the most important determinant of the timing of surgery.[4] As long as the maxillary sinus has not yet developed and the tooth germs have not yet grown caudally enough, the infraorbital horizontal osteotomy cannot be performed without damage to the tooth buds (Fig. 27–10). Therefore, the earliest age for hypertelorism correction is between 4 and 10 years, when the maxillary sinus is developing.

The development of the roots of the canines always merits special consideration. Often their apices are positioned far cranially in adolescents and even in adults because of missing space within the alveolar arch. It is imperative that the canines be preserved. Therefore, orthodontic treatment is often required after extraction of the first premolars in order to guide the eruption of the canines.

An exception to this is the facial bipartition procedure, in which no infraorbital horizontal osteotomy is performed. In this procedure there is less risk to the canines and premolars, but the molars may nonetheless be damaged, depending on the age of the patient.

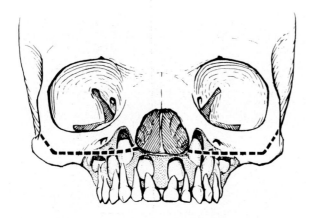

Figure 27–10. The drawing shows the state of tooth development in 4- to 5-year-old children and the infraorbital horizontal osteotomy that causes damage to the permanent dentition.

Craniomaxillofacial surgeons should always be aware that damage to the tooth buds results in growth impairment of the midface.[4] According to Enlow, the growth of the primary and the secondary dentition is also responsible for the development of the maxilla in all three dimensions.[5]

In some of the syndromes associated with hypertelorism (e.g., Crouzon and Apert syndromes), growth impairment of the midface is typical of the malformation; this is aggravated if tooth buds are damaged by early surgery as it is recommended by others.[6,7]

PLANNING

The surgical correction of hypertelorism is difficult and risky because of the highly important contiguous anatomic structures. The diagnostic and planning aspect of treatment are multidisciplinary tasks, but the surgeon should be the leader of the team because he or she is responsible for the result and for possible complications.

For planning, all modern diagnostic means should be available, including three-dimensional imaging and stereolithography. The most important rule gained by experience is that intercanthal distance reduction corresponds to only half of the amount of the removed bone; for example, interorbital bone resection of 30 mm results in a reduction of the ICD of about 15 mm. As mentioned, exact measurements in the posteroanterior cephalometric radiograph or in the computed tomographic scan (see Fig. 27–2) are necessary for preoperative assessment. Life-size photographs of the patient's face are beneficial (Fig. 27–11). Stereolithographic models allow the exact simulation of the surgical procedure (Fig. 27–12).

Every case of hypertelorism correction demonstrates profile alterations of various degrees (see Fig. 27–11*E,F*), necessitating simultaneous corrections of nasal form and of the projection of the zygomatic area as well as of the chin.

POSSIBILITIES IN SURGICAL CORRECTION

In the authors' department, correction of as much as possible in a single operation is the goal. The simultaneous transcranial and transoral approach is used in all hypertelorism corrections, and a higher incidence of infection has not been observed.

The correction of hypertelorism always involves hard and soft tissue procedures. Not only are the bony structures of the orbit, the maxilla, the nose, and the forehead involved; the soft tissues of the forehead, the nose, the cheek, the upper lip, the eyelids, and the medial and lateral canthi must also be restructured. In transcranial procedures, the cribriform plate is exposed and dissected, and consequently the olfactory nerve system may be damaged. The whole midface is degloved, including the zygomatic bone and arch, and the temporal muscles are elevated. The surgeon must therefore have experience in handling soft and hard tissue. He or she should also be accustomed to contemporary means of fixation such as micro- and miniplates in the treatment of maxillofacial trauma.

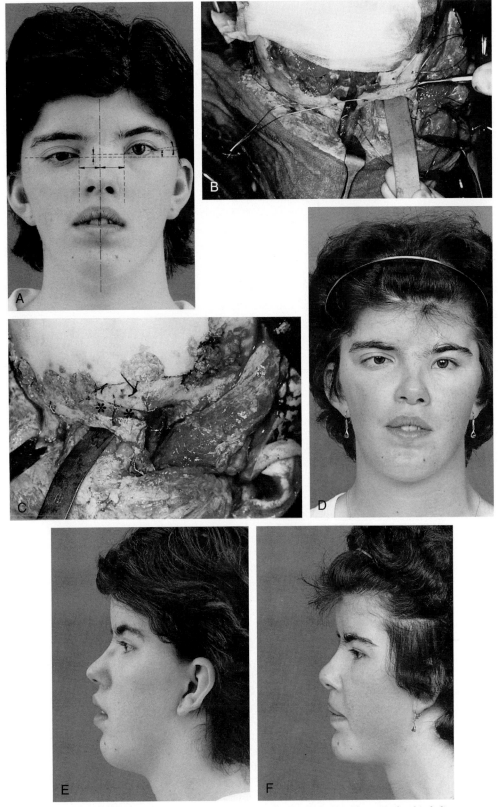

Figure 27–11. Planning and performance of a case of left unilateral hypertelorism with vertical orbital discrepancy. Exact measurements on the 1:1 life-size photograph *(A)* suggest removal of interorbital nasofrontal bone on the left, as seen in the intraoperative picture *(B)*, by lowering the left orbit *(C)* by interpositional bone graft *(asterisk)*. The result *(D)* shows both orbits on a horizontal level, but eyelid soft tissue differences remain. Simultaneous correction of the facial profile *(E, before surgery; F, after surgery)* is necessary.

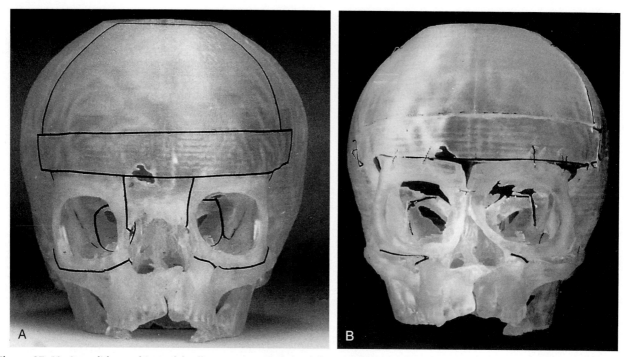

Figure 27–12. Stereolithographic models allow an exact analysis of the morphology of the malformation *(A)* and perfect simulation of the operation *(B)*.

Correction of hypertelorism can be accomplished subcranially or transcranially. There are many variations and modifications. The most common procedures used in the Department of Cranio-Maxillofacial Surgery, University Hospital Zurich, are presented and described step by step.

Subcranial Procedures

Subcranial correction of hypertelorism or pseudohypertelorism is indicated in mild forms only when the IOD is about 35 to 40 mm. This operation is indicated especially in posttraumatic cases or for tumors in which the lateral orbital walls are in a normal position. The procedure involves medial orbital wall approximation, including the nasal and lacrimal bones along with the medial canthi.

Another subcranial procedure involves orbital medialization without orbital roof osteotomy. In this procedure, both the medial and the lateral orbital walls and the orbital floor are shifted medially. Both subcranial operations can be simultaneously combined with a LeFort III osteotomy, if necessary.

The Medial Orbital Wall Approximation (Fig. 27–13A,B,C,D)

Step-by-Step Procedure

1. For the coronal incision, a 1.5-cm–wide strip of hair running from one ear to the other is removed; the remaining hair is disinfected, and the posterior part of the head is covered with a sterile cloth fixed to the galea by clamps. The anterior part of the hair-bearing scalp is covered with a cloth that is fixed by stitches, leaving the forehead free (Fig. 27–14). A local anesthetic containing epinephrine is injected, and an incision made along the hair-free strip of galea running from one ear to the other and, from there, forward and downward close to the helix. The wound edges are slightly mobilized on both sides. Hemostatic clips are applied along the posterior wound edge, and a hemostatic continuous running suture along the anterior wound edge is placed. Then a supraperiosteal dissection is performed, together with the dissection between the superficial and deep temporal fascia. The fat pad between both fasciae is dissected by knife to avoid damage to the facial nerve. About 2 cm above the supraorbital rims,

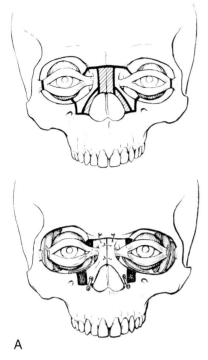

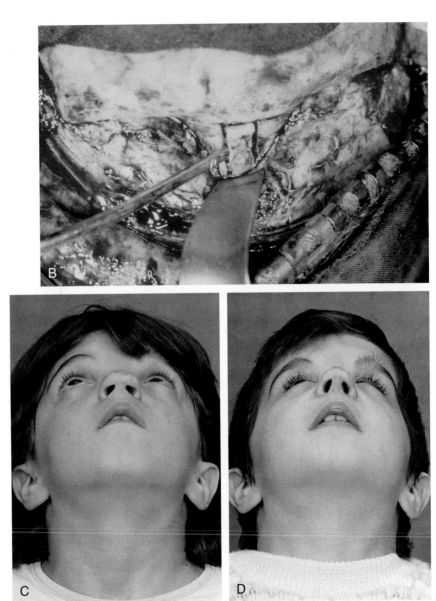

Figure 27–13. *A,* Schematic drawing of the medial orbital wall approximation as it is often used in cases of pseudo-hypertelorism. The osteotomy along the nasofrontal suture must be performed in a caudoposterior direction to avoid intracranial penetration. Along the pyriform aperture, some bone is removed to avoid nasal obstruction. The slight enlargement of the orbital volume is compensated by transplantation of bone or cartilage grafts to the lateral walls. The lateral canthal ligaments should also be repositioned. Orbital wall defects are bridged by grafts. *B,* The intraoperative photograph shows the amount of dissection and the osteotomies for interorbital nasal bone resection; patient with slight hypertelorism before *(C)* and after *(D)* medial orbital wall approximation and nasal correction.

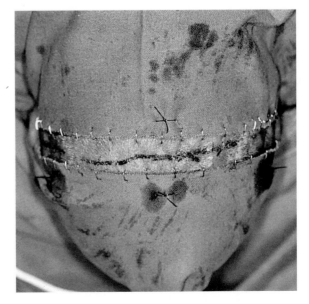

Figure 27–14. Preparation of the scalp. Only a 1.5-cm–wide strip of hair is removed, and the remaining hair anteriorly and posteriorly is disinfected and covered with a sterile cloth.

the pericranium is incised horizontally, and the bone around the supraorbital rims, the nasal bones, and the glabella are degloved. In most cases, the supraorbital neurovascular bundle must be removed from its canal on both sides.

2. The nasal bones, parts of the cartilaginous structures of the nose, the orbital roofs, and the medial, lateral, and inferior walls of the orbits are subperiosteally exposed, and the medial canthal ligaments (including the lacrimal duct) are dissected but not detached.

3. A horizontal bone cut is made along the nasofrontal suture running into the medial orbital wall on both sides and then downward behind the canthal ligaments and the lacrimal duct system, in the direction of the infraorbital rim. Two vertical cuts are then made through the nasal bones in front of the medial canthal ligaments. The distance between the cuts is coincident with the desired medial wall movement. A Toller bur is used for this osteotomy and helps to avoid damage to the underlying nasal mucosa. The interorbital nasal bone piece is now carefully removed without damaging the mucosa.

4. For the transoral osteotomies, a horizontal incision is made in the maxillary vestibule, and the canine fossa, including the infraorbital rims and the infraorbital foramen, is degloved. The nasal mucosa is elevated inside the pyriform aperture on both sides. An osteotomy beginning laterally is now performed through the infraorbital rim medially to the infraorbital foramen (but far enough laterally not to damage the lacrimal duct), running downward into the pyriform aperture beneath the inferior turbinate. With the use of chisels, the bony structures containing the medial canthal ligaments and the lacrimal ducts are mobilized medially and fixed into position with direct wiring (see Fig. 27–13). There is no absolute indication for the use of plates and screws in such a procedure.

5. The medial orbital wall approximation causes enlargement of the orbital volume, which necessitates compensation. Many surgeons use autologous rib grafts or split calvarial grafts placed onto the lateral orbital walls. The authors' material of choice is lyophilized cartilage.

6. If necessary, a strut of lyophilized cartilage can be placed to project the nasal dorsum. Other minor corrections are performed with the same biomaterial. In an alternative procedure, it is possible to detach the medial canthal ligaments to perform the osteotomies and replace the ligaments in the old or a new position. But usually the ligaments are left in place.

The Orbital Medialization Without Roof Osteotomy (Fig. 27–15)

This procedure is performed if a more extensive medial shifting of the orbits is necessary. This procedure allows 5- to 8-mm medial shifting of each side. It is possible only if the anterior cranial fossa with the cribriform plate does not extend downward between the orbits and is situated at the level of the orbital roofs. If the cribriform plate's position is farther downward, there is a high risk of entering the intracranial space and damaging the dura mater with the consequence of cerebrospinal fluid leakage and other complications.

Radiologic documentation (by computed tomography) is necessary to define the exact position of the cribriform plate and the anterior and medial cranial fossae. The authors recommend three-dimensional imaging for better evaluation. If there is any doubt about the extent of the cranial cavity, it is safer to make a bur hole in the temporal fossa and protect the cranial contents with a brain spatula than to perform a blind orbital osteotomy.

The transcranial procedure is the safer one.

Step-by-Step Procedure

1. Coronal approach and dissection of the periorbital and nasal bones are as described earlier; in addition, the zygomatic arch and complex are extensively exposed, and the anterior parts of the temporal muscles are elevated.

2. A horizontal osteotomy through the frontonasal suture is made. It is continued posteriorly beneath the cranial base and downward into the orbital floor through the infraorbital fissure, into the lateral orbital wall, and forward beneath the cranial base and through the frontozygomatic suture. The zygomatic complex, including the lower lateral orbital rim, is included in the osteotomy. This procedure is also performed on

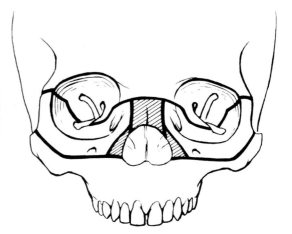

Figure 27–15. Osteotomy of the orbital walls, excluding the orbital roof, is shown. The lower part of the orbits is rotated to the midline after the nasal ostectomy.

the other side, and a strip of interorbital bone of the desired width is removed from the nasal structure.

3. The transoral approach is as described earlier. The zygomatic osteotomy is exposed, and a horizontal osteotomy running beneath the infraorbital foramen is made through the maxillary sinus into the pyriform aperture beneath the inferior turbinates. The orbital structures are then mobilized from intraoral and extraoral exposure. Triangular bone areas are removed along the pyriform margin to avoid nasal obstruction. The medially rotated midfacial structures are fixed with wires.

4. The defects within the lateral orbital walls and the orbital floor are bridged by lyophilized cartilage sheets (to be described). The nasal form is corrected by using a strut of lyophilized cartilage, which is fixed by a wire to the lacrimal bones or to the frontal bone. Wire fixation is also necessary at the lateral orbital rims and sometimes within the canine fossae.

5. The defects within the zygoma are bridged with lyophilized bone and microplates.

6. The lateral canthal ligaments are fixed inside the lateral orbital wall through bur holes.

Combination Procedure of Subcranial Hypertelorism Operation and LeFort III Osteotomy (see Fig. 27–23)

This procedure is indicated if the midface, including the zygomatic complex, has to be advanced.

Step-by-Step Procedure

1. The coronal approach and dissection of the periorbital soft tissues are as described earlier.

2. The osteotomy is performed as described earlier.

3. The connecting osteotomy is made between the infraorbital fissure and the pterygomaxillary suture on both sides; the pterygoid plates are separated from the maxillary tuberosity. An osteotomy of the zygomatic arch is also made.

4. The orbital walls are mobilized, and the orbital structure is approximated.

5. The midface is mobilized.

6. All bony structures are fixed according to the preoperative planning with wiring and mini- or microplates.

Combination Procedure of Subcranial Hypertelorism Operation and LeFort I Osteotomy (see Fig. 27–24)

This procedure is indicated only when the tooth-bearing part of the upper jaw has to be mobilized for occlusal reasons but the zygomatic complex does not.

The infraorbital horizontal osteotomy is connected to the LeFort I bone cut running under the zygomatic buttress to the tuberosity area, where the pterygomaxillary junction is separated by a chisel.

The Transcranial Hypertelorism Procedure

Tessier's Transcranial Hypertelorism Operation (THO) (Fig. 27–16)

Tessier's hypertelorism procedure[8] revolutionized the correction of monstrous cranio-facial malformations. Through this and other methods, Tessier inaugurated new dimensions of cranial base surgery; this transcranial approach to the orbits and cranial base has also widely influenced the field of craniofacial trauma and the treatment of craniofacial tumors. The THO allows movements of the orbits in all directions and also the correction of the hypotelorism by outward rotation of the orbits (Fig. 27–17). The procedure is not easy to understand; three-dimensional imagination is necessary in order to perform the cranial, orbital, and midfacial osteotomies and movements (Fig. 27–18).

Anesthetic Considerations

The transcranial hypertelorism procedure is one of the longest operations in the whole field of surgery. Operations lasting 8 to 15 hours and even longer are not rare. The anesthesiologist requires experience in delivering long-term anesthesia and must be equipped with all modern monitoring modalities. Blood loss during surgery can be severe, and in contrast to the subcranial procedures described earlier, it is usually not possible to avoid homologous blood transfusions. It is the surgeon's responsibility to reduce or avoid such transfusions; therefore, the hemodilution technique and intraoperative autotransfusion with the cell saver apparatus are routinely used.[9] The cell saver is also used in the oral cavity.

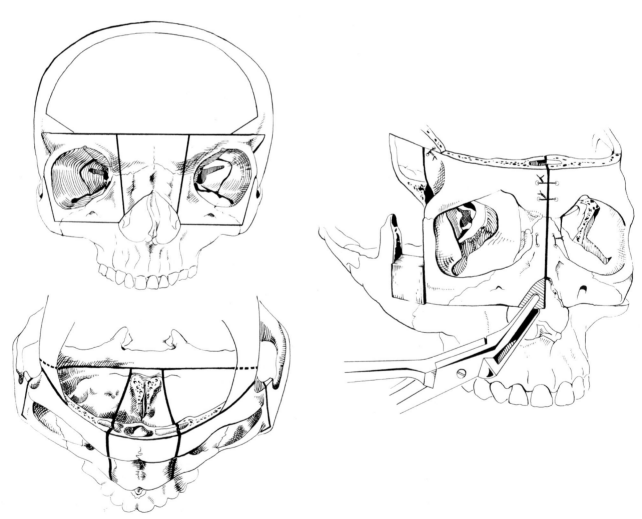

Figure 27–16. Tessier's transcranial hypertelorism procedure with resection of the cribriform plate.

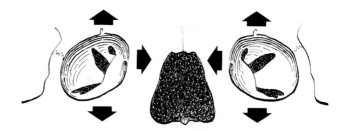

Figure 27-17. Tessier's THO procedure allows movements of the orbits in all necessary directions and also makes possible the correction of hypotelorism by lateralization of the orbits.

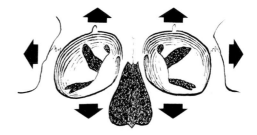

Neurosurgical Considerations

A transcranial procedure should be performed in collaboration with a neurosurgeon, especially when several malformations such as encephalomeningoceles or tumors such as neurofibromas are present. During elevation of the frontal lobe from the anterior cranial base, care should be taken not to damage the olfactory nerve filaments. Tessier's original hypertelorism procedure[8] includes the resection of the cribriform plate with the consequence of loss of olfaction (see Fig. 27-16). Soon they and others, such as Converse and colleagues[10] and Obwegeser and Farmand[11] attempted to preserve the cribriform plate by removing only a strip of bone laterally to the cribriform plate on each side (Fig. 27-19) to facilitate the rotation of the orbits. This is possible

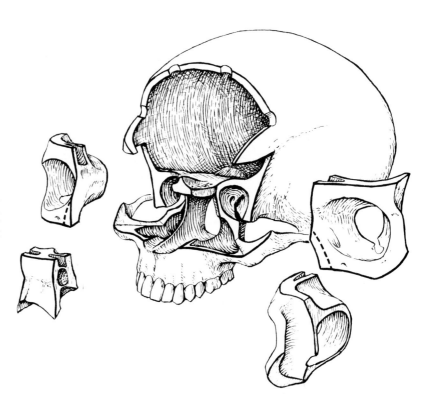

Figure 27-18. For three-dimensional understanding of the movements of the orbits, an explosion picture is presented. The cribriform plate in this picture is left in place but must be reduced or resected, as described in the next two figures.

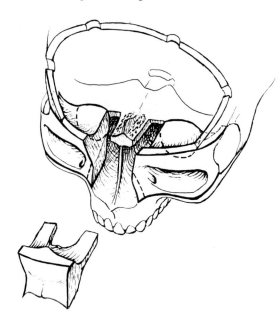

Figure 27–19. Transcranial hypertelorism procedure without resection of the cribriform plate. The osteotomy is performed laterally to the cribriform plate and allows medial orbital rotation (Converse method). This technique should be employed only in less severe cases.

only in cases of mild hypertelorism in which the cribriform plate is not too wide and especially not separated in the midline with dislocation of one or the other half. For severe cases, the authors have introduced their own method of preservation of the olfactory nerves[12, 13] by dissecting every nerve filament out of the cribriform plate (Fig. 27–20) to permit medial orbital rotation.

Ophthalmologic Aspects

As a member of the craniofacial team, the ophthalmologist is responsible for an extensive examination. It is important to recognize that all orbital movements can cause diplopia, especially in cases of hypertelorism in which binocular vision is present preoperatively. Experience indicates that when focusing was not possible

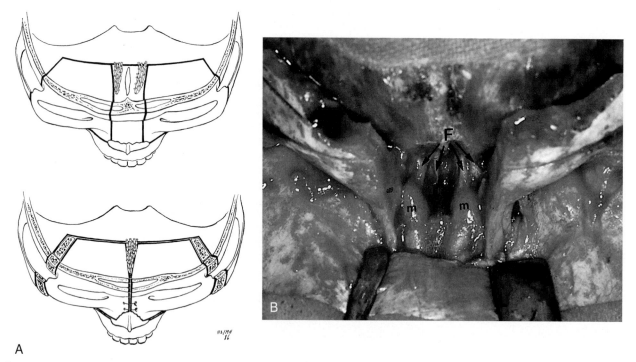

Figure 27–20. Sailer's transcranial hypertelorism procedure with resection of the cribriform plate but preservation of the olfactory nerve filaments (Sailer's method). The drawing (A) demonstrates nerve filaments assembled in the midline after orbital rotation (bottom); the intraoperative photograph (B) depicts the free filaments (F) running into the intact nasal mucosa (m).

preoperatively, the diplopia sometimes disappears after hypertelorism correction without further ophthalmologic measures.

Step-by-Step Procedure

1. The coronal approach is used; the skull, the orbital region, the nose, and the zygomatic area are dissected subperiosteally.

2. The anterior halves of the temporal muscles are elevated by freeing the temporal fossa.

3. The osteotomies and cranial bur holes are marked with methylene blue and bur lines (Fig. 27–21A,B).

4. The craniotomy is performed and the frontal bone removed (see Fig. 27–21C).

5. The frontal lobes of the brain are elevated, and the anterior cranial fossa and the cribriform plate are exposed as well as possible.

6. An osteotomy of the interorbital frontal and nasal bone (see Fig. 27–21D) is made, with preservation of the nasal mucosa. Now the access to the cribriform plate is free: With the use of magnifying glasses, the bone around the olfactory nerve filaments is removed (see Fig. 27–21E) with a mosquito clamp; this is usually necessary in the anterior and the lateral parts of the cribriform plate.

7. The ethmoids and the mucosal lining of the frontal sinus are removed.

8. A circular osteotomy of all orbital walls is made within the posterior part of the orbital pyramid just in front of the supraorbital fissure.

9. An osteotomy is made through the zygomatic complex.

10. The intraoral incision is made as described earlier, and the midface and the pyriform aperature are exposed subperiosteally.

11. A horizontal infraorbital connecting osteotomy is made between the zygomatic bone cut and the pyriform aperature; the osteotomy lies beneath the inferior turbinates.

12. Careful slow mobilization of both orbits is accomplished with the use of chisels.

13. A triangular bone piece along the pyriform aperature is removed to allow medial movements of the orbits without compromising the nasal airways.

14. Bur holes and wires are placed in the glabella region, and the orbits are slowly approximated by twisting the wires with direct control of the orbital contents and the olfactory nerve filaments. If bradycardia occurs because of compressing or pulling the orbital contents, mobilization is discontinued until normal heart rhythm returns. The process then continues.

15. The positions of the supraorbital and infraorbital rims are determined according to the preoperative planning, and lyophilized bone blocks are interpositioned into the defect. Adjustments of the orbital position can be made once the final position is achieved. The segments are fixed with wires, miniplates, or microplates.

16. Now the defects within the orbital walls are bridged with lyophilized cartilage slices, and those within the area of the cribriform plate are bridged with bone powder gained from the craniotomy plus lyophilized cartilage chips and bone morphogenetic proteins.

17. The frontal calvaria is then placed into the desired position, adapted by trimming edges, and fixed, preferably by wires (see Fig. 27–21F,G).

18. The temporal muscles are fully mobilized, advanced, and fixed to the lateral orbital walls and rims by sutures running through bur holes. The lateral canthal ligaments are now fixed into their new position through bur holes within the lateral orbital walls.

19. The surplus of skin in the nasal and forehead region is excised, preferably with the creation of a straight scar in the middle of the dorsum and the forehead (nasal reconstruction). When necessary, a forehead flap is harvested for construction of the columella and nasal tip.

20. Other nasal corrections are performed to achieve the best possible initial result (see Fig. 27–21G,H).

21. Two subgaleal Redon drains are placed under the temporal muscles on each side and led out through the *contralateral* retroauricular area.

22. Subcutaneous scalp stitches are placed, and the outer incision is closed by stapling.

23. The oral incision is closed with a continuous Supramid suture after additional miniplating or wiring of the infraorbital rim to its new position in relation to the maxilla.

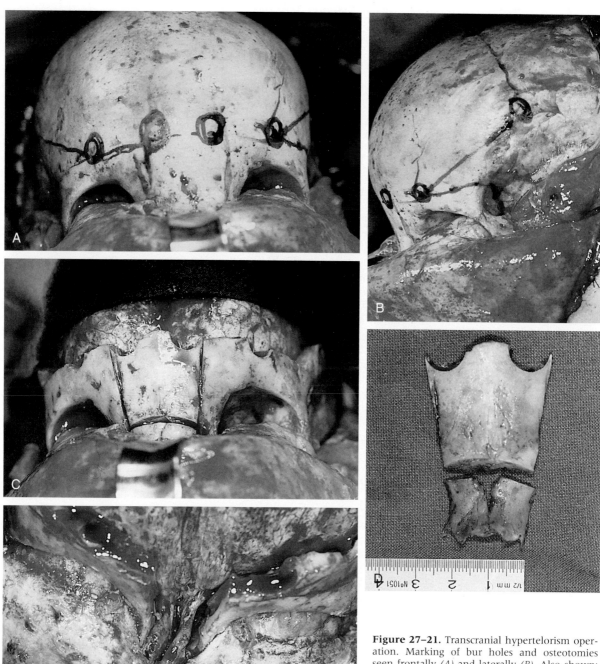

Figure 27–21. Transcranial hypertelorism operation. Marking of bur holes and osteotomies seen frontally *(A)* and laterally *(B)*. Also shown: removal of the frontal calvaria *(C)* and the interorbital bone structures *(D)*; freeing of the olfactory filaments *(E)*.

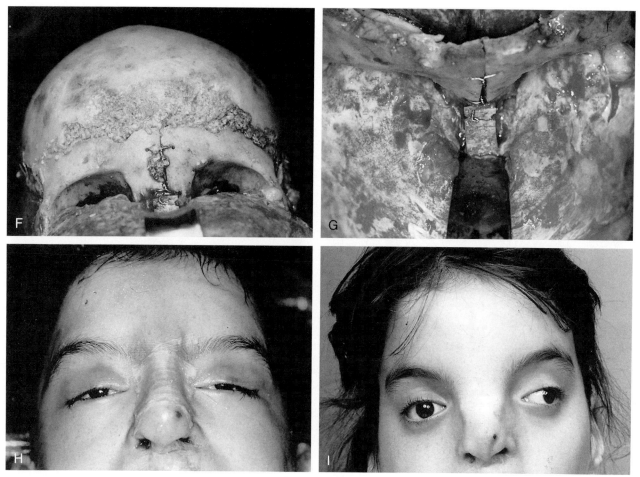

Figure 27-21. *Continued* and medial rotation and fixation of the orbits; the intraorbital osteotomies are clearly seen *(F)*. Nasal correction is by means of bone or lyocartilage struts *(G)* fixed by wires; at the end, a nasal acrylic stabilization dressing is applied *(H)*. *I*, preoperative condition of the same patient.

Remarks

When possible, the medial canthal ligaments are left in place in spite of the fact that this makes the intraorbital circular osteotomy more difficult. If the medial canthal ligaments require special movements, they are detached and placed into the correct position by twisted wires pulled through the approximated medial orbital walls to the opposite side and fixed there in the routine way.

The Facial Bipartition Procedure (Fig. 27-22)

This procedure is indicated in cases of cranial clefts No. 14 to 10 according to Tessier's classification[14] and also in cases of hypertelorism with "antimongoloid" orbital positions and an anterior open bite.

The procedure was initially described as facial bipartition[15-17] because both full halves of the face are mobilized, the orbits are tilted medially, and the dental arches are rotated downward. As a result of the downward rotation of the anterior maxilla, closure of the open bite occurs. The disadvantage is that the amount of the open bite influences the amount of the medial movements of the orbits. The same type of procedure had already been performed in the Department of Maxillofacial Surgery Zurich in 1970 in the famous case of Antonio, who presented with a double formation of the midface with two premaxillae and extreme hypertelorism.[18]

In the facial bipartition procedure, there is no infraorbital horizontal osteotomy. Instead, an osteotomy runs from the inferior orbital fissure through the posterior wall of the maxillary sinus into the pterygomaxillary junction, which is also separated. In addition, the zygomatic arch is dissected. The alveolar process is divided between both first incisors (if this is necessary), as is the whole palatal bone in the sagittal plane.

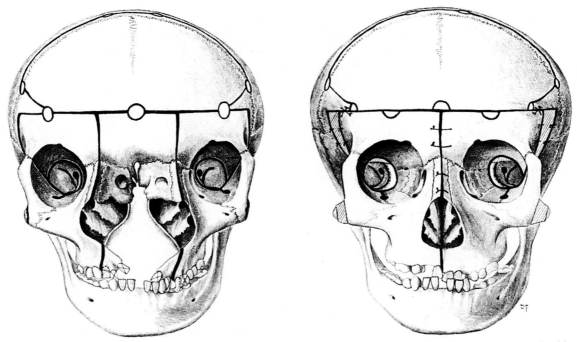

Figure 27–22. Facial bipartition, as it was performed in Zurich by Obwegeser in 1970 in the case of Antonio. No infraorbital horizontal osteotomy is performed; instead, an osteotomy is running from the infraorbital fissure through the posterior wall of the maxillary sinus to the pterygomaxillary junction, which is separated. (From Obwegeser HL, Weber G, Freihofer H-P, Sailer HF: Facial duplication—The unique case of Antonio. J Maxillofac Surg 1978; 6:179–198.)

After this, both halves of the face, including the orbits and the dentition, can be mobilized.

Combined Hypertelorism Operation and LeFort III Osteotomy
(Fig. 27–23)

Patients with some of the craniofacial syndromes (e.g., Crouzon and Apert syndromes) present with varying degrees of hypertelorism. Full correction of these syndromes therefore includes frontofacial advancement (forehead, orbital rims, zygomatic complex, and maxilla for occlusal correction) in combination with the normalization of the IOD.

The authors' original procedure for these cases includes the correction of the exorbitism together with the hypertelorism. It is most important in these patients that the intraorbital osteotomy is positioned not too far posteriorly but in the area of the largest circumference of the ocular globe. This makes it possible to advance the orbital walls, thus correcting the exorbitism as well as shifting the globes medially by approximation of the mobilized orbits. The reconstruction of the orbital walls is of great importance for ensuring the position of the globes. In order to move the zygomatic complex forward together with the maxilla, a connecting osteotomy is performed between the infraorbital fissure and the pterygomaxillary junction. The pteryoid plates are separated from the maxillary tuberosity. The zygomatic arch is osteotomized. Special care must be taken not to fracture the zygomatic complex during mobilization.

Important

If in cases of frontofacial advancement in combination with THO the circular intraorbital osteotomies are placed posteriorly as described for the routine THO, the eye globes are pulled forward with the optic nerves, and the protrusion of the eyes is not corrected.

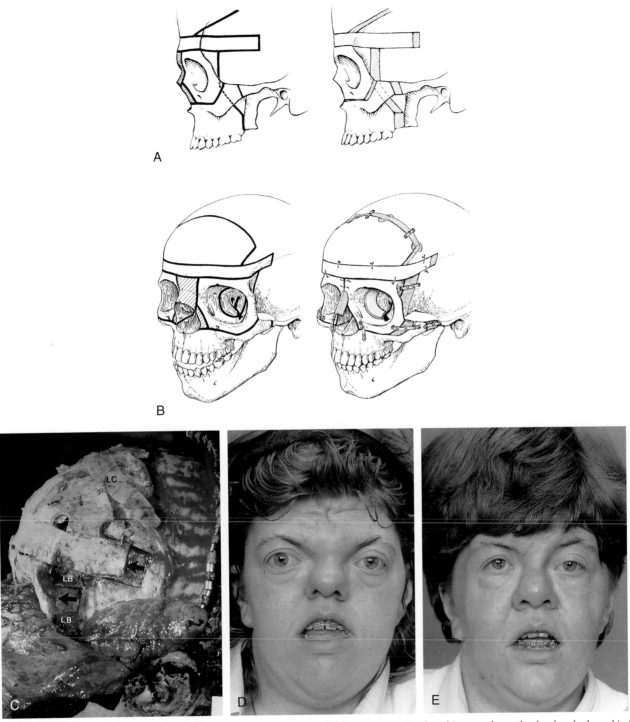

Figure 27–23. Combined THO and LeFort III osteotomy (frontofacial advancement). During this procedure, the forehead, the orbital rims, the zygomatic complex, and the dentition are advanced (A), and the orbits are simultaneously approximated. It is necessary to place the circular intraorbital osteotomies slightly farther forward (B) than in the routine hypertelorism correction. The defects within the frontal and parietal bones, the zygomatic bone, and the zygomatic arch are bridged by bone grafts (lyobone or autologous calvarial bone). Fixation is performed by miniplates and wiring. The intraoperative photograph (C) shows the amount of forward movement (arrows) of the forehead and orbits and the closure of the skull defect with lyocartilage (LC); also clearly visible is the stabilization of the orbital rims with lyobone (LB). The patient, who had Apert syndrome, is shown before (D) and after (E) this procedure.

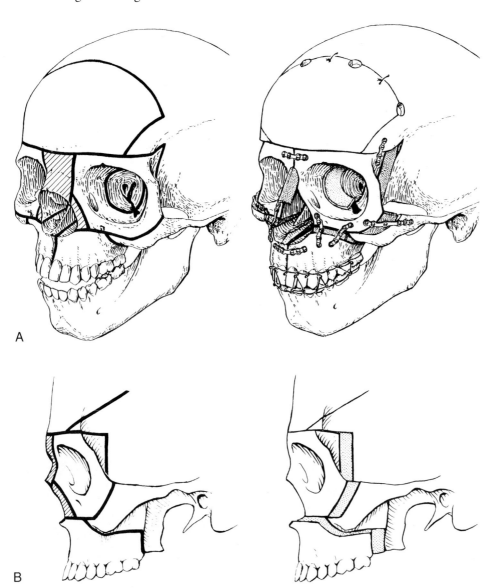

Figure 27–24. Combined THO and LeFort I osteotomy. The bone cut of the LeFort I osteotomy joins the infraorbital horizontal osteotomy. The upper jaw can be divided in the midline *(A)*. The procedure allows independent orbital and maxillary movements *(B)* and, at the same time, orbital approximation.

Combined Hypertelorism Operation and LeFort I Osteotomy
(Fig. 27–24)

The indication for this correction is hypertelorism and an occlusal disturbance, such as an open bite or class III occlusion, without the necessity to also advance the zygomatic complex (see Fig. 27–24A). A LeFort I osteotomy in one or more parts can be performed simultaneously with the THO. The whole zygomatic complex is then only "pedicled" to the zygomatic arch (see Fig. 27–24A,B).

If the orbits require advancement (see Fig. 27–25A), the circular intraorbital osteotomy should run more anteriorly than in the routine THO (as mentioned in the section "Combined Hypertelorism Operation and LeFort III Osteotomy"). Stabilization is accomplished by microplates and miniplates. Intermaxillary fixation is usually not necessary just during fixation of the segments by miniplates.

This procedure could also be used in cases of hypertelorism caused by a huge encephalocele extending to the oral cavity; in the patient shown in Figure 27–25, there was a palatal cleft with a width of 50 mm and a complete circular nonocclusion.

Nasal Reconstruction

Hypertelorism correction necessitates construction of the hard and soft nasal tissues. It is advisable to perform the best possible reconstruction of the nose simultaneously with the hypertelorism procedure; the patient will be grateful for this.

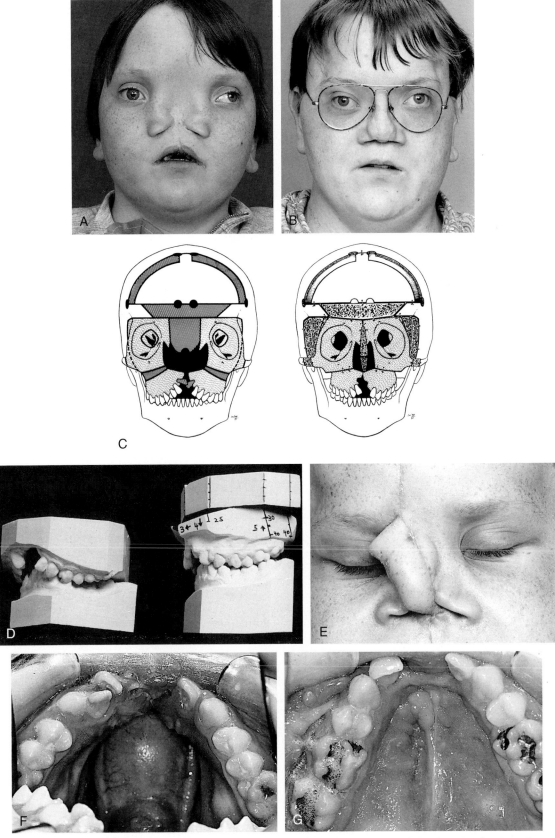

Figure 27–25. *A,* Monstrous hypertelorism with double nose formation caused by an encephalocele expanding into the oral cavity before correction; *B,* 10 years after correction. For correction of the nonocclusion, a bilateral LaFort I osteotomy was performed, and the maxillary segments were raised and narrowed according to the preoperative planning *(C)* and the model operation *(D).* Nasal reconstruction was achieved with a forehead flap *(E)* in combination with an L-shaped calvarial bone graft. The wide palatal cleft *(F)* that was narrowed by the LeFort I operation was closed in a second-stage procedure *(G)* with a cranially based pharyngeal flap. (From Sailer HF, Landolt AM: Hypertelorism with herniation of brain and pituitary gland into the oronasal cavity. *In* Marchac D [ed]: Craniofacial Surgery. Berlin: Springer, 1987.)

707

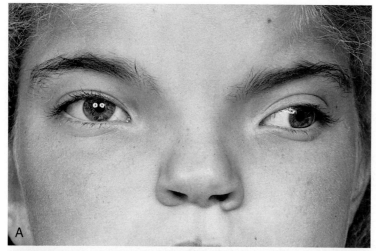

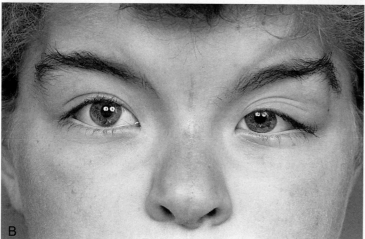

Figure 27–26. Patient with hypertelorism before *(A)* and after THO with median nasal scar *(B)*.

A new nasal dorsum is always constructed from homologous lyocartilage[19, 20] or calvarial bone, either of which is fixed to the lacrimal bone by wires. The surplus of skin in the glabella and the nasal area is excised, and this results in a midline scar running from the forehead along the nasal dorsum to the nasal tip. This scar is in most cases barely visible after some time and presents the best esthetic result (Fig. 27–26A,B). Less desirable is a Z-plasty in the area of the frontonasal angle, because the resulting scars are easily visible even if they are very fine. In cases of hypertelorism in which the dorsum and the columella are too short, good results are achieved with Sailer's original method of a caterpillar flap and a forked flap (Fig. 27–27; see also Fig. 27–3) or with their original intracolumellar forked-flap procedure (Fig. 27–28).

When the nasal tip and the columella require construction, the interorbital surplus of skin is used for a forehead flap, as in the patient shown in Figure 27–25, who had an encephalocele extending into the oral cavity. In cases of complex forms of hypertelorism combined with facial clefts (Fig. 27–29A; see also Fig. 27–6), a variety of nasal hard and soft tissue corrections are made in order to achieve an acceptable result in the first operation (see Fig. 27–29C,D). Additional revision, however, may be necessary.

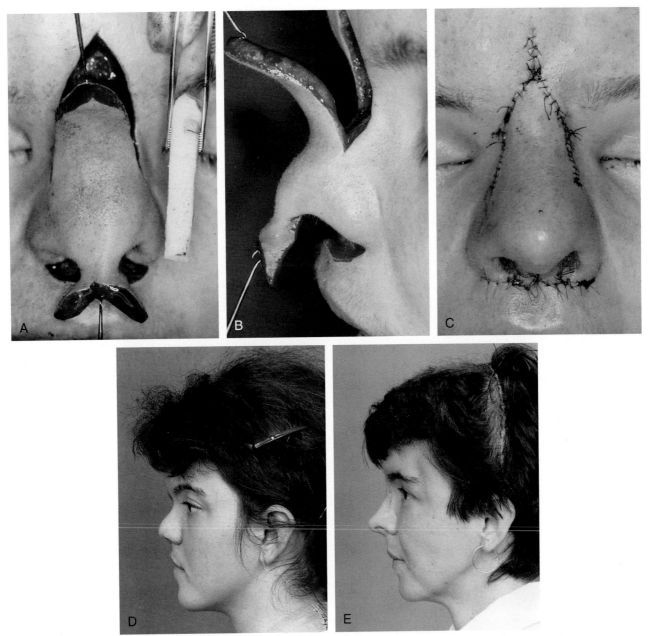

Figure 27–27. Sailer's method of increasing nasal length and projection. *A,* A caterpillar flap is designed along the dorsum, and a strut of lyocartilage is inserted. *B,* Blood supply is ensured over the nasal alae to the caterpillar flap and the columellar forked flap. *C,* Result after elongation of the dorsum and the columella. The result of this nasal and columellar elongation is seen in the profile of a patient with hypertelorism before *(D)* and after *(E)* surgery. The same patient is seen in Figure 27–3.

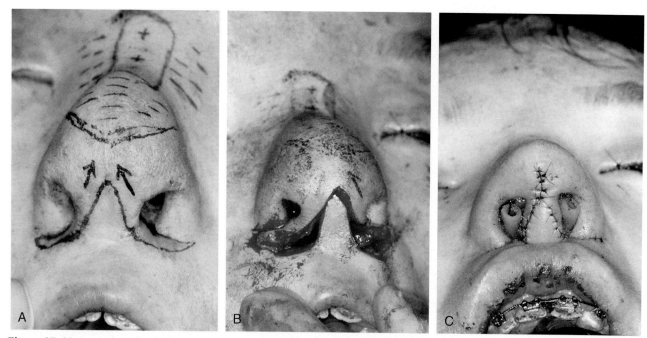

Figure 27–28. Intracolumellar forked-flap procedure (Sailer) in cases with a wide columella *(A).* The central part of the columella stays in place *(B);* the lateral parts plus the vestibular extensions move upward and give excellent tip projection *(C).*

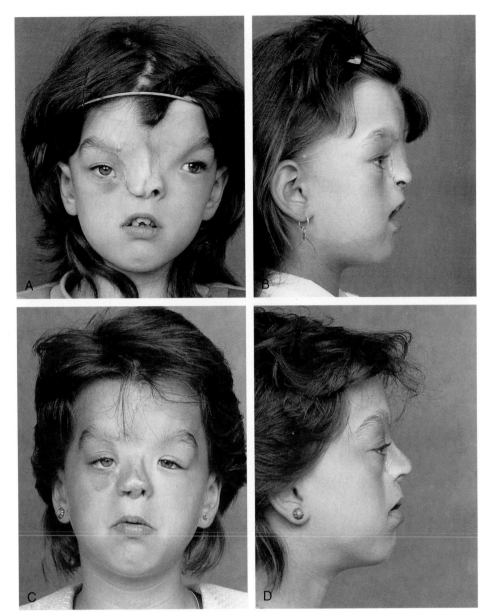

Figure 27–29. Asymmetric hypertelorism with several facial clefts *(A,B),* presenting a complex reconstructive nasal problem; the result *(C,D)* achieved in the first operation is acceptable, but revision is required.

RECONSTRUCTION MATERIAL IN CRANIOFACIAL SURGERY

All types of craniofacial surgery result in defects, and these must be filled or bridged by autologous or homologous hard tissue. Autologous split-thickness cranial bone is usually used.[2] Splitting of calvarial bone is possible only in older children and adults, not in infants. Splitting and forming the brittle calvarial bone is time consuming and prolongs surgery. In the authors' unit, the use of autologous bone in craniofacial surgery is obsolete. They have introduced and used for many years lyophilized homologous bone from different regions (sternum, calvaria, mandible, ribs, femur) as well as lyophilized homologous cartilage in craniomaxillofacial surgery.[19, 20] Since 1991, these materials have been combined with purified bovine bone morphogenetic proteins, which accelerate the incorporation of homologous lyophilized bone and cartilage.[21–23] Lyocartilage is the most suitable reconstructive material in craniofacial surgery. The lyocartilage from ribs is cut into slices by a dermatome. These slices are ideal for the reconstruction of the orbital walls as well as for the reconstruction of the cranial base (Fig. 27–30; see also Fig. 27–23C). The bridging of the defects within the zygomatic bone is also performed with lyophilized homologous calvarial bone (Fig. 27–31). Defects of the midface after the LeFort I operation are closed with

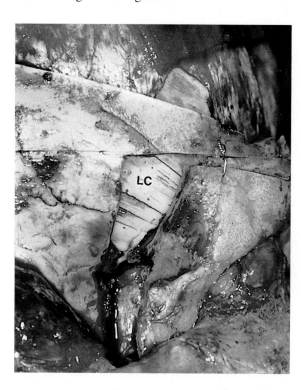

Figure 27–30. Reconstruction of the lateral anterior cranial base, using a slice of lyocartilage (LC).

Figure 27–31. Bridging a defect within the zygomatic complex after medial orbital rotation, using calvarial lyobone (LB).

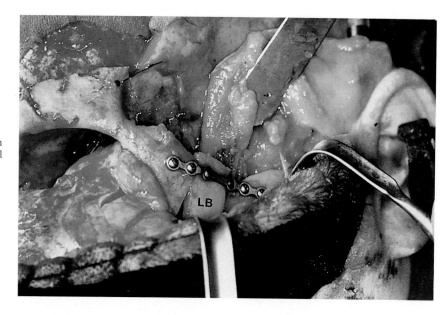

lyophilized sternum or iliac bone. The lyobones and the lyocartilage are loaded with bone morphogenic protein.

References

1. Tessier P: Experiences in treatment of orbital hypertelorism. Plast Reconst Surg 1974; 53:1–18.
2. Tessier P: Orbital hypertelorism: I. Successive surgical attempts; material and methods; causes and mechanisms. Scand J Plast Reconstr Surg 1972; 6:135–155.
3. Farkas LG, Kolar JC: Anthropometric guidelines in cranio-orbital surgery. Clin Plast Surg 1987; 14:1–16.
4. Sailer HF, Landolt AM: Treatment concepts for craniosynostosis and hypertelorism. *In* Pfeifer G (ed): Craniofacial Abnormalities and Clefts of the Lip, Alveolus and Palate, p 102. New York: Thieme, 1991.
5. Enlow DH: Handbook of Facial Growth, p 64. Philadelphia: WB Saunders, 1975.
6. Muhlbauer W, Anderl H, Ramatsch P, et al: Radical treatment of craniofacial anomalies in infancy and the use of miniplates in craniofacial surgery. Clin Plastic Surg 1987; 14:101–111.
7. McCarthy LG, La Trenta GS, Breitbart AS, et al: Hypertelorism correction in the young child. Plast Reconstr Surg 1990; 86:214–228.
8. Tessier P, Guiot G, Rougerie J, et al: Osteotomies cranio-naso-orbito-faciales hypertelorism. Ann Chir Plast 1967; 12:103–118.
9. Locher MC, Sailer HF: The use of the cell saver in transoral maxillofacial surgery: A preliminary report. J Maxillofac Surg 1992; 20:14.
10. Converse JM, Rassohoff J, Mathews ES, et al: Ocular hypertelorism and pseudohypertelorism: Advances in surgical treatment. Plast Reconstr Surg 1970; 45:1–13.
11. Obwegeser HL, Farmand M: Hypertelorbitism associated with other facial anomalies. *In* Caronni EP (ed): Craniofacial Surgery, pp 166–175. Boston: Little, Brown, 1985.
12. Sailer HF, Landolt AM: A new method for the correction of hypertelorism with preservation of the olfactory filaments. J Maxillofac Surg 1987; 3:122.
13. Sailer HF, Landolt AM: Hypertelorism with herniation of brain and pituitary gland into the oronasal cavity. *In* Marchac D (ed): Craniofacial Surgery. Berlin: Springer, 1987.
14. Tessier P: Anatomical classification of facial, craniofacial, and laterofacial clefts. J Maxillofac Surg 1976; 4:69.
15. Van der Meulen JC: Medial faciotomy. Br J Plast Surg 1979; 32:339.
16. Ortiz Monasterio F, Fuente del Campo A, Carillo A: Advancement of the orbit and the midface in one piece, combined with frontal repositioning for the correction of Crouzon deformity. Plast Reconstr Surg 1978; 61:507–516.
17. Oritz-Monasterio F, Media O, Musolas A: Geometrical planning for the correction of orbital hypertelorism. Plast Reconstr Surg 1990; 86(4):650–657.
18. Obwegeser HL, Weber G, Freihofer H-P, Sailer HF: Facial duplication—The unique case of Antonio. J Maxillofac Surg 1978; 6:179–198.
19. Sailer HF: Lyophilized Cartilage in Maxillo-Facial Surgery: Experimental Foundations and Clinical Success [Monograph]. Basel: Karger, 1983.
20. Sailer HF: Longterm results after implantation of different lyophilized bones and cartilage for reconstruction in craniofacial surgery. *In* Montoya AG (ed): Craniofacial Surgery, pp 69–72. Bologna: Monduzzi, 1992.
21. Sailer HF, Kolb E: Application of purified bone morphogenetic protein (BMP) preparations in cranio-maxillo-facial surgery: I. BMP in compromised surgical reconstructions using titanium implants. J Craniomaxillofac Surg 1994; 22:2–11.
22. Sailer HF, Kolb E: Application of purified bone morphogenetic protein (BMP) preparations in cranio-maxillo-facial surgery: II. Reconstruction in craniofacial malformations and posttraumatic or operative defects of the skull with lyophilized cartilage and BMP. J Craniomaxillofac Surg 1994; 22:191–199.
23. Kolb E, Sailer HF: Purification and application of bone morphogenetic protein: Preliminary clinical results. J Craniomaxillofac Surg 1992; 20(Suppl I):49–50.

Rhinoplasty for the Cleft Nasal Deformity

28

Clark O. Taylor

INTRODUCTION

Repair of the cleft nasal deformity has evolved with numerous methods of repair advocated over time. The diversity of approaches is testimonial to the enormous challenge and complexity of the problem. The current literature is inundated with papers describing additional modifications for correction. The basic pathology involved in the formation of the cleft nose deformity remains incompletely understood and, therefore, a significant challenge continues to exist when addressing the functional and cosmetic concerns of the cleft nose. This chapter focuses on the cleft nasal deformity and methods of improving it.

ANATOMIC CHARACTERISTICS

The aberration in normal anatomy of the cleft nose includes the lower lateral cartilages, upper lateral cartilages, and nasal dorsum, nasal septum, maxillary crest, vomer, columella, premaxilla, pyriform rim, as well as the sesamoid cartilages. Compounding the aberrant anatomy of the cleft nose is the almost universal finding of maxillary deficiency, especially in the paranasal regions. The recognition of maxillary deficiency in this population is critical because without adequate underlying structural support, even a perfectly shaped nose appears distorted and disproportionate relative to other facial features. This underscores the importance of adequately restoring the deficient maxillary tissues prior to or during cleft rhinoplastic surgery.

The deficiency and asymmetry of the pyriform rim in the cleft population accentuates the flattening and widening of the alar base on the cleft side. To fully correct the alar base deformity, it is necessary to restore the underlying deficient pyriform rim to provide adequate nasal support. If the maxilla, in addition, is deficient in projection or is asymmetric, it is impossible to establish adequate nasal projection relative to other facial features without reconstructing the underlying skeletal deficiency. When present, maxillary deficiency is addressed by maxillary advancement with additional grafting of the deficient nasal spine. Once this is accomplished, nasal projection may be reconstructed more appropriately, using the normalized skeletal base. Advancement of the deficient maxilla also improves lip support and allows the surgeon to more effectively restore lip symmetry and fullness.

The major clinical findings that reflect the anatomic abnormalities in the cleft nose consist of the following (Fig. 28–1A,B):

1. Displacement (posteriorly, laterally, and inferiorly) and malformation of the lower lateral cartilage on the cleft side
2. Caudal septum displacement toward the normal side following the deflection of the anterior nasal spine
3. Broad and flattened nasal tip, especially on the cleft side
4. Displacement of the alar base attachment laterally
5. Widened nostril on the cleft side with flattening of the "nasal wing"
6. Shortened columella on the cleft side
7. Bifid nasal tip because of increased interdomal width
8. Widened upper lateral nasal cartilages

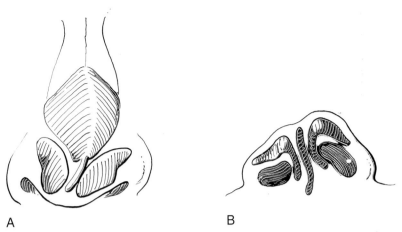

Figure 28–1. Frontal (*A*) and basal (*B*) views of the nose depicting the anatomic abnormalities associated with unilateral cleft nose. Unilateral cleft nose including displacement of the lower lateral cartilages on the cleft side; displacement of caudal septum; broad and flattened nasal tip; displacement of alar base attachment laterally; widened nostril on cleft side; shortened columella on cleft side; bifid nasal tip; widened upper lateral nasal cartilages.

HISTORY OF CLEFT NOSE RECONSTRUCTION

In 1898, Jacques Joseph described reduction of the nasal dorsum with minor revision of the alar cartilage.[1] Shortly thereafter, attention to the problems of the cleft nasal tip began to appear. Rethi and Gilles, in 1929 and 1932, respectively, described an open approach for reconstruction of the cleft nasal tip[2,3] (Fig. 28–2). In 1938, Humby described an operation to augment the tip by transposing the alar cartilage from the noncleft to the cleft side[4] (Fig. 28–3). Byars, in 1947, used the medial crus on the cleft side to accomplish the same outcome[5] (Fig. 28–4). Figi, in 1952, described the "baby flying bird incision" for access to the lower lateral cartilage[6] (Fig. 28–5). Erich described the "flying bird incision" with suturing of the domes to effect tip narrowing[7] (Fig. 28–6). In 1954, Potter modified the Gilles incision described in 1932 and added V-Y advancement of the columella[8] (Fig. 28–7). In 1956, Gelbke modified Figi's incision to include excision of excess dorsal nasal skin[9] (Fig. 28–8). Bardach, in 1967, modified Potter's incision to the skin from the cleft side into the columella[10] (Fig. 28–9). In 1970, Spira introduced a V-shaped modification of the flying bird incision to trim excess nostril skin on the cleft side[11] (Fig. 28–10).

In 1982, Goodman described a butterfly incision with a central notch[12] (Fig. 28–11). Nishimura in 1980 and Cronin in 1988 described their unique approaches.[13,14] Nishimura advanced the alar cartilage on the cleft side by freeing it from the underlying nasal mucosa and mobilized it medially to equalize the domes. Cronin described a mucochondral flap that included the underlying nasal mucosa to advance the cartilage on the cleft side. He closed the defect utilizing a V-Y–plasty.

Many other approaches have been described to address the cleft nasal problem, but the majority of these descriptions are modifications of the previously described procedures.

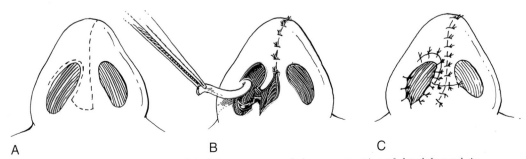

Figure 28–2. *A* to *C*, Gilles and Rethi's open approach for reconstruction of the cleft nasal tip.

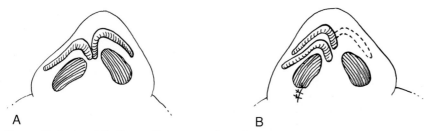

Figure 28–3. *A* and *B,* Alar cartilage transposition for reconstruction of the cleft nasal tip.

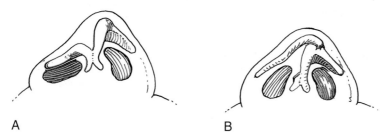

Figure 28–4. *A* and *B,* Byars transposition of the medial crus on the cleft side to accomplish tip augmentation.

Figure 28–5. Figi's "baby flying bird incision."

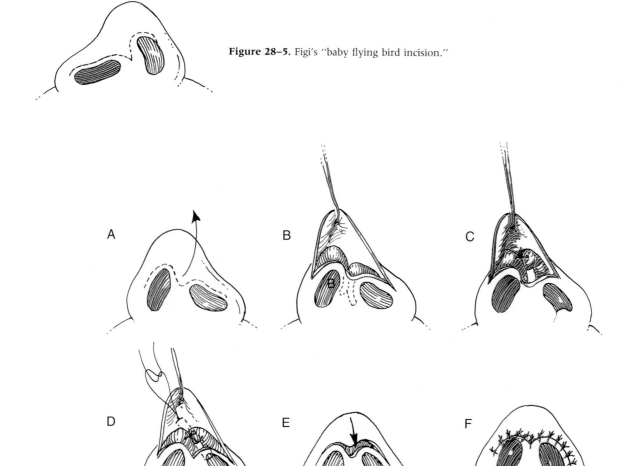

Figure 28–6. *A* to *F,* Erich's "flying bird incision" with suturing of the domes for cleft tip augmentation and narrowing.

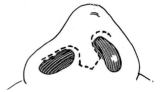

Figure 28–7. Potter's V columellar incision incorporated a V-Y advancement of the columellar skin for lengthening.

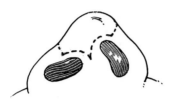

Figure 28–8. Gelbke's modification of Figi's incision to include an excision of excessive dorsal nasal skin.

Figure 28–9. Bardach's modification of Potter's incision to include advancement of skin from the cleft side into the columella.

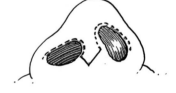

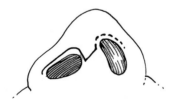

Figure 28–10. Spira's V-shaped modification of the "flying bird incision" to trim excess nostril skin on the cleft side.

Figure 28–11. Goodman's butterfly incision with a central notch.

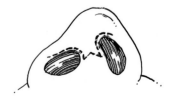

TIMING OF SURGERY

Early surgery for improvement of the nasal tip before cessation of growth is advocated. Many patients with clefts present for improvement of nasal deformities during adolescence or early adulthood before complete maturation. Weighing the psychosocial benefits of rhinoplastic surgery against the potential untoward growth effects must be done with the patient and parent included in the decision making. Although it is biologically sound to delay nasal reconstruction until complete maturation, the extent of deformation and its impact on socialization are important considerations in the timing of rhinoplasty, especially in the cleft population.

During primary unilateral lip closure, repositioning the alar cartilage on the cleft side, as suggested by McComb,[15] has the advantage of immediate cosmetic improvement and the potential for long-term growth benefits. The bilateral cleft lip nasal deformity may also be operated on early to minimize the stigma of the problem. However, several stages of nasal reconstruction are required in the bilateral cleft. Growth and development of the nasal complex do not appear to be adversely affected with these cartilage manipulation procedures, even when they are performed during primary lip closure.

PRINCIPLES OF CLEFT RHINOPLASTY

In general, it is desirable to correct all underlying skeletal deficiencies prior to nasal reconstruction whenever possible. In the adolescent and adult, maxillary advancement and contouring should precede definitive rhinoplastic surgery. In those patients who opt for early intervention nasal reconstructive surgery before maxillary reconstruction is indicated, full reconstruction of the underlying skeletal deficiency may not be possible. Future skeletal reconstruction in the form of osteotomies and/or augmentation bone grafting may further enhance the results. In all patients choosing early interventive nasal reconstructive surgery, the possibility of additional nasal surgery should be discussed, as should the importance of future normalization of their skeleton. Frequently, cleft nasal reconstruction is undertaken at the time of osseous reconstruction of the alveolar cleft. In these cases, onlay grafting of the deficient pyriform rim is simultaneously employed to optimize the symmetry of the nasal reconstruction.

Critical observation of previous results using traditional closed rhinoplastic techniques in the cleft population demonstrates an almost universal inability to fully correct the deformities associated with the cleft nose. Indeed, the nose frequently retains the major characteristics associated with the cleft nasal deformity. In large part, this is because of inability to visualize and fully correct the affected components of the nose. Using open rhinoplasty techniques, the operator immediately and clearly visualized the interrelationships of all deformed components of the nose. This allows more precise intraoperative treatment planning as well as more precise repositioning of the abnormal nasal structures.

The utilization of autogenous cartilaginous grafting, ideally obtained from the nasal septum, is recommended to obtain stable and symmetric reconstruction of the supporting elements of the nose. In addition, adequate nasal projection is difficult to achieve in the cleft nose without the utilization of augmentation grafts. Through the open rhinoplasty approach, grafted material can be precisely positioned and secured. Autogenous cartilage is readily available from the nasal septum, which is uniformly deviated to the cleft side and must be straightened to improve symmetry. In those cases in which septal cartilage is not available, Conchal cartilage is used. Conchal cartilage, because of its embryologic origin, is more brittle than septal cartilage and care must be taken in its manipulation.

The disadvantages of the open approach are the transcolumellar scar as well as slightly prolonged edema of the nose secondary to the widespread degloving. The transcolumellar scar is rarely noticeable and has never been a source of patient complaint. The prolonged tip edema is easily managed with subcutaneous steroid (Kenalog) injections when indicated. Visualization and precision maneuvering of cartilage and graft materials are the major advantages of the open rhinoplasty technique, and these far outweigh the relative disadvantages noted above.

The open rhinoplasty technique facilitates complete reconstruction of the cleft nasal deformity. The following are treatment goals: (1) maximizing nasal tip support by the utilization of the columellar strut graft placed between the medial crura and extending to just superior to the nasal spine; (2) cephalic volume reduction and sculpting of both lower lateral cartilages as needed; (3) advancement of the lower lateral cartilage on the cleft side with or without dome division to establish domal congruity and symmetry; (4) maximizing tip anatomy and projection utilizing autogenous onlay and/or shield tip grafts; (5) narrowing of the nasal dorsum by osteotomies, onlay grafting, or both; and (6) establishment of alar base symmetry using skeletal onlay grafts as well as alar base surgery to narrow the widened alar base component.

Mobilization of the lower lateral cartilage on the cleft side is usually accomplished by a mucochondral flap. The underlying vestibular mucosa remains attached to the cartilage to permit reconstruction of the collapsed nasal valve on the cleft side, as well as to prevent dead space between the advanced cartilage and the underlying vestibular mucosa. Advancement of cartilage alone leaves dead space between the cartilage and mucosa, which fills with scar tissue and frequently results in swelling and closure of the nasal valve on the cleft side. It is for this reason that the vestibular mucosa is included in the cartilaginous advancement, as described in the following technique section.

SURGICAL TECHNIQUE

The techniques described include a combination of those of Nishimura, Cronin, Johnson, and Sheen.[13, 14, 16, 17] Before the formal nasal reconstruction, the septal deformity must be corrected. Through a modified Killian incision, the septum is visualized and enough cartilage is removed to fabricate a columellar strut, tip graft, and, if necessary, a dorsal-only graft. Manipulation of the septum relative to the existing septal deformity is simultaneously performed. This may include excising areas of septal curvature or weakening the cartilage and straightening those sections exhibiting deformity. The intranasal incision is closed and attention directed to the formal nasal reconstruction via the external approach.

The columellar incision, as described by Potter,[8] permits complete skeletonization of the nose (Fig. 28–12). A vestibular incision on the cleft side is made continuous with the marginal incisions, and it outlines the border of the lateral crura (Fig. 28–13). Exposure is completed and the lateral crura on the cleft side is completely freed by incising through the nasal mucosa. This complex is mobilized as a medially based flap (Fig. 28–14). The cleft alar cartilage is advanced medially along with its nasal lining to establish domal congruity. The alar cartilage may be weakened by incising to facilitate domal curvature at the desired location relative to the adjacent normal dome (Fig. 28–15). An interdomal suture and a columellar strut of septal cartilage are

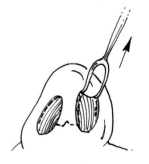

Figure 28–12. Modification of Potter's columellar incision is used for open approach to the nose. If columellar lengthening is needed, a modified "flying bird" incision is used.

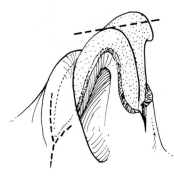

Figure 28–13. The columellar incision is connected to the marginal incision on both sides. On the cleft side, an intercartilaginous incision is joined at the hinge region of the lower lateral cartilage to mobilize the lateral crura on the cleft side.

Figure 28–14. The lateral crura on the cleft side is completely mobilized from the overlying cutaneous skin drape to allow medial rotation of the collapsed cleft dome.

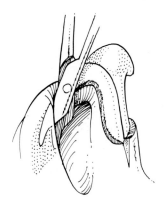

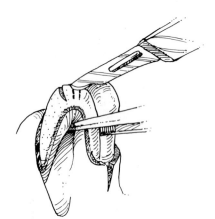

Figure 28–15. The dome is scored, morsalized, or divided to effect domal narrowing and congruity on the cleft side. The location of the weakening is determined relative to the adjacent normal dome.

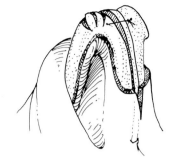

Figure 28–16. An interdomal suture and columellar strut of septal cartilage is employed to secure domal projection.

utilized to enhance domal projection (Fig. 28–16). This columellar strut is positioned just superior to the nasal spine, between the medial crura and extending to the tip-defining point. The strut is secured with horizontal mattress Vicryl sutures to the adjacent medial crura. Cephalic volume reduction of both lower lateral cartilages is performed to achieve symmetry, narrowing, and elevation of the tip, as needed. A tip graft of septal cartilage is routinely employed to project and define nasal tip anatomy. It is critical to structure this graft with beveled edges and to secure it with sutures to the underlying cartilaginous framework to prevent distortion and movement of the graft during healing (Fig. 28–17). Dorsal augmentation and/or reduction are used to narrow the dorsum and to form an appropriate supratip break. The cleft nose usually exhibits a wide nasal dorsum with or without overprojection. Narrowing the dorsal complex is required in almost all instances and can be achieved by either augmentation grafting, hump reduction along with medial and lateral osteotomies, or a combination of both.

V-Y closure of the mucosal defect resulting from the medial rotation of the lower lateral cartilage on the cleft side follows (Fig. 28–18). A buccal mucosal graft is utilized only when distortion of the alar rim from primary internal mucosal closure is observed.

Stable and satisfactory cosmetic and functional results have been observed utilizing the above technique. In addition to the described maneuvers affecting the underlying nasal skeleton, the tip and supratip skin are routinely thinned from the undersurface to allow more precise definition of tip anatomy. The utilization of ancillary procedures such as Weir excisions to effect alar base narrowing are employed along with the primary rhinoplasty, or they can be delayed and performed secondarily. The decision to augment or reduce the nasal dorsum is based upon the individual characteristics of the nose. Simultaneous augmentation of the pyriform rim on the cleft side is also a necessary maneuver to improve symmetry if this has not been performed previously. In the adolescent in need of lip revision, simultaneous lip/nose reconstruction is advocated and readily performed.

It is emphasized that precise reconstruction of the alar base on the cleft side is not possible in most instances without augmenting the deficient pyriform aperture. In many cases orthognathic correction of underlying facial skeletal imbalance is a prerequisite to maximize the cosmetic and functional results of cleft nasal reconstruction.

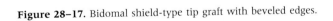

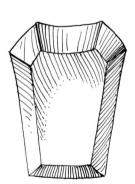

Figure 28–17. Bidomal shield-type tip graft with beveled edges.

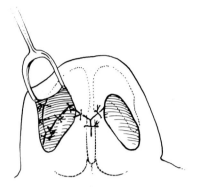

Figure 28–18. V-Y closure of a mucosal defect resultant from medial rotation of lateral crus and V-Y advancement of columellar skin.

CORRECTION OF THE BILATERAL CLEFT LIP/NOSE

In correcting the bilateral cleft nose deformity, the surgeon is rarely dealing with a situation in which there is excess tissue. The challenge is to rearrange and use all existing tissue, normal and cicatrix, rather than discarding it. Correction of the short columella, as seen in all bilateral cleft noses, should be completed at an early age (before school) to avoid ridicule by peers and to improve nasal breathing.

Virtually all cases of bilateral cleft nose deformity necessitate columellar lengthening, as well as narrowing of the nostril floor. Many techniques to lengthen the columella have been described, and the exact technique used depends upon the need for simultaneous lengthening of the philtrum of the lip and the position of existing scars. To lengthen the columella, tissue can be obtained from either the prolabium or the floor of the nose. Millard's forked-flap technique employs tissue from the lip scar to advance into the nostril floor and nasal sill area[18] (Fig. 28–19). The technique allows for columellar lengthening as well as simultaneous narrowing of the alar base

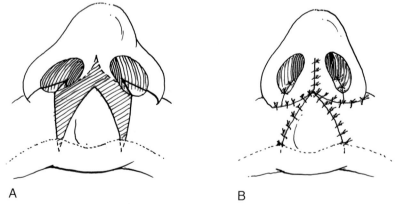

A   B

Figure 28–19. *A* and *B*, Millard forked-flap technique for lengthening columella and simultaneous alar base narrowing in bilateral cleft nose deformities.

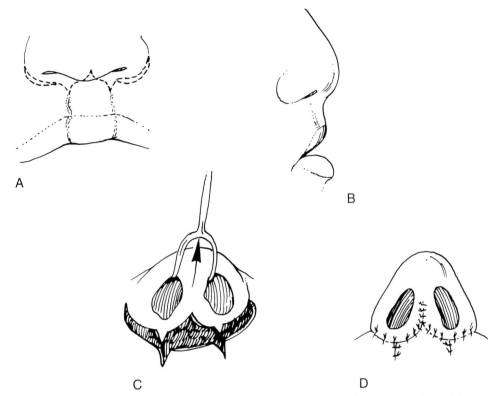

Figure 28–20. *A* to *D*, Brown and McDowell's V-Y advancement in the center of the prolabium with additional lateral wings along the nostril floor for narrowing of alar bases and lengthening of columella.

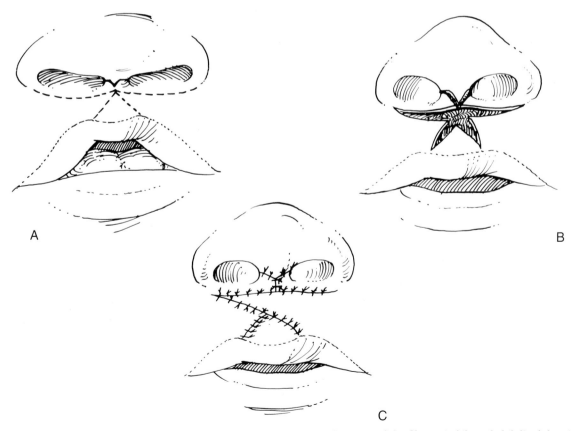

Figure 28–21. *A* to *C*, Bilateral crossover flaps for lengthening of the central portion of the filtrum in bilateral cleft lip deformity. This technique can be combined with either a Cronin or a V-Y advancement columellar incision for lengthening of such simultaneously.

while not imposing any new scars on the lip. The incisions can be extended to permit visualization of the lower lateral cartilages if done in conjunction with simultaneous rhinoplasty. Cronin described a bilobed incision along the alar base and below the nostril sill into which tissue may be advanced onto the columella.[19] Brown and McDowell describe a V-Y advancement in the center of the prolabium with additional lateral wings being developed along the nostril floor[20] (Fig. 28–20). Both of these approaches can also be extended to include complete visualization of the lower lateral cartilages if simultaneous open rhinoplasty is required. The general principles include bilateral mucochondral flaps with advancement of both lower lateral cartilages to effect domal projection. Frequently, buccal mucosal grafts are required rather than V-Y closures because of the inherent tissue deficiency.

In those cases in which simultaneous lengthening of the prolabium is required, tissue must be advanced into the area of the prolabium from the lateral lip. In these cases, bilateral crossover flaps are advanced into the midportion of the lip to allow lengthening of the prolabium while simultaneously permitting lengthening of the columella and narrowing of the alar base (Fig. 28–21).

CASE STUDIES

Case 1

A 14-year-old presented with a history of unilateral cleft lip and associated nasal deformity. The patient requested correction and was treated with an open septorhinoplasty using cartilaginous septal strut and autogenous septal cartilage shield tip grafts. Medial and lateral osteotomies were used to narrow the nose. Cephalic volume reduction of the lower lateral cartilages was performed bilaterally leaving a 5- to 6-mm intact strip, and the alar cartilage on the cleft side was advanced as a mucochondral flap (Figs. 28–22 to 28–26).

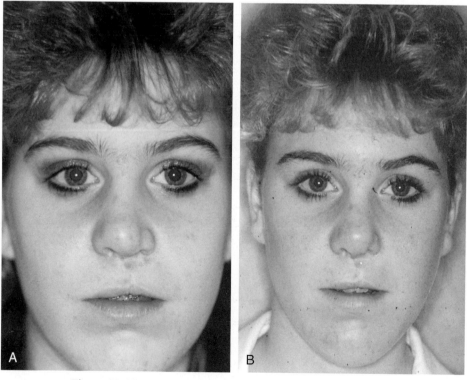

Figure 28–22. Preoperative (*A*) and postoperative (*B*) frontal views.

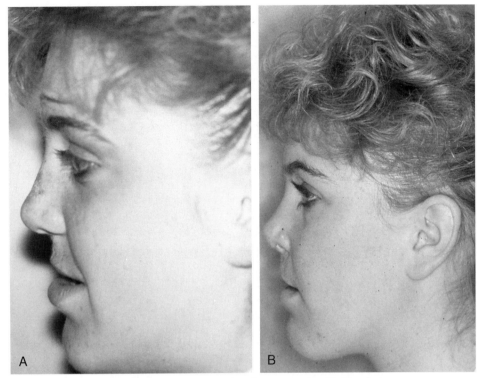

Figure 28–23. Preoperative (*A*) and postoperative (*B*) lateral views.

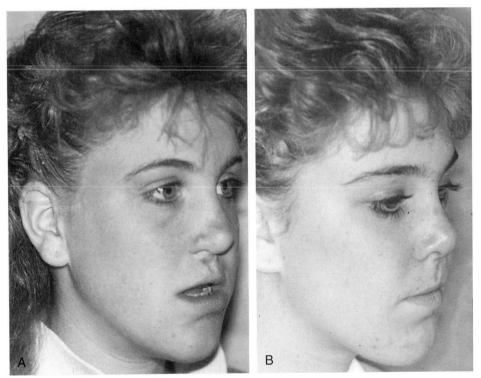

Figure 28–24. Preoperative (*A*) and postoperative (*B*) oblique views.

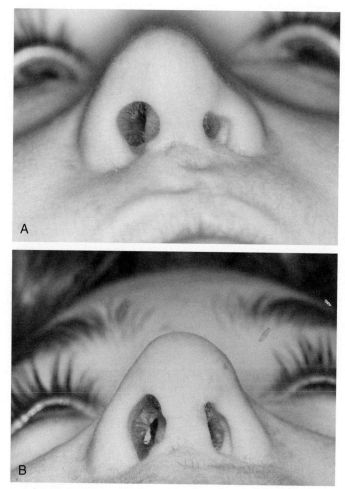

Figure 28–25. Preoperative (*A*) and postoperative (*B*) basal views.

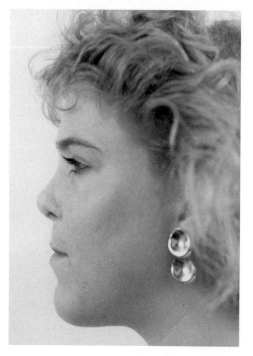

Figure 28–26. Five-year postoperative results showing good long-term stability utilizing open restructuring rhinoplasty. There have been no observed unfavorable effects on continued facial growth.

Case 2

A 13-year-old presented with cleft nose deformity treated with a procedure similar to that in Case 1. More aggressive weakening (by incising) of the domal region of the lower lateral cartilages was employed in this case to effect further tip narrowing. In addition, the existing scar was used to skeletonize the nose. The patient underwent secondary augmentation of the pyriform rim employing hydroxylapatite block. This case illustrates the importance of constructing adequate skeletal support for the nose (Figs. 28–27 to 28–30).

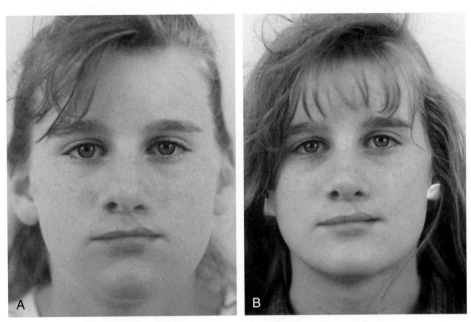

Figure 28–27. Preoperative (*A*) and postoperative (*B*) frontal views.

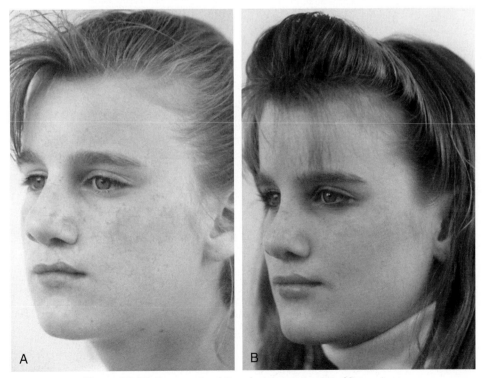

Figure 28–28. Preoperative (*A*) and postoperative (*B*) oblique views.

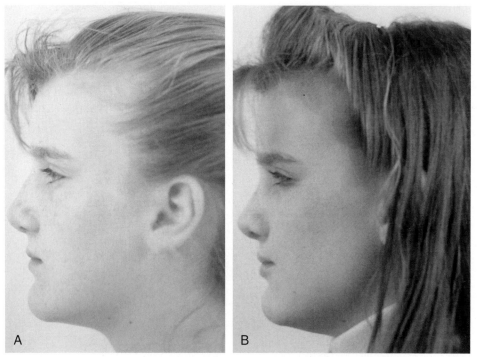

Figure 28–29. Preoperative (A) and postoperative (B) lateral views.

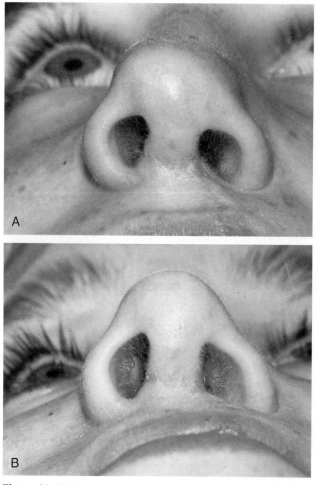

Figure 28–30. Preoperative (A) and postoperative (B) basal views.

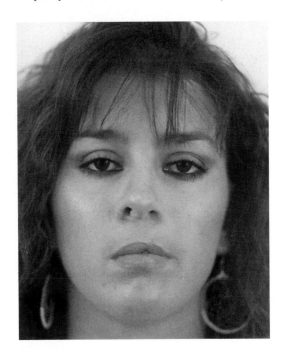

Figure 28–31. Preoperative frontal view.

Case 3

A 24-year-old presented with a chief complaint of cleft lip/nose deformity. Treatment consisted of open septorhinoplasty with simultaneous lip revision and reconstitution of the orbicularis muscle to eliminate a "whistle" deformity. This patient exhibited disarticulation of the medial crural footplates from the caudal edge of the nasal septum, resulting in some obstruction of nasal airflow. In addition, asymmetry of the nasal base was noted in part owing to the failure of the previous lip repair to approximate the orbicularis muscle and lend support to the ala on the cleft side. This patient underwent tip reconstruction using bilateral cephalic volume reductions along with autogenous septal cartilage shield tip graft. Flared medial crural footplates were narrowed with a horizontal mattress suture of 6–0 nylon placed submucosally as well as conservative trimming of the footplates themselves. The alar base symmetry was achieved with bilateral Weir excisions (Figs. 28–31 to 28–40).

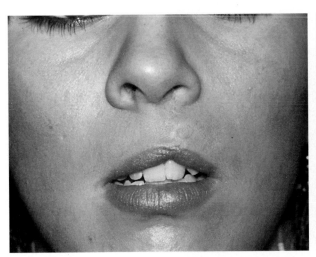

Figure 28–32. Close-up preoperative frontal view.

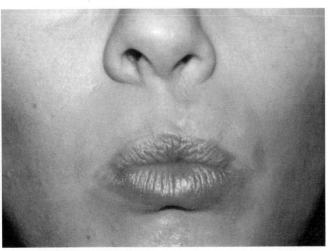

Figure 28–33. Functional preoperative close-up.

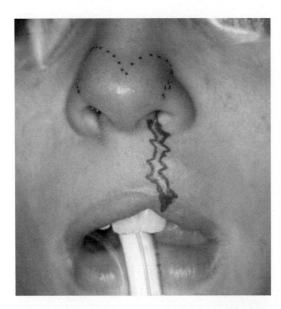

Figure 28–34. Incisions for lip revision simultaneous open rhinoplasty.

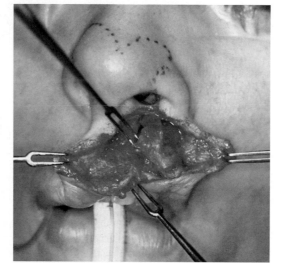

Figure 28–35. Orbicularis dissected free with reanastomosis across the midline of the cleft.

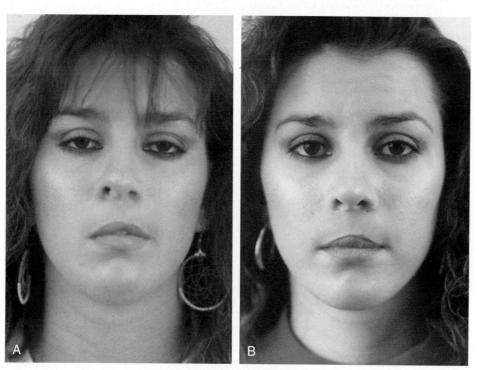

Figure 28–36. Preoperative (*A*) and postoperative (*B*) frontal views.

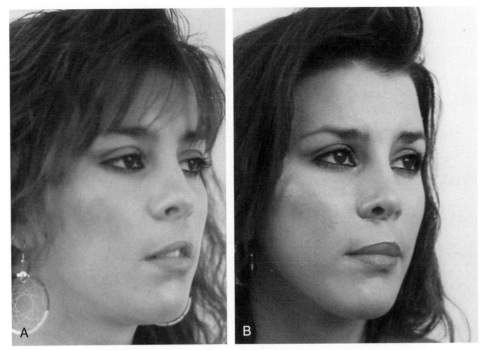

Figure 28–37. Preoperative (*A*) and postoperative (*B*) oblique views.

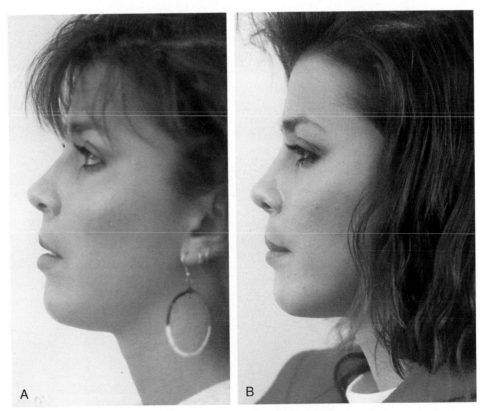

Figure 28–38. Preoperative (*A*) and postoperative (*B*) lateral views.

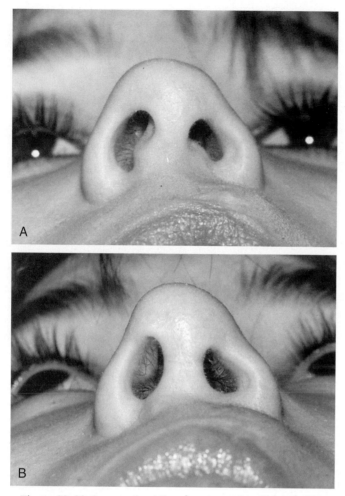

Figure 28–39. Preoperative (*A*) and postoperative (*B*) basal views.

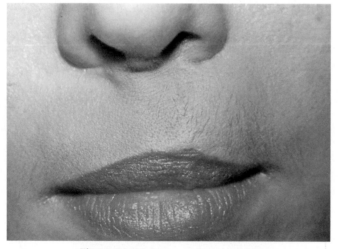

Figure 28–40. Postoperative view of lip.

Case 4

This 18-year-old presented with bilateral cleft nose deformity and maxillary deficiency. The patient was treated with LeFort I osteotomy as well as onlay grafting to the pyriform aperture. The patient's maxillary surgery was performed to improve the projection of her maxilla, restore support to the nasal base, and correct her malocclusion. Six months after her skeletal surgery the cleft nasal reconstruction was undertaken (Figs. 28–41 to 28–47).

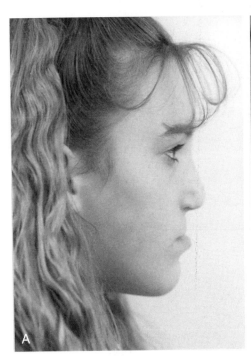

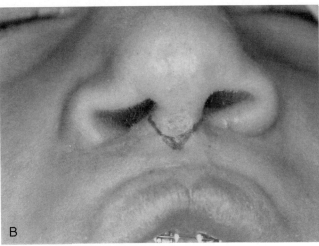

Figure 28–41. Preoperative lateral (*A*) and basal (*B*) views demonstrating the planned V-Y advancement flap for columellar lengthening.

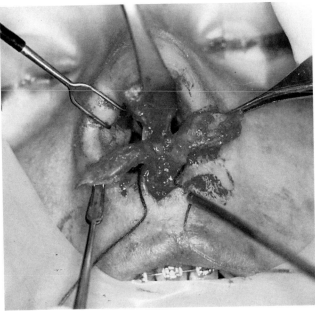

Figure 28–42. Exposure and mobilization of alar cartilages and underlying vestibular mucosa attached. After full mobilization of the cartilages, the domes were divided to allow maximal narrowing of the nasal tip.

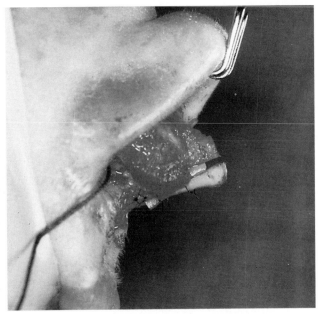

Figure 28–43. Lateral view showing intraoperative cartilaginous tip reconstruction. Note the columellar strut inserted between the medial crura and the tip graft sutured so that it projects above the dome. Conservative cephalic volume reduction was performed excising only cartilage and leaving intact the underlying vestibular mucosa.

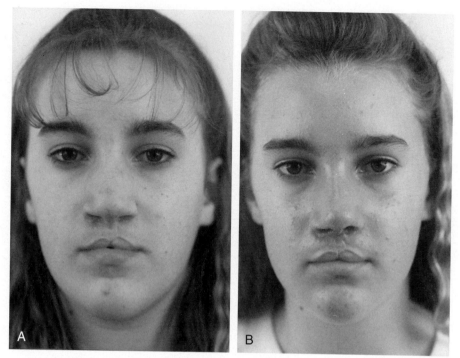

Figure 28–44. Preoperative (*A*) and postoperative (*B*) frontal views.

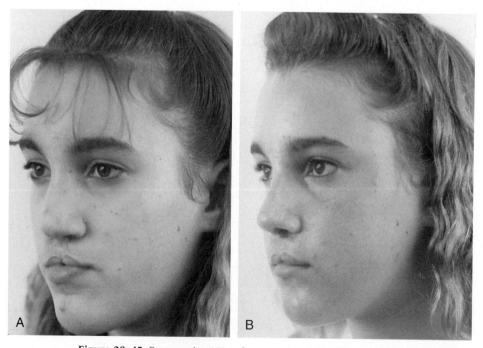

Figure 28–45. Preoperative (*A*) and postoperative (*B*) oblique views.

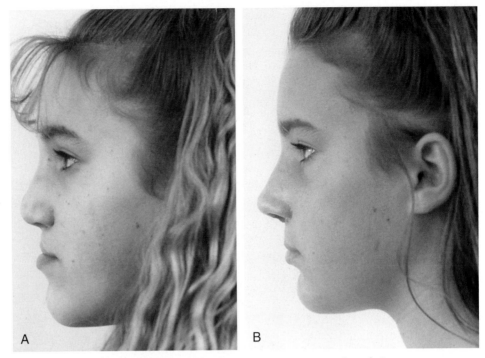

Figure 28–46. Preoperative (*A*) and postoperative (*B*) lateral views.

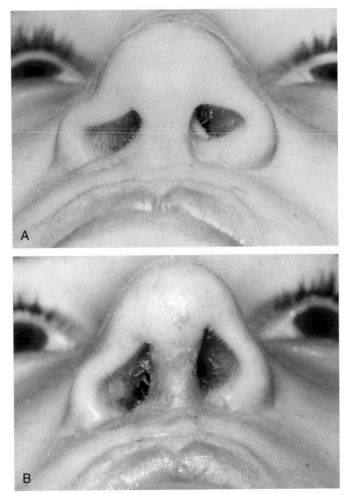

Figure 28–47. Preoperative (*A*) and postoperative (*B*) basal views. Although the bases were not narrowed, the additional projection of the tip yields a symmetric and triangular nasal base configuration.

Case 5

A 13-year-old presented with bilateral cleft lip/nose deformity and dehiscence of the orbicularis oris muscle at the philtrum. The patient had an extremely short columella and philtrum, necessitating lengthening not only of the columella but of the philtral tissue. This was accomplished by using bilateral crossover flaps advanced into the subcolumellar space and establishing muscle continuity (Figs. 28–48 to 28–58).

Text continued on page 741

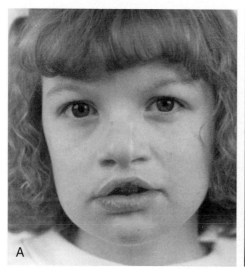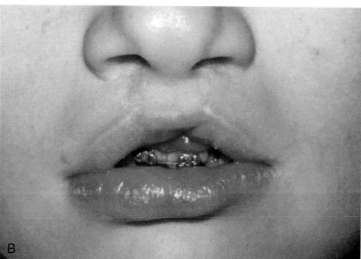

Figure 28–48. *A* and *B*, Preoperative frontal views.

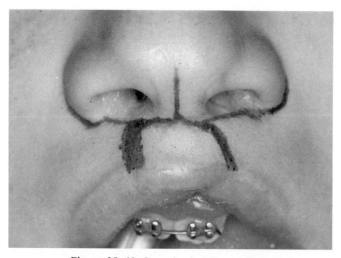

Figure 28–49. Operative incision marking.

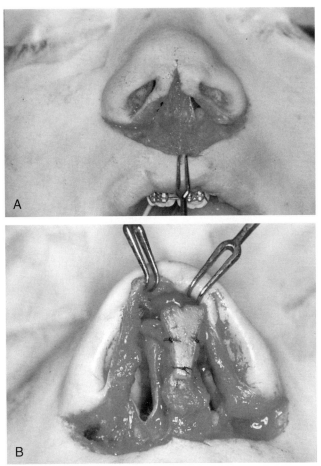

Figure 28–50. Intraoperative incisions (*A*) and tip reconstruction with autogenous cartilaginous shield graft (*B*). In addition, a columellar strut was employed between the medial crura.

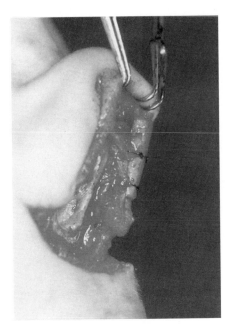

Figure 28–51. Lateral view of tip reconstruction with graft positioned above the domes. Although not shown, a conservative cephalic volume reduction was used as well as an interdomal suture of 6–0 nylon. Simultaneous augmentation of the columella to increase columellar show was possible with this technique, which also included a small segment of cartilage beneath the shield graft extending toward the nasal spine to add bulk at the subnasale point.

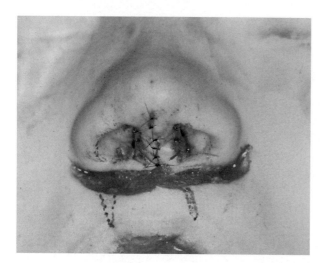

Figure 28–52. Intraoperative closure of columellar incision. Notice that columellar lengthening is achieved with this maneuver.

Figure 28–53. Mobilization of lateral flaps including the orbicularis oris muscle.

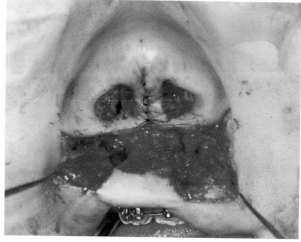

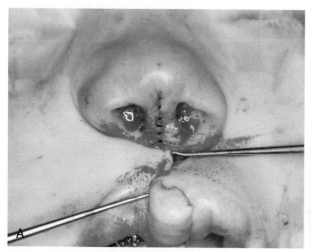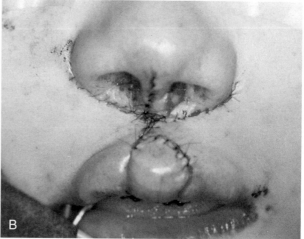

Figure 28–54. Transposition (*A*) and suturing (*B*) of lateral flaps to effect lip lengthening. The muscle layer must be sutured to establish orbicularis continuity. This maneuver also effectively narrows the alar width on both sides.

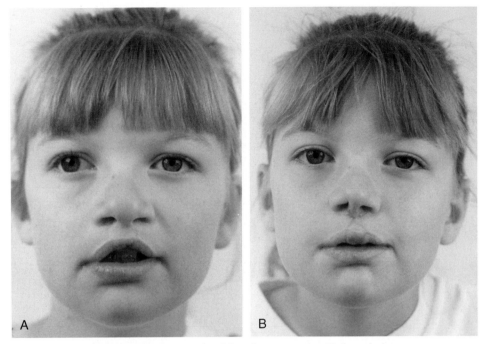

Figure 28–55. Preoperative (*A*) and postoperative (*B*) frontal views.

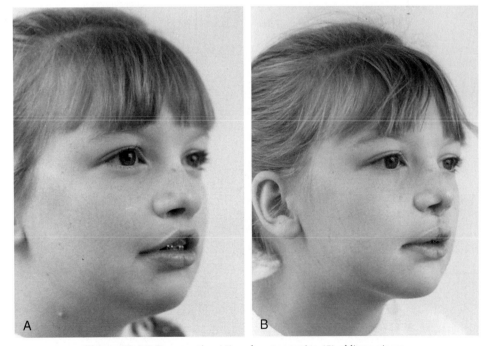

Figure 28–56. Preoperative (*A*) and postoperative (*B*) oblique views.

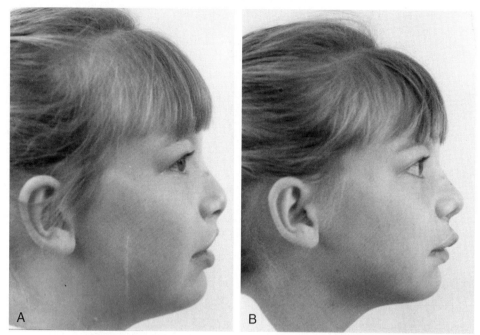

Figure 28–57. Preoperative (*A*) and postoperative (*B*) lateral views.

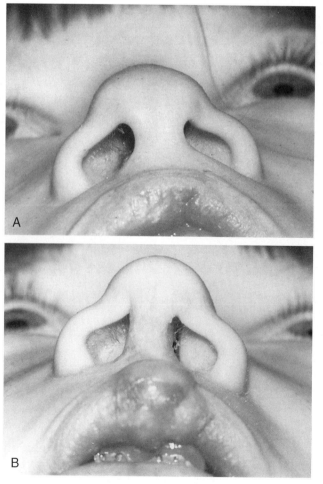

Figure 28–58. Preoperative (*A*) and postoperative (*B*) basal views.

These cases represent a variety of problems commonly encountered in dealing with the cleft lip/nose deformity. Utilization of the techniques represented has yielded stable long-term results.

CONCLUSIONS

A review of the history and evolution of the cleft nose operation indicates that the ideal mechanism of correction has yet to be described. Multiple maneuvers exist to assist in improving cleft rhinoplasty results, but the rhinoplastic surgeon must choose those techniques that will address the individual's needs rather than using a standard procedure. The standard closed rhinoplasty techniques almost universally fail to yield satisfactory cosmetic results and elimination of the cleft stigmata. The modified open rhinoplasty technique with extensive mobilization of abnormal tissue and augmentation with autogenous grafts is advocated to maximize functional as well as cosmetic reconstruction. Cleft lip/nose deformities represent a unique and ongoing challenge to the facial surgeon. Continued evolution and application of new techniques undoubtedly will yield increasingly improved results.

References

1. Joseph J: Operative reduction of the size of the nose (rhinomoisis). Berl Klin Wochenschr 1898; 40:882.
2. Gilles HD, Kilner TP: Harelip operation for the correction of the secondary deformities. Lancet 1932; 223:1369.
3. Rethi A: Uber die korrektiven operationen der nasendeformitaten. I. Die Hockerabtragung. Chirurgie 1929; 1:1103.
4. Humby G: The nostril in secondary hare-lip. Lancet 1938; 234:1276.
5. Byars L: Surgical correction of nasal deformities. Surg Gynecol Obstet 1947; 84:65–78.
6. Figi FA: The repair of secondary cleft lip and nasal deformity. J Int Coll Surg 1952; 17:297.
7. Erich JB: A technique for correction of a flat nostril in cases of repaired harelip. Plast Reconstr Surg 1953; 12:322.
8. Potter J: Some nasal tip deformities due to alar cartilage abnormalities. Plast Reconstr Surg 1954; 13:358.
9. Gelbke H: The nostril problem in unilateral harelips and its surgical management. Plast Reconstr Surg 1956; 18:65.
10. Bardach J: Rozszczepy wargi gornej podniebienig (Polish). Warsaw, Poland: Panstwowy Zaklad Wydawnictw Lekarskich, 1967.
11. Spira M, Hardy SB, Gerow FJ: Correction of nasal deformities accompanying unilateral cleft lip. Cleft Palate J 1970; 7:112.
12. Goodman WS, Zorn ML: The unilateral cleft lip nose. J Otolaryngol 1982; 11:198.
13. Nishimura Y: Transcolumellar incision for correction of unilateral cleft lip nose. Chir Plast (Berl) 1980; 5:169.
14. Cronin TD, Denkler KA: Correction of the unilateral cleft lip nose. Plast Reconstr Surg 1988; 82(3):419–432.
15. McComb H: Primary correction of unilateral cleft lip nasal deformity: A ten year review. Plast Reconstr Surg 1985; 75:91.
16. Johnson CM Jr, Toriumi DM: Open Structure Rhinoplasty. Philadelphia: WB Saunders, 1990.
17. Sheen JH, Sheen A: Aesthetic Rhinoplasty, 2nd ed. St Louis: CV Mosby, 1987.
18. Millard DR Jr: Columella lengthening by a forked flap. Plast Reconstr Surg 1958; 22:454.
19. Cronin TD: Lengthening columella by use of skin from nasal floor and alae. Plast Reconstr Surg 1958; 21:417–426.
20. Brown JB, McDowell F: Secondary repair to cleft lips and their nasal deformities. Am J Orthod 1941; 27:712.

IV | Outcome Assessment

29 | A Methodologic Approach to Outcome Assessment

J. F. Camilla Tulloch and Alexia A. Antczak-Bouckoms

The focus of this chapter is on the identification of suitable outcomes for the evaluation of treatment of facial clefts. Two specific issues will be addressed; first, the importance of the different perspectives that an evaluation may take, and second the levels at which the outcomes of treatment may be considered.

Outcome assessment has become an important focus for health care research. This is in part a result of the tremendous increase in the number of available treatments and practices, and in part to the perception that the health care system, at least in the United States, is a system in crisis. In the last decade, the cost of health care has increased well beyond the rate of inflation in other sectors of the U.S. economy. The need to control costs while maintaining quality and access has now become imperative. During the same period there has been a growing perception that a significant amount of money is being spent on health care that is either ill-suited to the needs of patients or at times even harmful. Current constraints require systematic evaluation of health practices including consideration of their health, economic, ethical, and social impact. By identifying less effective or even ineffective practices, such evaluations not only will help ensure the well-being of patients but also will maximize the benefits available from scarce health resources.

One of the major difficulties of health care research is the identification of an appropriate set of outcome measures that captures the essence of both the benefits and the risks of an intervention. There are many levels at which the outcomes of health care may be considered. These range from the immediate results of treatments, programs, or courses of action, defined in disease or condition-specific terms, to outcomes judged by their impact on the physical, social, and emotional health of a patient, or outcomes that may be used to formulate practice guidelines, make reimbursement decisions, and set national policy. The choice of outcomes for an evaluation then would depend not only upon the practice being evaluated and its anticipated benefit but also on the perspective of the evaluation and the purpose for which it is being conducted.

THE PERSPECTIVE OF THE EVALUATION

A general discussion of outcomes in health care may address some important questions that should be raised by the introduction of a new treatment or by the reassessment of existing practices or programs. These questions may be the following: How well does the treatment work under ideal conditions, and how well in day-to-day clinical practice? For whom does the treatment work best? Does the treatment make a difference? Should the treatment be available to all who might benefit?

The first question, whether the treatment will work under ideal conditions, relates to what is termed the *efficacy* of the practice. Efficacy has been defined as a measure of the probability of benefit to individuals in a defined population for a given medical problem under ideal conditions of use.[1] Advances in clinical care should always be evaluated by comparison with currently available practices. New systems should be adopted only if they achieve results that were not previously possible or reduce the failures, inconvenience, cost, or adverse consequences of existing systems.

Measures of efficacy generally result from studies undertaken under controlled situations with carefully chosen patient populations, indications, and settings. Rigorous and powerful research methods such as randomized controlled trials have been developed for clinical research, and are generally regarded as necessary when the differences in expected outcome are small as compared with the variation commonly seen among patients. Alternative assessment methods such as case series and cohort studies, although often used to evaluate new treatments, do not deal as well with the problems of placebo effect, confounding influence, and bias.[2,3] The outcomes of an efficacy study are frequently, although not always, measures of morphology or pathophysiology and should directly reflect the considerations that prompted the intervention. An example in cleft care is the carefully performed prospective trial by Marsh and colleagues[4] to examine the effect of intravelar veloplasty on velopharyngeal incompetence (VPI). In this study, the outcome of interest was the auditory symptom of VPI after palatoplasty. Additional but segregated measures of operating time, cost, and morbidity were also presented.

The next two related questions, whether the treatment works under day-to-day clinical practice and for whom the treatment works best, consider that which is termed the *effectiveness* of the treatment or practice. One of the initial objectives of effectiveness research was to measure how an intervention works under more general circumstances rather than under the ideal circumstances of a carefully controlled clinical trial. As such, these studies frequently draw on data from more than one source, and generally not only select those outcomes that reflect efficacy (as measured in a clinical trial) but also consider other outcomes relevant to patients and clinicians, such as levels of function, health status, quality of life, and adverse reactions.

The importance of identifying "what works in clinical practice" has been emphasized by the Health Care Financing Administration (HCFA), which adopted this as a special initiative.[5,6] Coupling the desire to improve patient care with increasing concern over widespread but unexplained variations in practice patterns,[7,8,9] the National Center for Health Services Research and Health Care Technology Assessment (NCHSR) established the Patient Outcome Assessment Research Program. This program has been expanded into the Medical Treatment Effectiveness Program (MEDTEP), now administered by the Public Health Service through the Agency for Health Care Policy and Research (AHCPR). A series of multidisciplinary studies, conducted by Patient Outcome Research Teams (PORTs) have been initiated to assess both the outcomes and the effectiveness of different interventions for specific clinical conditions. The goals of a PORT project are to identify and analyze the outcomes and costs of current alternative practice patterns to determine the best treatment strategy and develop and test methods for reducing inappropriate interventions. These effectiveness studies are generally multidisciplinary and make inferences from both experimental and nonexperimental data.

Many people believe that effectiveness research provides clinicians with the information needed to select those patients for whom a medical practice is most likely to provide the benefits that are important in day-to-day living.[10] As such, these studies are increasingly being employed to develop clinical practice guidelines.[11] An example of such guideline development is given by the AHCPR report on the management of cataracts in adults.[12] After reviewing the evidence from many sources, including evidence from nearly 8000 published studies, the researchers concluded that because there were as yet no objective independent measures of functional impairment that could serve as precise indicators of surgery, cataract surgery should not be recommended to improve vision if: (1) the patient did not desire surgery, (2) glasses or visual aids provided satisfactory vision, (3) the patient's lifestyle was not compromised, or (4) the patient was unfit medically. Although these recommendations, with hindsight, may seem somewhat prosaic, they should be reviewed in the context of more than 1.35 million cataract surgeries performed in the United States in 1991 at an approximate cost of $3.4 billion to Medicare. To date, no PORT study has been initiated to address the problems of cleft care, but the appropriateness of such an endeavor seems self-evident, because cleft lip and palate are such common conditions.

The last two questions, whether the intervention makes a difference and whether the treatment should be available to all, are generally considered under the rubric of technology assessment, and stem from the growing concern that the ever-increasing number of available treatments and practices are perhaps neither being used wisely nor producing the expected health benefits. Technology assessment in health care is a relatively new field, and as such is subject to some confusion about objectives, definitions, methods, and applications. The Office of Technology Assessment of the U.S. Congress defines medical technology broadly as "the set of techniques, drugs, equipment and procedures used by health care professionals in delivering medical care to individuals, and the systems within which such care is delivered.''[13] Technology assessment is a "comprehensive form of policy research that examines short and long-term social consequences (e.g., societal, economic, ethical, legal) of the application of technology.''[14] The intent is to consider the social impact of health care[15] and to provide guidance to practitioners and patients about clinical choices, to provide decision-makers with information on policy alternatives, to suggest appropriate allocation of research and development funds, and to aid in regulation and reimbursement decisions. *Technology assessment* is a term used to designate a conscious formal attempt to examine all relevant evidence needed to determine the optimal use, if any, of a technology.[16] As Relman noted,[5] to control costs without arbitrarily reducing access to health care, we need more information not only about the safety, effectiveness, and appropriateness of care but also about the way that care is provided.

The methods used to assess health care technologies are wide-ranging and have been well described in the Institute of Medicine's book *Assessing Medical Technologies*.[17] However, an important distinction should be made between the research studies used to provide data for a technology assessment and the assessment itself. Not every study of a health technology qualifies as a technology assessment. Because technology assessments examine the evidence from a broad perspective, they can seldom rely on a single study, but instead represent evidence from many sources.

The expansion of the scope of technology assessments led Fuchs and Garber[18] to draw a distinction between "old" assessments, which focus the choice of outcomes on features of safety and efficacy, and "new" assessments, which expand the outcomes to include consideration of costs and social issues, using a much broader perspective and drawing on multiple investigators, many data sets, and several analytic techniques. These "new" assessments have resulted in technology assessment now being considered a comprehensive form of research that provides the basis for the formulation of practice guidelines, policy decisions, and reimbursement recommendations.

LEVEL OF OUTCOME MEASURED

Turning to the selection of outcomes for a specific evaluation, an important if seldom discussed issue is the level at which the outcomes of health care should be measured. There are obviously many levels at which the effects of treatment programs or courses of action may be assessed. These can be considered as a hierarchy, ranging from the consequences defined in disease-specific terms to effects judged by their impact on the physical, social, and emotional health of a patient. As an example, the use of prolonged electrocardiographic monitoring can be considered in the treatment of patients with recurrent ventricular tachycardia and fibrillation.[19, 20, 21] The "outcome" considered may simply be the proportion of patients for whom an agent capable of suppressing provoked arrhythmias can be selected. A higher level of outcome, however, may include the effectiveness of the drug selected in preventing naturally occurring arrhythmias, the rates of drug-associated aggravation of arrhythmia, the rate or recurrence, the number of hospital days and number of trials needed to select a drug, and the cost of drug selection using this monitoring device. A third level of outcome may go further to include the effect of selected antiarrhythmic agent on relieving the symptoms of dizziness, syncope, and ventricular tachycardia. The fourth level may include the impact of drug selection on broader measures such as change in risk of myocardial infarction, days lost from work, other comorbidities, and death due to cardiovascular or other causes. Finally, the patients' value for these levels of outcomes may also be assessed.

Because most medical conditions are multidimensional in nature, with both the condition and the treatment affecting several aspects of a person's life, it is difficult to quantify the consequences of treatment using a single summary score. However, specifying a suitable set of outcomes that capture the essence of both the risks and the benefits of treatment can be extremely complex. Current clinical and administrative decisions are typically based on qualitative and subjective estimates that the risk of adverse outcomes is less than the potential benefit of the treatment, and that the risk-benefit ratio of one intervention is superior to that of another. Frequently, there is little objective evidence to support decisions either for individual patients or as the basis for practice guidelines or policy decisions.

Making quantitative assessments of health benefits accurately can be extremely difficult. The traditional approach usually involves collecting pieces of evidence about individual outcomes, implicitly weighing them, and synthesizing the results into a single subjective global statement about the effects of treatment. Rarely is there any explicit consideration of the way the evidence should be linked together, the magnitude or likelihood of the benefit, the range of uncertainty involved, or the patient's preferences for the outcomes or treatment. As an example in cleft care, the question of how to assess the benefits of infant presurgical orthopedics can be considered. The chain of events that needs to be integrated is the success or failure of the procedure itself in positioning the segments as desired, the impact of this on the surgical repair, the influence of the surgical repair on subsequent growth, the need for more or less orthodontic treatment and speech therapy, the impact of all of the above on the patient's psychosocial development, the need for later surgeries, and patient's and parents' preferences for any of these procedures and outcomes. Although circumstantial evidence and the clinician's past experience with presurgical orthopedics may suggest different approaches, it is clear from the literature that even this simple issue concerning the early management of patients with clefts is far from resolved.[22]

Much of the available evidence in health care has not dealt directly with the outcomes that are important to patients, such as improvement in symptoms, physical and psychosocial function, or costs associated with treatment. Instead, the evidence has tended to focus on outcomes measured in terms of morphology or pathophysiology. These measures can be thought of as *proximate outcomes,* in that they are the more immediate result of the intervention and are usually, although not always, measured relatively soon after a treatment or procedure has been carried out. Valuable though these measures may be, they do not capture the essence of why patients seek or why clinicians recommend treatment. Nor do they help in assessing the overall advantage of alternative health interventions. More global measures are needed to specify the success or failure of care, reflecting the specific factors that motivate patients to seek and clinicians to recommend a given treatment. These measures can be thought of as the *ultimate outcomes,* in that they somehow reflect the ultimate effects of the intervention.

The growing involvement of patients and consumer groups in treatment decisions has also created a need to broaden the way in which the effects of health care are described. The pressure for more global estimates of the impact of treatment raises important issues as to how a set of outcomes should be chosen, how several outcomes may be considered together, and how patients' preferences can be incorporated to give a summary measure of the impact of treatment. Some examples of more global outcome measures are presented to provide insight into their use and to provide a basis for discussion of some of the unresolved issues about their further application.

EXAMPLES

Developing a Summary Measure—The Extraction of Asymptomatic Third Molars

The first example examines the management of asymptomatic third molars or wisdom teeth.[23, 24] This illustrates one approach to the problem of combining multiple outcomes into a single summary measure of the impact of a health practice. The assessment method and results may be used for individual clinical decision making, as a basis for practice guidelines, or to formulate policy.

Third molars or wisdom teeth are the last of the teeth to develop and erupt. However, frequently there is insufficient growth of the jaw to allow space for these teeth to assume a satisfactory position in the mouth. Teeth that remain embedded or impacted in the jaw, covered by bone and/or soft tissue, are believed to pose a potential risk of subsequent disease including infection, damage to adjacent teeth, and the development of cysts or tumors. Additional support for this practice also comes from the belief that the early extraction (prior to complete root formation and eruption) of third molars in healthy young adults not only is easier but also carries less risk of operative morbidity than extraction in older patients. Accordingly, the early "prophylactic" removal of as yet asymptomatic third molars is both a long-standing and widespread practice. This analysis approached this controversial issue by suggesting that if the early removal of asymptomatic third molars is to be endorsed as a risk-minimizing option, it should be possible to show that the morbidity associated with this practice is less than the morbidity associated with delaying the extraction decision until the eruption status is clear or until pathology develops.

Although the complications of third molar extraction are diverse, each is associated with some pain, suffering, additional treatments, days lost from work, and cost, and thus all represent a measure of "disability" or "loss" to a patient. When the alternative managements are compared, the strategy with the least "expected disability or loss" should be the preferred option. To combine the disability associated with each of the several rather diverse complications of this surgery, some common measure was needed. In this analysis, disability was assessed as the equivalent number of days of standard discomfort (DSD) for each complication, using a modified time trade-off technique.[25]

In a modified time trade-off study, individuals are asked how much time they would be willing to undergo in one health state rather than suffer some other health state (complication). In the third molar study, clinicians (who make the bulk of all extraction recommendations) were asked how many additional days of the standard discomfort generally expected after an uncomplicated third molar extraction they would just be willing to undergo rather than suffer any of the complications of surgery. Fairly detailed clinical scenarios were used to describe each complication to the clinicians, who were already broadly familiar with these outcomes. Thus, if clinicians reported that they would rather undergo 7 additional days of standard discomfort rather than endure the complication of a dry socket, the complication of dry socket was assigned a value of 7 DSD.

Expected utility theory also suggests that clinicians, or patients, interested in minimizing disability should consider not only the magnitude but also the likelihood of the loss. In this way, complications that, no matter how disabling, almost never occur will contribute little to the overall assessment of the risks of treatment. Conversely, much less disabling complications that occur with great frequency should contribute more to an assessment. Because there were at that time no well-controlled studies available to suggest either the magnitude or the likelihood of any complications, expert panels were used to derive both of these estimates. This analysis was able to show that, if the experts were correct, contrary to many clinicians' beliefs and to accepted policy and practice, the early removal of all third molars is not a risk-minimizing policy. Instead, the policy of delaying the decision and then extracting only those teeth that both fail to erupt fully and also develop some pathology, under all likely assumptions, carries less "expected disability."

This example is of interest in that it demonstrates how the identification of a single "main effect" may be used to compare the outcomes of different management strategies. The use of the time trade-off technique allowed quantification and aggregation of diverse complications of surgery (proximate outcomes) into a single summary measure of disability (ultimate outcome), and thereby greatly facilitated the comparison of management strategies.

Patient Preference and Quality of Life—Surgery Versus Radiotherapy for the Treatment of Cancer

Two examples demonstrate the importance of taking patient preferences into account when evaluating the choice of treatments. Although it has long been argued that the value judgments underlying clinical decisions can and ought to be considered systematically and explicitly,[26, 27, 28] only recently have patients' values or preferences been formally included in clinical decisions.[29] In most clinical situations, competing concerns combine to determine the value of the outcome of care. In the past, professionals, who often have greater, albeit second-hand, experience with a particular illness or health state, have used their experience to implicitly weigh the risks and benefits of alternative treatments and make recommendations to patients.

Within the past two decades, two concepts—utilities and quality adjusted life years—have been increasingly incorporated into health care evaluations to address some of these complex issues. Although these two measures often appear together in health care analyses, they are in fact two distinctly different concepts.[30] Utilities are defined as numbers that represent the strength of an individual's preference for particular outcomes when faced with uncertainty. Utility theory and its methods of measurement were developed as a normative (prescriptive) model for individual decision making under uncertainty.[31] It is important to appreciate that this theory is intended as a description not of how people do make decisions when faced with uncertainty, but of how they ought to make decisions if they wish to act rationally. No one claims that people behave as they ought. The primary reason for adopting a prescriptive or normative theory is the observation that decisions left solely to unguided judgment are often made in an internally inconsistent fashion, and that perhaps consideration of utilities as an outcome would allow better decisions that really do maximize what people care about.

Quality adjusted life years, or QALYs, were developed as an outcome measure that would integrate both the quality and quantity of life by assigning weights to various health states. QALYs are based on the premise that a year in one state of health may not be judged equivalent to a year in a different state of health, and each should be weighted accordingly. Various weighting schemes have been suggested, but most frequently the weights assigned to each health state do reflect the preferences or "utility" of the individuals for that particular quality of life. The appeal and power of the QALY as an outcome measure is its ability to capture in a single summary measure the health improvement created, thereby allowing for broad comparison across different types of health care interventions.

Of importance, taking patients' preferences into account as well as considering the quality of life can have a significant impact on determining the preferred treatment option or management strategy. The two examples presented here illustrate this point.

In one example, the relative importance (utility) of immediate versus long-term survival is expressed by patients' willingness to trade off some later years of life in exchange for greater certainty of near-term survival. In the second, the influence of quality of life on attitudes toward survival is demonstrated by patients who would trade later years of life for better-quality near-term years.

The relative importance of immediate versus long-term survival to a patient was assessed in patients with lung cancer.[27] A utility curve for life-years was derived from patients' responses to a standard gamble[32, 33] between a fixed period of life for certain versus the choice of longer survival with a chance of immediate death. This gamble reflects the outcomes associated with a choice of treatments for lung cancer, namely, radiation or surgery. Radiation therapy has no practical risk of immediate death but is coupled with shorter long-term survival than is surgery. Surgery, on the other hand, entails greater long-term survival coupled with a risk of operative mortality. Because of the known difficulty untrained people have understanding odds other than 50:50, all gambles in this study were held at 50:50; this ratio is analogous to that of flipping a coin. The results of this analysis suggested that for a significant proportion of subjects with lung cancer (21% of 60-year-old men and 43% of 70-year-old men) radiation therapy is preferred to surgery because these individuals valued near-term more than long-term survival. If treatment had been evaluated on survival rates alone, surgery would have been recommended for all patients. This, however, would fail to maximize the benefit for patients for whom the risk of immediate death is associated with great disutility.

In the second example, patients' attitudes toward quality and quantity of survival were assessed, based on the clinical problem of T3 carcinoma of the larynx.[34] The treatment options were surgery with greater expected survival but loss of normal speech, and radiation therapy with lower expected survival but preservation of normal speech. In this analysis, radiation would be the preferred treatment for approximately 20% of subjects for whom the importance of the quality of life with speech was sufficient to overwhelm the reduction in life expectancy. These patients would choose preservation of speech at the expense of greater survival.

These two examples point to the need to integrate time, quality, and utility into the development of outcome measures used to compare treatments.

Multiattribute Utility Assessment—Cleft Lip and Palate Treatment

This example is drawn from the cleft palate literature and is one of the earliest attempts to formally and systematically integrate the multiple attributes of health care together with patient/parent preferences for the different outcomes of treatment.[35, 36] Because cleft lip and palate and its treatment affects so many aspects of an individual's life, and because patients may value these aspects differently, the comparison of alternative managements is unusually complex. If one treatment can clearly be shown to maximize all important outcomes, there is no difficulty in choosing a preferred treatment. However, more often, different treatments affect different aspects of the cleft condition in different ways. As an example, some types of palatal repair are thought to produce more aesthetic results in the short term, but cause undesirable interference with subsequent maxillary growth. Other procedures, although believed to disrupt growth less, are not considered able to produce such satisfactory speech outcomes. In such situations, trade-offs must be made between competing alternatives if one treatment is to be recommended over another.

In Krischer's example of multiattribute utility assessment,[35, 36] the focus of the analysis was on why the treatment offered by cleft teams can differ so widely, even when the disciplines represented within teams are substantially the same. Faced with the lack of any objective indices for the multiple outcomes of cleft care, Krischer suggested that the determination of the acceptability of the treatment result must involve an individual's relative utilities for the different benefits and risks of treatment. The analysis involved several steps, including a comprehensive review and synthesis of the then-available literature on the efficacy and effectiveness of different treatment procedures, an assessment of parents' and clinicians' utility for the different aspects of treatment together with their attitude toward risk, and the combination of the individual utility functions for different attributes of care into a multiattribute utility function that could be used to guide individual treatment decisions.

The aspects of cleft care that were chosen for this analysis were cosmetics, speech, hearing, and monetary expense. Although by no means comprehensive, these four attributes represent a major focus for cleft care. Utility functions for each of these four attributes were assessed by means of a series of standard gambles presented in a questionnaire that was completed at 17 treatment centers by 119 clinicians and parents of cleft children. Because the evaluation of alternative treatments must be made on the holistic basis of habilitation, and not on a checklist of attributes, the utility functions for each attribute needed to be aggregated according to an individual's preferences for each of the attributes. When a treatment has many outcomes, it is not sufficient to merely rank the outcomes. Instead, it needs to be specified how much better or worse one outcome is than another. A scale must be assessed for each attribute, and a weighting factor introduced that reflects true preferences for the combinations of attributes. In this way a multiattribute utility function can be interpreted as reflecting an individual's preference for combinations of each type of handicap associated with cleft lip and palate. The multiattribute utility function gives a single or summary measure for the various outcomes that reflects not only the different levels of each attribute but also the different combinations of all attributes, and thus the patient's value for the overall handicap of the condition.

In the cleft lip and palate example, a number of treatment alternatives were considered, including maxillary orthopedics, the timing of surgical repair, the type of surgical repair, and secondary procedures for the management of velopharyngeal insufficiency. Probabilistic data that described the results following each patient management decision were derived from the literature. Notwithstanding the generally weak research designs used at that time (largely case reports or case series with small sample sizes), there appeared to be broad agreement in the literature about the probable effects of different procedures when these were measured in terms of proximate outcomes, such as the position of the alveolar segments after presurgical orthopedics or the number of dental crossbites after different palatal procedures. However, major disagreements arose in determining the usefulness of alternative management in the overall rehabilitative process.

These disagreements were the result not only of the different effects of various treatments on the attributes of the cleft condition but also of the fact that no one treatment or series of treatments maximizes all attributes, leaving difficult trade-offs to be made in a subjective fashion by clinicians and parents. In 1974, apparently no available research existed to suggest how the proximate outcomes of care reported would translate into the outcomes of cosmetic improvement, speech intelligibility, and hearing ability desired by patients. Accordingly, subjective assessments had to be obtained from experts familiar with each problem. Even when there was general consensus about the level and likelihood of a particular outcome, when parents' or clinicians' utilities for these outcomes were incorporated in a multiattribute utility assessment, it became apparent that the preferred treatment depended not so much on the expected effect of the procedure as on the utility for the different attributes of the outcomes of care. Significant differences existed among clinicians grouped according to their specialty or the institution with which they were affiliated. These differences suggest that variation in patient management can at least be partially ascribed to variation in how the degrees of ''handicap'' are perceived. Clinicians may identify certain treatments as ''superior'' not because they differ in their estimates of what the proximate outcomes of care might be, but because they differ in the value they place on the resulting ''handicap.''

According to the then-available literature and the elicited expert opinion, the very small range in outcome expected suggested that no one treatment offered a major advantage over any other, yet there were marked differences in management protocols among different cleft palate teams. Within teams, similar preferences were found between teams and parents. It may be that team members influence parents' utilities, or that parents chose teams whose values correspond to their own. Families of patients with cleft lip and palate often travel great distances to receive treatment even when there is a treatment center nearby. It appeared in this analysis that treatment decisions are made on the basis of the values placed on the ultimate outcomes of rehabilitation, rather than on the basis of the beliefs about treatment efficacy as measured by conventional proximate outcomes.

An additional and important issue concerning the utility for the outcome versus the utility for the procedure is raised by this example. It is possible that parents or clinicians may value a particular outcome highly, but the treatment itself may be associated with greater disutility. If this were so, it may be perfectly appropriate to forego the treatment despite the desire to improve the level of a particular outcome. Thus, it appears to be important in any comprehensive evaluation to consider not only the value of the outcomes of the procedure but also the value of the procedure itself, because these can be at odds. This is particularly important when utilities are being considered or when a complete accounting of the costs, risks, and benefits is sought. Failure to include the value of the treatment itself is equivalent to saying that the actual means used to achieve the end is unimportant, which is clearly an untenable premise.

DISCUSSION

We have described here how the selection of different outcomes can be used to offer additional insight into the effects of health care. However, many difficulties remain before such measures can be widely adopted into the treatment of facial clefts. First, some agreement is needed as to which outcomes should be selected and how they should be prioritized so that comparisons can be made across common medical goals such as the prevention of illness and disability in the healthy or the preservation of life and relief of suffering in the sick.[37] Perhaps there are measures that do have universal applicability, but these may as yet be insufficiently refined to identify the increasingly subtle therapeutic benefits that are sought with the introduction of new techniques for cleft care. Direct extrapolation from the medical models of QALY and utility may pose some difficulties for the subtle rehabilitative improvements sought for children with cleft lip and palate. Yet the measures of preference and quality of life are the very measures that most parents would wish for their children. Perhaps there are some outcomes that have been successfully used for similar categories of disease or treatment that may be modified for broader comparison. The techniques of utility analysis and QALY assessment do show promise for addressing some of these issues. However, these techniques are extremely complex and are still in the early stages of development and refinement.[30, 33, 38-41]

Another issue is the difficulty of establishing the links between the outcomes a health intervention affects (proximate outcome) and the measures it is intended to influence (ultimate outcome). These links are difficult to establish even when they are both immediate and direct, as in the third molar example in which the complications of tooth extraction were directly translated into expected morbidity. In contrast, the ultimate outcomes of cosmetic improvement, speech, and hearing used in the cleft palate example must be related in a complex way to the events that occurred a considerable time before. In addition, ultimate outcomes are often influenced by events other than treatment. For example, speech intelligibility following palate repair is known to be influenced not only by the surgical repair but also by position of the teeth and the timing and intensity of speech therapy. Although these issues should ideally be resolved with a series of carefully conducted clinical trials, direct assessments span many years of a patient's and clinician's life. Such evidence is seldom available. Instead, clinicians must rely on less rigorous research designs or even subjective opinion for the basis of their treatment choices. Although clinicians are accustomed to making such decisions in an informal fashion, and often at a subconscious level, traditional medical education, with its preoccupation with deterministic explanations for disease, gives little emphasis to the probabilistic nature of much of the information on which health decisions are based. Clinicians have difficulty constructing and manipulating coherent sets of probabilities and with quantifying degrees of belief.[42, 43]

The problem of lack of data is neither new nor particular to cleft lip and palate treatment.[44] In 1976, the U.S. Office of Technology Assessment estimated that between 80% and 90% of all medical practices had had no formal evaluation of treatment efficacy or effectiveness.[13] A more recent (1990) analysis of the National Institutes of Health Medicare coverage assessment practices showed that fewer than 20% of all assessments relied on scientific evidence such as clinical trials, case control studies, or cohort studies. The remaining four fifths of the assessments relied only on expert opinion.[45] This is not to say that these practices are worse or better than any others, but simply that they have never been formally evaluated. The availability of systematic empirical evidence to aid the practitioner in clinical decisions has not been the standard situation in the medical profession, and this presents a considerable barrier to answering the challenge for a change toward evidence-based medicine.[46] When formal evaluations have been carried out, the results were often surprising and may have run counter to long-established beliefs and practices.[47, 48]

Notwithstanding the difficulties already present in clinical research, the failure to include more global estimates of treatment outcome may negate the usefulness of much careful work. In our recent analysis of the use of ambulatory cardiac monitoring to aid in the selection of antiarrhythmic agents,[20] we were unable to find any data from which to infer a relationship between the ability of the monitoring device to aid in selecting an antiarrhythmic agent and the impact such a selection would have on long-term clinical outcomes of morbidity and mortality, which are presumably of greater importance to patients and clinicians.

The use of utilities as a scale by which to measure the desirability of treatment and evaluate the outcomes of care may allow clinicians to reconsider treatment decisions and results in terms of their own expectations and the expectations of patients and their families. However, even when a benefit is highly valued by a patient, it is not clear whether it should be valued by society in the same way. Obviously, such desires should be considered within the context of available resources and the priorities assigned to various needs. Utility scales may help resolve questions about the significance of different aspects of cleft care and the primacy of various treatment methods. Cleft lip and palate care is widely valued, particularly in affluent societies. But how much is it worth, to whom, and how is this decided? Treatment strategies are based on the best judgment of the profession and, where possible, on the results of previous studies. Yet controversies about needs, benefits, risks, and optimal treatments continue, with major differences of opinion existing. There is an obvious need to find better methods to compare the relative benefits of treatment and better methods to select the most appropriate alternatives for care. The examples we have presented in this chapter are intended to show how the use of more global outcome measures may offer some further insight into evaluating the benefits of alternative managements for patients with facial clefts.

References

1. Banta DH, Behaney CJ, Willems JS: Toward Rational Technology in Medicine. New York: Springer, 1981.
2. Jaeschke R, Sackett DL: Research methods for obtaining primary evidence. Int J Technology Assessment in Health Care 1989; 5:503–519.
3. Moses LE: The series of consecutive cases as a device for assessing outcomes of interventions. In Bailar JC, Mosteller F (eds): Medical Uses of Statistics, 2nd ed. Boston: NEJM Books, 1992.

4. Marsh JL, Grames LM, Holtman B: Intravelar veloplasty: A prospective study. Cleft Palate J 1989; 26:46–50.

5. Relman AS: Assessment and accountability: The third revolution in medical care. N Engl J Med 1988; 319:1220–1222.

6. Roper WL, Winkenwerder W, Hackbarth GM, et al: Effectiveness in health care: An initiative to evaluate and improve medical practice. N Engl J Med 1988; 319:1197–1202.

7. Lewis CE: Variation in the incidence of surgery. N Engl J Med 1969; 281:880–885.

8. Wennberg JE, Gittelshon A: Small area variations in health care delivery. Science 1973; 142:1102–1108.

9. Wennberg JE, Gittelshon A: Variations in medical care among small areas. Sci Am 1982; 246:120–134.

10. Donaldson MS, Sox HC: Setting Priorities for Health Technology Assessment. Institute of Medicine. Washington, DC: National Academy Press, 1992.

11. McCormick KA, Flemming B: Clinical practice guidelines. Health Prog pp 30–34, 1990.

12. Cataract in Adults: Management of Functional Impairment. US Department of Health and Human Services. Public Health Service, AHCPR Research Activities No. 162; March 1993.

13. Office of Technology Assessment, US Congress: Development of Medical Technology: Opportunities for Assessment. US Government Printing Office, 1976.

14. Banta HD, Bekaney CJ: Policy formulation and technology assessment. Millbank Memorial fund Q 1981; 59:445–479.

15. Perry S, Pillar B: A national policy for health care technology assessment (editorial). Med Care Rev 1990; 47:401–416.

16. Bailar JC, Mosteller F: Medical Technology Assessment. In Bailar JC, Mosteller F (eds): Medical Uses of Statistics, 2nd ed. Boston: NEJM Books, 1992.

17. Institute of Medicine (US) Division of Health Sciences Policy: Assessing Medical Technologies. National Academy Press, 1985.

18. Fuchs VR, Garber AM: Sounding board: The new technology assessment. N Engl J Med 1990; 323:673–677.

19. Mason JW: A comparison of electrophysiologic testing with Holter monitoring to predict antiarrhythmic-drug efficacy for ventricular tachyarrhythmias. N Engl J Med 1993; 329:445–451.

20. Antczak-Bouckoms A, Tulloch JFC, Adams ME: Ambulatory cardiac monitoring for the evaluation of antiarrhythmic agents. Int J Technology Assessment in Health Care 1993; 9:124–139.

21. Ward DE, Camm AJ: Dangerous ventricular arrhythmias—can we predict drug efficacy? N Engl J Med 1993; 329:498–499.

22. Shaw WC, Asher-McDade C, Brattstrom V, et al: A six-center international study of treatment outcome in patients with clefts of the lip and palate: Part 1. Principles and study design. Cleft Palate J 1992; 29:393–397.

23. Tulloch JFC, Antczak-Bouckoms AA: Decision analysis in the evaluation of clinical strategies for the management of mandibular third molars. J Dent Ed 1987; 51:652–660.

24. Tulloch JFC, Antczak-Bouckoms AA, Ung N: Evaluation of the costs and relative effectiveness of alternate strategies for the removal of mandibular third molars. Int J Technology Assessment in Health Care 1990; 6:505–515.

25. Weinstein MC, Feinberg HV: Clinical Decision Analysis. Philadelphia: WB Saunders, 1980.

26. Pauker SP, Pauker SG: Prenatal diagnosis: A directive approach to genetic counseling using decision analysis. Yale J Biol Med 1977; 50:275–289.

27. McNeil BJ, Weichschelbaum R, Pauker SG: Fallacy of the five year survival in lung cancer. N Engl J Med 1978; 299:1397–1401.

28. McNeil BJ, Pauker SG, Sox HC, Taversky A: On the elicitation of preferences for alternative therapies. N Engl J Med 1982; 306:1259–1262.

29. Kassirer JP: Adding insult to injury: Usurping patients' perogatives. N Engl J Med 1983; 308:898–901.

30. Torrance GW, Feeny D: Utilities and quality-adjusted life years. Int J Technology Assessment in Health Care 1989; 5:559–575.

31. von Neumann J, Morganstern O: Theory of Games and Economic Behavior. Princeton, NJ: Princeton University Press, 1944.

32. Raiffa H: Decision Analysis. Introductory Lectures on Choices Under Uncertainty. Reading, MA: Addison-Wesley, 1968.

33. Keeney RL, Raiffa H: Decisions With Multiple Objectives: Preferences and Value Tradeoffs. New York: Wiley, 1976.

34. McNeil BJ, Weichschelbaum R, Pauker SG: Speech and survival tradeoffs between quality and quantity of life in laryngeal cancer. N Engl J Med 1981; 305:982–987.

35. Krischer JP: An analysis of patient management decisions as applied to cleft palate [Doctoral Dissertation]. Boston, Harvard University, 1974.

36. Krischer JP: The mathematics of cleft lip and palate treatment evaluation: Measuring the desirability of treatment outcomes. Cleft Palate J 1976; 14:165–180.

37. Black D: Expensive medical and surgical technology. Int J Technology Assessment in Health Care 1989; 5:308–312.

38. Pliskin JS, Shepherd DS, Weinstein MC: Utility functions for life years and health states. Operations Res 1980; 28:206–222.

39. Torrance GW, Boyle MH, Horwood SP: Application of multiattribute utility theory to measures of social preferences for health states. Operations Res 1982; 30:1043–1069.

40. Boyle MH, Torrance GW: Developing multiattribute health indexes. Med Care 1984; 22:1045–1057.

41. Nord E: Toward quality assurance in quality calculations. Int J Technology Assessment in Health Care 1993; 9:37–45.

42. Poses RM, Cebul RD, Collus M, Frazer SS: The accuracy of experienced physicians' probability estimates for patients with sore throats. Implications for decision making. JAMA 1985; 254:925–929.

43. Fryback DG: Decision maker, quantify thyself. Med Decision Making 1985; 5:51–60.

44. Semb G, Roberts CT, Shaw WC: Strategies for the advancement of surgical knowledge in cleft lip and palate. *In* Bader JD (ed): Risk Assessment in Dentistry. Chapel Hill: University of North Carolina Dental Ecology, 1987, pp 273–278.
45. Dubinsky M, Ferguson JH: Analysis of the National Institutes of Health Medicare coverage assessment. Int J Technology Assessment in Health Care 1990; 6:480–488.
46. Evidence-Based Medicine Working Group: Evidence-Based Medicine. A new approach to teaching the practice of medicine. JAMA 1992; 268:2420–2425.
47. Guyatt G, Drummond MF, Fenny D: Guidelines for Health Technology Assessment: Therapeutic Technologies. *In* Fenny D, Guyatt G, Tugwell P (eds.): Health Care Technology. Montreal: 1986.
48. Echt DS, Liebson PR, Mitchell LB, et al: Mortality and morbidity in patients receiving Encainide and Flecainide or placebo. The cardiac arrhythmia suppression trial. N Engl J Med 1991; 324:781–788.

Evaluating Treatment Alternatives: Measurement and Design

William C. Shaw, Christopher T. Roberts, and Gunvor Semb

A new era of assessment and accountancy in health care has resulted in the current need for systematic evaluation of health practices, including their health, economic, ethical, and social impact.

For cleft lip and palate care providers, there are some challenges ahead. The present scientific basis of the discipline is weak because virtually no elements of treatment have been subjected to the rigors of contemporary clinical trial design.[23] Thus, highly complex and varied protocols of care are practiced by different teams. In general, choices in surgical technique, timing and sequencing, and choices in ancillary procedures such as orthopedics, orthodontics, and speech therapy are derived following disappointment in the results of former practices rather than from firm evidence that the new protocol has succeeded elsewhere. As a consequence, the unsubstantiated testimony of enthusiasts for a particular treatment (often advocated with near religious zeal!) has done much to shape current practices. Typically, enthusiastic claims are made for a new type of therapy; the procedure is widely adopted; a flow of favorable clinical reports ensues; little or no positive evidence develops to support the desirability of the procedure; there is a sharp drop in the number of clinical reports of one favored practice, without evidence to support the change to another alternative method.[30]

Meaningful appraisal of the overall quality of care must include consideration of its therapeutic effectiveness, its financial cost, and the burden imposed upon the patient and family by the treatment process. All of these must be included in comparisons of different methods of care.

TREATMENT EFFECTIVENESS

The essential goal of cleft care is restoration of the patient to a ''normal'' life, unhindered by handicap or disability. However, the measurement of ''normalcy'' is a highly complex proposition; there is certainly no index at present that allows sufficiently sensitive comparison between alternative treatment protocols. Clinical research focuses more on ''proximate'' outcomes (as described in Chapter 29). These mainly represent different aspects of anatomic form and function in the parts affected by the clefting process, often reflecting the particular interests of individual disciplines and provider groups. In essence, most measures are an indication of the degree of handicap that persists despite (or as a result of) treatment, such as shortcomings in speech, hearing, and dentofacial development.

Outcome Measures

Proximate outcome measures must satisfy several criteria. The easiest to meet is that the measurement should be *reproducible* between and within examiners.

The most suitable statistic for comparing the reproducibility of different measurement scales is the intraclass correlation coefficient (ICC), also referred to as the reliability coefficient. In a research setting a measurement may be broken up into two components—first the ''true'' or ''error-free'' measurement of each case, and second the measurement error or ''noise'' in the measurement that is best to minimize. The ICC is a ratio of the variation of the error-free measurement to the total variation, including measurement error. As a ratio it is dimensionless and hence independent of the units of measurement, whether distances, angles, or scale points in a rating scale. Consequently, it allows cross-comparison of reproducibility between different methods of measurement.

In the unlikely circumstance that a measurement scale is applied without any measurement error, the variation of error-free measurement equals the total variation, and thus the ICC is one. On the other hand, a scale containing substantial error has a much smaller ICC. In the worst case, in which the measurement error is so great that the scale is unable to distinguish between cases, the ICC is equal to zero. At the design stage of a study, poor reproducibility of an outcome measure may be offset by an increase in sample size. The sample size required is increased (relative to that for an entirely reliable scale) by a factor $1/R$, where R is the ICC. It is generally estimated using analysis of variance. If the scale used is categorical, the weighted kappa statistic may be used.[8] This is equivalent to the ICC if squared weights are used.[9]

Another strategy to improve the reproducibility of a measure is to use the total or mean of a set of measurements from a panel of observers working independently. This also reduces any bias that may be related to the idiosyncratic perceptions of a particular observer. It is possible to estimate the reliability of such a pooled value by using the Spearman Brown formula.[10] If R is the ICC for a single observer, then the ICC for a measurement obtained by totaling the scores of m observers is given by the result of the following equation:

$$R_m = \frac{m \cdot R}{(1 + (m - 1) \cdot R)}$$

More difficult is the requirement of *validity*, meaning that the measure truly represents what it is supposed to. For example, do the results of a nasoendoscopy examination reflect how well the patient sounds to others? Or does a series of cephalometric measurements actually reflect how well the patient looks to others? External facial appearance is a crucial outcome for the patients, because this, after all, is what they and society around them actually see. Cephalometric analysis, with its central place in the thinking of orthodontists, is assumed to be an important outcome in its own right, if only as a *"surrogate"* measure.[12] It is, however, an invalid measure of many aspects of external facial appearance.

A particular problem in the study of a congenital condition such as cleft lip/palate (CLP) arises when outcomes are assessed in childhood, although eventual form and function will not be known until adulthood. This is especially true for aspects of facial growth such as maxillary prominence because this feature deteriorates steadily while growth is occurring (see Fig. 2–7; Chapter 2). A useful way to identify potential outcome measures that are valid and predictive is to examine longitudinal archives. The relative prominence of the maxilla in patients with complete clefts is an important outcome for evaluating the success of primary surgery (see Chapter 2). One common method for doing this is to measure angle A-N-B, the relationship of the anterior outlines of the maxilla and mandible to the frontonasal suture. However, identification of point A on the maxillary outline is difficult in early childhood because of the position of the unerupted permanent incisors. In the Eurocleft study,[19] soft tissue analysis at age 10 for unilateral cleft lip/palate (UCLP) was broadly consistent with that derived from hard tissues (Fig. 30–1), and if soft tissue A-N-B angle can be shown to be adequately predictive, it is a good alternative. Indeed, it has the further advantages of being measurable on photographs, obviating the need for irradiation, and reflecting the actual facial outline observable in everyday life.

Data from the Oslo archive[25] were examined at a number of age points to assess how well early measurement of A-N-B angle would predict the situation in adulthood. To assess the strength of any linear predictive relationship, r^2 was calculated between soft tissue A-N-B angle at age 6 ± 1 year and measurements at a later stage (Table 30–1). Small groups of 20 to 30 patients with UCLP from Manchester and Oslo have been compared in a number of studies at different ages. In Figure 30–2, average soft tissue A-N-B angles for each center in patients at ages 6, 9, and 12 years are shown. Although the levels of significance for the differences fall just below the 5% level, the differences between each center in children at different ages are of similar magnitude, reinforcing the predictive worth of soft tissue A-N-B angle at age 6 ± 1 year.

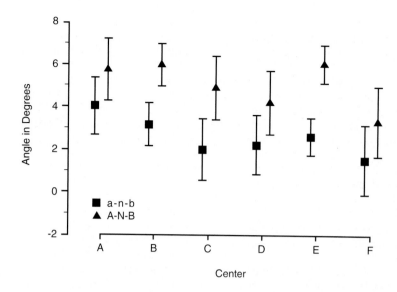

Figure 30–1. Comparison of maxillomandibular profile measurements for UCLP: hard tissue (a-n-b), soft tissue (A-N-B). Derived from data collected in the Eurocleft study.

Measurement Scales

The development of measurement scales that are both reproducible and valid for cleft outcomes is still at an early stage. Our preliminary experience derives from attempts to compare dentofacial form and relationships in the Eurocleft study using cephalometric analysis for skeletal form,[19] dental arch relationships,[15] and nasolabial appearance.[1,2]

Cephalometric measurements, although reproducible, suffer from a lack of *content validity,* because they measure three-dimensional structures in a two-dimensional way. Nonetheless, cephalometric relationships can tell a great deal about potential growth inhibition for structures undoubtedly affected by surgical procedures (see Chapter 2), and they successfully discriminated between results in different centers.[19]

To compare dental arch relationships, we applied the Goslon yardstick,[14] an index designed to systemize subjective perception. Originally a large sample of study casts was graded by a panel of orthodontists and a series of five groups containing representative cases ranging from the best (group 1) to the worst (group 5) dental arch relationships. These reference groups were subsequently used to assist in grading new cases.

In the Eurocleft study, five observers assessed a sample of 149 study casts using the yardstick, and a good level of reliability with an ICC of 0.80 was obtained (Table 30–2). The mean of the five measurements was then used as a summary score. Application of the Spearman Brown formula suggests that the reliability of this average score is excellent. From the formula above, the estimated value for the mean of five assessments was 0.95. The mean of the five examiners' scores was found to be sensitive to differences between treatment centers.[15]

In a subsequent study,[18] we attempted to discover whether certain measurements could be made directly without the need to assemble a panel of orthodontists. To relate the subjective assessment of the Goslon yardstick to objective measurement, overjet, overbite, incisor angulation, and various arch form and crossbite relationships were

Table 30–1. CORRELATION BETWEEN MEASUREMENT OF MAXILLOMANDIBULAR PROFILE AT AGE 6 AND SUBSEQUENTLY IN THE SAME CASES

	Strength of Linear Relationship with A-N-B at age 6 years (± 1) Measured by r^2 (n = 56)		
	12 Years	*15 Years*	*18 Years*
a-n-b	0.67	0.45	0.27
A-N-B	0.74	0.57	0.46

Data from the Oslo Archive.

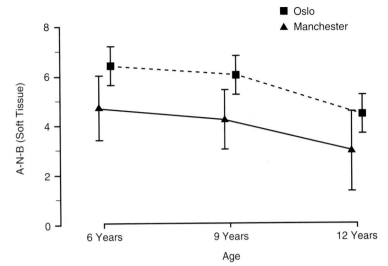

Figure 30–2. Comparison of Oslo and Manchester samples with UCLP for different age groups. Group means with 95% confidence limits.

measured on the same series of study casts with a reflex metrograph. These objective measurements were then used as predictors of the mean Goslon score in a multiple regression analysis. Overjet of the incisor on the unaffected side (all cases were UCLP) explained a substantial proportion of the variance ($r^2 = 0.87$). The other measures explained only an additional 3% of variance. Hence, we concluded that the mean Goslon score is essentially a measure of the overjet (prominence) of the incisor, so that in future assessments of dental arch relationships, panels and series of reference casts will not be necessary.

We sought to compare the nasolabial appearance of the patients in the Eurocleft study using photographs, but confronted several difficulties. Technical issues such as film quality, lighting, sharpness of image, the patients' facial expression, and the background general facial appearance were all factors that could influence an observer's opinion. To assess the influence of background appearance such as hair, eyes, and complexion, a panel of observers was asked to examine independently three frontal views, including the nasolabial area in isolation, the full face, and the surrounding features without the nasolabial part.[1] Each view was scored in terms of attractiveness using a visual analogue scale. There was found to be a strong correlation between the full face and surrounding area ($r = 0.53$, $p < 0.001$), indicating that, indeed, the nasolabial rating is likely to be influenced by surrounding features.

Consequently, we considered that a more valid measure would be based on restricting the areas under consideration to those directly affected by the anomaly and its repair. Thus, the Eurocleft examiners were asked to make assessments of a standardized view of the frontal and lateral view of the nasolabial area. We considered it important to break down the task into four components: (1) nasal form (frontal view);

Table 30–2. EVALUATION OF REPRODUCIBILITY FOR STUDY CAST (GOSLON) AND FEATURES OF NASOLABIAL APPEARANCE

	Goslon	Nasal	Symmetry	Vermilion	Profile	Total
Intra-class correlation coefficient	0.80	0.47	0.36	0.47	0.48	0.49
Lower 95% confidence limit	0.76	0.41	0.30	0.40	0.42	0.43
Sample size	149	115	115	115	115	115

Number of Examiners	Spearman Brown Estimates of Reliability of Total of Independent Scores by N Examiners					
3	0.92	0.73	0.62	0.72	0.74	0.75
5	0.95	0.82	0.73	0.81	0.82	0.83
6	0.96	0.84	0.77	0.84	0.85	0.85

All based on six observers except Goslon, which involved 5.
Derived from data from the Eurocleft study.

(2) deviation of the nose from the midline; (3) shape of the vermilion border; and (4) profile, including the upper lip. Each observer was asked to score each of the components with a five-point subjective scale with scale points ranging from very good appearance to very poor appearance. A total score was also computed by aggregation of the scores of the four components. The reliability of each component and the total score were rated from 0.47 for nasal form and vermilion border to 0.36 for symmetry (Table 30–2).

We found reproducibility poor compared with that obtained for dental arch relationships, and the reliability of the total score was little better than that for the component scores. In this case, the strategy of splitting the assessment into components appeared to have a limited ability to improve the quality of measurement. Detailed analysis of the data suggested that if one observer scored higher than another observer for one of the four components, the observer was likely to do so for the other three.

For future work, we will test whether the reproducibility is improved by reducing the subjective element by providing reference examples or "bench marks," as with the Goslon yardstick, or by the enumeration of specific features for rating. Elsewhere, we have found this to improve reproducibility. For example, rating of dental aesthetics is assisted by providing an illustrated ten-point scale, and orthodontic treatment need on dental health grounds is reproducibly rated when clear diagnostic categories are used.[6]

The provision of "bench marks" must be done with some caution, however, because the choice of categories for each scale and the subject of each subscale determine the content validity of the total measurement. Thus, there is a danger of imposing the researchers' perceptions of what is important.

An alternative strategy for rating appearance is to rank subjects pairwise against each other. All possible pairs of subjects may be compared,[32] and for each pair a score of one is allocated to the preferred photograph. The score for each case is then its total after comparison with all other cases. One practical difficulty, however, is that the number of comparisons escalates with sample size. The number of possible pairs is equal to $N(N - 1)/2$ for a sample of N cases. Therefore, for a sample of 10 subjects, 45 comparisons are needed; with 50 subjects the number rises to 1225. However, the pairwise technique may be modified by comparing each case with a random or systematic sample of other subjects. For example, the photographs for the complete sample may be arranged in a random sequence and then a score for each case obtained by comparing against a given number of subjects that follow. The reliability of the score for each case would be improved by increasing the size of the group against which comparison is made, but again, of course, the performance time is increased. A more fundamental limitation is that the scale is only meaningful as the relationship between subjects within the same sample since the comparison is not transferable from one study to another.

The static nature of a still photograph, of course, is a major weakness in respect of validity because the lip in function cannot be judged. Consequently, the use of video recording has been explored.[17] An edited sequence for a series of 30 subjects using a number of standardized views of the nasolabial area at rest and function was prepared. A panel of judges then rated the cases, using a scoring chart with nine responses for the lip and 10 for the nose.

Assessment was made of the nose and the lip separately with eight components and an overall score for lip and nine components and an overall score for the nasal area. For the nasal area, the ICC for individual components ranged from 0.40 to 0.27, with 0.52 for the overall score and 0.49 for the sum of the components. For the lip, the ICC ranged from 0.39 to 0.10, with 0.28 for the overall score and 0.34 for the sum of components.

Although such a dynamic view may be more valid, the interexaminer agreement was generally worse than that achieved from a static image. This may reflect the significantly higher content of information contained in the video format, and by further discussion of the items to be rated and possible provisions of improved descriptive categories or illustrated examples, an appearance scale of high validity seems feasible.

TREATMENT COSTS

In most developed countries, the high medical costs of rehabilitating the child with a cleft are borne, or at least supported in part, by the state. Economic pressures around the world now force a re-examination of the true financial costs of treatment. With reduced budgets, clinicians must either be involved in cost controls or have arbitrary choices imposed upon them. Surgical operations are invariably expensive treatment episodes, and successful primary operations that minimize the need for multiple secondary revisions are highly desirable. Furthermore, successful primary repairs are likely to reduce the duration and complexity of ancillary procedures such as speech therapy, orthodontics, and maxillary osteotomy.

In economic terms, the cheapest care will certainly be that which is provided with a high degree of planning and coordination. Common examples may be combining the placement of drainage tubes with another operation, timing alveolar bone grafting so that natural space closure is facilitated and the duration of subsequent orthodontics is minimized, and recognizing a later need for maxillary osteotomy so that inappropriate early orthodontics is avoided.

THE BURDEN OF CARE

Because the consequences of an orofacial cleft are apparent through every phase of childhood and adolescence, there is seldom a time when the disciplines involved in care could not recommend various interventions. The powerful desire of patients and parents to reach the point at which the stigma of clefting is completely eradicated makes it likely that they will accept most proposals. Most patients and parents willingly comply with protocols of care recommended by all members of their team, no matter how demanding they may be. They have little choice.

So far, "burden of care" has received little attention in cleft care, yet the combined total of operations, other treatment episodes, and review appointments for the first 20 years of life, including all the disciplines that may be involved, can easily exceed 100. Apart from pain and suffering and the disruption of family life and school attendance, the dependent role in which this places the patient may have an adverse effect on the patient's sense of self-determination or locus of control.

BALANCING OUTCOME, COST, AND BURDEN

The important concept of relative utilities and the techniques available to formulate global outcome measures more relevant to patients than the more short-sighted proximal outcomes that absorb clinicians has been discussed in the previous chapter. Clearly it behooves the providers of cleft care to seek better balance in the development of protocols of care spanning the years from birth until late adolescence.

Undoubtedly, there are intriguing discussions ahead. An example is the use of early orthopedics and delayed palatal closure. Patients receiving this treatment have to be brought on many additional visits to the treatment center during infancy and childhood and must endure the minor risk of impression-taking and the greater risk of some discomfort associated with the appliances. For the years until the hard palate is closed patients have to tolerate a fistula or an obturator, all the while having a rather clear sense of being an orthodontic *patient*. How much benefit does this additional treatment have to produce over treatment without early orthopedics to justify its inclusion in care—an average increase in angle S-N-A (maxillary prominence) of 1°, a 10% reduction in osteotomy rate in the teens, or a better cosmetic repair of the lip? If the latter, how would it be measured? Similar questions arise about other elements of care. How often should lip or nasal revision be attempted? When does the law of diminishing returns start to apply? Surgical management of velopharyngeal incompetence is not without some risk, so how bad does the problem have to be to justify the average gain from pharyngoplasty or flap? How much orthodontics should be performed in childhood if the duration and outcome of definitive treatment in the permanent dentition will not be radically altered?

MAKING COMPARISONS

Although measurement of outcomes, cost, and burden of care still requires much development in the field of clefts, strategies for comparing different treatments are more straightforward. The general rules of health technology assessment are well-established, and the quality of treatment comparisons conforms to a widely accepted hierarchy, from anecdotal reports to randomized trials.[7]

Anecdotal Case Reports

Although case reports may signal important new developments in surgical practice, the evidence they contain for a widespread change in practice remains generally unconvincing in the absence of subsequent confirmatory series. A positive example in our experience is secondary bone grafting, which was first reported on a small scale,[4,5] adopted elsewhere, and eventually the subject of published reports of large series of cases.[3]

Case Series

Reports of a series of cases treated by the same method provide more substantial evidence of the merits of a particular technique or program of treatment and provide the professional community with a general impression of relative efficacy. They are of particular value in demonstrating that new procedures can be reliably performed and have a low risk of serious morbidity. Rather commonly, however, outcome is measured in the short term, and the enthusiasm of the reporters may impair true objectivity. Thus, primary bone grafting, first heralded as an important breakthrough in case series reports, was later shown by randomized control trials to be harmful to facial growth.[13,22] On the other hand, case series of secondary bone grafting in which cancellous iliac crest grafts were used revealed persuasive evidence that one aspect of outcome, the patient's dentition, could be reliably restored beyond levels previously attainable.[3] The immediacy of these benefits ruled against the need for a randomized trial, although potential growth disturbances still deserved consideration.[24] Future trials of bone grafting may still be necessary to examine individual aspects of surgical technique or timing, or to test the suitability of alternative graft materials.

Case series rarely provide evidence of the superiority of one technique over others when a choice of broadly similar methods exists and in which any improvement may be incremental rather than dramatic. This is a major problem in the evaluation of primary surgical repair because this may be achieved with apparently similar success by methods that differ in technique, timing, and sequence. Meaningful comparison of reports of case series in the literature is often prohibited by methodologic inconsistencies in assessment and by the absence of strict and well-defined entry criteria such as consecutive cases with an equivalent prognosis.

Case series reports may include equivalent data for the noncleft population, the implication being that the closer the CLP data conform to normal, the better treatment has been. However, such bench marks do little to enhance comparability with other techniques. If samples are small, real differences between the cleft and noncleft patient may not be detected statistically.

Retrospective Comparative Studies

Opportunities for nonexperimental comparisons of therapies or programs of care can arise in several ways—through co-existing therapies at the same center, through the replacement of one therapy with a second, or by the comparison of treatment centers using different therapies. However, any lack of equivalence between the cases prior to treatment or lack of equivalence in the competence of the providers undermines the conclusions.

Comparison of Co-existing Therapies

In using retrospective material such as case notes or clinical databases, checks can be made on the equivalence of the groups, commonly in terms of gender, age, or cleft subtype. Preferably, they can be matched pairwise on these characteristics. Alternatively, adjustments can be made in the analysis by stratification or the use of multivariate statistical methods. In either case, doubt may remain that important prognostic factors have been masked, for if two or more therapies were being used concurrently within a single center, selective allocation to treatment must be suspected.

Factors that may have influenced clinical decision making may be unrecorded or unreliably recorded. For example, decisions as to when (at what age) to perform primary surgery may be influenced by unrecorded aspects of the morphology of the cleft, the availability of personnel, the health of the child, or parental attitudes toward the cleft. If these factors influence outcome, confounding would occur in any study of the effect of age on surgical outcome.

The possibility of confounding in this way is especially likely when treatment has been provided 5 or 10 years previously and different staff were involved. Retrospective ascertainment of details of primary surgery or cleft subtype is difficult, and descriptive terminology may have changed in subtle ways. It may be possible to match or adjust data to remove bias due to gender, age, or cleft subtype, but this gives no guarantee that some other prognostic factor that may affect outcome is not associated with choice of treatment. A critical factor in surgical outcome appears to be the competence of the surgeon, high-volume operators being apparently more likely to achieve good results.[26]

In certain circumstances the researcher has little alternative but to use retrospective data incorporating these potential biases, especially when multidimensional outcome is involved. When a procedure has shown clear benefit in one aspect of outcome, it may be inappropriate to withhold treatment to create a control group unless there is a dramatic adverse effect in another aspect.

Comparison with Historic Controls

These studies may arise as natural experiments by changes in therapy within a treatment center. Such research is particularly valuable when durable records (radiographs, study casts, speech recordings, photographs, and so forth) are obtained in a standardized way both for subjects treated by a previous method (the historic controls) and for subjects treated by the new method, allowing simultaneous unbiased evaluation. Data may already exist on two well-documented treatments that have been used in different time periods.

An alternative circumstance in which such studies arise is when data for a group of patients receiving a standard treatment already exist and can be gathered in a similar way when a new treatment is introduced. This design requires only half the number of patients to be gathered prospectively as a randomized clinical trial and is clearly attractive where recruitment of cases is slow. Furthermore, it has been argued that in circumstances of poor outcome, it may be unethical to withhold new treatment to create a control group.[11] Nevertheless, several biases and possibilities for confounding generally tend to favor the newly introduced procedure.

In practice, changes in technique at a treatment center often come about as a result of changes in personnel who may have performed differently in respect of the previous method. This leads to bias due to differences in skill of personnel associated with either treatment method. Even where there is stability of staff, bias reflecting gradual changes of ability and technique are highly likely, and definition or ascertainment of prognosis may change. New methods may be initially applied with some selectivity to "suitable" cases as experience is gained. A new method is likely to be tested by an experienced and innovative surgeon who may be expected to achieve better results than the average surgeon. This clearly introduces the confounding effect of operator skill with treatment. Other aspects of clinical management may have been altered with the intention of improving outcome, creating additional possibilities for bias in favor of the innovative procedure. Multivariate methods have been suggested as a way to adjust for these biases, but serial changes in treatment are likely to take place in parallel, resulting in a strong association between treatment variables. This is one reason why historic control design is generally unsuited to evaluating primary surgery because other changes in the total program of care are likely to have occurred during the extensive follow-up period.

The bias toward the innovative procedure is a major cause for concern with historic control studies because they either may fail to resolve a controversy or alternatively may create ethical concerns that preclude further more rigorous comparisons. Favorable outcomes suggested for a new procedure by historic control studies have been disputed by subsequent randomized controlled trials.[20, 21] The danger exists that historic control studies could set in motion an unwarranted cycle of change with no benefit to the patient, and consequently they may delay the process of development.

The reduction in recruitment time for a historic control study in which data is gathered prospectively on a new method is also less important when evaluating primary surgery because of the extended follow-up required of each case. If, for example, the proposed follow-up of a trial of two methods of primary surgery is 10 years and the recruitment time of patients sufficient for a randomized trial is 4 years, the total duration of the study is 14 years. The potential saving of time in a partially prospective historic control study would be only 2 years (14%).

Intercenter Audit

In even the busiest CLP treatment centers, the generation of adequate samples within specific cleft subtypes treated by contrasting treatment modalities is extremely difficult. Consequently, the multicenter approach offers distinct advantages. Prospectively planned recall of cases at participating centers allows data on outcome to be collected in a standardized way, and rigorous planning and execution across the centers can ensure consecutive case recruitment and unbiased evaluation.[27]

Provided that procedures for entry into the study are equivalent in all participating centers, this strategy is extremely valuable in assessing the outcome of primary surgery together with other major components of the treatment program at respective centers. However, it is difficult, if not impossible, to establish the key beneficial or harmful features of a specific treatment as a general scientific conclusion, because of the invariably complex and arbitrary mix of surgical technique, timing, and sequence, ancillary procedures, and surgical personnel.[26] For example, if two centers differ in the use of presurgical orthopedics and types of primary lip and palate surgery, there is no way to determine which of these procedures may be responsible for differences in outcome between centers, nor would a null result allow the conclusion that individual aspects of the treatment program are equivalent. The method is therefore better suited to comparative clinical audit than definitive clinical research. Nevertheless, the existence of significant disparities in outcome of the overall treatment process provides a basis for speculating about the possible cause, and intercenter studies should therefore be highly motivating toward the generation of specific hypotheses for subsequent more detailed testing.

Randomized Controlled Trials

For the comparison of therapies, there is little doubt that the randomized control trial is the epitome of scientific validity. Randomization avoids conscious or unconscious bias in treatment allocation. Prognostic factors, whether known or unknown to the investigator, tend to be balanced between treatment groups. Because patients are followed prospectively according to a clearly defined protocol, missing data are less likely because the potential loss to follow-up is reduced. If loss does occur, it may be possible to quantify any induced bias, in contrast with retrospective studies in which the researcher may be unaware of patients lost to follow-up, and hence unaware of the scale of bias this may have introduced into the results.

In 1973, Spriestersbach and coworkers[30] identified the need for prospective research to resolve central problems of cleft management, but remarkably few randomized trials have been performed in CLP surgery despite being the surest means of advancing the discipline in the face of overwhelming uncertainty about the relative efficacy of countless different programs of care around the world. In 25 years of publication of the *Cleft Palate Journal,* only five randomized clinical trials were identified with only one involving a follow-up of surgery for more than 4 years.[23]

The most common reasons cited for nonadoption of randomized trials are ethical objections and the specificity of surgical skill for a particular operation.

Ethical Objections

Ethical issues arise because the risk of surgery and its irreversibility demand as much certainty as possible that the operation prescribed is the correct one. Surgeons holding the opinion that their own favored method is at least as good as any other (usually formed on the testimonials of their own teachers, on theoretical appeal, or on clinical impressions) are disinclined to withhold their method from patients. Furthermore, surgeons have reported that their participation in a randomized controlled trial may jeopardize their credibility with patients by making them appear unsure and indecisive. It may be argued, however, that ethical issues do not go away in the absence of randomized trials. During a period of genuine uncertainty about any aspect of clinical practice, there is the same ethical imperative to inform patients of this uncertainty, whether they are treated within or outside a clinical trial. To do otherwise is exercising double standards, and, indeed, the irreversibility of surgery demands the highest order of evidence whether traditional procedures are being perpetuated or new ones introduced.

Entry into a clinical trial may be beneficial by itself to the patient. Well-conducted clinical trials require standardized treatment protocols and recall systems that tend to raise the quality of care. Evidence from studies of childhood cancers suggests that entry into a randomized clinical trial per se offers an immediate advantage to patients, becoming in itself a treatment of choice.[31] In a recent randomized trial of feeding methods for cleft lip and palate neonates, a standardized system of care provided by a health visitor (home visiting nurse) raised the general level of care while allowing appraisal of the feeding methods in the study.[28]

Specificity of Skill

A surgeon most familiar with one procedure is likely to attain better results with this than with an unfamiliar one, introducing systematic bias. Consequently it can be argued that where a new procedure is being compared against the standard, the methodology may create a bias weighted against innovation. This is a reversal of the probable bias with nonexperimental and retrospective studies, which tend, in the absence of any real effect, to be biased toward innovation and hence unnecessary change in clinical practice. It is, of course, unreasonable to expect surgeons to perform complex alternative operations with which they were unfamiliar. An appropriate standardization phase is essential in the prerandomization period before the commencement of the trial. In a recent prospective trial of palatoplasty, conducted with and without intravelar veloplasty, the two participating surgeons compared and standardized their techniques prior to the trial by direct observation of one another's procedures.[16] Similarly, standardization of surgical technique has been achieved in an international trial of sphincter pharyngoplasty and pharyngeal flap.[29] Removal of bias in surgical skill in this way, of course, is not possible in retrospective studies. Differences in surgical skill therefore must be seen as a stronger argument against retrospective than prospective studies.

It follows from this discussion that surgeons participating in trials should be actively involved in the surgical management of CLP with a substantial, regular caseload. This by itself may bring improvements in quality of outcome.[26]

Surgical training is a lengthy process, and the level of skill attained in performing a specific technique undoubtedly reflects the surgeon's familiarity and experience with that particular method. Thus, the design of randomized trials will tend to favor technically simple or more orthodox operations. However, this may be seen as a strength of the method, not a weakness. Trials whose outcome depends on attention to the minutiae of surgical detail by their very nature lack generalizability, whereas a pragmatic trial addresses the question in such a way that the outcome is more likely to relate to activity in the real world. If a complex high technology procedure can work in only two or three specialist centers in the world, it is of less value than a less complex procedure that produces better results in the hands of the majority of surgeons practicing in the field.

References

1. Asher-McDade C, Roberts CT, Shaw WC, Gallagher C: The development of a method for rating nasolabial appearance in patients with clefts of the lip and palate. Cleft Palate Craniofac J 1991; 28:385–391.
2. Asher-McDade C, Brattström V, Dahl E, et al: A six-centre international study of treatment outcome in patients with clefts of the lip and palate: Part 4. Assessment of nasolabial appearance. Cleft Palate Craniofac J 1992; 29:409–412.

3. Bergland O, Semb G, Åbyholm FE: Elimination of the residual alveolar cleft by secondary bone grafting and subsequent orthodontic treatment. Cleft Palate J 1986; 23:175–205.

4. Boyne PJ, Sands NR: Secondary bone grafting of residual alveolar and palatal clefts. J Oral Surg 1972; 30:87–92.

5. Boyne PJ, Sands NR: Combined orthodontic surgical management of residual alveolar cleft defects. J Oral Surg 1976; 70:20–37.

6. Brook PH, Shaw WC: The development of an index of orthodontic treatment priority. Eur J Orthop 1989; 11:309–320.

7. Byar DP: Why databases should not replace randomized clinical trials. Biometrics 1990; 31:337–342.

8. Cohen J: Weighted Kappa nominal scale agreement with provision for scaled disagreement or partial credit. Psychol Bull 1968; 70:213–220.

9. Fleiss JL, Cohen J: The equivalence of weighted Kappa and the intra-class correlation coefficient as a measure of reliability. Educ Psychol Meas 1973; 33:613–619.

10. Fleiss JL: Design and analysis of clinical experiment. New York: John Wiley, 1986.

11. Gehan AE: The evaluation of therapies: Historical control studies. Stat Med 1984; 3:315–324.

12. Herson J: The use of surrogate endpoints in clinical trials (an introduction to a series of four papers). Stat Med 1989; 8:403–404.

13. Jolleys A, Robertson NRE: A study of the effects of early bone grafting in complete clefts of the lip and palate—five year study. Br J Plast Surg 1972; 25:229–237.

14. Mars M, Plint DA, Houston WJB, et al: The Goslon yardstick: A new system of assessing dental arch relationships in children with unilateral clefts of the lip and palate. Cleft Palate J 1987; 24:314–322.

15. Mars M, Asher-McDade C, Brattström V, et al: A six-centre international study of treatment outcome in patients with clefts of the lip and palate. Part 3. Dental arch relationships. Cleft Palate Craniofac J 1992; 29:405–408.

16. Marsh JL, Grames LM, Holtman B: Intravelar veloplasty: A prospective study. Cleft Palate J 1989; 26:46–50.

17. Morrant DG: A method of assessing surgical outcome in unilateral cleft lip and nose repair using standardised video records [M.Sc. Thesis]. Manchester: University of Manchester, 1992.

18. Morris TA, Roberts CT, Shaw WC: Incisal overjet as an outcome measure in unilateral cleft lip and palate management. Cleft Palate Craniofac J 1994; 31:142–145.

19. Mølsted K, Asher-McDade C, Brattström V, et al: A six-centre international study of treatment outcome in patients with clefts of the lip and palate. Part 2. Craniofacial form and soft tissue profile. Cleft Palate Craniofac J 1992; 29:398–404.

20. Pinsky CA: Experience with historical control studies in cancer immunotherapy. Stat Med 1984; 3:325–329.

21. Pollock AV: Historical evolution: Method, attitudes, goals. In Troidl H, Spitzer WO, McPeak B, et al (eds): Principle and Practice of Research: Strategies for Surgical Investigators, pp 7–17. New York: Springer-Verlag, 1986.

22. Rehrmann AH, Koberg WR, Koch H: Long-term post-operative results of primary and secondary bone grafting in complete clefts of the lip and palate. Cleft Palate J 1970; 7:206–221.

23. Roberts CT, Semb G, Shaw WC: Strategies for the advancement of surgical methods in cleft lip and palate. Cleft Palate Craniofac J 1991; 28:141–149.

24. Semb G: Effect of alveolar bone grafting on maxillary growth in unilateral cleft lip and palate patients. Cleft Palate J 1988; 25:288–295.

25. Semb G: A study of facial growth in patients with unilateral cleft lip and palate treated by the Oslo CLP team. Cleft Palate J 1991; 28:1–21.

26. Shaw WC, Asher-McDade C, Brattström V, et al: A six-centre international study of treatment outcome in patients with clefts of the lip and palate. Part 5. General discussion and conclusions. Cleft Palate Craniofac J 1992; 29:413–418.

27. Shaw WC, Asher-McDade C, Brattström V, et al: A six-centre international study of treatment outcome in patients with clefts of the lip and palate. Part 1. Principles and study design. Cleft Palate Craniofac J 1992; 29:393–397.

28. Shaw WC, Bannister RP, Roberts CT: Randomized trial of feeding methods in cleft lip and palate (abstract 119). 7th International Congress on Cleft Palate and Related Craniofacial Anomalies, Brisbane, Australia, 1993.

29. Sloan GM, Abyholm F, D'Antonio LL, et al: A multicentre international trial of pharyngoplasty and pharyngeal flap (abstract 301). 7th International Congress on Cleft Palate and Related Craniofacial Anomalies, Brisbane, Australia, 1993.

30. Spriestersbach DC, Dickson DR, Fraser FC, et al: Clinical research in cleft lip and palate: The state of the art. Cleft Palate J 1973; 10:113–165.

31. Stiller CA: Survival of patients with cancer: Those included in clinical trials do better. Br Med J 1989; 299:1058–1059.

32. Tobiasen JM: Scaling facial impairment. Cleft Palate J 1989; 26:249–254.

Index

Note: Pages in *italics* indicate illustrations; those followed by t refer to tables.

A

Achondroplasia, 57
  fibroblast growth factor receptor gene mutations in, 90
Acrocephalosyndactyly. See also *Apert syndrome.*
  craniosynostosis in, 95
Acrocephaly, in craniosynostosis, 603
Adenoid, hypertrophy of, airway obstruction from, 517
Adenoidectomy, for middle ear disease, 217–219
  peritubal, 219
Adolescence, cleft lip-palate repair in, nursing care for, 158
  malocclusion in, psychological issues in, 148–149
  Treacher Collins syndrome in, psychological issues in, 147–148
Adulthood, ill-fitting appliance in, psychological issues in, 149–150
Airways, management of, 174–181
  in pre-existing pharyngeal flap, 518–519, *519*
  nasal, maxillary expansion effects on, 205–206
  obstruction of, adenoid hypertrophy and, 517
    causes of, 515
    inferior turbinate hyperplasia and, 516, *516*
    management of, *515*, 515–517, *516*
    maxillary sinus disease and, 517
    polyps and, 517
    septal deviation and, *515*, 515–516
  resistance in, facial growth and, 241, 263
    in cleft palate, 207
  size of, in adult cleft lip-palate, 204–205, 205t
    in child cleft lip-palate, 203t, 203–204, *204*
  speech effect of, 206–207
  surgical effects on, 205
  obstruction of, in cleft lip-palate, 39–40
  in mandibulofacial dysostosis, 67, *67*
  upper, deficiency of, in cleft lip-palate, 202–203
    obstruction of, adenoid hypertrophy and, 174
      allergic rhinitis and, 174
      anatomy and, 174–177, 175t
      causes of, 174–178, 175t, *175–176*, *178*
      continuous positive airway pressure for, 181

Airways *(Continued)*
      endotracheal intubation for, 180
      evaluation of, 179, *179*
      failure to thrive in, 165
      in microretrognathia, 165–166
      nasopharyngeal tube for, 166
      neurologic causes of, 178
      partial uvulopalatopharyngoplasty for, 181
      perioperative management of, 180
      physiologic causes of, 177–178
      prone positioning for, 165–166, 177
      sleep apnea and, 178
      tongue-lip adhesion for, 181
      tracheotomy for, 180–181
      treatment of, 179–181
      uvulectomy for, 181
Alar base, narrowing of, in bilateral cleft lip-nose correction, 722, *722*, *723*, 724
Alar base cinch suture, 513, *513*
Alloplastic materials, for facial augmentation, 334, *334*
Alveolar ridge, development of, 9
Alveolus, bone grafting of. See *Bone grafts, alveolar.*
  clefts of. See *Cleft alveolus.*
  prominence of, lip-palate repair and, 41, 41t
  surgery on, during lip repair, 42
Amniotic bands, phalangeal amputation from, 78, *79*
  swallowed, craniofacial disruption from, 78, *78*
Amputation, phalangeal, by amniotic bands, 78, *79*
A-N-B angle, in unilateral cleft lip-palate, 757, *758*, 758t, *759*
Anesthesia, in transcranial hypertelorism operation, 698
Anomaly (anomalies), major, 79–80
  minor, 79–80
  nonsyndromic, 80–81, 82, 86–91
    chance in, 87–88
    definition of, 86
    empiric recurrence risks for, 86, 87, 90
    familial, 87
    genetic counseling for, 87–91, *88*, *89*
    genetic predisposition to, 87–88, 89
    genomic imprinting in, *88*, 88–89, *89*
    Mendelian inheritance patterns in, 87
    multifactorial inheritance in, 87, 88, *88*
    nonfamilial, 87
    polygenic, 87, 88, *88*
  sequence in, 80
  syndromic, 80–81
Anophthalmia, ethanol exposure and, 18

Anterior chamber, cleavage anomalies of, ethanol exposure and, 18
Apert syndrome, 631
  as pedigree syndrome, 61
  autosomal dominant inheritance in, 85
  calvarial defect in, *70*, 70–71, 71t
  cleft palate in, 634
  cranial base in, 70–71, 72t
  cranial vault osteotomy for, 673–674, *674–675*, 678, *679–680*
  craniofacial growth in, 68–73
  craniosynostosis in, *68*, 70, *71*, 71t, 95
  extremity anomalies in, 634–635
  facial bipartition osteotomy for, 678, *679–680*
  fontanelles in, 70, *70*
  hearing loss in, 200, 635
  hydrocephalus in, 169
  hypertelorism in, 692
  in latency, psychological issues in, 146–147
  increased intracranial pressure in, 169
  intellectual development in, 200
  language development in, 199
  long-term care for, 169
  midface deformity in, bipartition osteotomy for, 642
  midface hypoplasia in, 176, 190, *191*
  newborn assessment in, 168–169
  nursing care in, 168–170
  ocular findings in, 190–191, *191*
  ocular malformations in, 189
  optic nerve atrophy in, 185
  orbits in, 190, *191*
  osteotomies for, 665, *666–667*
  parent education in, 168–169
  physical findings in, 631
  prelinguistic vocalizations in, 199
  reconstruction for, 631
    historical perspective on, 637–638
  skeletal findings in, 112, *112–115*, 114
  skull defect in, 73
  strabismus in, 189
  suture closure in, 71, *72*, *73*
  syndactyly in, *68*, 190, *191*
  treatment of, 73
Appelt-Gerken-Lenz syndrome, 57
Appliances, feeding, 161, 222, *223*
  in early adulthood, psychological issues over, 149–150
  palatal expansion, *224*, 225
  presurgical, 222, *223*
  quad-helix, for maxillary transverse expansion/protraction, 296, *297*, 298, *298*
  speech, 222–223, *224*, 225
    in velopharyngeal inadequacy, 445, *445*

ISBN 0-7216-3783-3